MW01531556

Patient Counseling Handbook

2nd Edition ‖ 1995

Published by
American Pharmaceutical Association
Washington, D.C.

NOTICE

This publication is intended to be a handy reference, not a complete drug information resource. It covers 800 commonly prescribed drugs and is specifically designed to present certain important aspects of drug data in a concise format.

Drug information is constantly evolving and is often subject to interpretation. Great care has been taken to ensure the accuracy of the information presented in this book. However, the reader is advised that the publisher cannot be responsible for the continued currency of the information or for any errors or omissions in this book or for any consequences arising therefrom. All decisions regarding drug therapy must be based on the independent judgment of the clinician.

Portions of this book have been copied from *USP DI®*, copyright The United States Pharmacopeial Convention, Inc. Permission granted.

Library of Congress Catalog Number: 94-73600
ISBN 0-917330-69-2

Table of Contents

Patient Counseling under OBRA '90*

In 1990, the U.S. Congress enacted legislation that, like the controlled substances law, directly affects the practice of pharmacy. Known as the Omnibus Budget Reconciliation Act of 1990 (OBRA '90),† this legislation mandated certain pharmacy services for Medicaid beneficiaries. The act applies only to outpatient dispensing to Medicaid patients, but "outpatient" covers more than community pharmacy practice. It applies to hospital outpatient pharmacies that dispense medications when patients are discharged, through the emergency room, or to employees, and it applies to extended care facilities when medications are dispensed to residents for their use while they are away from the nursing home.

On November 9, 1992, the U.S. Department of Health and Human Services, Health Care Financing Administration (HCFA), published an "interim final rule with comment period" to give specificity to OBRA '90.‡ Since the enactment of OBRA '90, individual states have passed laws containing the same provisions with respect to drug utilization review (DUR) and patient counseling. With rare exceptions, these laws have expanded the scope of OBRA '90, extending the requirements to almost all outpatients. Understanding the laws in your state is essential to ensure full compliance with their provisions.

You may find that your state law contains provisions that differ from those in the federal law, particularly the HCFA regulations. For example, at least one state includes the words

---

*Reprinted portions of Fitzgerald WL, "Legal Control of Pharmacy Services," in Canaday BR, ed., *OBRA '90: A Practical Guide to Effecting Pharmaceutical Care* (Washington, D.C.: American Pharmaceutical Association, 1994).

†Copies of OBRA '90 may be obtained for $1.50 each from the Government Printing Office (202-783-3238). Ask for *Federal Register,* Volume 57, Number 212, November 2, 1992, pp. 49397–49412.

‡On September 23, 1994, HCFA published the final rule, which took effect on October 24, 1994. It revises some of the regulatory requirements for the drug utilization review program. The final rule specifies several issues that state agencies must address when formulating counseling standards (e.g., whether the offer to counsel is required for new prescriptions only, whether auxiliary personnel may be authorized to make the offer to counsel, whether documentation of counseling is required). In addition, the standards must require mail order pharmacies to provide toll-free telephone service for long distance calls. See *Federal Register,* Volume 59, Number 184, September 23, 1994, pp. 48811–48825.

"face to face" in describing patient counseling. When conflict exists between federal and state law, federal law generally preempts state law; however, if state law is more stringent, you should follow the state law.

For the practicing pharmacist, three principal duties arise from OBRA '90, one implied and two stated. The implied duty is the *duty to warn*. The screening requirement does not specifically mention the pharmacist's duty to warn a prescriber or a patient about a potential drug-therapy-related problem, but if you discover a potential problem, it is logical and reasonable that you would take appropriate steps to resolve the problem.

The two specifically stated duties are the *duty to maintain patient profiles*, including documenting the pharmacist's observations about drug therapy, and *offering to counsel patients about their drug therapy*. The law provides significant detail as to what is required to fulfill each of these duties. (See OBRA '90 Patient Counseling Checklist, inside front cover.)

Patient counseling was included in OBRA '90 for the value it provides to the patient, but it benefits the pharmacist equally. In fact, the benefit is such that you may wish to personally counsel *all* patients, unless the patient objects. This approach will help to ensure that patients use their medication properly, to achieve the desired therapy outcome, to build patient loyalty and trust, and to avoid medication-related injuries that could lead to liability lawsuits.

Patient Counseling Tips*

Pharmacists should not sound like robots when they counsel patients or caregivers. The criteria of the American Pharmaceutical Association's National Patient Counseling Competition are designed to help the competitor avoid robot-like behavior and to improve the effectiveness of counseling. [The pharmacist]

1. Properly identifies self and purpose of the counseling session
2. Expresses concern for, and interest in, patient
3. Assesses patient's prior knowledge of the disease or treatment and any real or anticipated concerns or problems
4. Displays appropriate nonverbal behaviors (voice, eye contact, and body language)
5. Uses language the patient can understand
6. Maintains control and direction of counseling session
7. Makes appropriate use of patient profile information and checks for additions or changes
8. Presents facts and concepts in a logical, sequential order
9. Conveys complete and accurate information to the patient
10. Summarizes information presented
11. Checks to determine patient's understanding.

When dispensing a medicine for the first time, ask

1. What did your doctor tell you the medicine is for?
2. How did your doctor tell you to take the medicine?
3. What did your doctor tell you to expect?
4. (Verification, after counseling) Just to make sure I didn't leave anything out, please tell me how you are going to take your medicine.

When dispensing a refill, ask

1. What do you take the medicine for?
2. How do you take it?
3. What kind of problems are you having?

---

*Reprinted portions of Srnka QM, "Patient Counseling and Communication," in Canaday BR, ed., *OBRA '90: A Practical Guide to Effecting Pharmaceutical Care* (Washington, D.C.: American Pharmaceutical Association, 1994).

Recommended Patient Counseling Resources*

Agency for Health Care Policy and Research. *Clinical Practice Guidelines.* Guidelines have been developed on more than a dozen clinical conditions, including depression in primary care, management of cancer-related pain, and managing heart failure. An abbreviated version of each guideline, called a *Quick Reference Guide for Clinicians,* includes summary points on prevention, diagnosis, and treatment. To obtain copies of the complete or abbreviated guidelines, call toll-free (800) 358-9295 or write AHCPR Publications Clearinghouse, P.O. Box 8547, Silver Spring, MD 20907.

American Pharmaceutical Association. "One Minute Counselor" in *American Pharmacy.* Washington, D.C.: APhA, April 1992–present. A two-sided, tearout column that covers a different clinical condition each month. The front side contains information for the pharmacist; the back, for the patient. Information: (800) 237-APhA

_____. Patient Education Video Programs. Washington, D.C.: APhA. Four different programs for presentation to consumers, including presentation kits, are available: "National Medication Awareness Test" (1989), "Self-Medication Awareness Test" (1989), "Managing Your Medicines as You Grow Older" (1989), and "Your Pharmacist and You: A Health Partnership" (1993). Information: (800) 237-APhA

American Society of Health-System Pharmacists. *Medication Teaching Manual,* sixth edition. Bethesda, Md.: ASHP, 1994. A software product, MedTeach®, is also available. Information: (301) 657-3000

Canaday BR. *OBRA '90: A Practical Guide to Effecting Pharmaceutical Care.* Washington, D.C.: American Pharmaceutical Association, 1994. Information: (800) 237-APhA

Facts and Comparisons. *Patient Drug Facts.* St. Louis, Mo.: Facts and Comparisons, 1995. Yearly with quarterly updates. A software product, Patient Drug Facts—PC, is also available. Information: (800) 223-0554

Lem KW, ed. *Handbook of Nonprescription Drugs: Case Studies Workbook.* Washington, D.C.: American Pharmaceutical Association, 1993. Information: (800) 237-APhA

Tindall WN, Beardsley RS, Kimberlin CL. *Communication Skills in Pharmacy Practice.* Malvern, Pa.: Lea & Febiger, 1994. Information: (800) 638-0672

United States Pharmacopeial Convention. *USP DI® Vol. II, Advice for the Patient®.* Rockville, Md.: USP, 1995. Yearly with monthly updates. Information: (800) 227-8772

_____. *USP DI® Patient Education Leaflets®.* Rockville, Md.: USP, 1995. A software product, USP Leaflet Diskette, is also available. Information: (800) 227-8772

---

*For a comprehensive listing of patient counseling resources, see National Council on Patient Information and Education, *Directory of Prescription Medicine Information and Education Products, Programs, and Services,* 1994. Contact: NCPIE, 666 Eleventh Street, N.W., Suite 810, Washington, DC 20001; phone (202) 347-6711.

How to Use This Book

The information in this book is organized into monographs for each drug or family of drugs. These monographs are arranged alphabetically by the generic name of the drug or by the drug family name. Within family groupings, the generic drugs are listed immediately below the family monograph title. Although brand names are not included in the monographs, the index includes brand and generic names.

Each monograph has two major sections. The first section is entitled "For the Pharmacist." This section reflects the "Patient Consultation" section in the monographs in *USP DI® Volume I, Drug Information for the Health Care Professional*. Entries in this section that have greater importance are marked with a chevron (»).

The second section of each monograph is entitled "For the Patient." This section reproduces the *USP DI® Patient Education Leaflet®* for each drug or drug family. Written in language appropriate for the consumer, this information generally corresponds to the major points in the "Pharmacist" section. Chevroned (») entries in the "Pharmacist" section have corresponding lay language in the "Patient" section. In addition, some nonchevroned entries also appear in the "Patient" section, especially if the entries cover commonly asked questions.

The pharmacist should first refer to the "For the Pharmacist" section for consultation guidelines. Then, the pharmacist should use the "For the Patient" section for a more complete description and for language appropriate for the average consumer. In addition, the pharmacist may ask the patient to read the information in the "Patient" section.

Limitations of the information. The information provided is intended to enhance patient compliance and the effectiveness of the drug therapy. The information is not complete; it is intended to be a basic reminder or general guide to the pharmacist, who may vary or omit information in accordance with professional judgment. The information is not intended to substitute for professional judgment or to modify any legal requirements imposed on the pharmacist.

Some drugs are not amenable to general rules, since they may be prescribed for various purposes not necessarily known to the pharmacist; also, the differences in their use might affect the advice to be given. Occasionally, a pharmacist may have particular knowledge of problems specific to the patient that justifies giving exceptional instructions. The fact that this book makes no mention of such unusual or exceptional circumstances is not intended to limit or influence professional judgment in giving the patient information that is deemed to be correct and proper under the circumstances.

ACYCLOVIR   Systemic

■ For the Pharmacist ■

In providing consultation, consider emphasizing the following selected information (» = major clinical significance):

Before using this medication
» Conditions affecting use, especially:
    Hypersensitivity to acyclovir or ganciclovir
    Pregnancy—Acyclovir crosses the placenta
    Breast-feeding—Acyclovir is distributed into breast milk at concentrations from 0.6 to 4.1 times the corresponding plasma concentration
    In children—Neonates have an age-related decrease in acyclovir clearance
    Other medications, especially nephrotoxic medications
    Other medical problems, especially dehydration or pre-existing renal function impairment

Proper use of this medication
    Supplying patient information about herpes simplex or varicella-zoster infections
    For treatment of recurrent herpes simplex infections, initiating use of the medication as soon as possible after symptoms of recurrence begin to appear
    For treatment of chickenpox (varicella), initiating use of oral acyclovir at the earliest sign or symptom; it is most effective when started within 24 hours of the onset of a typical chickenpox rash
    Capsules, tablets, and oral suspension may be taken with meals
    Taking with full glass of water
    Proper administration technique for oral liquids
» Compliance with full course of therapy; not using more often or for longer than prescribed
» Proper dosing
    Missed dose: Taking as soon as possible; not taking if almost time for next dose; not doubling doses
» Proper storage

Precautions while using this medication
» Women with herpes genitalis may have an increased risk of developing cervical cancer; annual Pap tests may be required
    Checking with physician if no improvement within a few days
    Keeping affected areas as clean and dry as possible; wearing loose-fitting clothing to avoid irritation of lesions
» Use of acyclovir has not been shown to prevent the transmission of herpes simplex virus to sexual partners
» Herpes genitalis may be sexually transmitted even if partner is asymptomatic; sexual activity should be avoided if either partner has signs and symptoms of herpes genitalis; use of a condom may help prevent transmission of herpes; however, spermicidal jellies or diaphragms probably will not be adequately protective

Side/adverse effects
    Signs of potential side effects, especially phlebitis or inflammation at site of injection, acute renal failure, and encephalopathic changes

▲ For the Patient ▲

915530

ABOUT YOUR MEDICINE

Acyclovir (ay-SYE-kloe-veer) is used to prevent and treat the symptoms of herpes virus infections of the genitals (sex organs). It is also used to treat herpes infections of the skin (shingles) and chickenpox. Although acyclovir will not cure herpes, it does help relieve the pain and discomfort and helps the sores (if any) heal faster. Acyclovir may also be used for other virus infections as determined by your doctor. However, it does not work in treating certain viruses, such as the common cold.

If any of the information in this leaflet causes you special concern or if you want additional information about your medicine and its use, check with your doctor, nurse, or pharmacist. **Remember, keep this and all other medicines out of the reach of children and never share your medicines with others.**

BEFORE USING THIS MEDICINE

Tell your doctor, nurse, and pharmacist if you . . .
- are allergic to any medicine, either prescription or non-prescription (OTC);
- are pregnant or intend to become pregnant while using this medicine;
- are breast-feeding;
- are taking any other prescription or nonprescription (OTC) medicine, especially inflammation or pain medicine, except narcotics;
- have any other medical problems.

PROPER USE OF THIS MEDICINE

Acyclovir is best used as soon as possible after the symptoms of herpes infection (for example, pain, burning, blisters) begin to appear.

Acyclovir capsules, tablets, and oral suspension may be taken with meals.

For patients taking acyclovir for the treatment of chickenpox:
- Start using acyclovir as soon as possible after the first sign of the chickenpox rash, usually within one day.

For patients using acyclovir oral suspension:
- Use a specially marked measuring spoon or other device to measure each dose accurately. The average household teaspoon may not hold the right amount of liquid.

Do not use after the expiration date on the label. The medicine may not work as well. Check with your pharmacist if you have any questions about this.

To help clear up your herpes infection, **keep taking acyclovir for the full time of treatment,** even if your symptoms begin to clear up after a few days. **Do not miss any doses.** However, **do not use this medicine more often or for a longer time than your doctor ordered.**

If you do miss a dose of this medicine, take it as soon as possible. However, if it is almost time for your next dose, skip the missed dose and go back to your regular dosing schedule. Do not double doses.

PRECAUTIONS WHILE USING THIS MEDICINE

If your symptoms do not improve within a few days, or if they become worse, check with your doctor.

The areas affected by herpes should be kept as clean and dry as possible. Also, wear loose-fitting clothing to avoid irritating the sores (blisters).

It is important to remember that acyclovir will not keep you from spreading herpes to others.

For patients taking acyclovir for genital herpes:

- **Women with genital herpes may be more likely to get cancer of the cervix (mouth of the womb).** Therefore, it is very important that Pap tests be taken at least once a year to check for cancer. Cervical cancer can be cured if found and treated early.
- Herpes infection of the genitals can be caught from or spread to your partner during any sexual activity. Even though you may get herpes if your partner has no symptoms, the infection is more likely to be spread if sores are present. This is true until the sores are completely healed and the scabs have fallen off. **Therefore, it is best to avoid any sexual activity if either you or your sexual partner has any symptoms of herpes.** The use of a latex condom ('rubber') may help prevent the spread of herpes. However, spermicidal (sperm-killing) jelly or a diaphragm will probably not help.

This medicine must not be given to other people or used for other infections unless you are otherwise directed by your doctor.

POSSIBLE SIDE EFFECTS OF THIS MEDICINE
Side Effects That Usually Do Not Require Medical Attention

These possible side effects may go away during treatment; however, if they continue or are bothersome, check with your doctor, nurse, or pharmacist.

> *Less common (especially seen with long-term use or high doses)*—Diarrhea; headache; lightheadedness; nausea or vomiting

Other side effects not listed above may also occur in some patients. If you notice any other effects, check with your doctor, nurse, or pharmacist.

ACYCLOVIR   Topical

■For the Pharmacist■

In providing consultation, consider emphasizing the following selected information (**»** = major clinical significance):

Proper use of this medication
Reading patient information about herpes simplex infections
» Avoiding contact with eyes
» Using medication as soon as possible after symptoms of herpes begin to appear
» Proper administration technique:
Using a finger cot or rubber glove to prevent autoinoculation
Applying sufficient medication to cover affected areas; a 1.25-cm strip of ointment per 25 cm² of affected skin is usually sufficient
» Compliance with full course of therapy; not using more often or longer than prescribed
» Proper dosing
Missed dose: Applying as soon as possible; not applying if almost time for next dose
» Proper storage

Precautions while using this medication
» Women with herpes genitalis may be more likely to develop cervical cancer; annual or more frequent Pap tests may be required
Checking with physician if no improvement within 1 week
Keeping affected areas as clean and dry as possible; wearing loose-fitting clothing to avoid irritation of lesions
» Herpes genitalis may be sexually transmitted, even if sexual partner is asymptomatic; avoiding sexual activity if either partner has symptoms of herpes genitalis; use of condom may help prevent transmission of herpes; however, topical acyclovir or the use of spermicidal jellies or diaphragms will not prevent transmission of herpes to others

▲ For the Patient ▲

915541

ABOUT YOUR MEDICINE

Topical acyclovir (ay-SYE-kloe-veer) is used to treat the symptoms of herpes virus infections of genitals (sex organs) and mucous membranes (fever blisters, oral herpes). Although topical acyclovir will not cure herpes, it may help relieve the pain and discomfort and may help the sores (if any) heal faster.

If any of the information in this leaflet causes you special concern or if you want additional information about your medicine and its use, check with your doctor, nurse, or pharmacist. **Remember, keep this and all other medicines out of the reach of children and never share your medicines with others.**

BEFORE USING THIS MEDICINE

Tell your doctor, nurse, and pharmacist if you . . .
- are allergic to any medicine, either prescription or non-prescription (OTC);
- are pregnant or intend to become pregnant while using this medicine;
- are breast-feeding;
- are taking any other prescription or nonprescription (OTC) medicine;
- have any other medical problems.

PROPER USE OF THIS MEDICINE

Acyclovir may come with patient information about herpes simplex infections. Read this information carefully. If you have any questions, check with your doctor, nurse, or pharmacist.

Do not use this medicine in the eyes.

Acyclovir is best used as soon as possible after the symptoms of herpes infection (for example, pain, burning, blisters) begin to appear.

Use a finger cot or rubber glove when applying this medicine. This will help keep you from spreading the infection to other areas of your body. Apply enough medicine to completely cover all the sores (blisters). A 1.25–cm (approximately 1/2-inch) strip of ointment applied to each area of the affected skin measuring 5 × 5 cm (approximately 2 × 2 inches) is usually enough, unless otherwise directed by your doctor.

To help clear up your herpes infection, **continue using acyclovir for the full time of treatment,** even if your symptoms begin to clear up after a few days. **Do not miss any doses.** However, **do not use this medicine more often or for a longer time than your doctor ordered.**

If you do miss a dose of this medicine, apply it as soon as possible. However, if it is almost time for your next dose, skip the missed dose and go back to your regular dosing schedule.

PRECAUTIONS WHILE USING THIS MEDICINE

If your symptoms do not improve within 1 week, or if they become worse, check with your doctor.

It is important to remember that acyclovir will not keep you from spreading herpes to others.

For patients using acyclovir for genital herpes:
- **Women with genital herpes may be more likely to get cancer of the cervix (opening to the womb).** Therefore, it is very important that Pap tests be taken at least once a year to check for cancer. Cervical cancer can be cured if found and treated early.

- The areas affected by herpes should be kept as clean and dry as possible. Also, wear loose-fitting clothing to avoid irritating the sores (blisters).
- Herpes infection of the genitals can be caught from or spread to your partner during any sexual activity. Even though you may get herpes if your partner has no symptoms, the infection is more likely to be spread if sores are present. This is true until the sores are completely healed and the scabs have fallen off. **Therefore, it is best to avoid any sexual activity if either you or your sexual partner has any symptoms of herpes.** The use of a latex condom ('rubber') may help prevent the spread of herpes. However, spermicidal (sperm-killing) jelly or a diaphragm will probably not help.

This medicine must not be given to other people or used for other infections unless you are otherwise directed by your doctor.

POSSIBLE SIDE EFFECTS OF THIS MEDICINE
Side Effects That Usually Do Not Require Medical Attention

These possible side effects may go away during treatment; however, if they continue or are bothersome, check with your doctor, nurse, or pharmacist.

> *More common*—Mild pain, burning, or stinging

> *Less common or rare*—Itching; skin rash

Other side effects not listed above may also occur in some patients. If you notice any other effects, check with your doctor, nurse, or pharmacist.

ALLOPURINOL   Systemic

■ For the Pharmacist ■

In providing consultation, consider emphasizing the following selected information (» = major clinical significance):

Before using this medication
» Conditions affecting use, especially:
    Other medications, especially coumarin- or indandione-derivative anticoagulants, azathioprine, and mercaptopurine

Proper use of this medication
    Taking after meals, if necessary, to minimize gastrointestinal irritation
» Compliance with therapy
    Importance of high fluid intake during therapy and compliance with therapy for alkalinization of urine, if prescribed, to help prevent kidney stones
    Several months of continuous therapy may be required for maximum effectiveness in patients with chronic gout
» Medication helps prevent, but does not relieve, acute gout attacks; need to continue taking allopurinol with medication prescribed for gout attacks
» Proper dosing
    Missed dose: Taking as soon as possible; not taking if almost time for next dose; not doubling doses
» Proper storage

Precautions while using this medication
    Regular visits to physician to check progress during therapy; possible need for periodic blood tests to determine efficacy of therapy and/or occurrence of side effects
    Avoiding large amounts of alcohol, which may increase uric acid concentrations and reduce effectiveness of medication
    Possibility that vitamin C taken in large amounts may increase the potential for kidney stone formation
» Notifying physician immediately if skin rash occurs or if influenza-like symptoms (chills, fever, muscle aches and pains, or nausea or vomiting) occur concurrently with or shortly after skin rash; these symptoms may rarely indicate onset of severe hypersensitivity reaction
» Caution if drowsiness occurs

Side/adverse effects
    Signs of potential adverse effects, especially allergic dermatitis, agranulocytosis, anemia, angiitis, aplastic anemia, exfoliative dermatitis, erythema multiforme, hepatotoxicity, hypersensitivity reaction, loosening of fingernails, toxic epidermal necrolysis, peripheral neuritis, renal caluli, renal failure, Stevens-Johnson syndrome, thrombocytopenia, and unexplained nosebleeds

▲ For the Patient ▲

912033

ABOUT YOUR MEDICINE

Allopurinol (al-oh-PURE-i-nole) is used to treat chronic gout. It helps to prevent gout attacks, but will not relieve an attack that has already started. Allopurinol is also used to prevent or treat medical problems caused by too much uric acid in the body, including certain kinds of kidney stones or other kidney problems.

If any of the information in this leaflet causes you special concern or if you want additional information about your medicine and its use, check with your doctor, nurse, or pharmacist. **Remember, keep this and all other medicines out of the reach of children and never share your medicines with others.**

BEFORE USING THIS MEDICINE
Tell your doctor, nurse, and pharmacist if you . . .
- are allergic to any medicine, either prescription or non-prescription (OTC);
- are pregnant or intend to become pregnant while using this medicine;
- are breast-feeding;
- are taking any other prescription or nonprescription (OTC) medicine, especially anticoagulants, azathioprine, or mercaptopurine;
- have any other medical problems, especially diabetes mellitus (sugar diabetes), high blood pressure, or kidney disease.

PROPER USE OF THIS MEDICINE
If this medicine upsets your stomach, take it after meals. If stomach upset (nausea, vomiting, diarrhea, or stomach pain) continues, check with your doctor.

In order for this medicine to help you, it must be taken regularly as ordered.

If you are taking allopurinol to prevent gout attacks and they continue, **keep taking this medicine, even if you are taking another medicine for the attacks.**

To help prevent kidney stones while taking allopurinol, adults should drink at least 10 to 12 full glasses (8 ounces each) of fluids each day unless otherwise directed by their doctor. Check with your doctor about the amount of fluids to be taken each day by children being treated with this medicine. Also, your doctor may want you to take another medicine to make your urine less acid.

If you miss a dose of this medicine, take it as soon as possible. However, if it is almost time for your next dose, skip the missed dose and go back to your regular dosing schedule. Do not double doses.

PRECAUTIONS WHILE USING THIS MEDICINE
Drinking too much alcohol may increase the amount of uric acid in the blood and lessen the effects of allopurinol. Therefore, people with gout and other people with too much uric acid in the body should be careful to limit the amount of alcohol they drink.

Check with your doctor immediately if you notice a skin rash, hives, or itching while taking allopurinol or if chills, fever, joint pain, muscle aches or pains, sore throat, or nausea or vomiting occur, especially if they occur together with or shortly after a skin rash. Very rarely, these effects may be the first signs of a serious reaction to the medicine.

This medicine may cause some people to become drowsy or less alert than they are normally. **Make sure you know how you react to this medicine before you drive, use machines, or do other jobs that require you to be alert.**

POSSIBLE SIDE EFFECTS OF THIS MEDICINE
Side Effects That Should Be Reported To Your Doctor Immediately

Stop taking this medicine and check with your doctor immediately if you notice:

> *More common*—Skin rash or sores, hives, or itching

> *Rare*—Black, tarry stools; bleeding sores on lips; blood in urine or stools; chills, fever, muscle aches or pains, nausea, or vomiting, especially if occurring with or shortly after a skin rash; difficult or painful urination; pinpoint red spots on skin; red and/or irritated eyes; redness, tenderness, burning, or peeling of skin; red, thickened, or scaly skin; shortness of breath, troubled breathing, tightness in chest, or wheezing; sores, ulcers, or white spots in mouth or on lips; sore throat and fever; sudden decrease in urine; swelling in upper abdominal (stomach) area; swelling of face, feet, fingers, or lower legs; unusual bleeding or bruising; unusual weakness; weight gain (rapid); yellow eyes or skin

Other Side Effects That Should Be Reported To Your Doctor

> *Rare*—Loosening of fingernails; numbness, tingling, pain, or weakness in hands or feet; pain in lower back or side; unexplained nosebleeds

Other side effects not listed above may also occur in some patients. If you notice any other effects, check with your doctor, nurse, or pharmacist.

AMANTADINE   Systemic

■For the Pharmacist■

In providing consultation, consider emphasizing the following selected information (» = major clinical significance):

Before using this medication
» Conditions affecting use, especially:
  Hypersensitivity to amantadine
  Pregnancy—Amantadine crosses the placenta
  Breast-feeding—Amantadine is excreted in breast milk
  Use in the elderly—Geriatric patients may exhibit increased sensitivity to the anticholinergic-like side effects of amantadine
  Other medications, especially alcohol, anticholinergics or other medications with anticholinergic activity, or other CNS stimulation–producing medications
  Other medical problems, especially congestive heart failure, peripheral edema, renal function impairment, seizure disorders, or a history of epilepsy

Proper use of this medication
» Proper storage
» Proper dosing
  Missed dose: Taking as soon as possible; not taking if almost time for next dose; not doubling doses
For use as an antiviral
  Receiving a flu shot if have not already done so
» Taking before exposure or as soon as possible after exposure
» Compliance with full course of therapy
» Importance of not missing doses and taking at evenly spaced times
  Proper administration technique for oral liquid
For use as an antidyskinetic
» Not taking more medication than the amount prescribed; not missing doses
  May require up to 2 weeks for full benefit

Precautions while using this medication
» Avoiding alcoholic beverages
» Caution if mental acuity or eyesight is impaired
  Caution when getting up suddenly from a lying or sitting position
  Possible dryness of mouth, nose, and throat; using sugarless candy or gum, ice, or saliva substitute for relief of dry mouth; checking with physician or dentist if dry mouth continues for more than 2 weeks
  Possible appearance of livedo reticularis; gradual disappearance within 2 to 12 weeks after stopping medication
For use as an antiviral
  Checking with physician if no improvement within a few days
For use as an antidyskinetic
» Resuming physical activities gradually as condition improves
  Checking with physician if medication gradually loses its effectiveness
» Checking with physician before discontinuing medication; gradual dosage reduction may be necessary

Side/adverse effects
Signs of potential side effects, especially anticholinergic-like effects, orthostatic hypotension, CNS toxicity, congestive heart failure, corneal deposits, and skin rash

---

▲ For the Patient ▲

913218

ABOUT YOUR MEDICINE

Amantadine (a-MAN-ta-deen) is an antiviral. It is used to prevent or treat certain influenza (flu) infections (type A). It will not work for colds, other types of flu, or other virus infections. Amantadine is also used to treat Parkinson's disease (paralysis agitans or shaking palsy) and to treat stiffness and shaking caused by medicines used to treat nervous, mental, and emotional conditions. It may also be used for other conditions as determined by your doctor.

If any of the information in this leaflet causes you special concern or if you want additional information about your medicine and its use, check with your doctor, nurse, or pharmacist. **Remember, keep this and all other medicines out of the reach of children and never share your medicines with others.**

BEFORE USING THIS MEDICINE

Tell your doctor, nurse, and pharmacist if you . . .
- are allergic to any medicine, either prescription or nonprescription (OTC);
- are pregnant or intend to become pregnant while using this medicine;
- are breast-feeding;
- are taking **any** other prescription or nonprescription (OTC) medicine;
- have **any** other medical problems.

PROPER USE OF THIS MEDICINE

For patients taking amantadine to prevent or treat flu infections:
- Talk to your doctor about the possibility of getting a flu shot if you have not had one yet.
- This medicine is **best taken before exposure, or as soon as possible after exposure**, to people who have the flu.
- To help keep yourself from getting the flu, **keep taking this medicine for the full time of treatment.** Or if you already have the flu, continue taking this medicine for the full time of treatment.
- This medicine works best when there is a constant amount in the blood. **To help keep the amount constant, do not miss any doses. Also, it is best to take the doses at evenly spaced times day and night.**

For patients taking amantadine for Parkinson's disease or movement problems caused by certain medicines used to treat nervous, mental, and emotional conditions:
- **Take this medicine exactly as directed by your doctor.** Do not miss any doses and do not take more medicine than your doctor ordered.

If you do miss a dose of this medicine, take it as soon as possible. This will help to keep a constant amount of medicine in the blood. However, if it is almost time for your next dose, skip the missed dose and go back to your regular dosing schedule. Do not double doses.

PRECAUTIONS WHILE USING THIS MEDICINE

Drinking alcoholic beverages while taking this medicine may cause increased side effects such as circulation problems, dizziness, lightheadedness, fainting, or confusion. Therefore, **do not drink alcoholic beverages while you are taking this medicine.**

This medicine may cause some people to become dizzy, confused, or lightheaded, or to have blurred vision or trouble concentrating. **Make sure you know how you react to this medicine before you drive, use machines, or do other jobs that require you to be alert or to see clearly.**

For patients taking amantadine for Parkinson's disease or movement problems caused by certain medicines used to treat nervous, mental, and emotional conditions:
- **Be careful not to overdo physical activities as your condition improves and body movements become easier.** Injuries resulting from falls may occur.
- **Do not suddenly stop taking this medicine without first checking with your doctor.** Your doctor may want you to reduce your dose gradually before stopping the medicine completely.

POSSIBLE SIDE EFFECTS OF THIS MEDICINE
Side Effects That Should Be Reported To Your Doctor Immediately

   Less common—Blurred vision; confusion, especially in elderly patients; difficult urination, especially in elderly patients; fainting; hallucinations

   Rare—Convulsions (seizures); decreased vision or any change in vision; difficulty in coordination; irritation and swelling of the eye; mental depression; skin rash; swelling of feet or lower legs; unexplained shortness of breath

Side Effects That Usually Do Not Require Medical Attention

These possible side effects may go away during treatment; however, if they continue or are bothersome, check with your doctor, nurse, or pharmacist.

More common—Difficulty concentrating; dizziness or lightheadedness; headache; irritability; loss of appetite; nausea; nervousness; purplish red, blotchy spots on skin; trouble in sleeping or nightmares

Other side effects not listed above may also occur in some patients. If you notice any other effects, check with your doctor, nurse, or pharmacist.

AMIODARONE   Systemic

■ For the Pharmacist ■

In providing consultation, consider emphasizing the following selected
information (» = major clinical significance):

Before using this medication
» Conditions affecting use, especially:
  Sensitivity to amiodarone
  Pregnancy—Potential risk of bradycardia and iodine toxicity in
    fetus
  Breast-feeding—Excreted in breast milk
  Use in children—Shorter onset and duration of action
  Use in elderly—Increased sensitivity to effects on thyroid func-
    tion and increased incidence of ataxia and other neurotoxic
    effects
  Other medications, especially other antiarrhythmics, coumarin-
    derivative anticoagulants, digitalis glycosides, or phenytoin
  Other medical problems, especially pre-existing AV block with-
    out pacemaker, bradycardic episodes resulting in syncope
    (unless controlled by pacemaker), or severe sinus node func-
    tion impairment causing marked bradycardia (unless con-
    trolled by pacemaker)

Proper use of this medication
» Compliance with therapy; taking as directed even if feeling well
» Proper dosing
  Missed dose: Not taking at all; notifying physician if two or more
    doses in a row are missed; not doubling doses
» Proper storage

Precautions while using this medication
  Regular visits to physician to check progress
  Carrying medical identification card or bracelet
» Caution if any kind of surgery (including dental surgery) or emer-
    gency treatment is required
» Protecting skin from sunlight during and for several months follow-
    ing withdrawal of treatment; burns may occur even through win-
    dow glass and thin cotton clothing; use of protective clothing
    and barrier sunscreen; checking with physician if severe burn
    occurs
  Checking with physician if blue-gray discoloration of skin occurs

Side/adverse effects
  Signs of potential side effects, especially pulmonary fibrosis; inter-
    stitial pneumonitis/alveolitis; neurotoxicity; photosensitivity; blue-
    gray coloring of skin on face, neck, and arms; ocular toxicity;
    hypothyroidism; hyperthyroidism; new or exacerbated arrhyth-
    mias; noninfectious epididymitis; sinus bradycardia; congestive
    heart failure; allergic reaction; and hepatitis

▲ For the Patient ▲

915246

ABOUT YOUR MEDICINE
Amiodarone (am-ee-OH-da-rone) is an antiarrhythmic. It is
used to correct irregular heartbeats to a normal rhythm.

If any of the information in this leaflet causes you special concern or if you want additional information about your medicine and its use, check with your doctor, nurse, or pharmacist. **Remember, keep this and all other medicines out of the reach of children and never share your medicines with others.**

BEFORE USING THIS MEDICINE

Tell your doctor, nurse, and pharmacist if you . . .
- are allergic to any medicine, either prescription or non-prescription (OTC);
- are pregnant or intend to become pregnant while using this medicine;
- are breast-feeding;
- are taking any other prescription or nonprescription (OTC) medicine, especially anticoagulants, other heart medicine, or phenytoin;
- have any other medical problems.

PROPER USE OF THIS MEDICINE

Take amiodarone exactly as directed by your doctor even though you may feel well. Do not take more medicine than ordered and do not miss any doses.

If you do miss a dose of this medicine, do not take the missed dose at all and do not double the next one. Instead, go back to your regular dosing schedule. If you miss two or more doses in a row, check with your doctor.

PRECAUTIONS WHILE USING THIS MEDICINE

It is important that your doctor check your progress at regular visits to make sure the medicine is working properly.

Your doctor may want you to carry a medical identification card or bracelet stating that you are taking this medicine.

Before having any kind of surgery or dental or emergency treatment, tell the physician or dentist in charge that you are taking this medicine.

Amiodarone increases the sensitivity of your skin to sunlight; too much exposure could cause a serious burn. Your skin may continue to be sensitive to sunlight for several months after treatment with this medicine is stopped. A burn can occur even through window glass or thin cotton clothing. If you must go out in the sunlight, **cover your skin and wear a wide-brimmed hat. A special sun-blocking cream should also be used**; it must contain zinc or titanium oxide because other sunscreens will not work. **In case of a severe burn, check with your doctor.**

After you have taken this medicine for a long time, it may cause a blue-gray color to appear on your skin, especially in areas exposed to the sun, such as your face, neck, and arms. This color will usually fade after treatment with amiodarone has ended, although it may take several months. However, check with your doctor if this effect occurs.

POSSIBLE SIDE EFFECTS OF THIS MEDICINE
Side Effects That Should Be Reported To Your Doctor Immediately

> *More common*—Cough; painful breathing; shortness of breath

Other Side Effects That Should Be Reported To Your Doctor

> *More common*—Fever (slight); numbness or tingling in fingers or toes; sensitivity of skin to sunlight; trembling or shaking of hands; trouble in walking; unusual and uncontrolled movements of the body; weakness of arms or legs

> *Less common*—Blue-gray coloring of skin on face, neck, and arms; blurred vision or blue-green halos seen around objects; coldness; dry eyes; dry, puffy skin; fast or irregular heartbeat; nervousness; pain and swelling in scrotum; sensitivity of eyes to light; sensitivity to heat; slow heartbeat; sweating; swelling of feet or lower legs; trouble in sleeping; unusual tiredness; weight gain or loss

> *Rare*—Skin rash; yellow eyes or skin

Side Effects That Usually Do Not Require Medical Attention

These possible side effects may go away during treatment; however, if they continue or are bothersome, check with your doctor, nurse, or pharmacist.

> *More common*—Constipation; headache; loss of appetite; nausea and vomiting

Other side effects not listed above may also occur in some patients. If you notice any other effects, check with your doctor, nurse, or pharmacist.

After you stop using this medicine, your body may need time to adjust. The length of time this takes depends on the amount of medicine you were using and how long you used it. **During this time check with your doctor** if you notice cough, fever (slight), painful breathing, or shortness of breath.

AMLODIPINE   Systemic

■ For the Pharmacist ■

In providing consultation, consider emphasizing the following selected information (» = major clinical significance):

Before using this medication
» Conditions affecting use, especially:
    Use in the elderly—Half-life increased; increased sensitivity to hypotensive effects
    Dental—Risk of gingival hyperplasia
    Other medications
    Other medical problems, especially severe hypotension

Proper use of this medication
» Compliance with therapy; importance of not taking more medication than amount prescribed
» Proper dosing
    Missed dose: Taking as soon as possible; not taking if almost time for next scheduled dose; not doubling doses
» Proper storage
For use as an antihypertensive
    Possible need for control of weight and diet, especially sodium intake
» Patient may not experience symptoms of hypertension; importance of taking medication even if feeling well
» Does not cure, but helps control hypertension; possible need for lifelong therapy; serious consequences of untreated hypertension

Precautions while using this medication
    Regular visits to physician to check progress during therapy
    Checking with physician before discontinuing medication; gradual dosage reduction may be necessary
» Discussing exercise or physical exertion limits with physician; reduced occurrence of chest pain may tempt patient to be overactive
    Possible headache; checking with physician if continuing or severe
» Maintaining good dental hygiene and seeing dentist frequently for teeth cleaning to prevent tenderness, bleeding, and gum enlargement
For use as an antihypertensive
» Not taking other medications, especially nonprescription sympathomimetics, unless discussed with physician

Side/adverse effects
    Signs of potential side effects, especially peripheral edema, dizziness, palpitations, angina, bradycardia, hypotension, or orthostatic hypotension

▲ For the Patient ▲

919270

ABOUT YOUR MEDICINE
Amlodipine (am-LOE-di-peen) is a calcium channel blocker used to treat angina (chest pain) and high blood pressure.

If any of the information in this leaflet causes you special concern or if you want additional information about your

medicine and its use, check with your doctor, nurse, or pharmacist. **Remember, keep this and all other medicines out of the reach of children and never share your medicines with others.**

BEFORE USING THIS MEDICINE

Tell your doctor, nurse, and pharmacist if you . . .
- are allergic to any medicine, either prescription or nonprescription (OTC);
- are pregnant or intend to become pregnant while using this medicine;
- are breast-feeding;
- are taking any other prescription or nonprescription (OTC) medicine;
- have any other medical problems, especially very low blood pressure.

PROPER USE OF THIS MEDICINE

Take this medicine exactly as directed even if you feel well. Do not take more of it and do not take it more often than your doctor ordered. Do not miss any doses.

If you do miss a dose of this medicine, take it as soon as possible. However, if it is almost time for your next dose, skip the missed dose and go back to your regular dosing schedule. Do not double doses.

PRECAUTIONS WHILE USING THIS MEDICINE

If you have been taking this medicine regularly for several weeks, do not suddenly stop taking it. Stopping suddenly may bring on your previous problem. Check with your doctor for the best way to reduce gradually the amount you are taking before stopping completely.

Chest pain resulting from exercise or exertion is usually reduced or prevented by this medicine. This may tempt you to be overly active. **Make sure you discuss with your doctor a safe amount of exercise for your medical problem.**

In some patients, tenderness, swelling, or bleeding of the gums may occur. Brushing and flossing your teeth carefully and regularly and massaging your gums may help prevent this. **See your dentist regularly to have your teeth cleaned. Check with your physician or dentist if you notice any tenderness, swelling, or bleeding of your gums.**

POSSIBLE SIDE EFFECTS OF THIS MEDICINE
Side Effects That Should Be Reported To Your Doctor

More common—Swelling of ankles or feet

Less common—Dizziness; pounding heartbeat

Rare—Chest pain; dizziness or lightheadedness when getting up from a lying or sitting position

Side Effects That Usually Do Not Require Medical Attention

These possible side effects may go away during treatment; however, if they continue or are bothersome, check with your doctor, nurse, or pharmacist.

More common—Flushing; headache; nausea

Less common—Unusual tiredness or weakness

Other side effects not listed above may also occur in some patients. If you notice any other effects, check with your doctor, nurse, or pharmacist.

AMPHETAMINES   Systemic

Including Amphetamine; Amphetamine and
Dextroamphetamine Resin Complex; Dextroamphetamine;
Methamphetamine.

■ For the Pharmacist ■

In providing consultation, consider emphasizing the following selected
information (» = major clinical significance):

Before using this medication
» Conditions affecting use, especially:
  Sensitivity to amphetamines and other sympathomimetics
  Pregnancy—Increased risk of congenital malformations, espe-
    cially in cardiovascular system and biliary tract; potential
    embryotoxic and teratogenic effects in animals given large
    doses; risk of premature delivery and low birth weight may
    be increased; newborn may experience withdrawal symptoms
  Breast-feeding—Not recommended since amphetamines are dis-
    tributed into breast milk
  Use in children—May inhibit growth; may provoke motor and
    vocal tics and Tourette's syndrome; may exacerbate behavior
    problems and thought disorder in psychotic children
  Other medications, especially tricyclic antidepressants, beta-
    adrenergic blocking agents, digitalis glycosides, meperidine,
    monoamine oxidase inhibitors, other CNS stimulation–pro-
    ducing medications, or thyroid hormones
  Other medical problems, especially agitated states, advanced
    arteriosclerosis or symptomatic cardiovascular disease, his-
    tory of drug dependence, glaucoma, hypertension, hyperthy-
    roidism, or Tourette's syndrome or other tics

Proper use of this medication
  Taking the last dose of the day of the regular dosage form at least
    6 hours before bedtime and the daily dose of the extended-release
    dosage form about 10 to 14 hours before bedtime to minimize
    the possibility of insomnia
  Proper administration of extended-release dosage forms:
    Swallowing whole
    Not breaking, crushing, or chewing
» Importance of not taking more medication than the amount pre-
    scribed because of habit-forming potential
» Not increasing dose if medication becomes less effective after a few
    weeks; checking with physician
» Proper dosing
  Missed dose: If dosing schedule is—
    Once a day: Taking as soon as possible but not later than stated
      above; if remembered later, not taking until next day; not
      doubling doses
    Two or three times a day: Taking as soon as possible if remem-
      bered within an hour or so; not taking if remembered later;
      not doubling doses
» Proper storage

Precautions while using this medication
  Regular visits to physician to check progress during therapy
» Checking with physician before discontinuing medication after pro-
    longed high-dose therapy; gradual dosage reduction may be nec-
    essary to avoid possibility of withdrawal symptoms

» Caution if dizziness or euphoria occurs; not driving, using machinery, or doing other activities that are potentially hazardous

Caution if any laboratory tests required; possible interference with results of metyrapone test

» Suspected psychological or physical dependence; checking with physician

Side/adverse effects

Signs of potential side effects, especially irregular heartbeat; allergic reaction; chest pain; tics or other signs of severe CNS stimulation; hyperthermia; cardiomyopathy; increased blood pressure; psychotic reactions

Potential unwanted effects during long-term use in children

Possibility of withdrawal effects, especially mental depression, nausea, stomach cramps or pain, vomiting, trembling, or unusual tiredness or weakness

---

▲ For the Patient ▲

913240

ABOUT YOUR MEDICINE

Amphetamines (am-FET-a-meens) belong to the group of medicines called central nervous system (CNS) stimulants. They are used to treat attention-deficit hyperactivity disorder (ADHD). Amphetamine and dextroamphetamine are also used in the treatment of narcolepsy (uncontrollable desire for sleep or sudden attacks of deep sleep).

Amphetamines should not be used for weight loss or weight control or to combat fatigue or replace rest. When used for these purposes, they may be dangerous to your health.

If any of the information in this leaflet causes you special concern or if you want additional information about your medicine and its use, check with your doctor, nurse, or pharmacist. **Remember, keep this and all other medicines out of the reach of children and never share your medicines with others.**

BEFORE USING THIS MEDICINE

Tell your doctor, nurse, and pharmacist if you . . .

- are allergic to any medicine, either prescription or nonprescription (OTC);
- are pregnant or intend to become pregnant while using this medicine;
- are breast-feeding;
- are taking **any** other prescription or nonprescription (OTC) medicine;
- have **any** other medical problems;
- use cocaine.

PROPER USE OF THIS MEDICINE

For patients taking the short-acting form of this medicine:

- Take the last dose for each day at least 6 hours before bedtime to help prevent trouble in sleeping.

For patients taking the long-acting form of this medicine:
- Take the daily dose about 10 to 14 hours before bedtime to help prevent trouble in sleeping.
- These capsules or tablets should be swallowed whole. Do not break, crush, or chew them before swallowing.

Take this medicine only as directed by your doctor. Do not take more of it, do not take it more often, and do not take it for a longer time than your doctor ordered. If too much is taken, it may become habit-forming.

If you miss a dose of this medicine and your dosing schedule is:
- One dose a day—Take the missed dose as soon as possible, but not later than stated above. But if you do not remember until the next day, skip it and go back to your regular dosing schedule. Do not double doses.
- Two or three doses a day—If you remember within an hour or so of the missed dose, take it right away. But if you do not remember until later, skip it and go back to your regular dosing schedule. Do not double doses.

PRECAUTIONS WHILE USING THIS MEDICINE

Your doctor should check your progress at regular visits to make sure this medicine does not cause unwanted effects.

If you will be taking this medicine in large doses for a long time, **do not stop taking it without first checking with your doctor**. Your doctor may want you to reduce gradually the amount you are taking before stopping completely.

If you have been taking this medicine for a long time and you think you may have become mentally or physically dependent on it, check with your doctor. Some signs of dependence on amphetamines are:
- a strong desire or need to continue taking the medicine.
- a need to increase the dose to receive the effects of the medicine.
- withdrawal effects (for example, mental depression, nausea or vomiting, unusual tiredness or weakness) occurring after the medicine is stopped.

This medicine may cause some people to feel a false sense of well-being or to become dizzy, lightheaded, or less alert than they are normally. **Make sure you know how you react to this medicine before you drive, use machines, or do other jobs that require you to be alert.**

POSSIBLE SIDE EFFECTS OF THIS MEDICINE
Side Effects That Should Be Reported To Your Doctor

More common—Irregular heartbeat

Rare—Chest pain; fever (unusually high); skin rash or hives; uncontrolled movements of head, neck, arms, and legs

Side Effects That Usually Do Not Require Medical Attention

These possible side effects may go away during treatment; however, if they continue or are bothersome, check with your doctor, nurse, or pharmacist.

> *More common*—False sense of well-being; irritability; nervousness; restlessness; trouble in sleeping

Other side effects not listed above may also occur in some patients. If you notice any other effects, check with your doctor, nurse, or pharmacist.

After you stop using this medicine, your body may need time to adjust. The length of time this takes depends on the amount of medicine you were using and how long you used it. **Check with your doctor if you notice any unusual effects,** especially mental depression, nausea or vomiting, stomach cramps or pain, trembling, or unusual tiredness or weakness.

ANABOLIC STEROIDS   Systemic

Including Nandrolone; Oxandrolone; Oxymetholone; Stanozolol.

■For the Pharmacist■

In providing consultation, consider emphasizing the following selected information (» = major clinical significance):

Before using this medication
» Conditions affecting use, especially:

      Carcinogencity—Hepatocellular carcinoma associated with long-term, high-dose therapy

      Tumorigenicity—Hepatic neoplasms associated with long-term, high-dose therapy

      Pregnancy—Not recommended during pregnancy because of possible masculinization of fetus

      Use in children—Cautious use because of effects on growth and sexual development (precocious sexual development in males, virilization in females)

      Use in elderly—Increased risk of prostatic hypertrophy or prostatic carcinoma

      Other medications, especially anticoagulants (coumarin- or indandione-derivatives) or hepatotoxic medications

      Other medical problems, especially breast cancer, hepatic function impairment, hypercalcemia, nephrosis, nephrotic phase of nephritis, prostatic cancer, coronary artery disease, or myocardial infarction

Proper use of this medication
» Importance of not taking more medication than the amount prescribed; to do so may increase chance of side effects
» Importance of diet high in proteins and calories while taking this medication to achieve maximum therapeutic effect
» Proper dosing

    Missed dose: If dosing schedule is—

      Once daily: Taking as soon as possible; if not remembered until next day, not taking at all; not doubling doses

      More than once daily: Taking as soon as possible; not taking if almost time for next dose; not doubling doses
» Proper storage

Precautions while using this medication
    Regular visits to physician to check progress during therapy

    Diabetics: May decrease blood sugar concentrations

Side/adverse effects
    Signs of potential side effects, especially:

      In females only—Virilism, hypercalcemia

      In prepubertal males only—Virilism or unexplained darkening of skin

      In males only—Gynecomastia, priapism, or bladder irritability

      In geriatric males only—Prostatic carcinoma or hypertrophy

      In all patients, in addition to those side effects listed above—Leukemia; peliosis hepatis; anemia; edema; clotting factor suppression; and hepatic dysfunction, carcinoma, or necrosis

---

▲ For the Patient ▲

913251

ABOUT YOUR MEDICINE

Anabolic (an-a-BOL-ik) **steroids** are used to help patients gain weight after a severe illness, injury, or continuing infection; to treat certain types of anemia; to treat certain kinds of breast cancer in women; or to treat hereditary angioedema, which causes swelling of the face, arms, legs, throat, windpipe, bowels, or sexual organs. They may also be used for other conditions as determined by your doctor.

There is no good medical evidence to support the belief that use of these medicines by athletes will increase muscle strength. When used for this purpose, they may even be dangerous because of unwanted side effects. Also, anabolic steroid use can lead to disqualification of athletes in most athletic events.

If any of the information in this leaflet causes you special concern or if you want additional information about your medicine and its use, check with your doctor, nurse, or pharmacist. **Remember, keep this and all other medicines out of the reach of children and never share your medicines with others.**

BEFORE USING THIS MEDICINE

Tell your doctor, nurse, and pharmacist if you . . .
- are allergic to any medicine, either prescription or nonprescription (OTC);
- are pregnant or intend to become pregnant while using this medicine;
- are breast-feeding;
- are taking **any** other prescription or nonprescription (OTC) medicine;
- have **any** other medical problems.

PROPER USE OF THIS MEDICINE

Take this medicine only as directed. Do not take more of it and do not take it more often than ordered. To do so may increase the chance of side effects.

In order for this medicine to work properly, it is important that you follow a diet high in proteins and calories. If you have any questions about this, check with your doctor, nurse, or pharmacist.

If you miss a dose of this medicine and your dosing schedule is:
- One dose a day—Take the missed dose as soon as possible. However, if you do not remember it until the next day, skip it and go back to your regular dosing schedule. Do not double doses.
- More than one dose a day—Take the missed dose as soon as possible. However, if it is almost time for your

next dose, skip the missed dose and go back to your regular dosing schedule. Do not double doses.

PRECAUTIONS WHILE USING THIS MEDICINE
Your doctor should check your progress at regular visits to make sure that this medicine does not cause unwanted effects.

Anabolic steroids can decrease the amount of sperm made. Also, anabolic steroids may cause children to stop growing early or to develop too fast sexually.

POSSIBLE SIDE EFFECTS OF THIS MEDICINE
Tumors of the liver or liver disease have occurred during long-term, high-dose therapy with anabolic steroids. These effects are rare but can be very serious.

Side Effects That Should Be Reported To Your Doctor Immediately

For both females and males
  Less common—Yellow eyes or skin

   Rare (with long-term use)—Black, tarry, or light-colored stools; dark-colored urine; purple or red spots on body or inside the mouth or nose; sore throat and fever; vomiting of blood

Other Side Effects That Should Be Reported To Your Doctor

For both females and males
  Less common—Bone pain; nausea or vomiting; sore tongue; swelling of feet or lower legs; unusual bleeding; unusual weight gain

For females only
  More common—Acne or oily skin; enlarged clitoris; hair loss; hoarseness or deepening of voice; irregular periods; unnatural hair growth

   Less common—Mental depression; unusual tiredness

For young males (boys) only
  More common—Acne; enlarging penis; increased frequency of erections; unnatural hair growth

   Less common—Skin darkening

For sexually mature males only
  More common—Enlargement of breasts or breast soreness; frequent or continuing erections; frequent urge to urinate

For elderly males only
  Less common—Difficult or frequent urination; increase in sexual desire

Other side effects not listed above may also occur in some patients. If you notice any other effects, check with your doctor, nurse, or pharmacist.

ANDROGENS   Systemic

Including Fluoxymesterone; Methyltestosterone; Testosterone.

■For the Pharmacist■

In providing consultation, consider emphasizing the following selected information (» = major clinical significance):

Before using this medication
» Conditions affecting use, especially:
> Sensitivity to androgens or anabolic steroids
> Carcinogenicity—Hepatocellular carcinoma associated with long-term, high-dose therapy
> Tumorigenicity—Hepatic neoplasms associated with long-term, high-dose therapy
> Fertility—May be severely impaired in males
> Pregnancy—Contraindicated for use during pregnancy because of possible masculinization of female fetus
> Use in children—Cautious use due to effects on growth and sexual development (precocious sexual development in males, virilization in females)
> Use in the elderly—Increased risk of prostatic hypertrophy or prostatic carcinoma
> Other medications, especially anticoagulants (coumarin- or indandione-derivatives) or hepatotoxic medications
> Other medical problems, especially male breast cancer, possible prostate cancer, cardiac failure, cardio-renal disease, history of myocardial infarction, hepatic function impairment, hypercalcemia, nephritis, nephrosis, or prostatic hypertrophy

Proper use of this medication
For fluoxymesterone, and capsule and oral tablet dosage forms of methyltestosterone
> Taking with food to minimize possible stomach upset
For methyltestosterone buccal tablets
» Importance of not swallowing buccal tablets
For testosterone skin patch
> Applying to dry, clean, and hairless skin of scrotum; may be reapplied after bathing, swimming, or showering
For all androgens
» Importance of not taking more medication than the amount prescribed
» Proper administration
» Proper dosing
> Missed dose: Taking as soon as possible; not taking if almost time for next dose; not doubling doses
» Proper storage

Precautions while using this medication
> Regular visits to physician to check progress during therapy
> Diabetics: May alter blood sugar concentrations
> Checking with doctor if female sexual partner develops mild virilization

Side/adverse effects
> Signs of potential side effects, especially:
> In females only—Menstrual irregularities, virilism

In males only—Bladder irritability or urinary tract infection,
breast soreness, gynecomastia, priapism, epididymitis, prostatic carcinoma, prostatic hypertrophy
In prepubertal males only—Virilism
In all patients—Edema, erythrocytosis or polycythemia, gastrointestinal irritation, hepatic necrosis, hepatocellular tumor,
hepatic dysfunction, hypercalcemia, leukopenia, or peliosis
hepatis

▲ For the Patient ▲

913262

ABOUT YOUR MEDICINE

Androgens (AN-droe-jens) are male hormones which are necessary for the normal sexual development of males. Androgens are used for several reasons: to replace the hormone
when the body is unable to produce enough; to stimulate the
beginning of puberty in certain boys who are late starting
puberty naturally; to treat certain types of breast cancer in
females. Some of these medicines may also be used for other
conditions as determined by your doctor.

There is no good medical evidence to support the belief that
use of androgens in athletes will increase muscle strength.
When used for this purpose, they may even be dangerous
because of their side effects. Also, use of androgens can lead
to disqualification of athletes in most athletic events.

If any of the information in this leaflet causes you special
concern or if you want additional information about your
medicine and its use, check with your doctor, nurse, or pharmacist. **Remember, keep this and all other medicines out of
the reach of children and never share your medicines with
others.**

BEFORE USING THIS MEDICINE

Tell your doctor, nurse, and pharmacist if you . . .
- are allergic to any medicine, either prescription or nonprescription (OTC);
- are pregnant or intend to become pregnant while using
this medicine;
- are breast-feeding;
- compete in athletics;
- are taking **any** other prescription or nonprescription
(OTC) medicine;
- have **any** other medical problems.

PROPER USE OF THIS MEDICINE

**Take this medicine only as directed. Do not take more of it
and do not take it more often than ordered.** To do so may
increase side effects.

For patients taking the capsule or regular tablet form of this
medicine:
- Take this medicine with food to lessen possible stomach
upset.

For patients taking the buccal tablet form of methyltestosterone:

- **This medicine should not be swallowed whole.** Place the tablet in the upper or lower pouch between your gum and the side of your cheek. Let the tablet slowly dissolve there. Do not eat, drink, chew, or smoke while the tablet is dissolving.

If you miss a dose of this medicine and your dosing schedule is:

- One dose a day—Take the missed dose as soon as possible. However, if you do not remember it until the next day, skip the dose. Do not double doses.

- More than one dose a day—Take the missed dose as soon as possible. However, if almost time for your next dose, skip the missed dose. Do not double doses.

If you have any questions about this, check with your doctor.

PRECAUTIONS WHILE USING THIS MEDICINE
Your doctor should check your progress at regular visits to make sure this medicine does not cause unwanted effects.

Androgens can decrease the amount of sperm made. Also, androgens may cause children to stop growing early or to develop too fast sexually.

POSSIBLE SIDE EFFECTS OF THIS MEDICINE
Tumors of the liver or liver disease have occurred with long-term, high-dose therapy with androgens. These effects are rare but can be very serious.

Side Effects That Should Be Reported To Your Doctor Immediately

For both females and males
    Less common—Yellow eyes or skin

    Rare (with long-term use and/or high doses)—Black, tarry, or light-colored stools; dark-colored urine; purple or red spots on body or inside the mouth or nose; sore throat or fever; vomiting of blood

Other Side Effects That Should Be Reported To Your Doctor

For both females and males
    Less common—Changes in skin color; confusion; dizziness; flushing of skin; headache (frequent or continuing); mental depression; nausea or vomiting; shortness of breath; skin rash or itching; swelling of feet or lower legs; unusual bleeding; unusual tiredness; weight gain (rapid)

    Rare (with long-term use and/or high doses)—Hives; loss of appetite (continuing); pain, tenderness, or swelling in the abdominal or stomach area; unpleasant breath odor (continuing)

For females only
    More common—Acne or oily skin; enlarged clitoris; hair
    loss; hoarseness or deepening of voice; irregular pe-
    riods; unnatural hair growth

For sexually mature males only
    More common—Acne; breast soreness; frequent or con-
    tinuing erections; frequent urge to urinate; increased
    breast size

    Less common—Chills; pain in scrotum or groin

For elderly patients only
    Less common—Difficult or frequent urination (in males);
    increase in sexual desire

Other side effects not listed above may also occur in some
patients. If you notice any other effects, check with your
doctor, nurse, or pharmacist.

ANGIOTENSIN-CONVERTING ENZYME (ACE) INHIBITORS   Systemic
Including Benazepril; Captopril; Enalapril; Fosinopril; Lisinopril; Quinapril; Ramipril.

■ For the Pharmacist ■

In providing consultation, consider emphasizing the following selected information (» = major clinical significance):

Before using this medication
» Conditions affecting use, especially:
    Sensitivity to any ACE inhibitor
    Pregnancy—ACE inhibitors cross the placenta; ACE inhibitor–associated fetal hypotension, oliguria, and death reported in humans; fetotoxicity found in animals
    Breast-feeding—Benazepril, captopril, and fosinopril are distributed into breast milk
    Other medications, especially alcohol, diuretics (particularly potassium-sparing), potassium-containing medications, or potassium supplements
    Other medical problems, especially angioedema related to previous ACE inhibitor therapy, hyperkalemia, renal artery stenosis, renal transplant, renal function impairment, or sodium and volume depletion
    Use of low-salt milk or salt substitutes

Proper use of this medication
    Getting into the habit of taking at same time each day to help increase compliance
» Proper dosing
    Missed dose: Taking as soon as possible; not taking if almost time for next dose; not doubling doses
» Proper storage
For captopril
    For best results, taking on an empty stomach 1 hour before meals
For use as an antihypertensive
    Possible need for control of weight and diet, especially sodium intake; risks associated with sodium depletion; not taking salt substitutes or using low-salt milk unless approved by physician
» Patient may not experience symptoms of hypertension; importance of taking medication even if feeling well
» Does not cure, but helps control hypertension; possible need for lifelong therapy; checking with physician before discontinuing medication; serious consequences of untreated hypertension

Precautions while using this medication
    Regular visits to physician to check progress
    Caution when driving or doing other things requiring alertness, because of possible dizziness, especially after initial dose of ACE inhibitor in patients taking diuretics
    To prevent dehydration and hypotension, checking with physician if severe nausea, vomiting, or diarrhea occurs and continues
    Caution when exercising or during hot weather because of the risk of dehydration and hypotension due to reduced fluid volume
    Caution if any kind of surgery (including dental surgery) or emergency treatment is required

For use as an antihypertensive
» Not taking other medications, especially nonprescription sympatho-
    mimetics, unless discussed with physician
For captopril and fosinopril
    Caution if any laboratory tests required; possible interference with
    test results

Side/adverse effects
    Signs of potential side effects, especially hypotension, skin rash (with
    or without itching, fever, or joint pain), angioedema, chest pain,
    neutropenia or agranulocytosis, pancreatitis, and hyperkalemia

---

▲ For the Patient ▲

913014

ABOUT YOUR MEDICINE

ACE inhibitors are used to treat high blood pressure (hypertension). Some of these medicines are also used to treat
congestive heart failure. These medicines may also be used
for other conditions as determined by your doctor.

If any of the information in this leaflet causes you special
concern or if you want additional information about your
medicine and its use, check with your doctor, nurse, or pharmacist. **Remember, keep this and all other medicines out of
the reach of children and never share your medicines with
others.**

BEFORE USING THIS MEDICINE

Tell your doctor, nurse, and pharmacist if you . . .
  • are allergic to any medicine, either prescription or non-
    prescription (OTC);
  • are pregnant or intend to become pregnant while using
    this medicine;
  • are breast-feeding;
  • are taking any other prescription or nonprescription
    (OTC) medicine, especially diuretics (water pills) or po-
    tassium-containing medicines or supplements;
  • have any other medical problems, especially heart or
    blood vessel disease or kidney disease;
  • are on a strict low-sodium diet or dialysis, or use low-
    salt milk or salt substitutes;
  • have had a kidney transplant.

PROPER USE OF THIS MEDICINE

Even if you feel well and do not notice any signs of your
medical problem, **take this medicine exactly as directed.**

For patients taking captopril:
  • This medicine is best taken on an empty stomach 1 hour
    before meals, unless you are otherwise directed by your
    doctor.

For patients taking this medicine for high blood pressure:
  • This medicine will not cure your high blood pressure,
    but it does help control it. You must continue to take
    it—even if you feel well—if you expect to keep your

blood pressure down. **You may have to take high blood pressure medicine for the rest of your life.**

If you miss a dose of this medicine, take it as soon as possible. However, if it is almost time for your next dose, skip the missed dose and go back to your regular dosing schedule. Do not double doses.

PRECAUTIONS WHILE USING THIS MEDICINE

If you think that you may have become pregnant, check with your doctor immediately. Use of this medicine, especially during the second and third trimesters (after the first three months) of pregnancy, may cause serious injury or even death to the unborn child.

Check with your doctor if you become sick while taking this medicine, especially with severe or continuing vomiting or diarrhea. These conditions may cause you to lose too much water and lead to low blood pressure.

Dizziness, lightheadedness, or fainting may occur after the first dose, especially if you have been taking a diuretic (water pill). Make sure you know how you react to this medicine before you drive, use machines, or do other jobs that require you to be alert and clearheaded.

Avoid alcoholic beverages until you have discussed their use with your doctor. Alcohol may increase the low blood pressure effect and the possibility of dizziness and fainting.

POSSIBLE SIDE EFFECTS OF THIS MEDICINE

Side Effects That Should Be Reported To Your Doctor Immediately

>   *Rare*—Fever and chills; hoarseness; swelling of face, mouth, hands, or feet; trouble in swallowing or breathing (sudden)

Other Side Effects That Should Be Reported To Your Doctor

>   *Less common*—Dizziness, lightheadedness, or fainting; skin rash, with or without itching, fever, or joint pain

>   *Rare*—Chest pain; fever, nausea, stomach bloating, stomach pain, or vomiting

>   *Signs of too much potassium in the body*—Confusion; irregular heartbeat; nervousness; numbness or tingling in hands, feet, or lips; shortness of breath or difficulty breathing; weakness or heaviness of legs

Side Effects That Usually Do Not Require Medical Attention

These possible side effects may go away during treatment; however, if they continue or are bothersome, check with your doctor, nurse, or pharmacist.

More common—Cough (dry)

Less common—Diarrhea; headache; loss of taste; nausea; unusual tiredness

Other side effects not listed above may also occur in some patients. If you notice any other effects, check with your doctor, nurse, or pharmacist.

ANGIOTENSIN-CONVERTING ENZYME (ACE) INHIBITORS AND HYDROCHLOROTHIAZIDE   Systemic

Including Captopril and Hydrochlorothiazide; Enalapril and Hydrochlorothiazide; Lisinopril and Hydrochlorothiazide.

■ For the Pharmacist ■

In providing consultation, consider emphasizing the following selected information (» = major clinical significance):

Before using this medication
» Conditions affecting use, especially:
Sensitivity to any ACE inhibitor, thiazide diuretic, carbonic anhydrase inhibitor, or other sulfonamide-type medications
Pregnancy—ACE inhibitor–associated fetal hypotension, oliguria, and death reported in humans; and fetotoxicity found in animals; hydrochlorothiazide may cause jaundice, thrombocytopenia, hypokalemia in infant
Breast-feeding—Captopril and hydrochlorothiazide are distributed into breast milk
Use in children—Caution if giving to infants with jaundice
Use in the elderly—May be more sensitive to hypotensive and electrolyte effects
Other medications, especially alcohol, cholestyramine, colestipol, diuretics (particularly potassium-sparing), potassium-containing medications, potassium supplements, low salt milk, salt substitutes, digitalis glycosides, lithium, cocaine, norepinephrine, or phenylephrine
Other medical problems, especially angioedema related to previous ACE inhibitor therapy, hereditary angioedema, idiopathic angioedema, hyperkalemia, renal artery stenosis, renal transplant, renal function impairment, or sodium and volume depletion

Proper use of this medication
Getting into the habit of taking at same time each day to help increase compliance
Diuretic effects of the medication and timing of doses to minimize inconvenience of diuresis
» Proper dosing
Missed dose: Taking as soon as possible; not taking if almost time for next dose; not doubling doses
» Proper storage
For captopril and hydrochlorothiazide
For best results, taking on an empty stomach 1 hour before meals
For use as an antihypertensive
Possible need for control of weight and diet, especially sodium intake; risks associated with sodium depletion; not taking salt substitutes or using low-salt milk unless approved by physician
» Patient may not experience symptoms of hypertension; importance of taking medication even if feeling well
» Does not cure, but helps control hypertension; possible need for lifelong therapy; checking with physician before discontinuing medication; serious consequences of untreated hypertension

Precautions while using this medication

Regular visits to physician to check progress

Caution when driving or doing other things requiring alertness, because of possible dizziness, especially with initial dose

To prevent dehydration and hypotension, checking with physician if severe nausea, vomiting, or diarrhea occurs and continues

Caution when exercising or during hot weather because of the risk of dehydration and hypotension due to reduced fluid volume

Caution if any kind of surgery (including dental surgery) or emergency treatment is required

Caution in using alcohol

Diabetics: May increase blood sugar levels

Possible photosensitivity; avoiding unprotected exposure to sun; using protective clothing and sun block product; avoiding use of sunlamp

Caution if any laboratory tests required; possible interference with test results

For use as an antihypertensive

» Not taking other medications, especially nonprescription sympathomimetics, unless discussed with physician

Side/adverse effects

Signs of potential side effects, especially hypotension, skin rash (with or without itching, fever, or joint pain), angioedema, chest pain, neutropenia or agranulocytosis, hyperuricemia or gout, cholecystitis or pancreatitis, thrombocytopenia, hepatic function impairment, and electrolyte imbalance

---

▲ For the Patient ▲

913025

ABOUT YOUR MEDICINE

ACE inhibitors and **hydrochlorothiazide** combinations are used to treat high blood pressure (hypertension). They may also be used for other conditions as determined by your doctor.

If any of the information in this leaflet causes you special concern or if you want additional information about your medicine and its use, check with your doctor, nurse, or pharmacist. **Remember, keep this and all other medicines out of the reach of children and never share your medicines with others.**

BEFORE USING THIS MEDICINE

Children and infants may be especially sensitive to the blood pressure–lowering effect of ACE inhibitors. **Discuss with the child's doctor the possible side effects that may be caused by this medicine.** Some of them may be serious.

Tell your doctor, nurse, and pharmacist if you . . .

- are allergic to any medicine, either prescription or non-prescription (OTC);
- are pregnant or intend to become pregnant while using this medicine;
- are breast-feeding;
- are taking any other prescription or nonprescription (OTC) medicine, especially cholestyramine, colestipol,

digitalis glycosides (heart medicine), diuretics (water pills), lithium, potassium-containing medicines or supplements, or salt substitutes or low-salt milk;
- have any other medical problems, especially kidney disease;
- are on a strict low-sodium diet or dialysis;
- have had a kidney transplant.

PROPER USE OF THIS MEDICINE

Even if you feel well and do not notice any signs of your medical problem, **take this medicine exactly as directed.**

For patients taking this medicine for high blood pressure:
- This medicine will not cure your high blood pressure, but it does help control it. You must continue to take it—even if you feel well—if you expect to keep your blood pressure down. **You may have to take high blood pressure medicine for the rest of your life.**

If you miss a dose of this medicine, take it as soon as possible. However, if it is almost time for your next dose, skip the missed dose and go back to your regular dosing schedule. Do not double doses.

PRECAUTIONS WHILE USING THIS MEDICINE

If you think that you may have become pregnant, check with your doctor immediately. Use of this medicine, especially during the second and third trimesters (after the first three months) of pregnancy, may cause serious injury or even death to the unborn child.

Dizziness or lightheadedness may occur, especially after the first dose of this medicine. Make sure you know how you react to the medicine before you drive, use machines, or do other things that require you to be alert and clearheaded.

Check with your doctor if you become sick while taking this medicine, especially with severe or continuing vomiting or diarrhea. These conditions may cause you to lose too much water and lead to low blood pressure.

Dizziness, lightheadedness, or fainting may occur if you exercise or if the weather is hot. Use extra care during exercise or hot weather.

Avoid acoholic beverages until you have discussed their use with your doctor. Alcohol may increase the low blood pressure effect and the possibility of dizziness and fainting.

POSSIBLE SIDE EFFECTS OF THIS MEDICINE

Side Effects That Should Be Reported To Your Doctor Immediately

> *Rare*—Fever and chills; hoarseness; swelling of face, mouth, hands, or feet; trouble in swallowing or breathing (sudden)

Other Side Effects That Should Be Reported To Your Doctor

> *Less common*—Dizziness, lightheadedness, or fainting; skin rash, with or without itching, fever, or joint pain

> *Rare*—Chest pain; joint pain; lower back or side pain; severe stomach pain with nausea and vomiting; unusual bleeding or bruising; yellow eyes or skin

> *Signs of too much or too little potassium in the body*— Dryness of mouth; increased thirst; irregular heartbeats; mood or mental changes; muscle cramps or pain; numbness or tingling in hands, feet, or lips; weakness or heaviness of legs; weak pulse

Side Effects That Usually Do Not Require Medical Attention

These possible side effects may go away during treatment; however, if they continue or are bothersome, check with your doctor, nurse, or pharmacist.

> *More common*—Cough (dry, continuing)

> *Less common*—Diarrhea; headache; increased sensitivity of skin to sunlight; loss of appetite; loss of taste; stomach upset; unusual tiredness

Other side effects not listed above may also occur in some patients. If you notice any other effects, check with your doctor, nurse, or pharmacist.

ANTICOAGULANTS Systemic
Including Anisindione; Dicumarol; Warfarin.

■For the Pharmacist■

In providing consultation, consider emphasizing the following selected information (» = major clinical significance):

Before using this medication
» Conditions affecting use, especially:
   Sensitivity to the anticoagulant considered for therapy
   Pregnancy—Not becoming pregnant during therapy without first discussing plans with physician, or informing physician immediately if any suspicion of pregnancy; these medications should not be used during the first trimester because of their teratogenic effects or after the 37th week of pregnancy because of the risk of fetal and neonatal bleeding
   Use in children—Infants, especially neonates, are especially sensitive to effects because of vitamin K deficiency
   Use in the elderly—Increased risk of bleeding
   Other medications
   Other medical problems, especially bleeding or clotting defects, or history of; recent surgery or childbirth; diabetes mellitus; severe renal or hepatic function impairment; active gastrointestinal, respiratory, or urinary tract ulceration; malignancy; recent spinal puncture; subacute bacterial endocarditis; or polyarthritis

Proper use of this medication
» Taking medication only as directed
» Regular prothrombin-time tests and regular visits to physician or clinic to check progress
» Proper dosing
» Missed dose: Taking as soon as possible; not taking if not remembered until next day; not doubling doses; keeping a record of doses taken to avoid mistakes; keeping record of missed doses to give physician
» Proper storage

Precautions while using this medication
» Need for patient to inform all physicians, dentists, and pharmacists that this medication is being used
» Not taking or discontinuing any other medication, including salicylates or any other over-the-counter (OTC) medications, without physician's permission
» Carrying identification indicating use of an anticoagulant
   Not engaging in activities that may lead to injuries
   Using care in activities that may cause a cut or bleeding (such as shaving)
   Minimizing alcohol consumption; i.e., not consuming more than an occasional drink or two
   Eating a normal, balanced diet; not changing dietary habits, taking vitamins, or using nutritional supplements without first seeking professional advice because of possible alteration of anticoagulant effect by substantial changes in intake of Vitamin K (present in some multiple vitamins and nutritional supplements as well as foods, including green, leafy vegetables [such as broccoli, cabbage, collard greens, kale, lettuce, spinach], and, to a lesser extent, meats and dairy products)

Checking with physician if unable to eat for several days or if continuing gastric upset, diarrhea, or fever occurs

Caution following cessation of therapy while body is recovering bloodclotting abilities

Side/adverse effects
» Checking with physician immediately if any symptoms of bleeding occur

Checking with physician if anisindione turns urine orange

Signs and symptoms of potential side effects, especially bleeding, agranulocytosis, renal damage, hepatotoxicity, and "purple toes" syndrome

---

▲ For the Patient ▲

912226

ABOUT YOUR MEDICINE

Oral anticoagulants decrease the clotting ability of the blood and therefore help prevent harmful clots from forming in the blood vessels. These medicines are sometimes called "blood thinners," although they do not actually thin the blood. They will not dissolve clots that already have formed. However, they may prevent clots from becoming larger and causing more serious problems.

If any of the information in this leaflet causes you special concern or if you want additional information about your medicine and its use, check with your doctor, nurse, or pharmacist. **Remember, keep this and all other medicines out of the reach of children and never share your medicines with others.**

BEFORE USING THIS MEDICINE

In order for an anticoagulant to help you without causing serious bleeding, it must be used properly and all of the precautions concerning its use must be followed exactly. Be sure that you have discussed the use of this medicine with the doctor or pharmacist who is following your treatment. It is very important that you understand all directions and that you are willing and able to follow them exactly.

Tell your doctor, nurse, and pharmacist if you . . .
- are allergic to any medicine, either prescription or nonprescription (OTC);
- are pregnant or intend to become pregnant while using this medicine;
- are breast-feeding;
- are taking **any** other prescription or nonprescription (OTC) medicine;
- have **any** other medical problems.

PROPER USE OF THIS MEDICINE

Take this medicine exactly as directed. Do not take more or less of it, do not take it more often, and do not take it for a longer time than ordered. This is especially important for elderly patients, who are especially sensitive to the effects of anticoagulants. **Your blood must be checked regularly.**

If you miss a dose of this medicine, take it as soon as possible if you remember the same day. However, if you do not remember until the next day, do not take the missed dose at all and do not double the next one. **Doubling the dose may cause bleeding.** Be sure to give the doctor or pharmacist who is following your treatment a record of any doses you miss.

PRECAUTIONS WHILE USING THIS MEDICINE

Tell all physicians, dentists, and pharmacists you go to that you are taking this medicine. You should also carry identification stating that you are taking it.

Always check with your doctor or pharmacist before you start or stop taking any other medicine. This includes any nonprescription medicine, even aspirin, acetaminophen, and diet supplements or vitamins. Many medicines change the way this medicine affects your body. In addition, drinking too much alcohol or changing your diet may change the way this medicine works.

POSSIBLE SIDE EFFECTS OF THIS MEDICINE
Side Effects That Should Be Reported Immediately

> *Less common or rare*—Blue or purple color and pain in toes; cloudy or dark urine; difficult or painful urination; sores, ulcers, or white spots in mouth or throat; sore throat, fever, chills, or unusual tiredness or weakness; sudden decrease in amount of urine; swelling of face, feet, or lower legs; unusual weight gain; yellow eyes or skin

> *Signs of bleeding inside the body*—Abdominal pain or swelling; back pain; bloody or black, tarry stools; bloody urine; constipation; coughing up blood; dizziness; headache (severe or continuing); joint pain, stiffness, or swelling; vomiting blood or material that looks like coffee grounds

> *Signs of overdose*—Bleeding from gums when brushing teeth; unexplained bruising or purplish areas on skin; unexplained nosebleeds; unusually heavy bleeding from cuts; unusually heavy or unexpected menstrual bleeding

Other Side Effects That Should Be Reported

> *Less common or rare*—Diarrhea; itching, skin rash, or hives; nausea or vomiting; stomach cramps or pain

Side Effects That Usually Do Not Require Medical Attention

These possible side effects may go away during treatment; however, if they continue or are bothersome, check with your doctor, nurse, or pharmacist.

> *More common*—Bloated stomach or gas

Less common—Loss of appetite; unusual hair loss

Depending on your diet, anisindione may cause your urine to turn orange. Since it may be hard to tell the difference between blood in the urine and this color change, check with your doctor if you notice any color change in your urine.

Other side effects not listed above may also occur in some patients. If you notice any other effects, check with your doctor, nurse, or pharmacist.

ANTICONVULSANTS, DIONE   Systemic
Including Paramethadione; Trimethadione.

■For the Pharmacist■

In providing consultation, consider emphasizing the following selected
information (» = major clinical significance):

Before using this medication
» Conditions affecting use, especially:
    Sensitivity to dione anticonvulsants
    Pregnancy and delivery—Risk of congenital malformations in
      the fetus; women of child-bearing potential advised to use an
      effective method of birth control during therapy, and to no-
      tify physician immediately if pregnancy occurs; bleeding
      problems may occur in mother during delivery and in baby
      immediately after delivery.
    Dental—Risk of bleeding and infections due to dione-induced
      blood dyscrasias
    Other medications, especially CNS depressants
    Other medical problems, especially blood dyscrasias and hepatic
      function impairment

Proper use of this medication
    Proper administration:
    For paramethadione capsules
      Swallowing whole; not breaking, chewing, or crushing before
        swallowing
    For trimethadione tablets
      Chewing, or crushing and dissolving in small amount of water,
        if necessary
    For all dosage forms
      Taking with a small amount of food or milk to reduce gastric
        irritation
» Compliance with therapy; taking every day as directed by physician
» Proper dosing
    Missed dose: Taking as soon as possible; not taking if almost time
      for next scheduled dose; one missed dose may be added at bed-
      time
» Proper storage

Precautions while using this medication
» Regular visits to physician to check progress of therapy
» Checking with physician before discontinuing medication; gradual
    dosage reduction is usually needed
    Possible vision changes, especially intolerance to bright light; wear-
      ing sunglasses and avoiding bright light; caution when driving
      at night
» Avoiding use of alcohol and other CNS depressants
» Caution if drowsiness occurs; not driving or doing jobs requiring
    alertness
» Caution if any kind of surgery, dental treatment, or emergency
    treatment is required
» Reporting sore throat, fever, and any unusual bleeding or bruising
    to physician as soon as possible
» Informing physician as soon as possible if pregnancy occurs during
    therapy

Side/adverse effects
> Signs of potential side effects, especially allergic reaction; blood dyscrasias; confusion; convulsions; hemeralopia, scotomata, or diplopia; hepatitis; myasthenia gravis–like syndrome; nephrosis; skin rash or hives; and SLE-like syndrome

---

▲ For the Patient ▲

913750

ABOUT YOUR MEDICINE

Dione anticonvulsants are used to control certain types of seizures in the treatment of epilepsy.

If any of the information in this leaflet causes you special concern or if you want additional information about your medicine and its use, check with your doctor, nurse, or pharmacist. **Remember, keep this and all other medicines out of the reach of children and never share your medicines with others.**

BEFORE USING THIS MEDICINE

Tell your doctor, nurse, and pharmacist if you . . .
- are allergic to any medicine, either prescription or non-prescription (OTC);
- are pregnant or intend to become pregnant while using this medicine;
- are breast-feeding;
- compete in athletics;
- are taking any other prescription or nonprescription (OTC) medicine, especially CNS depressants;
- have any other medical problems, especially blood disease or liver or kidney disease.

PROPER USE OF THIS MEDICINE

For patients taking paramethadione capsules:
- Swallow whole. Do not crush, chew, or break before swallowing.

For patients taking trimethadione tablets:
- The tablets may be chewed or crushed and dissolved in a small amount of water before they are swallowed.

If this medicine upsets your stomach, take it with a small amount of food or milk unless otherwise directed by your doctor.

This medicine must be taken every day in regularly spaced doses as ordered.

If you miss a dose of this medicine, take it as soon as possible. However, if it is almost time for your next dose, skip the missed dose and go back to your regular dosing schedule. If only one dose is missed, it may be taken at bedtime.

PRECAUTIONS WHILE USING THIS MEDICINE

It is very important that your doctor check your progress at regular visits, especially during the first few months of treatment with this medicine.

If you have been taking this medicine regularly, do not stop taking it without first checking with your doctor. Your doctor may want you to reduce gradually the amount you are taking before stopping completely.

This medicine may cause your eyes to become more sensitive to bright light than they are normally, making it difficult for you to see well. Wearing sunglasses may help. It may also be difficult to see in light that changes in brightness. If you notice this effect, be especially careful when driving at night.

This medicine will add to the effects of alcohol and other CNS depressants (medicines that slow down the nervous system). **Check with your doctor before taking any such depressants while you are using this medicine.**

This medicine may cause some people to become drowsy or less alert than they are normally. **Make sure you know how you react before you drive, use machines, or do other jobs that require you to be alert.**

Before having any kind of surgery or dental or emergency treatment, tell the physician or dentist in charge that you are taking this medicine.

Be sure to tell your doctor as soon as possible if you have a sore throat, fever, or general feeling of tiredness, or if you notice any unusual bleeding or bruising, such as reddish or purplish spots on the skin, or recurring nosebleeds or bleeding gums.

Check with your doctor as soon as possible if you suspect you are pregnant.

POSSIBLE SIDE EFFECTS OF THIS MEDICINE
Side Effects That Should Be Reported To Your Doctor

> *More common*—Changes in vision, such as glare or snowy image caused by bright light, or double vision

> *Rare*—Confusion; convulsions (seizures); dark or cloudy urine; fever; loss of appetite or weight; muscle weakness (severe), especially drooping eyelids, difficulty in chewing, swallowing, talking, or breathing, and unusual tiredness; nausea or vomiting; pain in abdomen or joints; skin rash or itching; sore throat and fever; swelling of face, hands, legs, and feet; swollen glands; unusual bleeding or bruising, such as recurring nosebleeds, bleeding gums, or vaginal bleeding, or red or purple spots on skin; unusual tiredness or weakness; yellow eyes or skin

Side Effects That Usually Do Not Require Medical Attention

These possible side effects may go away during treatment; however, if they continue or are bothersome, check with your doctor, nurse, or pharmacist.

>   *More common*—Dizziness; drowsiness; headache; increased sensitivity of eyes to light; irritability

Other side effects not listed above may also occur in some patients. If you notice any other effects, check with your doctor, nurse, or pharmacist.

ANTICONVULSANTS, HYDANTOIN Systemic
Including Ethotoin; Mephenytoin; Phenytoin.

■For the Pharmacist■

In providing consultation, consider emphasizing the following selected information (» = major clinical significance):

Before using this medication
» Conditions affecting use, especially:
   Sensitivity to hydantoin anticonvulsants
   Pregnancy—Hydantoin anticonvulsants cross placenta; risk-benefit should be considered because of possibility of increased birth defects; seizures may increase during pregnancy with need for dose increase; bleeding problems may occur in mother during delivery and in baby immediately after delivery
   Breast-feeding—Ethotoin and phenytoin distributed into breast milk
   Use in children—Bleeding, tender, and enlarged gums more common in children; unusual and excessive hair growth, more noticeable in young girls; decreased performance in school (cognitive impairment) may occur with long-term use of high doses
   Use in the elderly—Side effects more likely to occur in the elderly; hydantoin anticonvulsants metabolized more slowly in elderly, possibly leading to toxicity
   Dental—Gingival hyperplasia may appear; good dental hygiene and visits to dentist every 3 months for cleaning recommended; agranulocytosis or thrombocytopenia may cause gingival bleeding, slowed healing, and infections
   Other medications, especially estrogen-containing oral contraceptives, estrogens, aminophylline, amiodarone, antacids, anticoagulants, caffeine, CNS depressants, alcohol, chloramphenicol, cimetidine, corticosteroids, diazoxide, disulfiram, isoniazid, calcium-containing medicine, fluconazole, fluoxetine; lidocaine, methadone, oxtriphylline, phenacemide, phenylbutazone, rifampin, streptozocin, sucralfate, sulfonamides, theophylline, or valproic acid
   Other medical problems, especially blood dyscrasias, cardiac function impairment, hepatic function impairment, history of hydantoin hypersensitivity, porphyria, or renal function impairment

Proper use of this medication
   Proper administration:
   For liquid dosage forms—Shaking well; using an accurate measuring device, such as a specially marked measuring spoon, a plastic syringe, or a small graduated cup
   For chewable tablet dosage form—Chewing or crushing tablets or swallowing them whole
   For capsule dosage form—Swallowing capsule whole
   Taking with food to reduce gastrointestinal irritation
» Compliance with therapy; taking every day exactly as directed
» Proper dosing

» Missed dose: If dosing schedule is—
> One dose a day: Taking as soon as possible unless next day, then continuing on schedule; not doubling doses
>
> Several doses a day: Taking as soon as possible unless within 4 hours of next scheduled dose, then continuing on regular schedule; not doubling doses
>
> Checking with doctor if doses are missed for 2 or more days in a row

» Proper storage

Precautions while using this medication
» Regular visits to physician to check progress of therapy
» Not taking other medication without physician's advice
» Avoiding the use of alcoholic beverages and other CNS depressants while taking this medicine
> Not taking within 2 to 3 hours of taking antacids or medication for diarrhea
>
> Not changing brands or dosage forms of phenytoin without checking with physician or pharmacist

» Checking with physician before discontinuing medication; gradual dosage reduction is usually needed to maintain seizure control
> Carrying medical identification card or bracelet during therapy
>
> Diabetic patients: Checking blood or urine sugar concentrations
>
> Caution if any laboratory tests required; possible interference with test results of dexamethasone, metyrapone, or Schilling tests, thyroid function tests, or gallium citrate Ga 67 imaging

» Caution if any kind of surgery, dental treatment, or emergency treatment is required
» Caution when driving, using machines, or doing other jobs requiring alertness
» Using different or additional means of birth control than estrogen-containing oral contraceptives

For phenytoin or mephenytoin only
» Maintaining good dental hygiene and seeing dentist every 3 months for teeth cleaning, to prevent tenderness, bleeding, and enlargement of gums

Side/adverse effects
> Increased incidence of gingival hyperplasia in children and young adults taking phenytoin or mephenytoin
>
> Unusual and excessive hair growth more noticeable in young girls
>
> Signs of potential side effects, especially blood dyscrasias, CNS toxicity, cholestatic jaundice, cognitive impairment, hepatitis, an increase in seizures, lupus erythematosus, phenytoin hypersensitivity syndrome, periarteritis nodosa, Peyronie's disease, pulmonary infiltrates or fibrosis, Stevens-Johnson syndrome, toxic epidermal necrolysis, transient choreoathetoid movements, or vitamin D and/or calcium imbalance

---

▲ For the Patient ▲

912328

ABOUT YOUR MEDICINE

Hydantoin anticonvulsants (hye-DAN-toyn an-tye-kon-VUL-sants) are used to control certain types of seizures in the treatment of epilepsy. Phenytoin may also be used for other conditions as determined by your doctor.

If any of the information in this leaflet causes you special concern or if you want additional information about your

medicine and its use, check with your doctor, nurse, or pharmacist. **Remember, keep this and all other medicines out of the reach of children and never share your medicines with others.**

BEFORE USING THIS MEDICINE
Tell your doctor, nurse, and pharmacist if you . . .
- are allergic to any medicine, either prescription or nonprescription (OTC);
- are pregnant or intend to become pregnant while using this medicine;
- are breast-feeding;
- are taking **any** other prescription or nonprescription (OTC) medicine;
- have any other medical problems, especially blood, heart, kidney, or liver disease; or porphyria.

PROPER USE OF THIS MEDICINE
Take this medicine every day exactly as ordered by your doctor in order to control your medical problem. If it upsets your stomach, take it with food.

If you miss a dose of this medicine and your schedule is:
- One dose a day—Take it as soon as possible. However, if you do not remember until the next day, skip the missed dose. Do not double doses.
- More than one dose a day—Take it as soon as possible unless your next scheduled dose is within 4 hours. Do not double doses.

If you miss doses for 2 or more days in a row, check with your doctor.

PRECAUTIONS WHILE USING THIS MEDICINE
Your doctor should check your progress at regular visits, especially during the first few months of treatment with this medicine since your dose may have to be adjusted. Also, do not change brands or dosage forms of phenytoin without first checking with your doctor. Different products may not work the same way.

If you have been taking this medicine for several weeks or more, do not suddenly stop taking it. Your doctor may want you to reduce your dose gradually.

Before having any kind of surgery or dental or emergency treatment, tell the physician or dentist in charge that you are taking this medicine.

Taking other medicines or drinking alcohol may change the way this medicine works. Check with your doctor before you stop or start taking other medicines or before drinking alcoholic beverages while you are taking this medicine.

Oral contraceptives containing estrogen may not work as well if you take them while taking this medicine. Unplanned pregnancies may occur. Use different or additional birth control while taking this medicine.

Do not take this medicine within 2 to 3 hours of taking antacids or medicine for diarrhea. Taking them too close together may make this medicine less effective.

This medicine may cause some people to become dizzy, drowsy, lightheaded, or less alert than they are normally. **Make sure you know how you react before you drive or do jobs that require you to be alert.**

In some patients (usually younger ones), tenderness, swelling, or bleeding of the gums (gingival hyperplasia) may appear soon after taking phenytoin. Brushing and flossing your teeth carefully and regularly and massaging your gums may help prevent this. **If you have questions about how to take care of your teeth and gums or if you notice problems,** check with your physician or dentist.

POSSIBLE SIDE EFFECTS OF THIS MEDICINE
Side Effects That Should Be Reported To Your Doctor

More common—Bleeding, tender, or enlarged gums; clumsiness or unsteadiness; confusion; enlarged glands in neck or underarms; fever; increase in seizures; mood or mental changes; muscle weakness; skin rash or itching; slurred speech; stuttering; trembling of hands; unusual excitement, nervousness, or irritability

Rare—Bone malformations; chest discomfort; dark urine; frequent breaking of bones; headache; joint pain; learning difficulties (in children taking high doses for a long time); light-colored stools; loss of appetite; pain of penis on erection; restlessness or agitation; slowed growth; soreness of muscles; sore throat, chills, and fever; stomach pain (severe); troubled or quick, shallow breathing; uncontrolled jerking or twisting movements of hands, arms, or legs; uncontrolled movements of lips, tongue, or cheeks; unusual bleeding (such as nosebleeds) or bruising; unusual weight loss; unusual tiredness or weakness; yellow eyes or skin

Signs of overdose—Blurred or double vision; continuous, uncontrolled back and forth and/or rolling eye movements; dizziness or drowsiness (severe); staggering walk; trembling

Side Effects That Usually Do Not Require Medical Attention

These possible side effects may go away during treatment; however, if they continue or are bothersome, check with your doctor, nurse, or pharmacist.

More common—Constipation; dizziness or drowsiness; nausea and vomiting

Other side effects not listed above may also occur in some patients. If you notice any other effects, check with your doctor, nurse, or pharmacist.

ANTICONVULSANTS, SUCCINIMIDE   Systemic

Including Ethosuximide; Methsuximide; Phensuximide.

■ For the Pharmacist ■

In providing consultation, consider emphasizing the following selected information (» = major clinical significance):

Before using this medication
» Conditions affecting use, especially:
> Sensitivity to succinimide anticonvulsants
> Pregnancy—Possible birth defects
> Other medications, especially CNS depressants or haloperidol
> Other medical problems, especially blood dyscrasias, hepatic function impairment, severe renal function impairment, or intermittent porphyria

Proper use of this medication
» Compliance with therapy; taking daily in regularly spaced doses as ordered
> Taking with food or milk to reduce gastric irritation
» Proper dosing
> Missed dose: Taking as soon as possible; if remembered within 4 hours of next dose, skipping missed dose and continuing on regular dosing schedule; not doubling doses
» Proper storage

Precautions while using this medication
» Regular visits to physician to check progress of therapy
» Checking with physician before discontinuing this medication; gradual dosage reduction may be necessary
» Not starting or stopping other medication without physician's advice
» Avoiding the use of alcoholic beverages and other CNS depressants while taking this medication
» Possibility of drowsiness; caution if driving or doing jobs requiring alertness
» Caution if any kind of surgery, dental treatment, or emergency treatment is required
> Carrying medical identification card or bracelet
For methsuximide
> Not taking capsules that are melted or not full; effectiveness may be reduced

Side/adverse effects
> Signs of potential side effects, especially Stevens-Johnson syndrome, systemic lupus erythematosus, aggressiveness, difficulty in concentration, mental depression, nightmares, blood dyscrasias, tonic-clonic convulsions, paranoid psychosis, or pruritic erythematous rash
> Phensuximide may cause harmless discoloration of urine (pink, red, or red-brown)

▲ For the Patient ▲

914902

ABOUT YOUR MEDICINE

Succinimide (suk-SIN-i-mide) **anticonvulsants** are used to control certain seizures in the treatment of epilepsy.

If any of the information in this leaflet causes you special concern or if you want additional information about your medicine and its use, check with your doctor, nurse, or pharmacist. **Remember, keep this and all other medicines out of the reach of children and never share your medicines with others.**

BEFORE USING THIS MEDICINE

Tell your doctor, nurse, and pharmacist if you . . .
- are allergic to any medicine, either prescription or non-prescription (OTC);
- are pregnant or intend to become pregnant while using this medicine;
- are breast-feeding;
- compete in athletics;
- are taking any other prescription or nonprescription (OTC) medicine, especially haloperidol or CNS depressants;
- have any other medical problems.

PROPER USE OF THIS MEDICINE

This medicine must be taken every day in regularly spaced doses as ordered by your doctor. Do not take more or less of it than your doctor ordered.

If this medicine upsets your stomach, take it with food or milk unless otherwise directed by your doctor.

If you miss a dose of this medicine and remember within 4 hours, take it as soon as possible. Then go back to your regular dosing schedule. Do not double doses.

PRECAUTIONS WHILE USING THIS MEDICINE

Your doctor should check your progress at regular visits, especially during the first few months of treatment with this medicine. During this time the amount of medicine you are taking may have to be changed often to meet your individual needs.

If you have been taking this medicine regularly, do not stop taking it without first checking with your doctor. Your doctor may want you to reduce gradually the amount you are taking before stopping completely. Stopping this medicine suddenly may cause seizures.

Do not start or stop taking any other medicine without your physician's advice. Other medicines may affect the way this medicine works.

This medicine will add to the effects of alcohol and other CNS depressants (medicines that slow down the nervous system). **Check with your doctor before taking any such depressants while you are using this medicine.**

This medicine may cause some people to become drowsy or less alert than they are normally. **Make sure you know how you react to this medicine before you drive, use machines, or do other jobs that require you to be alert.** After you have taken this medicine for a while, this effect may lessen.

Before having any kind of surgery, dental treatment, or emergency treatment, tell the physician or dentist in charge that you are taking this medicine.

Your doctor may want you to carry a medical identification card or bracelet stating that you are taking this medicine.

For patients taking methsuximide:
- Do not use capsules that are not full or in which the contents have melted, because they may not work as well.

POSSIBLE SIDE EFFECTS OF THIS MEDICINE
Side Effects That Should Be Reported To Your Doctor

More common—Muscle pain; skin rash and itching; sore throat and fever; swollen glands

Less common—Aggressiveness; difficulty in concentration; mental depression; nightmares

Rare—Chills; increased chance of certain types of seizures; mood or mental changes; nosebleeds or other unusual bleeding or bruising; shortness of breath; sores, ulcers, or white spots on lips or in mouth; unusual tiredness or weakness; wheezing, tightness in chest, or troubled breathing

Side Effects That Usually Do Not Require Medical Attention

These possible side effects may go away during treatment; however, if they continue or are bothersome, check with your doctor, nurse, or pharmacist.

More common—Clumsiness or unsteadiness; dizziness; drowsiness; headache; hiccups; loss of appetite; nausea or vomiting; stomach cramps

Phensuximide may cause the urine to turn pink, red, or red-brown. This is harmless and is to be expected while you are taking this medicine.

Other side effects not listed above may also occur in some patients. If you notice any other effects, check with your doctor, nurse, or pharmacist.

ANTIDEPRESSANTS, MONOAMINE OXIDASE (MAO) INHIBITOR   Systemic

Including Isocarboxazid; Phenelzine; Tranylcypromine.

■ For the Pharmacist ■

In providing consultation, consider emphasizing the following selected information (**»** = major clinical significance):

Before using this medication
» Conditions affecting use, especially:
Sensitivity to any MAO inhibitor, including furazolidone or procarbazine
Pregnancy—MAO inhibitors cross placenta; no appropriate human studies done; animal studies have shown hyperexcitability and reduced growth rate in neonates
Breast-feeding—Not known if distributed into human breast milk; animal studies have shown distribution into milk
Use in the elderly—Increased sensitivity to hypotensive effects
Other medications, especially CNS depressants, tricyclic antidepressants, oral antidiabetic agents, insulin, bupropion, buspirone, caffeine in high doses, carbamazepine, cyclobenzaprine, cocaine, maprotiline, dextromethorphan, fluoxetine, paroxetine, or sertraline, trazodone, guanadrel, guanethidine, rauwolfia alkaloids, levodopa, meperidine, methyldopa, methylphenidate, sympathomimetics, tryptophan, or foods and beverages containing tyramine
Other medical problems, especially alcoholism (active), congestive heart failure, hepatic function impairment, pheochromocytoma, renal function impairment, cardiac arrhythmias, cardiovascular disease, coronary insufficiency, severe or frequent headaches, hypertension, schizophrenia, or suicidal tendencies

Proper use of this medication
» May require up to 3 or 4 weeks of therapy to obtain signs of improvement; regular visits to physician, especially during first few months of therapy, to check progress of therapy and to check for unwanted effects
» Taking exactly as directed by physician
» Importance of not taking more medication than the amount prescribed
» Proper dosing
Missed dose: Taking as soon as possible within 2 hours of next dose; going back to regular dosing schedule; not doubling doses
» Proper storage

Precautions while using this medication
» Avoiding tyramine-containing foods, alcoholic beverages, and large quantities of caffeine-containing beverages, over-the-counter cold and cough medicines, and other medications, unless prescribed; having list of such for reference
» Checking with hospital emergency room or physician if symptoms of hypertensive crisis develop
» Checking with physician before discontinuing medication; gradual reduction may be needed to prevent withdrawal effects
» Dizziness may occur; caution when getting up suddenly from a lying or sitting position

» Drowsiness and blurred vision may occur; caution when driving or doing things requiring alertness or clear vision
» Caution if any kind of surgery, dental treatment, or emergency treatment is required
Carrying medical identification card
» Patients with angina: Not increasing physical activities without consulting physician
Diabetic patients: Carefully checking urine or blood sugar; results may be lowered by this medication
» Obeying rules of caution for 14 days after discontinuing medication

Side/adverse effects
» Signs of potential side effects, especially symptoms of hypertensive crisis, severe orthostatic hypotension, diarrhea, peripheral edema, sympathetic stimulation, hepatitis, leukopenia, or parkinsonian syndrome

---

▲ For the Patient ▲

913116

ABOUT YOUR MEDICINE

Monoamine oxidase (MAO) inhibitors are used to relieve certain types of mental depression. These medicines may also be used for other conditions as determined by your doctor.

If any of the information in this leaflet causes you special concern or if you want additional information about your medicine and its use, check with your doctor, nurse, or pharmacist. **Remember, keep this and all other medicines out of the reach of children and never share your medicines with others.**

BEFORE USING THIS MEDICINE

Tell your doctor, nurse, and pharmacist if you . . .
• are allergic to any medicine, either prescription or nonprescription (OTC);
• are pregnant or intend to become pregnant while using this medicine;
• are breast-feeding;
• are taking **any** other prescription or nonprescription (OTC) medicine;
• have **any** other medical problems.

PROPER USE OF THIS MEDICINE

MAO inhibitors may be taken with or without food. Take them as directed.

Sometimes this medicine must be taken for several weeks before you begin to feel better. Your doctor should check your progress at regular visits to make sure that this medicine is working properly.

Take this medicine only as directed. Do not take more of it, do not take it more often, and do not take it for a longer time than ordered.

If you miss a dose of this medicine, take it as soon as possible. However, if it is within 2 hours of your next dose, skip the

missed dose and go back to your regular dosing schedule.
Do not double doses.

PRECAUTIONS WHILE USING THIS MEDICINE

**Do not stop taking this medicine without checking with your
doctor.** You may have to reduce gradually the amount you
are using before stopping completely.

This medicine may cause blurred vision or make some people
drowsy or less alert than they are normally. **Make sure you
know how you react before you drive, use machines, or do
other jobs that require you to be alert.**

**Before having any kind of surgery or dental or emergency
treatment, tell the physician or dentist in charge that you are
using this medicine or have used it within the past 2 weeks.**

When taken with certain foods, drinks, or other medicines,
**MAO inhibitors can cause very dangerous reactions such as
sudden high blood pressure** (also called hypertensive crisis).
To help avoid such reactions:
  • Do not eat foods that are aged or fermented to increase
    their flavor, such as cheeses; fava or broad bean pods;
    yeast or meat extracts; smoked or pickled meat, poultry,
    or fish; fermented sausage (bologna, pepperoni, salami,
    and summer sausage) or other fermented meat; sauer-
    kraut; or any overripe fruit. Ask your doctor, nurse, or
    pharmacist for a list of these foods and beverages.
  • Do not drink alcoholic beverages or alcohol-free or re-
    duced-alcohol beer and wine or eat or drink large amounts
    of caffeine-containing food or beverages such as coffee,
    tea, cola, or chocolate.
  • Do not take any other medicine unless prescribed by
    your doctor.

**After you stop using this medicine, you must continue to obey
the rules of caution** concerning food, drink, and other medicine for at least 2 weeks since those substances may continue
to react with MAO inhibitors.

POSSIBLE SIDE EFFECTS OF THIS MEDICINE
*Side Effects That Should Be Reported To Your Doctor
Immediately*

**Stop taking this medicine and get emergency help immedi-
ately** if any of the following signs of unusually high blood
pressure (hypertensive crisis) occur:

> Chest pain (severe); enlarged pupils; fast or slow heart-
> beat; headache (severe); increased sensitivity of eyes
> to light; increased sweating (possibly with fever or cold,
> clammy skin); nausea and vomiting; stiff or sore neck

*Other Side Effects That Should Be Reported To Your
Doctor*

> *More common*—Dizziness or lightheadedness (severe)

Less common—Diarrhea; fast or pounding heartbeat; swelling of feet or lower legs; unusual excitement or nervousness

Rare—Dark urine; fever; skin rash; slurred speech; sore throat; staggering walk; yellow eyes or skin

Side Effects That Usually Do Not Require Medical Attention

These possible side effects may go away during treatment; however, if they continue or are bothersome, check with your doctor, nurse, or pharmacist.

More common—Blurred vision; decreased amount of urine; decreased sexual ability; dizziness or lightheadedness (mild); drowsiness; headache (mild); increased appetite (especially for sweets) or weight gain; increased sweating; muscle twitching during sleep; restlessness; shakiness or trembling; tiredness and weakness; trouble in sleeping

Other side effects not listed above may also occur in some patients. If you notice any other effects, check with your doctor, nurse, or pharmacist.

ANTIDEPRESSANTS, TRICYCLIC Systemic

Including Amitriptyline; Amoxapine; Clomipramine; Desipramine; Doxepin; Imipramine; Nortriptyline; Protriptyline; Trimipramine.

■For the Pharmacist■

In providing consultation, consider emphasizing the following selected information (» = major clinical significance):

Before using this medication
» Conditions affecting use, especially:
   Sensitivity to tricyclic antidepressants, maprotiline, or trazodone
   Pregnancy—Clinical reports of fetal malformations with imipramine; animal sudies have shown some tricyclics to cause embryotoxic or fetotoxic effects, and decreased rate of conception; when tricyclics taken by mother immediately before delivery, clinical reports of newborns suffering from muscle spasms, and heart, breathing, and urinary problems
   Breast-feeding—Pass into breast milk and may cause drowsiness in nursing baby
   Use in children—Children and adolescents more sensitive to effects, requiring lower doses; may cause nervousness, sleeping problems, tiredness, mild stomach upset; generally not recommended for depression in children
   Use in elderly—Elderly more sensitive to effects; lower doses and more gradual increases required
   Dental—Decreased salivary flow contributes to caries, periodontal disease, candidiasis, and discomfort; blood dyscrasias may cause increased infections, delayed healing, and gingival bleeding; increased extrapyramidal motor activity of head, face, and neck with amoxapine may cause difficulty with occlusal and other procedures
   Other medications, especially CNS depressants, antithyroid agents, cimetidine, clonidine, guanadrel, guanethidine, phenothiazines, extrapyramidal reaction–causing medications, MAO inhibitors, metrimazide, or sympathomimetics
   Other medical problems, especially alcoholism (active), asthma, bipolar disorder, blood disorders, cardiovascular disorders, gastrointestinal disorders, glaucoma or increased intraocular pressure, hepatic function impairment, hyperthyroidism, prostatic hypertrophy, renal function impairment, schizophrenia, seizure disorders, or urinary retention

Proper use of this medication
   Taking with food to reduce gastrointestinal irritation
» Compliance with therapy; not taking more or less medicine than prescribed
» May require from 1 to 6 weeks of therapy to obtain antidepressant effects
   Proper administration of doxepin oral solution
      Using dropper provided by manufacturer for accurate measurement
      Diluting medication in one-half glass of recommended beverage (water, milk, or fruit juice, but not grape juice or carbonated beverages) immediately before use
      Not preparing or storing bulk solutions

» Proper dosing
Missed dose: If dosing schedule is—
More than one dose a day: Taking as soon as possible unless almost time for next dose; not doubling doses
One dose at bedtime: Not taking in morning because of side effects; checking with physician
» Proper storage

Precautions while using this medication
Regular visits to physician to check progress of therapy
» Avoiding the use of alcoholic beverages; not taking other medication unless prescribed by physician
» Possible drowsiness; caution when driving or doing things requiring alertness
» Possible dizziness or lightheadedness; caution when getting up suddenly from a lying or sitting position
» Possible dryness of mouth; using sugarless gum or candy, ice, or saliva substitute for relief; checking with physician or dentist if dry mouth continues for more than 2 weeks
» Possible skin photosensitivity; avoiding unprotected exposure to sun; using protective clothing; using a sun block product that includes protection against both UVA-caused photosensitivity reactions and UVB-caused sunburn reactions; avoiding use of sunlamp, tanning bed, or tanning booth
Caution if any laboratory tests required; possible interference with results of metyrapone test.
» Caution if any kind of surgery, dental treatment, or emergency treatment is required
» Checking with physician before discontinuing medicine; gradual dosage reduction may be needed to avoid worsening of condition or withdrawal symptoms
» Observing precautions for 3 to 7 days after stopping medication
For protriptyline
Possibility of sleep interference if taken late in the day

Side/adverse effects
Signs of potential side effects, especially anticholinergic effects; hypotension; fast, slow, or irregular heartbeat; Parkinsonian syndrome; nervousness or restlessness; sexual function impairment; shakiness or tremors; neuroleptic malignant syndrome (NMS) or tardive dyskinesia (with amoxapine only); anxiety; breast enlargement in males and females; galactorrhea; testicular swelling; alopecia; allergic reactions; blood dyscrasias; cholestatic jaundice; seizures; SIADH; tinnitus; or trouble with teeth or gums

---

▲ For the Patient ▲

912736

ABOUT YOUR MEDICINE

Tricyclic antidepressants are used to relieve mental depression and depression that sometimes occurs with anxiety. One form of this medicine (imipramine) may also be used to treat enuresis (bedwetting). Another form (clomipramine) is used to treat obsessive-compulsive disorders. Tricyclic antidepressants may also be used for other conditions as determined by your doctor.

If any of the information in this leaflet causes you special concern or if you want additional information about your

medicine and its use, check with your doctor, nurse, or pharmacist. **Remember, keep this and all other medicines out of the reach of children and never share your medicines with others.**

BEFORE USING THIS MEDICINE

Tell your doctor, nurse, and pharmacist if you . . .
- are allergic to any medicine, either prescription or non-prescription (OTC);
- are pregnant or intend to become pregnant while using this medicine;
- are breast-feeding;
- are taking **any** other prescription or nonprescription (OTC) medicine;
- have **any** other medical problems.

PROPER USE OF THIS MEDICINE

Take this medicine only as directed by your doctor. Sometimes tricyclic antidepressants must be taken for several weeks before you feel better.

If you miss a dose of this medicine, take it as soon as possible. However, if it is almost time for your next dose, skip the missed dose. Do not double doses. If a once-a-day bedtime dose is missed, do not take that dose in the morning since it may cause disturbing side effects during waking hours.

PRECAUTIONS WHILE USING THIS MEDICINE

Do not stop taking this medicine without first checking with your doctor.

This medicine will add to the effects of alcohol and other CNS depressants (medicines that make you drowsy or less alert). **Check with your doctor before taking any such depressants while you are taking this medicine.**

This medicine may cause some people to become drowsy or less alert than they are normally. **Make sure you know how you react before you drive, use machines, or do other jobs that require you to be alert.**

Dizziness, lightheadedness, or fainting may occur, especially when getting up from a lying or sitting position. Getting up slowly may help.

Before having any kind of surgery or dental or emergency treatment, tell the physician or dentist in charge that you are taking this medicine.

The effects of this medicine may last for 3 to 7 days after you stop taking it. Make sure you continue to follow the precautions during this time.

POSSIBLE SIDE EFFECTS OF THIS MEDICINE
Side Effects That Should Be Reported To Your Doctor

Less common—Blurred vision; confusion or delirium; constipation (especially in the elderly); decreased sexual ability (more common with amoxapine and clomipramine); difficulty in swallowing or speaking; eye pain; fainting; fast or irregular heartbeat; hallucinations; loss of balance control; mask-like face; nervousness or restlessness; problems in urinating; shakiness or trembling; shuffling walk; slowed movements; stiff arms and legs

Rare—Breast enlargement; hair loss; inappropriate secretion of milk (in females); increased sensitivity to sunlight; irritability; muscle twitching; red or brownish spots on skin; ringing, buzzing, or other unexplained noises in the ears; seizures (more common with clomipramine); skin rash and itching; sore throat and fever; swelling of face and tongue; swelling of testicles (more common with amoxapine); trouble with teeth or gums (more common with clomipramine); unusual bleeding or bruising; yellow eyes or skin

For amoxapine only (in addition to the above)—**Stop taking this medicine and get emergency help immediately** if any of the following side effects occur: Convulsions (seizures); fever with increased sweating; high or low blood pressure; loss of bladder control; muscle stiffness (severe); tiredness or weakness; troubled breathing; unusually pale skin. Other side effects of amoxapine that need medical attention include: Lip smacking or puckering; puffing of cheeks; rapid or worm-like movements of the tongue; uncontrolled chewing movements; uncontrolled movements of hands, arms, or legs

Side Effects That Usually Do Not Require Medical Attention

These possible side effects may go away during treatment; however, if they continue or are bothersome, check with your doctor, nurse, or pharmacist.

More common—Dizziness or lightheadedness; drowsiness (mild); dryness of mouth; headache; increased appetite (may include craving for sweets); nausea; unpleasant taste; weight gain

Other side effects not listed above may also occur in some patients. If you notice any other effects, check with your doctor, nurse, or pharmacist.

After you stop taking this medicine, your body may need time to adjust. Check with your doctor if you notice headache; irritability; nausea, vomiting, or diarrhea; restlessness;

trouble in sleeping, with vivid dreams; uncontrolled movements of mouth, tongue, jaw, arms, or legs; or unusual excitement.

ANTIDIABETIC AGENTS, ORAL   Systemic
Including Acetohexamide; Chlorpropamide; Glipizide; Glyburide; Tolazamide; Tolbutamide.

■ For the Pharmacist ■

In providing consultation, consider emphasizing the following selected information (» = major clinical significance):

Before using this medication
» Conditions affecting use, especially:
   Sensitivity to oral antidiabetic agents, sulfonamides, or thiazides
   Pregnancy—Should not be used during pregnancy
   Breast-feeding—Because chlorpropamide is distributed into breast milk, its use while breast-feeding is not recommended
   Use in the elderly—May be more susceptible to hypoglycemia and neurological effects associated with hypoglycemia
   Dental—Caution advised in dental care if leukopenia or thrombocytopenia occurs
   Other medications, especially coumarin- or indandione-derivative anticoagulants; chloramphenicol; guanethidine; MAO inhibitors including furazolidone, pargyline, and procarbazine; salicylates; sulfonamides; or beta-adrenergic blocking agents, including ophthalmics
   Other medical problems, especially acute medical conditions requiring use of insulin, adrenal insufficiency, high fever, nausea, vomiting, pituitary insufficiency, thyroid function impairment, or conditions in which increased susceptibility to hypoglycemia occurs; in addition, for chlorpropamide only—cardiac function impairment or fluid retention

Proper use of this medication
» Importance of following prescribed diet; necessary to allow medicine to work properly
» Compliance with therapy; not taking more or less medicine than directed; taking at same time each day
» Proper dosing
   Missed dose: Taking as soon as possible; not taking if almost time for next dose; not doubling doses
» Proper storage

Precautions while using this medication
   Regular visits to physician to check progress
   Testing for sugar in blood or urine as ordered by physician
» Avoiding use of other medication unless prescribed or approved by physician
» Possible disulfiram-like reactions may occur when alcohol is ingested (less likely with glipizide and glyburide)
   Possibility of photosensitivity
» Taking sugar and notifying physician if symptoms of hypoglycemia occur; also caution patients taking chlorpropamide for diabetes insipidus
   Caution if any kind of surgery, dental treatment, or emergency treatment is required
   Carrying medical identification card or bracelet

Side/adverse effects
   Signs of potential side effects, especially aplastic anemia, eosinophilia, porphyria cutanea tarda, hepatic function impairment,

bone marrow depression, agranulocytosis, infection, thrombocytopenia, or hemolytic anemia; in addition, for chlorpropamide
only—antidiuretic effect and congestive heart failure

▲ For the Patient ▲

912044

ABOUT YOUR MEDICINE

Oral antidiabetics (diabetes medicine you take by mouth)
are used to treat certain types of diabetes mellitus (sugar
diabetes). Chlorpropamide may also be used for other conditions as determined by your doctor.

If any of the information in this leaflet causes you special
concern or if you want additional information about your
medicine and its use, check with your doctor, nurse, or pharmacist. **Remember, keep this and all other medicines out of
the reach of children and never share your medicines with
others.**

BEFORE USING THIS MEDICINE

Tell your doctor, nurse, and pharmacist if you . . .
- are allergic to any medicine, either prescription or nonprescription (OTC);
- are pregnant or intend to become pregnant while using
  this medicine;
- are breast-feeding;
- are taking any other prescription or nonprescription
  (OTC) medicine, especially anticoagulants (blood thinners); aspirin or other salicylates; beta-blockers; chloramphenicol; guanethidine; MAO inhibitors; medicines
  for coughs, colds, asthma, hay fever, or appetite control;
  or sulfonamides (sulfa drugs);
- have any other medical problems, especially kidney, liver,
  or thyroid disease; severe infection; or underactive adrenal or pituitary glands.

PROPER USE OF THIS MEDICINE

Follow carefully the special meal plan your doctor gave you.
This is the most important part of controlling your condition,
and is necessary if the medicine is to work properly. Also,
test for sugar in your blood or urine as directed.

Take this medicine only as directed. Do not take more or
less of it than your doctor ordered, and take it at the same
time each day.

If you miss a dose of this medicine, take it as soon as possible.
However, if it is almost time for your next dose, skip the
missed dose and go back to your regular dosing schedule.
Do not double doses.

PRECAUTIONS WHILE USING THIS MEDICINE

**Avoid drinking alcoholic beverages until you have discussed
their use with your doctor.** They may affect diet, produce
low blood sugar, and cause other side effects.

Eat or drink something containing sugar and check with your doctor right away if mild symptoms of low blood sugar (hypoglycemia) appear. Good sources of sugar are glucose tablets or gel, fruit juice, corn syrup, honey, regular (non-diet) soft drinks, or sugar dissolved in water. It is a good idea to check your blood sugar to confirm that it is low.

If severe symptoms such as convulsions (seizures) or unconsciousness occur, diabetics should not eat or drink anything. There is a chance that they could choke from not swallowing correctly. Emergency medical help should be obtained immediately.

Symptoms of low blood sugar include abdominal or stomach pain (mild); anxious feeling; chills (continuing); cold sweats; confusion; convulsions (seizures); cool pale skin; difficulty in thinking; drowsiness; excessive hunger; headache (continuing); nausea or vomiting (continuing); nervousness; rapid heartbeat; shakiness; unconsciousness; unsteady walk; unusual tiredness or weakness; or vision changes. **These symptoms may occur if you** delay or miss a meal or snack, exercise much more than usual, cannot eat because of nausea and vomiting, or drink a significant amount of alcohol. **Tell someone to take you to your doctor or to a hospital right away if the symptoms do not improve after eating or drinking a sweet food.**

POSSIBLE SIDE EFFECTS OF THIS MEDICINE
Side Effects That Should Be Reported To Your Doctor

> *Rare*—Chest pain; chills; coughing up blood; dark urine; fatigue; fever; general feeling of illness; increased sweating; increased amounts of sputum (phlegm); itching of the skin; light-colored stools; sore throat; troubled breathing; unusual bleeding or bruising; unusual tiredness or weakness (continuing and unexplained); yellow eyes or skin

Side Effects That Usually Do Not Require Medical Attention

These possible side effects may go away during treatment; however, if they continue or are bothersome, check with your doctor, nurse, or pharmacist.

> *More common*—Changes in taste (for tolbutamide); constipation; diarrhea; dizziness; drowsiness (mild); headache; heartburn; increased or decreased appetite; nausea; stomach pain, fullness, or discomfort; vomiting

> *Less common*—Hives; increased sensitivity of skin to sun; skin redness, itching, or rash

Other side effects not listed above may also occur in some patients. If you notice any other effects, check with your doctor, nurse, or pharmacist.

ANTIDYSKINETICS Systemic

Including Benztropine; Biperiden; Ethopropazine;
Procyclidine; Trihexyphenidyl.

■For the Pharmacist■

In providing consultation, consider emphasizing the following selected
information (» = major clinical significance):

Before using this medication
» Conditions affecting use, especially:
  Sensitivity to antidyskinetics (history of)
  Breast-feeding—May inhibit lactation
  Use in children—Increased susceptibility to anticholinergic ef-
    fects
  Use in the elderly—Predisposition to glaucoma with chronic use;
    increased risk of mental confusion and other psychotic-like
    symptoms; impairment of memory
  Dental problems—Decrease or inhibition of salivary flow
  Other medications, especially other anticholinergics and CNS
    depressants
  Other medical problems, especially cardiovascular instability,
    tardive dyskinesia, glaucoma, intestinal obstruction, myas-
    thenia gravis, or urinary retention

Proper use of this medication
» Importance of not taking more medication than the amount pre-
    scribed
  Taking with food to relieve gastric irritation
» Proper dosing
  Missed dose: Taking as soon as possible; not taking if within 2 hours
    of next dose; not doubling doses
» Proper storage

Precautions while using this medication
  Regular visits to physician to check progress during prolonged ther-
    apy; eye examination may also be needed
» Checking with physician before discontinuing medication; gradual
    dosage reduction may be necessary
» Avoiding use of alcohol or other CNS depressants
  Avoiding use of antidiarrheal medications within 1 or 2 hours of
    taking this medication
  Suspected overdose: Getting emergency help at once
  Possible increased eye sensitivity to bright light
» Caution if drowsiness or blurred vision occurs
  Caution when getting up suddenly from a lying or sitting position
» Caution during exercise and hot weather
  Possible dryness of mouth; using sugarless gum or candy, ice, or
    saliva substitute for relief; checking with physician or dentist if
    dry mouth continues for more than 2 weeks

Side/adverse effects
  Signs of potential side effects, especially allergic reaction, confusion,
    increased intraocular pressure, anticholinergic effects, or CNS
    depression or stimulation

▲ For the Patient ▲

912055

ABOUT YOUR MEDICINE

Antidyskinetics (an-tye-dis-kin-ET-iks) are used to treat Parkinson's disease, sometimes referred to as "shaking palsy." Antidyskinetics are also used to control certain side effects of other medicines. Antidyskinetics may also be used for other conditions as determined by your doctor.

If any of the information in this leaflet causes you special concern or if you want additional information about your medicine and its use, check with your doctor, nurse, or pharmacist. **Remember, keep this and all other medicines out of the reach of children and never share your medicines with others.**

BEFORE USING THIS MEDICINE

Tell your doctor, nurse, and pharmacist if you . . .

- are allergic to any medicine, either prescription or nonprescription (OTC);
- are pregnant or intend to become pregnant while using this medicine;
- are breast-feeding;
- are taking any other prescription or nonprescription (OTC) medicine, especially antacids, anticholinergics (medicine for abdominal or stomach spasms or cramps), CNS depressants, or tricyclic antidepressants;
- have any other medical problems, especially difficult urination; glaucoma; heart or blood vessel disease; intestinal blockage; myasthenia gravis; or uncontrolled movements of hands, mouth, or tongue.

PROPER USE OF THIS MEDICINE

Take this medicine only as directed. Do not take more of it, do not take it more often, and do not take it for a longer period of time than your doctor ordered. To lessen stomach upset, take this medicine with meals or right after meals.

If you miss a dose of this medicine, take it as soon as possible. However, if it is within 2 hours of your next dose, skip the missed dose and go back to your regular dosing schedule. Do not double doses.

PRECAUTIONS WHILE USING THIS MEDICINE

Your doctor should check your progress at regular visits, especially for the first few months you take this medicine. Your doctor may also want you to have your eyes examined before and also sometime later during treatment.

Do not stop taking this medicine without first checking with your doctor. Your doctor may want you to reduce your dose gradually.

This medicine will add to the effects of alcohol and other CNS depressants (medicines that slow down your nervous system). **Check with your doctor before taking any such depressants while you are using this medicine.**

Antidyskinetics may cause some people to have blurred vision or to become drowsy, dizzy, or less alert than they are normally. **Make sure you know how you react to this medicine before you drive, use machines, or do other jobs that require you to be alert or able to see well.**

Antidyskinetics will often reduce your tolerance to heat, since they make you sweat less, causing your body temperature to increase. **Use extra care not to become overheated during exercise or hot weather while you are taking this medicine as this could possibly result in heat stroke.** Also, hot baths or saunas may make you feel dizzy or faint while you are taking this medicine.

If you think you or anyone else has taken an overdose of this medicine, get emergency help at once. Overdose may lead to unconsciousness. Some signs of an overdose are clumsiness; hallucinations; seizures; severe drowsiness; severe dryness of mouth, nose, and throat; troubled breathing; unusually fast heartbeat; or unusual warmth, dryness, and flushing of the skin.

POSSIBLE SIDE EFFECTS OF THIS MEDICINE
Side Effects That Should Be Reported To Your Doctor

   Rare—Confusion; eye pain; skin rash

Side Effects That Usually Do Not Require Medical Attention

These possible side effects may go away during treatment; however, if they continue or are bothersome, check with your doctor, nurse, or pharmacist.

   More common—Blurred vision; constipation; decreased sweating; difficult or painful urination; drowsiness; dryness of mouth, nose, or throat; increased sensitivity of eyes to light; nausea or vomiting

Other side effects not listed above may also occur in some patients. If you notice any other effects, check with your doctor, nurse, or pharmacist.

After you stop using this medicine, your body may need time to adjust. The length of time this takes depends on how long you used this medicine. **During this period of time, check with your doctor** if you have anxiety; difficulty in speaking or swallowing; loss of balance control; muscle spasms, especially of face, neck, and back; restlessness; shuffling walk; trembling and shaking of hands and fingers; or unusually fast heartbeat.

ANTIFUNGALS, AZOLE Systemic

*Including Fluconazole (Injection); Fluconazole (Oral);
Itraconazole (Oral); Ketoconazole (Oral); Miconazole
(Injection).*

■For the Pharmacist■

In providing consultation, consider emphasizing the following selected
information (» = major clinical significance):

Before using this medication
» Conditions affecting use, especially:
   Hypersensitivity to azole antifungals
   Fertility—High doses of ketoconazole have been shown to cause
      menstrual irregularities, oligospermia, azoospermia, and im-
      potence
   Pregnancy—High doses of azole antifungals may cause maternal
      toxicity, embryotoxicity, and teratogenicity in animals
   Other medications, especially alcohol, antacids, anticholiner-
      gics/antispasmodics, oral antidiabetic agents, astemizole,
      carbamazepine, cyclosporine, didanosine, digoxin, hepato-
      toxic medications, histamine H_2-receptor antagonists, isoni-
      azid, omeprazole, phenytoin, rifampin, sucralfate, terfena-
      dine, or warfarin
   Other medical problems, especially achlorhydria, alcoholism, he-
      patic function impairment, hypochlorhydria, or renal func-
      tion impairment

Proper use of this medication
» Taking itraconazole and ketoconazole with food to increase absorp-
   tion
   Proper administration technique for oral liquids
   Proper administration technique in achlorhydria
» Compliance with full course of therapy
» Importance of not missing doses and taking at evenly spaced times
» Proper dosing
   Missed dose: Taking as soon as possible; not taking if almost time
      for next dose; not doubling doses
» Proper storage

Precautions while using this medication
   Checking with physician if no improvement within a few days
» Not taking itraconazole or ketoconazole with terfenadine or astemizole; concurrent use may cause cardiac arrhythmias
» Avoiding alcoholic beverages or other alcohol-containing preparations while taking ketoconazole because of increased risk of hepatotoxicity
» Avoiding antacids and other medications that increase gastrointestinal pH while taking itraconazole or ketoconazole; concurrent
   use may decrease the absorption of itraconazole or ketoconazole
   Possible photophobic reactions when taking ketoconazole; wearing
      sunglasses and avoiding bright light to minimize potential eye
      discomfort

Side/adverse effects
   Phlebitis, hypersensitivity, agranulocytosis, anemia, exfoliative skin
      disorders, hepatotoxicity and thrombocytopenia

▲ For the Patient ▲

910468

AZOLE ANTIFUNGALS (Injection): *Including Fluconazole; Miconazole.*

ABOUT YOUR MEDICINE

Azole (AY-zole) **antifungals** are used to treat serious fungus infections that may occur in different parts of the body. These medicines may also be used for other conditions as determined by your doctor.

If any of the information in this leaflet causes you special concern or if you want additional information about your medicine and its use, check with your doctor, nurse, or pharmacist. **Remember, keep this and all other medicines out of the reach of children and never share your medicines with others.**

BEFORE USING THIS MEDICINE

Tell your doctor, nurse, and pharmacist if you . . .
- are allergic to any medicine, either prescription or non-prescription (OTC);
- are pregnant or intend to become pregnant while using this medicine;
- are breast-feeding;
- are taking **any** other prescription or nonprescription (OTC) medicine;
- have any other medical problems, especially alcohol abuse (or history of), or kidney or liver disease.

PROPER USE OF THIS MEDICINE

Some medicines given by injection may sometimes be given at home to patients who do not need to be in the hospital for the full time of treatment. If you are using this medicine at home, **make sure you clearly understand and carefully follow your doctor's instructions.**

Put used syringes and needles in a covered container that the needles cannot punch through, then throw the container away. Otherwise, throw away used syringes as directed by your doctor, nurse, or pharmacist.

To help clear up your infection completely, **it is very important that you keep using this medicine for the full time of treatment,** even if your symptoms begin to clear up or you begin to feel better after a few days. Since fungus infections may be very slow to clear up, you may have to continue using this medicine every day for as long as 6 months to a year or more. Some fungus infections never clear up completely and require continuous treatment. If you stop using this medicine too soon, your symptoms may return.

This medicine works best when there is a constant amount in the blood. **To help keep the amount constant, do not miss** any doses. Also, it is best to use each dose at the same time every day. If you need help in planning the best time to use your medicine, check with your doctor, nurse, or pharmacist.

If you do miss a dose of this medicine, use it as soon as possible. However, if it is almost time for your next dose, skip the missed dose and go back to your regular dosing schedule. Do not double doses.

PRECAUTIONS WHILE USING THIS MEDICINE

It is important that your doctor check your progress at regular visits. This will allow your doctor to check for any unwanted effects.

If your symptoms do not improve within a few weeks (or months for some infections), or if they become worse, check with your doctor.

POSSIBLE SIDE EFFECTS OF THIS MEDICINE

Side Effects That Should Be Reported To Your Doctor Immediately

> *More common*—Redness, swelling, or pain at place of injection (miconazole only)

> *Less common*—Fever and chills; skin rash or itching

> *Rare*—Dark or amber urine; fever and sore throat; loss of appetite; pale stools; reddening, blistering, peeling, or loosening of skin and mucous membranes; stomach pain; unusual bleeding or bruising; unusual tiredness or weakness; yellow skin or eyes

Side Effects That Usually Do Not Require Medical Attention

These possible side effects may go away during treatment; however, if they continue or are bothersome, check with your doctor, nurse, or pharmacist.

> *Less common*—Constipation; diarrhea; dizziness; drowsiness; flushing or redness of the face or skin; headache; nausea; vomiting

Other side effects not listed above may also occur in some patients. If you notice any other effects, check with your doctor, nurse, or pharmacist.

▲ For the Patient ▲

910457

Azole Antifungals (Oral): *Including Fluconazole; Itraconazole; Ketoconazole.*

ABOUT YOUR MEDICINE

Azole (AY-zole) **antifungals** are used to treat serious fungus infections that may occur in different parts of the body. These medicines may also be used for other problems as determined by your doctor.

If any of the information in this leaflet causes you special concern or if you want additional information about your medicine and its use, check with your doctor, nurse, or pharmacist. **Remember, keep this and all other medicines out of the reach of children and never share your medicines with others.**

BEFORE USING THIS MEDICINE
Tell your doctor, nurse, and pharmacist if you . . .
* are allergic to any medicine, either prescription or nonprescription (OTC);
* are pregnant or intend to become pregnant while using this medicine;
* are breast-feeding;
* are taking **any** other prescription or nonprescription (OTC) medicine;
* have any other medical problems, especially achlorhydria (absence of stomach acid), alcohol abuse (or history of), hypochlorhydria (decreased amount of stomach acid), or kidney or liver disease.

PROPER USE OF THIS MEDICINE
Itraconazole and ketoconazole should be taken with a meal or snack.

For patients taking the oral liquid form of ketoconazole:
* Use a specially marked measuring spoon or other device to measure each dose. The average household teaspoon may not hold the right amount.

If you have achlorhydria or hypochlorhydria and you are taking itraconazole or ketoconazole, your doctor may have special instructions for you. Your doctor may want you to take your medicine with an acidic drink, such as cola or seltzer water, or mixed into a special solution of weak hydrochloric acid. Be sure to follow your doctor's instructions carefully.

To help clear up your infection completely, **it is very important that you keep taking this medicine for the full time of treatment.**

This medicine works best when there is a constant amount in the blood. **To help keep this amount constant, do not miss any doses. Also, it is best to take each dose at the same time every day.** If you need help in planning the best time to take your medicine, check with your doctor, nurse, or pharmacist.

If you do miss a dose of this medicine, take it as soon as possible. However, if it is almost time for your next dose, skip the missed dose and go back to your regular dosing schedule. Do not double doses.

PRECAUTIONS WHILE USING THIS MEDICINE
It is important that your doctor check your progress at regular visits.

If your symptoms do not improve within a few weeks (or months for some infections), or if they become worse, check with your doctor.

Itraconazole and ketoconazole should not be taken with astemizole (e.g., Hismanal) or terfenadine (e.g., Seldane). Doing so may increase the risk of serious side effects affecting the heart.

Liver problems may be more likely to occur if you drink alcoholic beverages while you are taking ketoconazole. Alcoholic beverages may also cause stomach pain, nausea, vomiting, headache, or flushing or redness of the face. Other alcohol-containing preparations (for example, elixirs, cough syrups, tonics) may also cause problems. These problems may occur for at least a day after you stop taking ketoconazole. Therefore, **you should not drink alcoholic beverages while you are taking ketoconazole and for at least a day after you stop taking it.**

If you are taking antacids, cimetidine, famotidine, nizatidine, ranitidine, or omeprazole while you are taking itraconazole or ketoconazole, take them at least 2 hours after you take itraconazole or ketoconazole.

Ketoconazole may cause your eyes to become more sensitive to light than they are normally. Wearing sunglasses and avoiding too much exposure to bright light may help lessen the discomfort.

POSSIBLE SIDE EFFECTS OF THIS MEDICINE
Side Effects That Should Be Reported To Your Doctor Immediately

> *Less common or rare*—Dark or amber urine; fever, chills, or sore throat; loss of appetite; pale stools; reddening, blistering, peeling, or loosening of skin and mucous membranes; skin rash or itching; stomach pain; unusual bleeding or bruising; unusual tiredness or weakness; yellow eyes or skin

Side Effects That Usually Do Not Require Medical Attention

These possible side effects may go away during treatment; however, if they continue or are bothersome, check with your doctor, nurse, or pharmacist.

> *Less common*—Constipation; diarrhea; dizziness; drowsiness; flushing or redness of the face or skin; headache; nausea; vomiting

> *Rare (for ketoconazole only—in addition to above)*— Decreased sexual ability or enlarged breasts in males; increased sensitivity of eyes to light; menstrual irregularities

Other side effects not listed above may also occur in some patients. If you notice any other effects, check with your doctor, nurse, or pharmacist.

ANTIFUNGALS, AZOLE   Vaginal

Including Butoconazole; Clotrimazole; Econazole;
Miconazole; Terconazole; Tioconazole.

■ For the Pharmacist ■

In providing consultation, consider emphasizing the following selected
   information (» = major clinical significance):

Before using this medication
» Conditions affecting use, especially:
      Allergy to azoles
      Pregnancy—Some animal studies have shown that vaginal azoles
         may be embryotoxic or fetotoxic, however, problems have
         not been documented in humans
      Labor—Vaginal azoles have been shown to cause dystocia in
         some studies when given through labor

Proper use of this medication
   Reading patient instructions before using medication
   Using at bedtime, unless otherwise directed by physician; retaining
      miconazole vaginal tampons overnight and removing them the
      following morning
   Checking with physician before using applicator if pregnant
» Compliance with full course of therapy, even if menstruation begins
» Proper dosing
   Missed dose: Inserting as soon as possible; not inserting if almost
      time for next dose
» Proper storage

Precautions while using this medication
   Checking with physician if no improvement within a few days
   Protecting clothing because of possible soiling with vaginal azoles;
      avoiding the use of unmedicated tampons
» Using hygienic measures to cure infection and prevent reinfection
   Wearing cotton panties instead of synthetic underclothes
   Wearing only freshly washed underclothes
» Use of condom by partner to prevent reinfection; possible need for
      concurrent treatment of male partner; continuing medication if
      intercourse occurs during treatment
» Using douche prior to next dose; not overfilling vagina with douche
      solution; avoiding use of a douche during pregnancy

Side/adverse effects
   Signs of potential side effects, especially hypersensitivity, and va-
      ginal burning, itching, or other irritation not present before ther-
      apy

▲ For the Patient ▲

916158

ABOUT YOUR MEDICINE

Vaginal azole (AZ-ole) **antifungals** are used to treat fungus
(yeast) infections of the vagina.

If any of the information in this leaflet causes you special
concern or if you want additional information about your

medicine and its use, check with your doctor, nurse, or pharmacist. **Remember, keep this and all other medicines out of the reach of children and never share your medicines with others.**

BEFORE USING THIS MEDICINE

Tell your doctor, nurse, and pharmacist if you . . .
- are allergic to any medicine, either prescription or nonprescription (OTC);
- are pregnant or intend to become pregnant while using this medicine;
- are breast-feeding;
- are taking any other prescription or nonprescription (OTC) medicine;
- use condoms, a cervical cap, or a diaphragm for birth control;
- have any other medical problems.

PROPER USE OF THIS MEDICINE

Vaginal azole antifungals usually come with patient directions. Read them carefully before using this medicine.

Use this medicine at bedtime, unless otherwise directed by your doctor. The vaginal tampon form of miconazole should be left in the vagina overnight and removed the next morning.

To help clear up your infection completely, **it is very important that you keep using this medicine for the full time of treatment,** even if your symptoms begin to clear up after a few days. If you stop using this medicine too soon, your symptoms may return. **Do not miss any doses.** Also, **do not stop using this medicine if your menstrual period starts during the time of treatment.**

If you do miss a dose of this medicine, insert it as soon as possible. However, if it is almost time for your next dose, skip the missed dose and go back to your regular dosing schedule.

PRECAUTIONS WHILE USING THIS MEDICINE

If your symptoms do not improve within a few days, or if they become worse, check with your doctor.

Vaginal medicines usually will come out of the vagina during treatment. To keep the medicine from getting on your clothing, wear a minipad or sanitary napkin. The use of non-medicated tampons (like those used for menstrual periods) is not recommended since they may soak up the medicine.

To help clear up your infection completely and to help make sure it does not return, good health habits are also required.
- Wear cotton panties (or panties or pantyhose with cotton crotches) instead of synthetic (for example, nylon or rayon) panties.
- Wear only clean panties.

Many vaginal infections are spread by having sex. A male sexual partner may carry the fungus on or in his penis. While you are using this medicine, it may be a good idea for your partner to wear a condom during sex to avoid reinfection. Also, it may be necessary for your partner to be treated. **Do not stop using this medicine if you have sex during treatment.**

Some women may want to use a douche before the next dose. Some doctors will allow the use of a vinegar and water douche or other douche. However, others do not allow any douching. If you do use a douche, **do not overfill the vagina.** To do so may push the douche up into the uterus and possibly cause inflammation or infection. Also, **do not douche if you are pregnant since this may harm the fetus.** If you have any questions about this, check with your doctor, nurse, or pharmacist.

This medicine must not be given to other people or used for other infections unless otherwise directed by your doctor.

POSSIBLE SIDE EFFECTS OF THIS MEDICINE
Side Effects That Should Be Reported To Your Doctor

> *Less common*—Vaginal burning, itching, discharge, or other irritation not present before use of this medicine

> *Rare*—Skin rash or hives

Side Effects That Usually Do Not Require Medical Attention

These possible side effects may go away during treatment; however, if they continue or are bothersome, check with your doctor, nurse, or pharmacist.

> *Less common or rare*—Abdominal or stomach cramps or pain; burning or irritation of penis of sexual partner; headache

Other side effects not listed above may also occur in some patients. If you notice any other effects, check with your doctor, nurse, or pharmacist.

ANTIGLAUCOMA AGENTS, CHOLINERGIC, LONG-ACTING Ophthalmic

Including Demecarium; Echothiophate; Isoflurophate.

■For the Pharmacist■

In providing consultation, consider emphasizing the following selected information (» = major clinical significance):

Before using this medication
» Conditions affecting use, especially:
   Sensitivity to demecarium, echothiophate, or isoflurophate
   Pregnancy—Because of the toxicity of cholinesterase inhibitors in general, these medications are not recommended during pregnancy
   Breast-feeding—Medications may be absorbed into the body and are not recommended during breast-feeding, since they may cause adverse effects in nursing infants; a decision should be made whether to discontinue nursing or discontinue the medication
   Use in children—The iris cysts that may occur following prolonged use of these medications occur frequently in children
   Other medications, especially antimyasthenics; anticholinergics or other medications with anticholinergic activity; or other cholinesterase inhibitors, possibly including topical malathion
   Recent exposure to pesticides or insecticides
   Other medical problems, especially glaucoma associated with iridocyclitis, predisposition to or history of retinal detachment, or active uveitis

Proper use of this medication
   Proper administration technique for ophthalmic solution; removing excess solution around eye with clean tissue, being careful not to touch eye; washing hands immediately after application to avoid possible systemic absorption; not touching applicator tip to any surface; keeping container tightly closed
   Proper administration technique for ophthalmic ointment; washing hands immediately after application to avoid possible systemic absorption; not washing tip of ointment tube or allowing it to touch moist surface, since medication loses efficacy when exposed to moisture; not touching applicator tip to any surface, wiping tip of ointment tube with clean tissue; keeping container tightly closed; applying at bedtime, since ointment causes blurred vision after administration
» Importance of not using more medication than the amount prescribed
» Proper dosing
   Missed dose: If dosing schedule is—
      Every other day: Applying as soon as possible if remembered same day; if not remembered until the next day, applying it at that time, then skipping a day; not doubling doses
      Once a day: Applying as soon as possible; if not remembered until next day, skipping missed dose and going back to regular dosing schedule; not doubling doses

More than once a day: Applying as soon as possible; if almost time for next dose, skipping missed dose and going back to regular dosing schedule; not doubling doses

» Proper storage

Precautions while using this medication

Regular visits to physician during therapy to check eye pressure and, for patients on prolonged therapy, to examine eyes

» Caution if any kind of surgery is required

» Caution in exposure to carbamate- or organophosphate-type insecticides or pesticides during therapy

» Making sure vision is clear before driving, using machines, or doing anything else that could be dangerous if not able to see well; caution because of possibility of decreased night vision, blurred vision or change in near or distance vision, or blurred vision for short time if using ointment

Side/adverse effects

Signs of potential side effects, especially burning, redness, stinging, or other symptoms of systemic absorption; irritation of the eyes; eye pain; and retinal detachment

---

▲ For the Patient ▲

912838

ABOUT YOUR MEDICINE

Long-acting cholinergic (ko-lin-ER-jik) **glaucoma eye medicines** are used in the eye to treat certain types of glaucoma and other eye conditions. They may also be used in the diagnosis of other eye conditions.

If any of the information in this leaflet causes you special concern or if you want additional information about your medicine and its use, check with your doctor, nurse, or pharmacist. **Remember, keep this and all other medicines out of the reach of children and never share your medicines with others.**

BEFORE USING THIS MEDICINE

Tell your doctor, nurse, and pharmacist if you . . .

• are allergic to any medicine, either prescription or non-prescription (OTC);
• are pregnant or intend to become pregnant while using this medicine;
• are breast-feeding;
• are taking **any** other prescription or nonprescription (OTC) medicine;
• have any other medical problems, especially other eye disease.

PROPER USE OF THIS MEDICINE

It is very important that you use this medicine only as directed. Do not use more of it or use it more often than ordered. To do so may increase the chance of too much medicine being absorbed into the body and the chance of side effects.

To use the ophthalmic solution (eye drops) form of this medicine:

- First, wash your hands. Tilt the head back and, pressing your finger gently on the skin just beneath the lower eyelid, pull the lower eyelid away from the eye to make a space. Drop the medicine into this space. Let go of the eyelid and gently close the eyes. Do not blink. Keep the eyes closed and apply pressure to the inner corner of the eye with your finger for 1 or 2 minutes to allow the medicine to be absorbed by the eye.
- Remove excess solution around the eye with a clean tissue, being careful not to touch the eye.
- Wash hands to remove any medicine that may be on them.

To use the ophthalmic ointment (eye ointment) form of this medicine:

- First, wash your hands. Tilt the head back and, pressing your finger gently on the skin just beneath the lower eyelid, pull the lower eyelid away from the eye to make a space. Squeeze a thin strip of ointment into this space. A 1/2-cm (approximately 1/4-inch) strip of ointment is usually enough, unless you have been told by your doctor to use a different amount. Let go of the eyelid and gently close the eyes. Keep the eyes closed for 1 or 2 minutes to allow the medicine to be absorbed by the eye.
- Wash hands to remove any medicine that may be on them.
- Do not wash the tip of the ointment tube or allow it to touch any moist surface (including the eye). Wipe it with a clean tissue.

To keep the medicine as germ-free as possible do not touch the applicator tip to any surface (including the eye) and keep the container tightly closed.

If you miss a dose of this medicine, use the missed dose as soon as possible. However, if it is almost time for your next dose, skip the missed dose and go back to your regular dosing schedule. Do not double doses.

PRECAUTIONS WHILE USING THIS MEDICINE

Before having any kind of surgery (including eye surgery) or dental or emergency treatment, tell the physician or dentist in charge and the anesthesiologist or anesthetist (the person who puts you to sleep) that you are using this medicine or that you have used it within the past month.

Avoid breathing in carbamate- or organophosphate-type insecticides or pesticides. They may add to the effects of this medicine.

Make sure your vision is clear before you drive, use machines, or do other jobs that require you to see well.

POSSIBLE SIDE EFFECTS OF THIS MEDICINE

Side Effects That Should Be Reported To Your Doctor Immediately

Rare—Veil or curtain appearing across part of vision

Possible signs of too much medicine being absorbed into the body—Increased sweating; loss of bladder control; muscle weakness; nausea, vomiting, diarrhea, or stomach cramps or pain; shortness of breath, tightness in chest, or wheezing; slow or irregular heartbeat; unusual tiredness or weakness; watering of mouth

Other Side Effects That Should Be Reported To Your Doctor

Rare—Burning, redness, stinging, or other eye irritation; eye pain

Side Effects That Usually Do Not Require Medical Attention

These possible side effects may go away during treatment; however, if they continue or are bothersome, check with your doctor, nurse, or pharmacist.

Blurred vision or change in near or distance vision; difficulty in seeing at night or in dim light; headache or browache; twitching of eyelids; watering of eyes

Other side effects not listed above may also occur in some patients. If you notice any other effects, check with your doctor, nurse, or pharmacist.

ANTIHISTAMINES   Systemic

Including Acrivastine; Astemizole; Azatadine; Bromodiphenhydramine; Brompheniramine; Carbonoxamine; Cetirizine; Chlorpheniramine; Clemastine; Cyproheptadine; Dexchlorpheniramine; Dimenhydrinate; Diphenhydramine; Diphenylpyraline; Doxylamine; Hydroxyzine; Loratadine; Phenindamine; Pyrilamine; Terfenadine; Tripelennamine; Triprolidine.

■ For the Pharmacist ■

In providing consultation, consider emphasizing the following selected information (» = major clinical significance):

Before using this medication

» Conditions affecting use of most antihistamines (to a lesser extent with astemizole, loratadine, and terfenadine), especially:

Sensitivity to any antihistamine

Pregnancy—Not taking during early months of pregnancy because of fetal abnormalities in studies in animals (for hydroxyzine only); risk-benefit should be considered because of fetal abnormalities in studies in animals with doses above the human therapeutic range (for astemizole and terfenadine only)

Breast-feeding—Use not recommended; may cause unusual excitement or irritability in nursing infant

Use in children—Increased susceptibility to anticholinergic side effects in newborn or premature infants; hyperexcitability (paradoxical reaction) may occur in children

Use in geriatric patients—Increased susceptibility to anticholinergic side effects; hyperexcitability (paradoxical reaction) may occur

Dental—Increased risk of dental problems because of decrease or inhibition of salivary flow

Other medications, especially alcohol or other CNS depressants; anticholinergics; calcium channel blocking agents, disopyramide, maprotiline, phenothiazines, pimozide, procainamide, quinidine, and tricyclic antidepressants (with astemizole and terfenadine); erythromycin and other macrolide antibiotics (with astemizole and terfenadine only); itraconazole and ketoconazole (with astemizole and terfenadine); or MAO inhibitors

Other medical problems, especially angle-closure glaucoma, hepatic function impairment (with astemizole or terfenadine only), hypokalemia (with astemizole or terfenadine only), prostatic hypertrophy, or urinary retention

Proper use of this medication

» Importance of not taking more medication than the amount recommended

» Proper dosing

Missed dose: If on scheduled dosing regimen—Using as soon as possible; not using if almost time for next dose; not doubling doses

» Proper storage

For oral dosage forms
> Taking with food, water, or milk to minimize gastric irritation; taking astemizole and loratadine on an empty stomach to minimize absorption problems
> Swallowing extended-release dosage forms whole

For injection dosage forms
> Knowing correct administration technique for self-administration; checking with physician if necessary

For rectal dosage forms
> Proper administration technique

For dimenhydrinate and diphenhydramine when used as antivertigo agent
> Taking at least 30 minutes (preferably 1 to 2 hours) before traveling

Precautions while using this medication
> Possible interference with skin tests using allergens; need to inform physician if using medication
> May mask ototoxic effects of large doses of salicylates
» Avoiding use of alcohol or other CNS depressants
» Caution if drowsiness occurs
> Possible dryness of mouth; using sugarless gum or candy, ice, or saliva substitute for relief; checking with physician or dentist if dry mouth continues for more than 2 weeks

For dimenhydrinate, diphenhydramine, or hydroxyzine
> Need to inform physician of use: Possible interference with diagnosis of appendicitis; may mask signs of toxicity from overdosage of other drugs

For diphenhydramine and doxylamine when used in the treatment of insomnia
» Not using concurrently with other sedatives or tranquilizers

Side/adverse effects
> Signs of potential side effects, especially blood dyscrasias and cardiac arrhythmias (with astemizole and terfenadine only)

▲ For the Patient ▲

912066

ABOUT YOUR MEDICINE

Antihistamines (an-tye-HIST-a-meens) are used to relieve or prevent the symptoms of hay fever and other types of allergy. Some of the antihistamines are also used to prevent motion sickness, nausea, vomiting, and dizziness. In patients with Parkinson's disease, diphenhydramine may be used to decrease stiffness and tremors. In addition, since antihistamines may cause drowsiness as a side effect, some of them may be used to help people go to sleep. Hydroxyzine is used in the treatment of nervous and emotional conditions to help control anxiety. It can also be used to help control anxiety and produce sleep before surgery. Antihistamines may also be used for other conditions as determined by your doctor.

If this medicine was prescribed for you and any of the information in this leaflet causes you special concern or if you want additional information about your medicine and its use, check with your doctor, nurse, or pharmacist. **Remember, keep this and all other medicines out of the reach of children and never share your medicines with others.**

BEFORE USING THIS MEDICINE

If you are taking this medicine without a prescription, carefully read and follow any precautions on the label. You should be especially careful if you . . .

- are allergic to any medicine, either prescription or nonprescription (OTC);
- are pregnant, intend to become pregnant, or are breast-feeding;
- are taking any other prescription or nonprescription (OTC) medicine, especially CNS depressants, MAO inhibitors, or anticholinergics (medicine for abdominal or stomach spasms or cramps);
- are taking erythromycin or ketoconazole and are also taking astemizole or terfenadine;
- have any other medical problems, especially difficult urination, enlarged prostate, glaucoma, liver disease (for astemizole and terfenadine only), or urinary tract blockage.

If you have any questions, check with your doctor, nurse, or pharmacist.

PROPER USE OF THIS MEDICINE

Antihistamines are used to relieve or prevent the symptoms of your medical problem. Take them only as directed. Do not take more of them and do not take them more often than your doctor ordered. To do so may increase the chance of side effects.

Antihistamines can be taken with food or a glass of water or milk to lessen stomach irritation if necessary.

If you are taking the extended-release tablet form of this medicine, swallow the tablets whole. Do not break, crush, or chew before swallowing.

If you must take this medicine regularly and you miss a dose, take it as soon as possible. However, if it is almost time for your next dose, skip the missed dose and go back to your regular dosing schedule. Do not double doses.

PRECAUTIONS WHILE USING THIS MEDICINE

Antihistamines will add to the effects of alcohol and other CNS depressants (medicines that slow down the nervous system). **Check with your doctor before taking any such depressants while you are using this medicine.**

This medicine may cause some people to become drowsy or less alert than they are normally. Even if taken at bedtime, it may cause some people to feel drowsy or less alert on arising. This side effect is less likely to occur with astemizole, loratadine, and terfenadine; however, **make sure you know how you react to any antihistamine before you drive, use machines, or do other jobs that require you to be alert.**

POSSIBLE SIDE EFFECTS OF THIS MEDICINE

Side Effects That Should Be Reported To Your Doctor Immediately

 Less common or rare (with high doses of astemizole and terfenadine only)—Fast or irregular heartbeat

Other Side Effects That Should Be Reported To Your Doctor

 Less common or rare—Sore throat and fever; unusual bleeding or bruising; unusual tiredness or weakness

Side Effects That Usually Do Not Require Medical Attention

These possible side effects may go away during treatment; however, if they continue or are bothersome, check with your doctor, nurse, or pharmacist.

 More common (rare with astemizole, loratadine, and terfenadine)—Drowsiness; thickening of mucus

Other side effects not listed above may also occur in some patients. If you notice any other effects, check with your doctor, nurse, or pharmacist.

ANTIHISTAMINES AND DECONGESTANTS Systemic

■For the Pharmacist■

In providing consultation, consider emphasizing the following selected information (» = major clinical significance):

Before using this medication

» Conditions affecting use, especially:

Sensitivity to any of the antihistamines or sympathomimetic amines

Pregnancy—Concern for the fetus and/or newborn infant only with high doses and long-term therapy; psychiatric disorders more likely with use of phenylpropanolamine in postpartum women

Breast-feeding—Antihistamines may cause excitement or irritability in nursing infants; high risk for infants from sympathomimetic amines

Use in children—Increased susceptibility to anticholinergic effects of antihistamines and to vasopressor effects of sympathomimetic amines; psychiatric disorders more likely with use of phenylpropanolamine in children under 6 years of age; hyperexcitability (paradoxical reaction) may occur

Use in the elderly—Anticholinergic and CNS stimulant effects more likely to occur

Other medications, especially anticholinergics; CNS depressants or stimulants; erythromycin and other macrolide antibiotics (with terfenadine-containing combination only); itraconazole and ketoconazole (with terfenadine-containing combination only); or medicine for high blood pressure or depression

Other medical problems, especially cardiovascular disease, diabetes, hepatic function impairment (with terfenadine-containing combination only), hypertension, hyperthyroidism, or prostatic hypertrophy

Proper use of this medication

» Importance of not taking more medication than the amount recommended

Taking with food, water, or milk to minimize gastric irritation

Swallowing extended-release dosage form whole

» Proper dosing

Missed dose: If on scheduled dosing regimen—Taking as soon as possible; not taking if almost time for next dose; not doubling doses

» Proper storage

Precautions while using this medication

Caution if skin tests using allergens required; possible interference with test results

May mask ototoxic effects of large doses of salicylates

» Avoiding use of alcohol or other CNS depressants

» Caution if drowsiness or dizziness occurs

» Caution if taking phenylpropanolamine-containing appetite suppressants

» Possible insomnia; taking the medication a few hours before bedtime

Possible dryness of mouth; using sugarless gum or candy, ice, or saliva substitute for relief; checking with dentist if dry mouth continues for more than 2 weeks.

For promethazine
  Possible interference with diagnosis of intestinal obstruction, brain
    tumor, or overdosage of toxic drugs; need to inform physician
    of use

Side/adverse effects
  Signs of potential side effects, especially blood dyscrasias, cardiac
    arrhythmias, psychotic episodes, and tightness in chest

▲ For the Patient ▲

912077

ABOUT YOUR MEDICINE

Antihistamine (an-tye-HIST-a-meen) and **decongestant** (dee-
kon-JES-tant) combinations are used to treat the nasal
congestion (stuffy nose), sneezing, and runny nose caused
by colds and hay fever.

If this medicine was prescribed for you and any of the information in this leaflet causes you special concern or if you
want additional information about your medicine and its use,
check with your doctor, nurse, or pharmacist. **Remember,
keep this and all other medicines out of the reach of children
and never share your medicines with others.**

BEFORE USING THIS MEDICINE

If you are taking this medicine without a prescription, carefully read and follow any precautions on the label. You should
be especially careful if you . . .
  • are allergic to any medicine, either prescription or non-
    prescription (OTC);
  • are pregnant, intend to become pregnant, or are breast-
    feeding;
  • compete in athletics;
  • are taking any other prescription or nonprescription
    (OTC) medicine, especially beta-blockers, CNS de-
    pressants and stimulants, MAO inhibitors, medicine for
    abdominal or stomach spasms or cramps, phenothia-
    zines, rauwolfia alkaloids, or tricyclic antidepressants
    (medicine for depression);
  • are taking erythromycin or ketoconazole and are also
    taking the combination that contains terfenadine;
  • have any other medical problems, especially high blood
    pressure, liver disease (for terfenadine-containing com-
    bination only), or urinary tract blockage.

If you have any questions, check with your doctor, nurse,
or pharmacist.

PROPER USE OF THIS MEDICINE

**Take this medicine only as directed. Do not take more of it
and do not take it more often than recommended on the label,
unless otherwise directed by your doctor. To do so may increase the chance of side effects.**

Antihistamine and decongestant combinations may be taken with food or a glass of water or milk to lessen stomach irritation, if necessary.

For patients taking the extended-release capsule or tablet form of this medicine:
- Swallow it whole.
- Do not crush, break, or chew before swallowing.
- If the capsule is too large to swallow, you may mix the contents of the capsule with applesauce, jelly, honey, or syrup and swallow without chewing.

If you must take this medicine regularly and you miss a dose, take it as soon as possible. However, if it is almost time for your next dose, skip the missed dose and go back to your regular dosing schedule. Do not double doses.

PRECAUTIONS WHILE USING THIS MEDICINE

The antihistamine in this medicine will add to the effects of alcohol and other CNS depressants (medicines that slow down the nervous system). **Check with your doctor before taking any such depressants while you are taking this medicine.**

The antihistamine may also cause some people to become drowsy, dizzy, or less alert than they are normally. This side effect is less likely to occur with the terfenadine-containing combination; however, **make sure you know how you react to this medicine before you drive, use machines, or do other jobs that require you to be alert.**

The decongestant in this medicine may add to the effects of phenylpropanolamine-containing diet aids. **Do not use medicines for diet or appetite control while taking this medicine unless you have first checked with your doctor.**

The decongestant may also cause some people to be nervous or restless or to have trouble in sleeping. If you have trouble in sleeping, **take the last dose of this medicine for each day a few hours before bedtime.**

POSSIBLE SIDE EFFECTS OF THIS MEDICINE

Although serious side effects occur rarely when this medicine is taken as recommended, they may be more likely to occur if too much medicine is taken or if it is taken in large doses, or for a long period of time.

Side Effects That Should Be Reported To Your Doctor Immediately

    Rare—Fast or irregular heartbeat

Other Side Effects That Should Be Reported To Your Doctor

    Rare—Mood or mental changes; sore throat and fever; tightness in chest; unusual bleeding or bruising; unusual tiredness or weakness

Side Effects That Usually Do Not Require Medical Attention

These possible side effects may go away during treatment; however, if they continue or are bothersome, check with your doctor, nurse, or pharmacist.

> *More common (rare with terfenadine-containing combination)*—Drowsiness; thickening of the bronchial secretions

Other side effects not listed above may also occur in some patients. If you notice any other effects, check with your doctor, nurse, or pharmacist.

ANTIHISTAMINES, DECONGESTANTS, AND ANALGESICS Systemic

■ For the Pharmacist ■

In providing consultation, consider emphasizing the following selected information (» = major clinical significance):

Before using this medication
» Conditions affecting use, especially:

Sensitivity to any of the medications in the combination being taken

Pregnancy—Concern for the fetus and/or newborn infant only with high doses and long-term therapy; psychiatric disorders more likely with use of phenylpropanolamine in postpartum women; use of aspirin-containing combinations not recommended during third trimester

Breast-feeding—Antihistamines may cause excitement or irritability in nursing infant; high risk for infants from sympathomimetic amines; also, concern with high doses and chronic use because of high salicylate intake by infant

Use in children—Increased susceptibility to anticholinergic effects of antihistamines and to vasopressor effects of sympathomimetic amines; psychiatric disorders more likely with use of phenylpropanolamine in children under 6 years of age; hyperexcitability (paradoxical reaction) may occur; also, increased susceptibility to toxic effects of salicylates, especially if fever and dehydration present; possible association between aspirin usage and Reye's syndrome

Use in adolescents—Possible association between aspirin usage and Reye's syndrome

Use in the elderly—Anticholinergic and CNS stimulant effects more likely to occur; increased susceptibility to toxic effects of salicylates

Other medications, especially anticholinergics, medicine for high blood pressure or depression, or CNS depressants or stimulants

Other medical problems, especially alcoholism, cardiovascular disease, diabetes, gastritis or peptic ulcer (with salicylate-containing), hypertension, hyperthyroidism, or prostatic hypertrophy

Proper use of this medication
» Importance of not taking more medication than the amount recommended

Taking with food, water, or milk to minimize gastric irritation

Swallowing extended-release dosage form whole
» Not taking combinations containing aspirin if a strong vinegar-like odor is present
» Proper dosing

Missed dose: If on scheduled dosing regimen—Taking as soon as possible; not taking if almost time for next dose; not doubling doses
» Proper storage

Precautions while using this medication

Caution if skin tests using allergens required; possible interference with test results

Checking with physician if symptoms persist or become worse, or if high fever is present

» Avoiding alcoholic beverages or other CNS depressants while taking these medications; also, alcohol consumption may increase risk of salicylate-induced gastrointestinal toxicity and acetaminophen-induced liver toxicity

» Caution if drowsiness or dizziness occurs

» Possible insomnia; taking the medication a few hours before bedtime

» Caution if taking phenylpropanolamine-containing appetite suppressants

Need to inform physician or dentist of use of medication if any kind of surgery (including dental surgery) or emergency treatment is required

Possible dryness of mouth; using sugarless gum or candy, ice, or saliva substitute for relief; checking with dentist if dry mouth continues for more than 2 weeks

» Caution if other medications containing acetaminophen, aspirin, or other salicylates (including diflunisal) are used

» Suspected overdose: Getting emergency help at once

Not taking products containing aspirin for 5 days prior to any kind of surgery, unless otherwise directed by physician

Diabetics: Aspirin present in some combination formulations may cause false urine sugar test results with prolonged use of 8 or more 325-mg (5-grain) doses per day

Side/adverse effects

Signs of potential side effects, especially allergic reactions, anticholinergic effects, blood dyscrasias, jaundice (with acetaminophen-containing), and signs of gastrointestinal irritation or bleeding (with salicylate-containing)

▲ For the Patient ▲

916704

ABOUT YOUR MEDICINE

Antihistamine, decongestant, and **analgesic** combinations are taken by mouth to relieve the sneezing, runny nose, sinus and nasal congestion (stuffy nose), fever, headache, and aches and pain, of colds, influenza, and hay fever. These combinations do not contain any ingredient to relieve coughs.

Some of these medicines are available without a prescription. However, your doctor may have special instructions for your medical condition.

If any of the information in this leaflet causes you special concern or if you want additional information about your medicine and its use, check with your doctor, nurse, or pharmacist. **Remember, keep this and all other medicines out of the reach of children and never share your medicines with others.**

BEFORE USING THIS MEDICINE

Do not give a medicine containing aspirin or other salicylates to a child or a teenager with a fever or other symptoms of a virus infection, especially flu or chickenpox, without first discussing this with your child's doctor.

If you are taking this medicine without a prescription, carefully read and follow any precautions on the label. You should be especially careful if you. . .
- are allergic to any medicine, either prescription or non-prescription (OTC);
- are pregnant, intend to become pregnant, or are breast-feeding;
- are taking **any** other prescription or nonprescription (OTC) medicine;
- have **any** other medical problems.

If you have any questions, check with your doctor, nurse, or pharmacist.

PROPER USE OF THIS MEDICINE

Take this medicine only as directed. Do not take more of it and do not take it more often than recommended on the label, unless otherwise directed by your doctor. To do so may increase the chance of side effects.

If this medicine irritates your stomach, you may take it with food or a glass of water or milk to lessen the irritation.

If you must take this medicine regularly and you miss a dose, take it as soon as possible. However, if it is almost time for your next dose, skip the missed dose and go back to your regular dosing schedule. Do not double doses.

PRECAUTIONS WHILE USING THIS MEDICINE

Check with your doctor if your symptoms do not improve or become worse, or if you have a high fever.

This medicine will add to the effects of alcohol and other CNS depressants (medicines that slow down the nervous system). **Check with your doctor before taking any such depressants while you are taking this medicine.**

Do not drink alcoholic beverages while taking this medicine. To do so may increase the chance of serious side effects.

The antihistamine in this medicine may cause some people to become drowsy, dizzy, or less alert than they are normally. **Make sure you know how you react before you drive, use machines, or do other jobs that require you to be alert.**

The decongestant in this medicine may cause some people to become nervous or restless or to have trouble in sleeping. If you have trouble in sleeping, **take the last dose of this medicine for each day a few hours before bedtime.** If you have any questions about this, check with your doctor.

POSSIBLE SIDE EFFECTS OF THIS MEDICINE
Side Effects That Should Be Reported To Your Doctor

More common—Nausea or vomiting; stomach pain (mild)

Less common or rare—Bloody or black tarry stools; changes in urine or problems with urination; skin rash, hives, or itching; sore throat and fever; swelling of face, feet, or lower legs; tightness in chest; unusual bleeding or bruising; unusual tiredness or weakness; vomiting of blood or material that looks like coffee grounds; weight gain (unusual); yellow eyes or skin

Side Effects That Usually Do Not Require Medical Attention

These possible side effects may go away during treatment; however, if they continue or are bothersome, check with your doctor, nurse, or pharmacist.

More common—Drowsiness; heartburn or indigestion (for salicylate-containing medicines); thickening of mucus

Other side effects not listed above may also occur in some patients. If you notice any other effects, check with your doctor, nurse, or pharmacist.

ANTIHISTAMINES, DECONGESTANTS, AND ANTICHOLINERGICS Systemic

■ For the Pharmacist ■

In providing consultation, consider emphasizing the following selected information (» = major clinical significance):

Before using this medication
» Conditions affecting use, especially:
    Sensitivity to any of the medications in the combination being taken
    Pregnancy—Postpartum women are particularly susceptible to psychiatric disorders that may be caused by phenylpropanolamine
    Breast-feeding—Antihistamines may cause excitement or irritability in nursing infant; high risk to infants from sympathomimetic amines; possible inhibition of lactation
    Use in children—Increased susceptibility to anticholinergic effects and to vasopressor effects; children under 6 years of age may be particularly susceptible to psychiatric disorders that may be caused by phenylpropanolamine; hyperexcitability (paradoxical reaction) may occur; increased response to anticholinergics in infants and children with spastic paralysis or brain damage
    Use in the elderly—Anticholinergic and CNS stimulant effects more likely to occur in older patients; danger of precipitating undiagnosed glaucoma; possible impairment of memory
    Dental—Possible development of dental problems because of decreased salivary flow
    Other medications, especially alcohol, other anticholinergics, beta-adrenergic blocking agents, medicine for high blood pressure or depression, CNS depressants or stimulants, digitalis glycosides, and potassium chloride
    Other medical problems, especially cardiovascular disease, diabetes mellitus, hemorrhage, severe hypertension, hyperthyroidism, memyasthenia gravis, obstruction in gastrointestinal or urinary tract, prostatic hypertrophy, tachycardia, urinary retention, and xerostomia

Proper use of this medication
» Importance of not taking more medication than the amount recommended
    Taking with food, water, or milk to minimize gastric irritation
    Swallowing extended-release dosage form whole
» Proper dosing
    Missed dose: Taking as soon as possible; not taking if almost time for next dose; not doubling doses
» Proper storage

Precautions while using this medication
    Checking with physician if symptoms persist or become worse, or if high fever is present
    Caution if skin tests using allergens required; possible interference with test results
» Caution during exercise or hot weather; overheating may result in heat stroke
» Possible increased sensitivity of eyes to light
» Caution if blurred vision occurs

» Caution if drowsiness or dizziness occurs
» Possible insomnia; taking the medication a few hours before bedtime
» Caution if taking phenylpropanolamine-containing appetite suppressants
  Need to inform physician or dentist of use of medication if any kind of surgery (including dental surgery or emergency treatment) is required
  Possible dryness of mouth; using sugarless gum or candy, ice, or saliva substitute for relief; checking with dentist if dry mouth continues for more than 2 weeks
» Suspected overdose: Getting emergency help at once

Side/adverse effects
  Signs of potential side effects, especially allergic reactions, severe anticholinergic effects, blood dyscrasias, CNS stimulation, severe drowsiness, hypertension, psychotic episodes, and tightness in chest

---

▲ For the Patient ▲

919214

ABOUT YOUR MEDICINE

Antihistamine (an-tye-HIST-a-meen), **decongestant** (dee-kon-JES-tant), and **anticholinergic** (an-tye-koh-li-NER-jik) combinations are used to treat the nasal congestion (stuffy nose), and runny nose caused by allergies.

If any of the information in this leaflet causes you special concern or if you want additional information about your medicine and its use, check with your doctor, nurse, or pharmacist. **Remember, keep this and all other medicines out of the reach of children and never share your medicines with others.**

BEFORE USING THIS MEDICINE

Tell your doctor, nurse, and pharmacist if you . . .
  • are allergic to any medicine, either prescription or non-prescription (OTC);
  • are pregnant or intend to become pregnant while using this medicine;
  • are breast-feeding;
  • are taking any other prescription or nonprescription (OTC) medicine, especially other anticholinergics, beta-blockers, CNS depressants and stimulants, digitalis glycosides (heart medicine), MAO inhibitors, potassium chloride, rauwolfia alkaloids, or tricyclic antidepressants (medicine for depression);
  • have any other medical problems, especially diabetes mellitus, dryness of mouth (severe and continuing), enlarged prostate, heart or blood vessel disease, high blood pressure, intestinal blockage or other intestinal problems, myasthenia gravis, overactive thyroid, or urinary tract blockage.

PROPER USE OF THIS MEDICINE

Use this medicine only as directed by your doctor. Do not use more of it, do not use it more often, and do not use it for a longer time than your doctor ordered. To do so may increase the chance of side effects.

If this medicine irritates your stomach, you may take it with food or a glass of water or milk to lessen the irritation.

For patients taking the extended-release capsule or tablet form of this medicine:
- Swallow it whole.
- Do not crush, break, or chew before swallowing.
- If the capsule is too large to swallow, you may mix the contents of the capsule with applesauce, jelly, honey, or syrup and swallow without chewing.

If you miss a dose of this medicine, take it as soon as possible. However, if it is almost time for your next dose, skip the missed dose and go back to your regular dosing schedule. Do not double doses.

PRECAUTIONS WHILE USING THIS MEDICINE

This medicine may make you sweat less, causing your body temperature to increase. **Use extra care not to become overheated during exercise or hot weather while you are taking this medicine,** since overheating may result in heat stroke. Also, hot baths or saunas may make you dizzy or faint while you are taking this medicine.

This medicine may cause some people to become dizzy, drowsy, or less alert than they are normally, or to have blurred vision. **Make sure you know how you react to this medicine before you drive, use machines, or do other jobs that require you to be alert and able to see well.**

The decongestant in this medicine may add to the effects of phenylpropanolamine-containing diet aids. **Do not use medicines for diet or appetite control while taking this medicine unless you have first checked with your doctor.**

The decongestant may also cause some people to be nervous or restless or to have trouble in sleeping. If you have trouble in sleeping, **take the last dose of this medicine for each day a few hours before bedtime.**

If you think you or someone else may have taken an overdose, get emergency help at once. Taking an overdose of this medicine or taking this medicine with alcohol or CNS depressants may lead to unconsciousness and possibly death.

POSSIBLE SIDE EFFECTS OF THIS MEDICINE
Side Effects That Should Be Reported To Your Doctor

Rare—Mood or mental changes; skin rash, hives, or itching; sore throat and fever; tightness in chest; unusual bleeding or bruising; unusual tiredness or weakness

Side Effects That Usually Do Not Require Medical Attention

These possible side effects may go away during treatment; however, if they continue or are bothersome, check with your doctor, nurse, or pharmacist.

More common—Drowsiness; thickening of the bronchial
   secretions

Other side effects not listed above may also occur in some
patients. If you notice any other effects, check with your
doctor, nurse, or pharmacist.

ANTIHISTAMINES, PHENOTHIAZINE-DERIVATIVE   Systemic

Including Methdilazine; Promethazine; Trimeprazine.

■For the Pharmacist■

In providing consultation, consider emphasizing the following selected information (**》** = major clinical significance):

Before using this medication

》 Conditions affecting use of most antihistamines, especially:

Sensitivity to the antihistamine used or to phenothiazine medications

Pregnancy—Not taking during the 2 weeks before delivery, to avoid possible inhibition of platelet aggregation in newborn; also, jaundice and extrapyramidal effects may occur in infant

Breast-feeding—Use not recommended; may cause unusual excitement or irritability in nursing infant; possible association with sudden infant death syndrome (SIDS) and sleep apnea

Use in children—Increased susceptibility to anticholinergic side effects in newborn or premature infants; hyperexcitability (paradoxical reaction) may occur in children; possible association with sudden infant death syndrome (SIDS) and sleep apnea; diagnosis of Reye's syndrome may be obscured if extrapyramidal effects occur

Use in adolescents—Diagnosis of Reye's syndrome may be obscured if extrapyramidal effects occur

Use in the elderly—Increased susceptibility to CNS and anticholinergic side effects; hyperexcitability (paradoxical reaction) may occur; extrapyramidal symptoms more likely to occur

Dental—Increased risk of dental problems with prolonged use because of decrease or inhibition of salivary flow; involuntary orofacial muscle movements may result from extrapyramidal effects

Other medications, especially alcohol or other CNS depressants, anticholinergics, epinephrine, extrapyramidal reaction–causing medications, levodopa, MAO inhibitors, or metrizamide (intrathecal)

Other medical problems, especially angle-closure glaucoma (or predisposition to), bladder neck obstruction, prostatic hypertrophy, or urinary retention; jaundice (for parenteral promethazine)

Proper use of this medication

》 Importance of not taking more medication than the amount recommended

》 Proper dosing

Missed dose: If on scheduled dosing regimen—Using as soon as possible; not using if almost time for next dose; not doubling doses

》 Proper storage

For oral dosage forms

Taking with food, water, or milk to minimize gastric irritation

Swallowing extended-release dosage forms whole

For injection dosage forms

Knowing correct administration technique for self-administration; checking with physician if necessary

For rectal dosage forms
Proper administration technique
For promethazine when used to prevent motion sickness
Taking 30 minutes to 1 hour before traveling

Precautions while using this medication
Possible interference with skin tests using allergens; need to inform physician of using medication
May mask ototoxic effects of large doses of salicylates
» Avoiding use of alcohol or other CNS depressants
» Caution if drowsiness occurs
Possible dryness of mouth; using sugarless gum or candy, ice, or saliva substitute for relief; checking with physician or dentist if dry mouth continues for more than 2 weeks
Need to inform physician of use: Possible interference with diagnosis of appendicitis; may mask signs of toxicity from overdosage of other drugs

Side/adverse effects
Signs of potential side effects, especially blood dyscrasias

▲ For the Patient ▲

914797

ABOUT YOUR MEDICINE

Phenothiazine (FEE-noe-THYE-a-zeen) antihistamines are used to relieve or prevent the symptoms of hay fever and other types of allergy. Some are also used to prevent motion sickness, nausea, vomiting, and dizziness. In addition, some of them may be used to help people go to sleep and control their anxiety before or after surgery. Phenothiazine antihistamines may also be used for other conditions as determined by your doctor.

If any of the information in this leaflet causes you special concern or if you want additional information about your medicine and its use, check with your doctor, nurse, or pharmacist. **Remember, keep this and all other medicines out of the reach of children and never share your medicines with others.**

BEFORE USING THIS MEDICINE

Tell your doctor, nurse, and pharmacist if you . . .
- are allergic to any medicine, either prescription or nonprescription (OTC);
- are pregnant or intend to become pregnant while using this medicine;
- are breast-feeding;
- are taking **any** other prescription or nonprescription (OTC) medicine;
- have any other medical problems, especially asthma, difficult urination, enlarged prostate, glaucoma, or jaundice.

PROPER USE OF THIS MEDICINE

Antihistamines are used to relieve or prevent the symptoms of your medical problem. Take them only as directed. Do not take more of them and do not take them more often than directed by your doctor. To do so may increase the chance of side effects.

This medicine may be taken with food or a full glass (8 ounces) of water or milk to reduce stomach irritation.

If you are taking the **extended-release capsule** form of this medicine, swallow it whole. Do not break, crush, or chew before swallowing.

If you are taking promethazine for motion sickness, take it 30 minutes to 1 hour before you begin to travel.

If you are taking this medicine regularly and you miss a dose, take it as soon as possible. However, if it is almost time for your next dose, skip the missed dose and go back to your regular dosing schedule. Do not double doses.

PRECAUTIONS WHILE USING THIS MEDICINE

Tell the doctor in charge that you are taking this medicine before you have any skin tests for allergies. The results of the test may be affected by this medicine.

When taking phenothiazine antihistamines on a regular basis, make sure your doctor knows if you are taking large amounts of aspirin at the same time (as in arthritis or rheumatism). Effects of too much aspirin, such as ringing in the ears, may be covered up by the antihistamines.

This medicine will add to the effects of alcohol and other CNS depressants (medicines that slow down the nervous system). **Check with your doctor before taking any such depressants while you are using this medicine.**

This medicine may cause some people to become drowsy or less alert than they are normally. Even if taken at bedtime, it may cause some people to feel drowsy or less alert on arising. **Make sure you know how you react before you drive, use machines, or do other jobs that require you to be alert.**

Phenothiazine antihistamines may cause dryness of the mouth, nose, and throat. For temporary relief of mouth dryness, use sugarless candy or gum, melt bits of ice in your mouth, or use a saliva substitute. However, if your mouth continues to feel dry for more than 2 weeks, check with your medical doctor or dentist. Continuing dryness of the mouth may increase the chance of dental disease, including tooth decay, gum disease, and fungus infections.

This medicine controls nausea and vomiting. For this reason, it may cover up the signs of overdose caused by other medicines or the symptoms of appendicitis. This will make it difficult for your doctor to diagnose these conditions. Make sure your doctor knows that you are taking this medicine if you have other symptoms of appendicitis such as stomach or lower abdominal pain, cramping, or soreness. Also, if you think you may have taken an overdose of any medicine, tell your doctor that you are taking this medicine.

POSSIBLE SIDE EFFECTS OF THIS MEDICINE
Side Effects That Should Be Reported To Your Doctor

Less common or rare—Sore throat and fever; unusual bleeding or bruising; unusual tiredness or weakness

Side Effects That Usually Do Not Require Medical Attention

These possible side effects may go away during treatment; however, if they continue or are bothersome, check with your doctor, nurse, or pharmacist.

More common—Drowsiness (less common with methdilazine); thickening of mucus

Other side effects not listed above may also occur in some patients. If you notice any other effects, check with your doctor, nurse, or pharmacist.

ANTIMYASTHENICS Systemic
Including Ambenonium; Neostigmine; Pyridostigmine.

■For the Pharmacist■

In providing consultation, consider emphasizing the following selected
  information (» = major clinical significance):

Before using this medication
» Conditions affecting use, especially:
      Sensitivity to antimyasthenics or to bromides
      Pregnancy—Possible transient muscle weakness in newborns
        whose mothers received antimyasthenics during pregnancy
      Geriatrics—In one study in a limited number of patients, du-
        ration of antagonism of neuromuscular blockade by neostig-
        mine and pyridostigmine was prolonged
      Other medications, especially other cholinesterase inhibitors,
        guanadrel, guanethidine, mecamylamine, procainamide, or
        trimethaphan
      Other medical problems, especially intestinal or urinary tract
        blockage or urinary tract infection

Proper use of this medication
      Taking with food or milk to decrease possibility of side effects
» Importance of not taking more medication than the amount pre-
        scribed
      For use in myasthenia gravis: Keeping daily record of dosing and
        effects on condition during initial therapy
      Missed dose: Taking as soon as possible; not taking if almost time
        for next dose; not doubling doses
» Proper dosing
» Proper storage

Side/adverse effects
      Signs of potential side effects, especially thrombophlebitis at injec-
        tion site (for pyridostigmine only), and sensitivity

▲ For the Patient ▲

913284

ABOUT YOUR MEDICINE
Antimyasthenics are given by mouth to treat myasthenia
gravis.

If any of the information in this leaflet causes you special
concern or if you want additional information about your
medicine and its use, check with your doctor, nurse, or pharmacist. **Remember, keep this and all other medicines out of
the reach of children and never share your medicines with
others.**

BEFORE USING THIS MEDICINE
Tell your doctor, nurse, and pharmacist if you . . .
  • are allergic to any medicine, either prescription or non-
    prescription (OTC);
  • are pregnant or intend to become pregnant while using
    this medicine;

- are breast-feeding;
- are using any other prescription or nonprescription (OTC) medicine, especially demecarium, echothiophate, guanadrel, guanethidine, isoflurophate, malathion, mecamylamine, procainamide, or trimethaphan;
- have any other medical problems, especially intestinal blockage, urinary tract blockage, or urinary tract infection.

PROPER USE OF THIS MEDICINE

Your doctor may want you to take this medicine with food or milk to help lessen the chance of side effects. If you have any questions about how you should be taking this medicine, check with your doctor.

Take this medicine only as directed. Do not take more of it, do not take it more often, and do not take it for a longer period of time than your doctor ordered. To do so may increase the chance of side effects.

When you first begin taking this medicine, your doctor may want you to keep a daily record of:
  —the time you take each dose.
  —how long you feel better after taking each dose.
  —how long you feel worse.
  —any side effects that occur.
This is to help your doctor decide whether the dose of this medicine should be increased or decreased and how often the medicine should be taken, in order for it to be most effective in your condition.

If you miss a dose of this medicine, take it as soon as possible. However, if it is almost time for your next dose, skip the missed dose and go back to your regular dosing schedule. Do not double doses.

POSSIBLE SIDE EFFECTS OF THIS MEDICINE

Side Effects That Should Be Reported To Your Doctor

   Rare—Skin rash

Side Effects That Usually Do Not Require Medical Attention

These possible side effects may go away during treatment; however, if they continue or are bothersome, check with your doctor, nurse, or pharmacist.

   More common—Diarrhea; increased sweating; increased watering of mouth; nausea or vomiting; stomach cramps or pain

Other side effects not listed above may also occur in some patients. If you notice any other effects, check with your doctor, nurse, or pharmacist.

ANTITHYROID AGENTS   Systemic

Including Methimazole; Propylthiouracil.

■ For the Pharmacist ■

In providing consultation, consider emphasizing the following selected information (» = major clinical significance):

Before using this medication
» Conditions affecting use, especially:
  Allergies to any thioamide
  Pregnancy—May be used but careful monitoring is necessary
  Breast-feeding—Distributed into breast milk, although propylthiouracil is distributed in much lesser amounts; may continue breast-feeding with low doses and monitoring of infant
  Other medications, especially iodides, coumarin- or indandione-derivative anticoagulants, amiodarone, digitalis glycosides, or radioiodide
  Other medical problems, especially hepatic function impairment

Proper use of this medication
» Importance of not taking more or less medication than the amount prescribed
» Importance of not missing doses and, if taking more than one dose per day, of taking at evenly spaced intervals
  Taking methimazole at same time in relation to meals every day
» Proper dosing
  Missed dose: Taking as soon as possible; taking both doses together if almost time for next dose; checking with physician if more than one dose is missed
» Proper storage

Precautions while using this medication
» Importance of close monitoring by the physician
» Checking with physician before discontinuing medication
» Caution if any kind of surgery (including dental surgery) or emergency treatment is required, because of the risk of thyroid storm
» Checking with physician immediately if injury, infection, or other illness occurs, because of the risk of thyroid storm
  Caution if any laboratory tests required; possible interference with test results

Side/adverse effects
  Signs of potential side effects, especially fever, skin rash or itching, bone marrow depression, hepatic dysfunction, lupus-like syndrome, arthralgias, arthritis, nephritis (for methimazole), vasculitis, pneumonitis, lymphadenopathy, sialadenopathy, hypoprothrombinemia (for propylthiouracil), or peripheral neuropathy

▲ For the Patient ▲

913309

ABOUT YOUR MEDICINE

Methimazole (meth-IM-a-zole) and **propylthiouracil** (proe-pill-thye-oh-YOOR-a-sill) are used to treat conditions in which the thyroid gland produces too much thyroid hormone.

If any of the information in this leaflet causes you special concern or if you want additional information about your medicine and its use, check with your doctor, nurse, or pharmacist. **Remember, keep this and all other medicines out of the reach of children and never share your medicines with others.**

BEFORE USING THIS MEDICINE

Tell your doctor, nurse, and pharmacist if you . . .

- are allergic to any medicine, either prescription or non-prescription (OTC);
- are pregnant or intend to become pregnant while using this medicine;
- are breast-feeding;
- are taking any other prescription or nonprescription (OTC) medicine, especially amiodarone, anticoagulants (blood thinners), digitalis medicines, iodinated glycerol, or potassium iodide;
- have any other medical problems, especially liver disease.

PROPER USE OF THIS MEDICINE

Use this medicine only as directed by your doctor. Do not use more or less of it and do not use it more often or for a longer time than your doctor ordered.

In order for it to work properly, **this medicine must be taken every day in regularly spaced doses, as ordered by your doctor.**

Food in your stomach may change the amount of methimazole that is able to enter the bloodstream. To make sure that you always get the same effects, try to take methimazole at the same time in relation to meals every day. That is, always take it with meals or always take it on an empty stomach.

If you miss a dose of this medicine, take it as soon as possible. If it is almost time for your next dose, take both doses together. Then go back to your regular dosing schedule. If you miss more than one dose or if you have any questions about this, check with your doctor.

PRECAUTIONS WHILE USING THIS MEDICINE

It is very important that your doctor check your progress at regular intervals in order to make sure that this medicine is working properly and to check for unwanted effects.

It may take several days or weeks for this medicine to work. However, **do not stop taking this medicine without first checking with your doctor.** Some medical problems may require several years of continuous treatment.

Before having any kind of surgery or dental or emergency treatment, **tell the physician or dentist in charge that you are taking this medicine.**

Check with your doctor right away if you get an injury, infection, or illness of any kind. Your doctor may want you to stop taking this medicine or change the amount you are taking.

POSSIBLE SIDE EFFECTS OF THIS MEDICINE
Side Effects That Should Be Reported To Your Doctor Immediately

Less common—Cough; fever or chills (continuing or severe); general feeling of discomfort, illness, or weakness; hoarseness; mouth sores; pain, swelling, or redness in joints; throat infection

Rare—Yellow eyes or skin

Other Side Effects That Should Be Reported To Your Doctor

More common—Fever (mild and temporary); skin rash or itching

Rare—Backache; black, tarry stools; blood in urine or stools; changes in menstrual periods; coldness; constipation; diarrhea; dry, puffy skin; fast or irregular heartbeat; headache; increase in bleeding or bruising; increase or decrease in urination; listlessness or sleepiness; muscle aches; numbness or tingling of fingers, toes, or face; pinpoint red spots on skin; shortness of breath; swelling of feet or lower legs; swollen lymph nodes; swollen salivary glands; unusual tiredness or weakness; weight gain (unusual)

Side Effects That Usually Do Not Require Medical Attention

These possible side effects may go away during treatment; however, if they continue or are bothersome, check with your doctor, nurse, or pharmacist.

Less common—Dizziness; loss of taste (for methimazole); nausea; stomach pain; vomiting

Other side effects not listed above may also occur in some patients. If you notice any other effects, check with your doctor, nurse, or pharmacist.

APPETITE SUPPRESSANTS   Systemic
Including Benzphetamine; Diethylpropion; Fenfluramine;
Mazindol; Phendimetrazine; Phentermine.

■ For the Pharmacist ■

In providing consultation, consider emphasizing the following selected
information (» = major clinical significance):

Before using this medication
» Conditions affecting use, especially:
  Sensitivity to appetite suppressants or other sympathomimetics
  Pregnancy—Benzphetamine is contraindicated in human preg-
    nancy (FDA Category X); in animal studies, fenfluramine
    was shown to be embryotoxic and to reduce rate of concep-
    tion; mazindol was shown to increase the incidence of neo-
    natal mortality and possibly to increase the incidence of rib
    anomalies when given in relatively high doses
  Breast-feeding—Benzphetamine and diethylpropion are distrib-
    uted into breast milk
  Use in children—Not recommended for appetite suppression in
    children up to 12 years of age
  Other medications, especially alcohol, MAO inhibitors, other
    CNS stimulants (with all appetite suppressants except fen-
    fluramine), or CNS depressants (with fenfluramine)
  Other medical problems, especially agitated states, alcoholism,
    advanced arteriosclerosis, symptomatic cardiovascular dis-
    ease including arrhythmias, cerebral ischemia, history of drug
    abuse or dependence, glaucoma, hypertension, hyperthyroid-
    ism, psychosis, or uremia

Proper use of this medication
  Taking the last dose of the regular dosage form for each day about
    4 to 6 hours before bedtime (does not apply to fenfluramine)
» Importance of not taking more medication than the amount pre-
    scribed, because of habit-forming potential
» Not increasing dose if medication is not effective after a few weeks;
    checking with physician
» Proper dosing
» Proper storage
For extended-release and long-acting dosage forms only
  Proper administration: Swallowing whole; not breaking, crushing, or
    chewing
  Taking the daily dose about 10 to 14 hours before bedtime to min-
    imize the possibility of insomnia (does not apply to fenfluramine)
For mazindol
  1-mg tablet—Taking last dose 4 to 6 hours before bedtime
  2-mg tablet—Taking once-a-day dose 10 to 14 hours before bedtime

Precautions while using this medication
  Regular visits to physician to check progress during therapy
  Possible dryness of mouth; using sugarless candy or gum, ice, or
    saliva substitute for relief; checking with physician or dentist if
    dry mouth continues for more than 2 weeks
» Caution if dizziness, drowsiness, lightheadedness, or elated mood or
    euphoria occurs; not driving or using machines or doing other
    things that require alertness
» Caution if any kind of surgery, dental treatment, or emergency
    treatment is required

» Suspected physical or psychological dependence: checking with physician

» Not increasing dosage if tolerance develops; checking with physician
  Diabetic patients: Insulin or oral antidiabetic–agent requirements may be altered

» Checking with physician before discontinuing medication after prolonged high-dose therapy; gradual dosage reduction may be necessary to avoid possibility of withdrawal symptoms

For fenfluramine

» Avoiding the use of alcoholic beverages or other CNS depressants

Side/adverse effects

Symptoms of potential side effects, especially increased blood pressure, allergic reaction, blood dyscrasias (with diethylpropion), confusion or mental depression, psychotic episodes, or pulmonary hypertension (with fenfluramine)

▲ For the Patient ▲

912099

ABOUT YOUR MEDICINE

Appetite suppressants are used in the short-term treatment of obesity. For a few weeks these medicines in combination with dieting and exercise can help obese patients lose weight. However, since their appetite-reducing effect is only temporary, they are useful only for the first few weeks of dieting until new eating habits are established.

If any of the information in this leaflet causes you special concern or if you want additional information about your medicine and its use, check with your doctor, nurse, or pharmacist. **Remember, keep this and all other medicines out of the reach of children and never share your medicines with others.**

BEFORE USING THIS MEDICINE

Tell your doctor, nurse, and pharmacist if you . . .

* are allergic to any medicine, either prescription or nonprescription (OTC);
* are pregnant or intend to become pregnant while using this medicine;
* are breast-feeding;
* are taking any other prescription or nonprescription (OTC) medicine, especially MAO inhibitors;
* have any other medical problems, especially alcoholism, drug abuse or dependence (or history of), glaucoma, heart or blood vessel disease, high blood pressure, kidney disease, mental illness (severe), or overactive thyroid.

PROPER USE OF THIS MEDICINE

Take this medicine only as directed by your doctor. Do not take more of it, do not take it more often, and do not take it for a longer period of time than your doctor ordered. If too much is taken, it may become habit-forming.

If you think this medicine is not working properly after you have taken it for a few weeks, do not increase the dose. Instead, check with your doctor.

For patients taking the short-acting form of this medicine (effects last only a few hours):

- Take the last dose for each day about 4 to 6 hours before bedtime to help prevent trouble in sleeping.

For patients taking the long-acting form of this medicine (effects last 8 hours or more):

- Take the daily dose about 10 to 14 hours before bedtime to help prevent trouble in sleeping.
- The capsules or tablets are to be swallowed whole. Do not break, crush, or chew before swallowing.

PRECAUTIONS WHILE USING THIS MEDICINE

If you have taken this medicine for a while, do not stop taking it without first checking with your doctor. Your doctor may want you to reduce gradually the amount you are taking before stopping completely.

This medicine may cause some people to become dizzy, light-headed, drowsy, or less alert than they are normally. **Make sure you know how you react to this medicine before you drive, use machines, or do other jobs that require you to be alert.**

Before having any kind of surgery or dental or emergency treatment, tell the physician or dentist in charge that you are using this medicine.

If you have been taking this medicine for a long time or in large doses and **you think you may have become mentally or physically dependent on it, check with your doctor.**

POSSIBLE SIDE EFFECTS OF THIS MEDICINE
Side Effects That Should Be Reported To Your Doctor

   More common—Increased blood pressure

   Less common or rare—Confusion; mental depression; skin rash or hives; sore throat and fever; unusual bleeding or bruising

Side Effects That Usually Do Not Require Medical Attention

These possible side effects may go away during treatment; however, if they continue or are bothersome, check with your doctor, nurse, or pharmacist.

   False sense of well-being; irritability; nervousness; restlessness; trouble in sleeping

After the stimulant side effects have worn off, drowsiness, trembling, unusual tiredness or weakness, or mental depression may occur.

Other side effects not listed above may also occur in some patients. If you notice any other effects, check with your doctor, nurse, or pharmacist.

After you stop using this medicine, your body may need time to adjust. This may take several days or more. **Check with your doctor if you experience** mental depression, nausea or vomiting, stomach cramps or pain, trembling, or unusual tiredness or weakness.

110

BACLOFEN   Systemic

■ For the Pharmacist ■

In providing consultation, consider emphasizing the following selected information (» = major clinical significance):

Before using this medication
» Conditions affecting use, especially:
 Sensitivity to baclofen
 Use in the elderly—Increased risk of adverse CNS effects
 Other medications, especially other CNS depression–producing medications

Proper use of this medication
 Missed dose: Taking if remembered within an hour or so; not taking if not remembered within an hour; not doubling doses
» Proper storage

Precautions while using this medication
» Checking with physician before discontinuing medication; gradual dosage reduction is necessary
» Avoiding alcohol or other CNS depressants
» Caution if drowsiness, dizziness, visual disturbances, or impaired coordination occur
 Diabetics: May increase blood sugar concentrations

Side/adverse effects
» Convulsions, hallucinations, mood or mental changes, increased spasticity, or unusual nervousness or restlessness may occur following abrupt withdrawal
 Signs and symptoms of potential side effects, especially CNS effects, allergic dermatitis, bloody or dark urine, chest pain, and syncope

▲ For the Patient ▲

913320

ABOUT YOUR MEDICINE

Baclofen (BAK-loe-fen) is used to help relax certain muscles in your body. It relieves the spasms, cramping, and tightness of muscles caused by medical problems such as multiple sclerosis or certain injuries to the spine. Baclofen does not cure these problems, but it may allow other treatment, such as physical therapy, to be more helpful in improving your condition. Baclofen may also be used to relieve other conditions as determined by your doctor.

If any of the information in this leaflet causes you special concern or if you want additional information about your medicine and its use, check with your doctor, nurse, or pharmacist. **Remember, keep this and all other medicines out of the reach of children and never share your medicines with others.**

BEFORE USING THIS MEDICINE

Tell your doctor, nurse, and pharmacist if you . . .

- are allergic to any medicine, either prescription or non-prescription (OTC);
- are pregnant or intend to become pregnant while using this medicine;
- are breast-feeding;
- compete in athletics;
- are taking any other prescription or nonprescription (OTC) medicine, especially other CNS depressants;
- have any other medical problems.

PROPER USE OF THIS MEDICINE

If you miss a dose of this medicine, and you remember within an hour or so of the missed dose, take it as soon as you remember. However, if you do not remember until later, skip the missed dose and go back to your regular dosing schedule. Do not double doses.

PRECAUTIONS WHILE USING THIS MEDICINE

Do not suddenly stop taking this medicine. Unwanted effects may occur if the medicine is stopped suddenly. Check with your doctor for the best way to reduce gradually the amount you are taking before stopping completely.

This medicine will add to the effects of alcohol and other CNS depressants (medicines that slow down the nervous system). **Check with your doctor before taking any such depressants while you are using baclofen.**

This medicine may cause drowsiness, dizziness, vision problems, or clumsiness or unsteadiness in some people. **Make sure you know how you react to this medicine before you drive, use machines, or do other jobs that require you to be alert, well-coordinated, and able to see well.**

POSSIBLE SIDE EFFECTS OF THIS MEDICINE

Side Effects That Should Be Reported To Your Doctor

> *Rare*—Bloody or dark urine; chest pain; fainting; hallucinations; mental depression or other mood changes; ringing or buzzing in the ears; skin rash or itching

> *Signs of overdose*—Blurred or double vision; convulsions (seizures); muscle weakness (severe); shortness of breath or unusually slow or troubled breathing; vomiting

Side Effects That Usually Do Not Require Medical Attention

These possible side effects may go away during treatment; however, if they continue or are bothersome, check with your doctor, nurse, or pharmacist.

> *More common*—Confusion; dizziness or lightheadedness; drowsiness; nausea; unusual weakness, especially muscle weakness

Other side effects not listed above may also occur in some patients. If you notice any other effects, check with your doctor, nurse, or pharmacist.

Some side effects may occur after you have stopped taking this medicine, especially if you stop taking it suddenly. **Check with your doctor immediately** if any of the following effects occur: convulsions (seizures); hallucinations; increase in muscle spasm, cramping, or tightness; mood or mental changes; or unusual nervousness or restlessness.

BARBITURATES   Systemic

Including Amobarbital; Aprobarbital; Butabarbital;
Mephobarbital; Metharbital; Pentobarbital; Phenobarbital;
Secobarbital; Secobarbital and Amobarbital.

■ For the Pharmacist ■

In providing consultation, consider emphasizing the following selected
information (» = major clinical significance):

Before using this medication
» Conditions affecting use, especially:
   Sensitivity to barbiturates
   Pregnancy—Barbiturates readily cross placenta; increase in in-
      cidence of fetal abnormalities (FDA Pregnancy Category D);
      use during third trimester of pregnancy may cause physical
      dependence with resulting withdrawal symptoms in neonate;
      long-acting barbiturates associated with neonatal coagulation
      defect that may cause bleeding during early neonatal period;
      use during labor may cause respiratory depression in neonate
   Breast-feeding—Barbiturates distributed into breast milk; use
      by nursing mothers may cause CNS depression in infant
   Use in children—Children may react to barbiturates with par-
      adoxical excitement
   Use in the elderly—Elderly patients may react to usual doses
      of barbiturates with excitement, confusion, or mental depres-
      sion; risk of barbiturate-induced hypothermia may be in-
      creased in elderly patients; elderly patients more likely to
      have age-related hepatic or renal function impairment, which
      may require a dosage reduction of barbiturates
   Other medications, especially alcohol, adrenocorticoids, corti-
      cotropin, other CNS depression–producing medications, cou-
      marin- or indandione-derivative anticoagulants, carbamaze-
      pine, divalproex sodium, estrogen-containing contraceptives,
      or valproic acid
   Other medical problems, especially history of drug abuse or de-
      pendence, premonitory signs of hepatic coma, acute or chronic
      pain, or respiratory disease involving dyspnea or obstruction
      (particularly status asthmaticus)
   Caution if any laboratory tests required; possible interference
      with results of metyrapone test.

Proper use of this medication
» Importance of not using more medication than the amount pre-
   scribed because of habit-forming potential
» Not increasing dose if medication appears less effective after a few
   weeks; checking with physician
» For anticonvulsant use: Compliance with therapy; not missing any
   doses
» Proper dosing
   Missed dose: If on scheduled dosing regimen—Taking as soon as
      possible; not taking if almost time for next dose; not doubling
      doses
   Proper administration:
   For extended-release dosage form
      Swallowing capsule or tablet whole
      Not breaking, crushing, or chewing

For suppository dosage form
    Proper administration technique
» Proper storage

Precautions while using this medication
    Regular visits to physician to check progress during prolonged therapy
    Checking with physician before discontinuing medication after prolonged use; gradual dosage reduction may be necessary to avoid the possibility of withdrawal symptoms
» Avoiding use of alcohol or other CNS depressants
» Suspected psychological or physical dependence: Checking with physician
» Suspected overdose: Getting emergency help at once
» Caution if dizziness, lightheadedness, or drowsiness occurs
» Use of another or additional method of contraception if taking estrogen-containing oral contraceptives concurrently

Side/adverse effects
    Signs of potential side effects, especially allergic reaction or intolerance to barbiturate, blood dyscrasias, exfoliative dermatitis, hallucinations, hepatic damage (with prolonged or chronic use), mental depression, paradoxical reaction, osteopenia or rickets (with prolonged or chronic use), or Stevens-Johnson syndrome
    Unusual excitement may be more likely to occur in children and in elderly or very ill patients
    Confusion and mental depression may be more likely to occur in elderly or very ill patients

---

▲ For the Patient ▲

912102

ABOUT YOUR MEDICINE

Barbiturates belong to the group of medicines called central nervous system (CNS) depressants. Some barbiturates may be used before surgery to relieve anxiety. In addition, some are also used to help control seizures in certain disorders, such as epilepsy. Barbiturates may also be used for other conditions as determined by your doctor.

If any of the information in this leaflet causes you special concern or if you want additional information about your medicine and its use, check with your doctor, nurse, or pharmacist. **Remember, keep this and all other medicines out of the reach of children and never share your medicines with others.**

BEFORE USING THIS MEDICINE

Tell your doctor, nurse, and pharmacist if you . . .
- are allergic to any medicine, either prescription or nonprescription (OTC);
- are pregnant or intend to become pregnant while using this medicine;
- are breast-feeding;
- are taking **any** other prescription or nonprescription (OTC) medicine;
- have **any** other medical problems.

PROPER USE OF THIS MEDICINE

Use this medicine only as directed. If too much is used, it may become habit-forming. Even if you think this medicine is not working, **do not increase the dose.** Instead, check with your doctor.

If you are taking this medicine for epilepsy, it must be taken every day in regularly spaced doses in order for it to control your seizures.

If you are taking this medicine regularly and you miss a dose, take it as soon as possible. However, if it is almost time for your next dose, skip the missed dose and go back to your regular dosing schedule. Do not double doses.

PRECAUTIONS WHILE USING THIS MEDICINE

If you will be taking this medicine regularly for a long time, do not stop taking it without first checking with your doctor.

Barbiturates will add to the effects of alcohol and other CNS depressants. **Check with your doctor before taking any such depressants while taking this medicine.**

This medicine may cause some people to become dizzy, light-headed, drowsy, or less alert than they are normally. Even if taken at bedtime, it may cause these effects on arising. **Make sure you know how you react before you drive, use machines, or do other jobs that require you to be alert.**

Birth control pills containing estrogen may not work properly if you take them while taking barbiturates. Unplanned pregnancies may occur. Use a different or additional means of birth control while you are taking barbiturates. If you have any questions about this, check with your doctor or pharmacist.

If you have been using this medicine for a long time and you think that you may have become mentally or physically dependent on it, check with your doctor. Some signs of mental or physical dependence are:
—a strong desire or need to continue taking the medicine.
—a need to increase the dose to receive the effects of the medicine.
—withdrawal side effects after the medicine is stopped.

If you think you or someone else may have taken an overdose, get emergency help at once. Taking an overdose of a barbiturate or taking alcohol or other CNS depressants with it may lead to death. Some signs of overdose are decrease in reflexes; severe drowsiness, confusion, or weakness; shortness of breath or slow or troubled breathing; slurred speech; staggering; and slow heartbeat.

POSSIBLE SIDE EFFECTS OF THIS MEDICINE

Side Effects That Should Be Reported To Your Doctor Immediately

> *Rare*—Bleeding sores on lips; chest pain; fever; muscle or joint pain; red, thickened, or scaly skin; skin rash or hives; sores or white spots in mouth (painful); sore throat; swelling of eyelids, face, or lips; wheezing or tightness in chest

Other Side Effects That Should Be Reported To Your Doctor

> *Less common*—Confusion; mental depression; unusual excitement
>
> *Rare*—Hallucinations; unusual bleeding, bruising, tiredness, or weakness
>
> *With long-term or chronic use*—Bone pain or aching; loss of appetite; muscle weakness; weight loss (unusual); yellow eyes or skin

Side Effects That Usually Do Not Require Medical Attention

These possible side effects may go away during treatment; however, if they continue or are bothersome, check with your doctor, nurse, or pharmacist.

> *More common*—Clumsiness or unsteadiness, dizziness or lightheadedness, drowsiness, "hangover" effect

Other side effects not listed above may also occur in some patients. If you notice any other effects, check with your doctor, nurse, or pharmacist.

After you stop using this medicine, your body may need time to adjust. If you took this medicine in high doses or for a long time, this may take up to about 15 days. Check with your doctor **if you experience anxiety; convulsions (seizures); dizziness or lightheadedness; faint feeling; hallucinations; muscle twitching; nausea or vomiting; trembling of hands; trouble in sleeping, increased dreaming, or nightmares; vision problems; or weakness.**

BENZODIAZEPINES   Systemic

Including Alprazolam; Bromazepam; Chlordiazepoxide; Clonazepam; Clorazepate; Diazepam; Estazolam; Flurazepam; Halazepam; Ketazolam; Lorazepam; Nitrazepam; Oxazepam; Prazepam; Quazepam; Temazepam; Triazolam.

■ For the Pharmacist ■

In providing consultation, consider emphasizing the following selected information (» = major clinical significance):

Before using this medication
» Conditions affecting use, especially:
Sensitivity to benzodiazepines
Pregnancy—Benzodiazepines reported to increase risk of congenital malformations when used during first trimester of pregnancy; chronic use may cause physical dependence in the neonate with resulting withdrawal symptoms; use during last weeks of pregnancy may cause neonatal CNS depression; use just prior to or during labor may cause neonatal flaccidity
Breast-feeding—Some benzodiazepines and their metabolites distributed into breast milk and others may be distributed into breast milk; use by nursing mothers may cause sedation, and possibly feeding difficulties and weight loss in the infant
Use in children—Children, especially the very young, usually more sensitive to CNS effects of benzodiazepines
Use in the elderly—Elderly patients usually more sensitive to CNS effects of benzodiazepines
Other medications, especially other CNS depression–producing medications
Other medical problems, especially acute angle-closure glaucoma, myasthenia gravis, or severe chronic obstructive pulmonary disease

Proper use of this medication
Proper administration:
For extended-release dosage form of diazepam
Swallowing capsule whole
Not crushing, breaking, or chewing
For oral solution dosage form of lorazepam
Dose may be diluted with liquid or semisolid food such as water, soda or soda-like beverages, applesauce, or pudding
For sublingual tablet dosage form of lorazepam
Not chewing or swallowing tablet whole
Dissolving slowly under tongue; not swallowing for at least 2 minutes to allow sufficient absorption
» Importance of not taking more medication than the amount prescribed because of habit-forming potential
» Not increasing dose if medication is less effective after a few weeks; checking with physician
» Proper dosing
Missed dose: If on scheduled dosing regimen (e.g., for epilepsy)—Taking right away if remembered within an hour or so; if remembered later, not taking at all; not doubling doses
» Proper storage

For anticonvulsant use of clonazepam, clorazepate, diazepam, or nitrazepam
» Compliance with therapy; not missing any doses
For flurazepam only
» Maximum effectiveness of medication may not occur for 2 or 3 nights after initiation of therapy

Precautions while using this medication
Regular visits to physician to check progress during prolonged therapy (and during initial therapy with clonazepam)
Checking with physician before discontinuing medication after prolonged use; gradual dosage reduction may be necessary to avoid the possibility of withdrawal symptoms and, in patients with epilepsy or history of seizures, the possibility of precipitating seizures
» Avoiding use of alcohol or other CNS depressants during therapy
» Suspected overdose: Getting emergency help at once
Caution if any laboratory tests required; possible interference with results of metyrapone test
» Caution if drowsiness, dizziness, lightheadedness, or clumsiness or unsteadiness occurs, especially in the elderly
For anticonvulsant use of clonazepam, clorazepate, diazepam, or nitrazepam
Carrying medical identification card or bracelet during therapy

Side/adverse effects
Signs of potential side effects, especially allergic reaction, blood dyscrasias, CNS effects, extrapyramidal symptoms, hepatic dysfunction, muscle weakness, and paradoxical reaction
Most of side/adverse effects more likely to occur in children, especially the very young, and in elderly patients; these patients are usually more sensitive to effects of benzodiazepines
For patients receiving chlordiazepoxide, diazepam, or lorazepam injection: Checking with physician if redness, swelling, or pain at injection site occurs

---

▲ For the Patient ▲

912124

ABOUT YOUR MEDICINE

Benzodiazepines (ben-zoe-dye-AZ-e-peens) are used to relieve nervousness or tension, and to treat insomnia (trouble in sleeping). For these conditions, benzodiazepines are used only for a short time. Some benzodiazepines may also be used to relax muscles or relieve muscle spasm, and to treat panic disorders and certain convulsive disorders, such as epilepsy. Benzodiazepines may also be used for other conditions as determined by your doctor. Benzodiazepines should not be used for nervousness or tension caused by the stress of everyday life.

If any of the information in this leaflet causes you special concern or if you want additional information about your medicine and its use, check with your doctor, nurse, or pharmacist. **Remember, keep this and all other medicines out of the reach of children and never share your medicines with others.**

BEFORE USING THIS MEDICINE

Tell your doctor, nurse, and pharmacist if you . . .
- are allergic to any medicine, either prescription or non-prescription (OTC);
- are pregnant or intend to become pregnant while using this medicine;
- are breast-feeding;
- are taking any other prescription or nonprescription (OTC) medicine, especially other CNS depressants;
- have any other medical problems, especially asthma, bronchitis, emphysema, or other chronic lung disease; or myasthenia gravis.

PROPER USE OF THIS MEDICINE

Take this medicine only as directed by your doctor. Do not take more of it, do not take it more often, and do not take it for a longer time than your doctor ordered. If too much is taken, it may become habit-forming.

If you think this medicine is not working properly after you have taken it for a few weeks, **do not increase the dose**. Instead, check with your doctor.

If you are taking this medicine for epilepsy, it must be taken every day in regularly spaced doses in order for it to control your seizures.

If you are taking this medicine for insomnia, do not take it if you cannot get a full night's sleep (7 to 8 hours). Otherwise, you may feel drowsy and have memory problems because the effects of the medicine have not worn off.

If you are taking this medicine regularly (for example, every day) and you miss a dose, take it right away if you remember within an hour or so of the missed dose. However, if you do not remember until later, skip the missed dose and go back to your regular dosing schedule. Do not double doses.

PRECAUTIONS WHILE USING THIS MEDICINE

This medicine will add to the effects of alcohol and other CNS depressants (medicines that slow down the nervous system). **Check with your doctor before taking any such depressants while you are taking this medicine.**

Benzodiazepines may cause some people to become drowsy. **Make sure you know how you react to this medicine before you drive, use machines, or do other jobs that require you to be alert.**

If you think you or someone else may have taken an overdose, get emergency help at once. Some signs of an overdose are continuing slurred speech or confusion, severe drowsiness, severe weakness, and staggering.

POSSIBLE SIDE EFFECTS OF THIS MEDICINE
Side Effects That Should Be Reported To Your Doctor

Less common or rare—Behavior problems, including difficulty in concentrating and outbursts of anger; confusion or mental depression; convulsions (seizures); hallucinations; impaired memory; muscle weakness; skin rash or itching; sore throat, fever, and chills; ulcers or sores in mouth or throat (continuing); uncontrolled movements of body, including the eyes; unusual bleeding or bruising; unusual excitement, nervousness, or irritability; unusual tiredness or weakness; yellow eyes or skin

Signs of overdose—Confusion (continuing); drowsiness (severe); shakiness; shortness of breath or troubled breathing; slow heartbeat; slow reflexes; slurred speech (continuing); staggering; weakness (severe)

Side Effects That Usually Do Not Require Medical Attention

These possible side effects may go away during treatment; however, if they continue or are bothersome, check with your doctor, nurse, or pharmacist.

More common—Clumsiness or unsteadiness; dizziness or lightheadedness; drowsiness; slurred speech

Other side effects not listed above may also occur in some patients. If you notice any other effects, check with your doctor, nurse, or pharmacist.

After you stop using this medicine, your body may need time to adjust. If you took this medicine in high doses or for a long time, this may take up to 3 weeks. **During this time, check with your doctor if you experience** fast or pounding heartbeat; increased sense of hearing; increased sensitivity to touch and pain; increased sweating; mental depression; muscle or stomach cramps; nausea or vomiting; sensitivity of eyes to light; tingling, burning, or prickly sensations; trembling; trouble in sleeping; or if you are unusually irritable, nervous, or confused.

BETA-ADRENERGIC BLOCKING AGENTS   Ophthalmic

Including Betaxolol; Carteolol; Levobunolol; Metipranolol; Timolol.

■ For the Pharmacist ■

In providing consultation, consider emphasizing the following selected information (» = major clinical significance):

Before using this medication
» Conditions affecting use, especially:
    Allergy to any of the beta-adrenergic blocking agents, either ophthalmic or systemic, such as acebutolol, atenolol, betaxolol, bisoprolol, carteolol, labetalol, levobunolol, metipranolol, metoprolol, nadolol, oxprenolol, penbutolol, pindolol, propranolol, sotalol, or timolol
    Pregnancy—Ophthalmic beta-adrenergic blocking agents may be absorbed into the body. Studies in animals have not shown that betaxolol, levobunolol, metipranolol, or timolol causes birth defects. However, very large doses of carteolol given by mouth to pregnant rats have been shown to cause wavy ribs in rat babies. In addition, some studies in animals have shown that beta-adrenergic blocking agents increase the chance of death in the animal fetus
    Use in children—Infants may be especially sensitive to the effects of ophthalmic beta-adrenergic blocking agents, thus increasing the risk of side effects
    Use in the elderly—If significant systemic absorption of ophthalmic beta-adrenergic blocking agents occurs, the chance of side effects during treatment may be increased, since elderly people are especially sensitive to the effects of these medications
    Other medical problems, especially bronchial asthma, or history of, severe chronic obstructive pulmonary disease, overt cardiac failure, 2nd- or 3rd-degree atrioventricular (AV) heart block, cardiogenic shock, sinus bradycardia, nonallergenic or chronic bronchitis, emphysema or other pulmonary function impairment, congestive heart failure, history of cardiac failure, diabetes mellitus, spontaneous hypoglycemia, or hyperthyroidism

Proper use of this medication
» Proper administration technique; using nasolacrimal occlusion is especially important in infants and children
    Preventing contamination: Not touching applicator tip to any surface; keeping container tightly closed
    Proper use of medication having compliance cap
» Importance of not using more medication than the amount prescribed
» Proper dosing
    Missed dose: If dosing schedule is—
        Once a day: Applying as soon as possible; not applying if not remembered until next day; applying regularly scheduled dose
        More than once a day: Applying as soon as possible; not applying if almost time for next dose; applying next dose at regularly scheduled time
» Proper storage

Precautions while using this medication
Regular visits to physician to check eye pressure during therapy
» Caution if any kind of surgery (including dental surgery) or emergency treatment is required
» Diabetics: May mask some signs of hypoglycemia, such as increased pulse rate and trembling, but not dizziness and sweating; also, may cause decreased or sometimes increased blood glucose concentrations
Possible photophobia: Wearing sunglasses and avoiding too much exposure to bright light

Side/adverse effects
Signs of potential side effects, especially conjunctival hyperemia, anisocoria, blepharitis, blepharoconjunctivitis, conjunctivitis, corneal punctate keratitis, dermatitis of eyelid, edema, iridocyclitis, keratitis, blepharoptosis, corneal staining, decreased corneal sensitivity, diplopia, eye pain, glossitis, vision disturbances, or symptoms of systemic absorption

---

▲ For the Patient ▲

913058

ABOUT YOUR MEDICINE

Ophthalmic **beta-blockers** are used to treat certain types of glaucoma.

If any of the information in this leaflet causes you special concern or if you want additional information about your medicine and its use, check with your doctor, nurse, or pharmacist. **Remember, keep this and all other medicines out of the reach of children and never share your medicines with others.**

BEFORE USING THIS MEDICINE

Tell your doctor, nurse, and pharmacist if you . . .
• are allergic to any medicine, either prescription or nonprescription (OTC);
• are pregnant or intend to become pregnant while using this medicine;
• are breast-feeding;
• are taking any other prescription or nonprescription (OTC) medicine;
• have any other medical problems, especially asthma (or history of), chronic bronchitis, emphysema, or other lung disease; diabetes mellitus (sugar diabetes); heart or blood vessel disease; hypoglycemia (low blood sugar); or overactive thyroid.

PROPER USE OF THIS MEDICINE

To use: First, wash hands. With middle finger, apply pressure to the inside corner of the eye (and continue to apply pressure for 1 or 2 minutes after the medicine has been placed in the eye). **This is especially important if this medicine is used to treat infants and children.** Tilt head back and with the index finger of the same hand, pull lower eyelid away from eye to form a pouch. Drop the medicine into the pouch and gently close eyes. Do not blink. Keep eyes closed for 1 or 2 minutes to allow the medicine to be absorbed.

Immediately after using the eye drops, wash your hands to remove any medicine that may be on them.

To help keep the medicine germ-free, do not touch the applicator tip to any surface (including the eye) and keep the container tightly closed.

Use this medicine only as directed. Do not use more of it and do not use it more often than your doctor ordered. To do so may increase the chance of too much medicine being absorbed into the body and the chance of side effects.

If you miss a dose of this medicine and your schedule is one dose to be applied:

- Once a day—Use the missed dose as soon as possible. However, if you do not remember the missed dose until the next day, skip the missed dose and go back to your regular dosing schedule. Do not double doses.
- More than once a day—Use the missed dose as soon as possible. However, if it is almost time for your next dose, skip the missed dose and go back to your regular dosing schedule. Do not double doses.

PRECAUTIONS WHILE USING THIS MEDICINE

Your doctor should check your eye pressure at regular visits to make certain your glaucoma is being controlled.

Before having any kind of surgery or dental or emergency treatment, tell the physician or dentist in charge that you are using this medicine.

Diabetics—This medicine may affect blood sugar levels. Also, this medicine may cover up some signs of hypoglycemia (low blood sugar), such as trembling or increase in pulse rate or blood pressure. However, other signs of low blood sugar, such as dizziness or sweating, are not affected. If you have any questions about this, check with your doctor.

POSSIBLE SIDE EFFECTS OF THIS MEDICINE
Side Effects That Should Be Reported To Your Doctor

More common—Redness of eyes or inside of eyelids

Less common or rare—Blurred vision or other change in vision; different size pupils of the eyes; discoloration of the eyeball; droopy upper eyelid; eye pain; redness or irritation of the tongue; seeing double; swelling, irritation, or inflammation of eye or eyelid (severe)

Possible signs of too much medicine being absorbed into the body—Anxiety or nervousness; burning or prickling feeling on body; change in taste; chest pain; clumsiness or unsteadiness; confusion or mental depression; coughing, wheezing, or troubled breathing; decreased sexual ability; diarrhea; dizziness or feeling faint; drowsiness; hair loss; hallucinations; headache; irregular, slow, or pounding heartbeat; muscle or joint aches or pain; nausea or vomiting; raw or red areas of the skin; runny, stuffy, or bleeding nose; skin rash, hives, or itching; swelling of feet, ankles, or lower legs; trouble in sleeping; unusual tiredness or weakness

Side Effects That Usually Do Not Require Medical Attention

These possible side effects may go away during treatment; however, if they continue or are bothersome, check with your doctor, nurse, or pharmacist.

   More common—Decreased night vision; stinging of eye or other eye irritation (when medicine is applied)

Other side effects not listed above may also occur in some patients. If you notice any other effects, check with your doctor, nurse, or pharmacist.

BETA-ADRENERGIC BLOCKING AGENTS   Systemic

Including Acebutolol; Atenolol; Betaxolol; Bisoprolol; Carteolol; Labetalol; Metoprolol; Nadolol; Oxprenolol; Penbutolol; Pindolol; Propranolol; Sotalol; Timolol.

■For the Pharmacist■

In providing consultation, consider emphasizing the following selected information (» = major clinical significance):

Before using this medication
» Conditions affecting use, especially:
Sensitivity to the beta-blocker prescribed
Pregnancy—Beta-adrenergic blocking agents cross the placenta; risk of hypoglycemia, respiratory depression, bradycardia, and hypotension in the fetus and neonate
Breast-feeding—Beta-adrenergic blocking agents pass into breast milk; bradycardia, cyanosis, hypotension, and tachypnea have been reported in breast-fed infants whose mothers ingested atenolol or acebutolol
Use in the elderly—Older patients may be more susceptible to some side/adverse effects; increased risk of beta-blocker–induced hypothermia
Other medications, especially allergen immunotherapy and allergenic extracts used for skin testing, oral antidiabetic agents, insulin, calcium channel blocking agents, clonidine, guanabenz, cocaine, MAO inhibitors, sympathomimetics, or xanthines
Other medical problems, especially overt cardiac failure, cardiogenic shock, 2nd or 3rd degree AV block, sinus bradycardia, hypotension (when used in myocardial infarction), history of allergy, bronchial asthma, emphysema or nonallergenic bronchitis, congestive heart failure, diabetes mellitus, hyperthyroidism, or mental depression

Proper use of this medication
Proper administration of extended-release dosage forms: Swallowing whole without crushing, breaking (except with metoprolol succinate), or chewing
Proper use of concentrated oral propranolol solution:
Measuring with calibrated dropper
Mixing with liquid or semi-solid food such as water, juices, soda or soda-like beverages, applesauce, and puddings; making sure entire dose is taken
Not storing after mixing
Checking pulse as directed (checking with physician if less than 50 beats per minute)
Getting into habit of taking at same time each day to help increase compliance
» Importance of not missing doses, especially with schedules of one dose per day
» Proper dosing
Missed dose: Taking as soon as possible; not taking at all if within 4 hours of next scheduled dose (8 hours for atenolol, betaxolol, carteolol, labetalol, nadolol, penbutolol, sotalol, or extended-release oxprenolol or propranolol); not doubling doses
» Proper storage

For use as an antihypertensive
Possible need for control of weight and diet, especially sodium intake
» Compliance with therapy; patient may not experience symptoms of
  hypertension; importance of taking medication only as directed
  and keeping appointments with physician, even if feeling well
» Does not cure, but helps control hypertension; possible need for
  lifelong therapy; checking with physician before discontinuing
  medication; serious consequences of untreated hypertension

Precautions while using this medication
Regular visits to physician to check progress
» Checking with physician before discontinuing medication; gradual
  dosage reduction may be necessary
Having enough medication on hand to get through weekends, holidays, and vacations; possibly carrying second written prescrip-
  tion for emergency use
Carrying medical identification card during therapy
» Caution if any kind of surgery (including dental surgery) or emer-
  gency treatment is required
» Diabetics: May mask signs and symptoms of hypoglycemia or may
  cause increased blood glucose concentrations or prolong hypo-
  glycemia
» Caution when driving or doing things requiring alertness, because
  of possible drowsiness, dizziness, or lightheadedness
Caution during exposure to cold weather because of possible in-
  creased sensitivity to cold
» Caution against overexertion in response to decreased chest pain
Caution if any laboratory tests required; possible interference with
  test results
Patients with allergies to foods, medications, or stinging insect venom:
  Possible increase in severity of allergic reactions; checking with
  physician immediately if severe allergic reaction occurs
For use as an antihypertensive
» Not taking other medications, especially nonprescription sympatho-
  mimetics, unless discussed with physician
For oral labetalol only
» Caution when getting up suddenly from a lying or sitting position,
  especially during initiation of therapy or when dosage is in-
  creased
» Caution in using alcohol, while standing for long periods or exercising, and during hot weather because of enhanced orthostatic
  hypotensive effects
For parenteral labetalol only
» Lying down during injection and for up to 3 hours after getting
  injection, then getting up gradually

Side/adverse effects
Signs of potential side effects, especially bradycardia, breathing
  difficulty and/or wheezing, congestive heart failure, mental
  depression, reduced peripheral circulation, allergic reaction, arrhythmias, back pain or joint pain, chest pain, confusion, hallucinations, hepatotoxicity, leukopenia, psoriasiform eruption,
  thrombocytopenia, and withdrawal reaction
For labetalol: Transient scalp tingling may occur, usually at beginning of treatment

▲ For the Patient ▲

912135

ABOUT YOUR MEDICINE

Beta-blockers are used to treat high blood pressure. Some are also used in the relief of angina (chest pain) and in heart attack patients to help prevent additional heart attacks. Some beta-blockers are also used to correct irregular heartbeats, prevent migraine headaches, and treat tremors. Beta-blockers may also be used for other conditions as determined by your doctor.

If any of the information in this leaflet causes you special concern or if you want additional information about your medicine and its use, check with your doctor, nurse, or pharmacist. **Remember, keep this and all other medicines out of the reach of children and never share your medicines with others.**

BEFORE USING THIS MEDICINE

Tell your doctor, nurse, and pharmacist if you . . .
- are allergic to any medicine, either prescription or non-prescription (OTC);
- are pregnant or intend to become pregnant while using this medicine;
- are breast-feeding;
- are taking any other prescription or nonprescription (OTC) medicine, especially allergy shots or allergy skin testing; aminophylline; caffeine; calcium channel blockers; clonidine; diabetes medicine; dyphylline; guanabenz; insulin; MAO inhibitors; oxtriphylline; theophylline; or medicines for appetite control, asthma, colds, cough, hay fever, or sinus;
- have any other medical problems, especially allergy, asthma or other lung disease, diabetes, heart or blood vessel disease, mental depression, or overactive thyroid;
- use cocaine.

PROPER USE OF THIS MEDICINE

Even if you feel well, **take this medicine exactly as directed.**

Ask your doctor about your pulse rate before and after taking beta-blockers. Then, while you are taking this medicine, check your pulse regularly. If it is much slower than your usual rate (or less than 50 beats per minute), check with your doctor. A pulse rate that is too slow may cause circulation problems.

If you are taking this medicine for high blood pressure, remember that it will not cure your high blood pressure, but it does help control it. You must continue to take it—even if you feel well—if you expect to keep your blood pressure down. **You may have to take medicine for the rest of your life.**

Do not miss any doses, especially if you are taking only one dose a day. Some conditions may become worse when this medicine is not taken regularly.

If you do miss a dose of this medicine, take it as soon as possible. However, if it is within 4 hours of your next dose (8 hours when taking atenolol, betaxolol, carteolol, labetalol, nadolol, penbutolol, sotalol, or extended-release oxprenolol or propranolol), skip the missed dose and go back to your regular dosing schedule. Do not double doses.

PRECAUTIONS WHILE USING THIS MEDICINE

Do not stop taking this medicine without first checking with your doctor.

For diabetic patients:
- **This medicine may cause your blood sugar levels to fall. Also, this medicine may cover up signs of hypoglycemia (low blood sugar).**

This medicine may cause some people to become dizzy, drowsy, or lightheaded. **Make sure you know how you react before you drive, use machines, or do other jobs that require you to be alert.**

Chest pain resulting from exercise or physical exertion is usually reduced or prevented by this medicine. This may tempt a patient to be overly active. **Make sure you discuss with your doctor a safe amount of exercise for you.**

POSSIBLE SIDE EFFECTS OF THIS MEDICINE
Side Effects That Should Be Reported To Your Doctor

Less common—Breathing difficulty; cold hands and feet; mental depression; shortness of breath; slow heartbeat (especially less than 50 beats per minute); swelling of ankles, feet, and/or lower legs

Rare—Back pain or joint pain; chest pain; confusion (especially in elderly); dark urine (for acebutolol, bisoprolol, or labetalol); dizziness or lightheadedness when getting up from a lying or sitting position; fever and sore throat; hallucinations; irregular heartbeat; red, scaling, or crusted skin; skin rash; unusual bleeding and bruising; yellow eyes or skin (for acebutolol, bisoprolol, or labetalol)

Side Effects That Usually Do Not Require Medical Attention

These possible side effects may go away during treatment; however, if they continue or are bothersome, check with your doctor, nurse, or pharmacist.

More common—Decreased sexual ability; dizziness or lightheadedness; drowsiness (slight); trouble in sleeping; unusual tiredness or weakness

After you have been taking a beta-blocker for a while, it may cause unpleasant or even harmful effects if you stop taking it too suddenly. Check with your doctor right away if you notice chest pain, fast or irregular heartbeat, general feeling of body discomfort or weakness, shortness of breath (sudden), sweating, or trembling.

Other side effects not listed above may also occur in some patients. If you notice any other effects, check with your doctor, nurse, or pharmacist.

BETA-ADRENERGIC BLOCKING AGENTS AND THIAZIDE DIURETICS   Systemic

Including Atenolol and Chlorthalidone; Bisoprolol and Hydrochlorothiazide; Labetalol and Hydrochlorothiazide; Metoprolol and Hydrochlorothiazide; Nadolol and Bendroflumethiazide; Pindolol and Hydrochlorothiazide; Propranolol and Hydrochlorothiazide; Timolol and Hydrochlorothiazide.

■For the Pharmacist■

In providing consultation, consider emphasizing the following selected information (» = major clinical significance):

Before using this medication
» Conditions affecting use, especially:

Sensitivity to the beta-adrenergic blocking agent prescribed, or to any thiazide diuretic or other sulfonamide-type medications

Pregnancy—Risk of hypoglycemia, respiratory depression, bradycardia, and hypotension with beta-adrenergic blocking agents; thiazide diuretics may cause jaundice, thrombocytopenia, hypokalemia in infant

Breast-feeding—Distributed into breast milk; not known for bisoprolol

Use in the elderly—Increased sensitivity to effects; increased risk of beta-blocker–induced hypothermia

Other medications, especially allergen immunotherapy or skin testing, oral antidiabetic agents, calcium channel blocking agents, clonidine, cocaine, digitalis glycosides, guanabenz, insulin, lithium, MAO inhibitors, synmpathomimetics, or xanthines

Other medical problems, especially anuria or severe renal function impairment, bronchial asthma, cardiogenic shock, congestive heart failure, diabetes mellitus, emphysema or nonallergenic bronchitis, history of allergy, hyperthyroidism, hypotension, mental depression, overt cardiac failure, second or third degree AV block, or sinus bradycardia

Proper use of this medication
Possible need for control of weight and diet, especially sodium intake
» Compliance with therapy; patient may not experience symptoms of hypertension; importance of taking medication only as directed and keeping appointments with physician, even if feeling well
» Does not cure, but helps control hypertension; possible need for lifelong therapy; serious consequences of untreated hypertension
Proper administration of extended-release dosage forms: Swallowing whole without crushing, breaking, or chewing
Getting into habit of taking at same time each day to help increase compliance
Checking pulse as directed (checking with physician if less than 50 beats per minute)
Diuretic effects of the medication and timing of doses to minimize inconvenience of diuresis
» Importance of not missing doses, especially with schedules of one dose per day
» Proper dosing

Missed dose: Taking as soon as possible; not taking at all if within 4 hours of next scheduled dose (8 hours for atenolol and chlorthalidone, nadolol and bendroflumethiazide, or extended-release propranolol and hydrochlorothiazide); not doubling doses
» Proper storage

Precautions while using this medication
Regular visits to physician to check progress
» Checking with physician before discontinuing medication; gradual dosage reduction may be necessary
Having enough medication on hand to get through weekends, holidays, and vacations; possibly carrying second written prescription for emergency use
Carrying medical identification during therapy
» Not taking other medications, especially nonprescription sympathomimetics, unless discussed with physician
» Caution if any kind of surgery (including dental surgery) or emergency treatment is required
» Diabetics: May mask signs and symptoms of hypoglycemia or cause increased blood glucose concentrations
» Possibility of hypokalemia; possible need for additional potassium in diet; not changing diet without first checking with physician
To prevent dehydration, checking with physician if severe nausea, vomiting, or diarrhea occurs and continues
» Caution when driving or doing things requiring alertness, because of possible drowsiness, dizziness, or lightheadedness
Caution during exposure to cold weather because of possible increased sensitivity to cold
Possible skin photosensitivity; avoiding unprotected exposure to sun; using protective clothing and sun block product; avoiding use of sunlamp, tanning bed, or tanning booth
Caution if any laboratory tests required; possible interference with test results
Patients with allergies to foods, medications, or stinging insect venom: Possible increase in severity of allergic reactions; checking with physician immediately if severe allergic reaction occurs

Side/adverse effects
Signs of potential side effects, especially electrolyte imbalance, bradycardia, bronchospasm, congestive heart failure, mental depression, reduced peripheral circulation, allergic reaction, arrhythmias, agranulocytosis, back pain, joint pain, chest pain, cholecystitis, pancreatitis, confusion (especially in elderly), hallucinations, hepatotoxicity, hyperuricemia, gout, leukopenia, psoriasiform eruption, and thrombocytopenia

---

▲ For the Patient ▲

912146

ABOUT YOUR MEDICINE

Beta-blocker and **thiazide diuretic** combinations belong to the group of medicines known as antihypertensives (high blood pressure medicine). They are used to treat high blood pressure.

If any of the information in this leaflet causes you special concern or if you want additional information about your medicine and its use, check with your doctor, nurse, or pharmacist. **Remember, keep this and all other medicines out of**

the reach of children and never share your medicines with
others.

BEFORE USING THIS MEDICINE

Tell your doctor, nurse, and pharmacist if you . . .
- are allergic to any medicine, either prescription or non-prescription (OTC);
- are pregnant or intend to become pregnant while using this medicine;
- are breast-feeding;
- compete in athletics;
- are taking any other prescription or nonprescription (OTC) medicine, especially aminophylline; caffeine; clonidine; cortisone-like medicines; diabetes medicine; digitalis glycosides (heart medicine); diltiazem; dyphylline; guanabenz; lithium; MAO inhibitors; medicines for appetite control, asthma, colds, cough, hay fever, or sinus; methenamine; nicardipine; nifedipine; nimodipine; oxtriphylline; theophylline; or verapamil;
- have any other medical problems, especially allergies; asthma or other lung disease; diabetes; heart, blood vessel, or kidney disease; mental depression; or overactive thyroid;
- use cocaine.

PROPER USE OF THIS MEDICINE

This medicine will not cure your high blood pressure but it does help control it. You must continue to take it—even if you feel well—if you expect to keep your blood pressure down. **You may have to take high blood pressure medicine for the rest of your life.**

This medicine may cause an unusual feeling of tiredness when you begin to take it. You may also notice an increase in urine or in frequency of urination. To keep this from affecting nighttime sleep:
- if you are to take a single dose a day, take it in the morning after breakfast.
- if you are to take more than one dose, take the last one no later than 6 p.m.

Ask your doctor about your pulse rate before and after taking beta-blockers. Then, while you are taking this medicine, check your pulse regularly. If it is much slower than your usual rate (or less than 50 beats per minute), check with your doctor. A pulse rate that is too slow may cause circulation problems.

Do not miss any doses, especially if you are taking only one dose per day. Some conditions may become worse when this medicine is not taken regularly.

If you do miss a dose of this medicine, take it as soon as possible. However, if the next scheduled dose is to be taken

within 4 hours (8 hours for atenolol and chlorthalidone, labetalol and hydrochlorothiazide, nadolol and bendroflumethiazide, or extended-release propranolol and hydrochlorothiazide), skip the missed dose and go back to your regular
dosing schedule. Do not double doses.

PRECAUTIONS WHILE USING THIS MEDICINE

This medicine may cause some people to become dizzy,
drowsy, or lightheaded. **Make sure you know how you react
to this medicine before you drive, use machines, or do other
jobs that require you to be alert.**

**Do not stop taking this medicine without checking with your
doctor.** Your doctor may want you to reduce gradually the
amount you are taking before stopping.

POSSIBLE SIDE EFFECTS OF THIS MEDICINE
Side Effects That Should Be Reported To Your Doctor

> *Less common*—Breathing difficulty and/or wheezing; cold
> hands and feet; hallucinations; irregular heartbeat;
> mental confusion or depression; slow pulse

> *Rare*—Chest pain; dark urine; fever and sore throat; joint
> pain; lower back or side pain; red, scaling, or crusted
> skin; severe stomach pain with vomiting; skin rash or
> hives; swelling of ankles, feet, and/or lower legs; un-
> usual bleeding or bruising; yellow eyes or skin

> *Signs of too much potassium loss*—Dryness of mouth;
> increased thirst; mood changes; muscle cramps or pain;
> weak or irregular heartbeat

Side Effects That Usually Do Not Require Medical Attention

These possible side effects may go away during treatment;
however, if they continue or are bothersome, check with your
doctor, nurse, or pharmacist.

> *More common*—Decreased sexual ability; dizziness or
> lightheadedness; drowsiness (slight); trouble in sleep-
> ing; unusual tiredness or weakness

After you have taken this medicine for a while, it may cause
unpleasant or harmful effects if you stop taking it suddenly.
Check with your doctor right away if you notice chest pain,
fast or irregular heartbeat, general feeling of body discomfort or weakness, headache, shortness of breath (sudden),
sweating, or trembling.

Other side effects not listed above may also occur in some
patients. If you notice any other effects, check with your
doctor, nurse, or pharmacist.

BETA-CAROTENE (Systemic)

Including Beta-carotene (For Dietary Supplement—Oral);
Beta-carotene (For Photosensitivity—Oral).

■For the Pharmacist■

In providing consultation, consider emphasizing the following selected
information (» = major clinical significance):

Description of use
Description should include function in the body; indications for use;
signs of deficiency; medical conditions requiring additional beta-
carotene; and unproven uses

Importance of diet
For use as a dietary supplement
Diet as treatment of choice
Food sources of beta-carotene; effects of processing
Not using vitamins as substitute for balanced diet
Supplement may be needed because of inadequate dietary intake
or increased requirements

Before using this medication
» Conditions affecting use, especially:
Sensitivity to beta-carotene

Proper use of this medication
For use as a dietary supplement
Function of beta-carotene in body; megadoses not recommended
without first checking with physician
» Proper dosing
Missed dose: No cause for concern because of length of time nec-
essary for depletion; remembering to take as directed
For use in photosensitivity
» Proper dosing
Missed dose: Taking as soon as possible; not taking if almost time
for next dose; not doubling doses
» Proper storage

Side/adverse effects
Yellow discoloration of skin is to be expected; if taking as nutritional
supplement, may be a sign that the dose is too high

▲ For the Patient ▲

918608

BETA-CAROTENE (For Dietary Supplement—Oral)

ABOUT YOUR DIETARY SUPPLEMENT

Vitamins (VYE-ta-mins) are compounds that you *must* have
for growth and health. They are needed in small amounts
only and are usually available in the foods that you eat.
Beta-carotene (bay-ta-KARE-oh-teen) is converted in the
body to vitamin A, which is necessary for normal growth
and health and for healthy eyes and skin.

If you do not get enough vitamin A in your diet, a rare
condition called night blindness (problems seeing in the dark)

may develop. Lack of vitamin A may also cause dry eyes, eye infections, skin problems, and slowed growth. Your doctor may treat these problems by prescribing beta-carotene or vitamin A for you.

Beta-carotene or vitamin A supplements may be needed in patients with the following conditions: continuing diarrhea; cystic fibrosis; liver disease; long-term illness; malabsorption problems; pancreas disease; or serious injury. If any of these conditions apply to you, you should take beta-carotene only on the advice of your doctor after need has been established.

Claims that beta-carotene is effective as a sunscreen have not been proven. Although beta-carotene is being studied for its ability to prevent certain types of cancer, there is not enough information to show that this treatment is effective.

If any of the information in this leaflet causes you special concern or if you want additional information about your dietary supplement and its use, check with your doctor, nurse, or pharmacist. **Remember, keep this and all other medicines out of the reach of children and never share your medicines with others.**

BEFORE USING THIS DIETARY SUPPLEMENT

Importance of diet—Vitamin supplements should be taken only if you cannot get enough vitamins in your diet; however, some diets may not contain all of the vitamins you need. Follow carefully any diet program your doctor may recommend. For your specific vitamin and/or mineral needs, ask your doctor for a list of appropriate foods. Beta-carotene is found in carrots; dark-green leafy vegetables, such as spinach and green leaf lettuce; tomatoes; sweet potatoes; broccoli; cantaloupe; and winter squash.

If you are taking this dietary supplement without a prescription, carefully read and follow any precautions on the label. You should be especially careful if you . . .
- are allergic to any medicine, either prescription or non-prescription (OTC);
- are pregnant, intend to become pregnant, or are breast-feeding;
- are taking any other prescription or nonprescription (OTC) medicine;
- have any other medical problems.

If you have any questions, check with your doctor, nurse, pharmacist, or dietitian.

PROPER USE OF THIS DIETARY SUPPLEMENT

Beta-carotene is safer than vitamin A (retinol) because vitamin A can be harmful in high doses. If you have a high level of vitamin A in your blood, then your body will convert less beta-carotene to vitamin A. However, you should take large doses of beta-carotene only under the direction of your doctor after need has been identified.

If you miss taking a vitamin for one or more days, there is no cause for concern, since it takes some time for your body to become seriously low in vitamins. However, if your doctor has recommended that you take this vitamin, try to remember to take it as directed every day.

POSSIBLE SIDE EFFECTS OF THIS DIETARY SUPPLEMENT

Side Effects That Usually Do Not Require Medical Attention

These possible side effects may go away during treatment; however, if they continue or are bothersome, check with your doctor, nurse, or pharmacist.

> *More common*—Yellowing of palms, hands, soles of feet, or face (this may be a sign that your dose of beta-carotene as a dietary supplement is too high)

> *Rare*—Diarrhea; dizziness; joint pain; unusual bleeding or bruising

Other side effects not listed above may also occur in some patients. If you notice any other effects, check with your doctor, nurse, or pharmacist.

▲ For the Patient ▲

918357

BETA-CAROTENE (For Photosensitivity—Oral)

ABOUT YOUR MEDICINE

Beta-carotene (bay-ta-KARE-oh-teen) is used to prevent or treat sun reaction (photosensitivity) in patients with a disease called erythropoietic protoporphyria.

It may also be used to treat other conditions as determined by your doctor. However, beta-carotene has not been shown to be useful as a sunscreen.

If any of the information in this leaflet causes you special concern or if you want additional information about your medicine and its use, check with your doctor, nurse, or pharmacist. **Remember, keep this and all other medicines out of the reach of children and never share your medicines with others.**

BEFORE USING THIS MEDICINE

If you are taking this medicine without a prescription, carefully read and follow any precautions on the label. You should be especially careful if you . . .

- are allergic to any medicine, either prescription or nonprescription (OTC);
- are pregnant, intend to become pregnant, or are breastfeeding;
- are taking any other prescription or nonprescription (OTC) medicine;

- have any other medical problems.

If you have any questions, check with your doctor, nurse, or pharmacist.

PROPER USE OF THIS MEDICINE

If you miss a dose of this medicine, take it as soon as possible. However, if it is almost time for your next dose, skip the missed dose and go back to your regular dosing schedule. Do not double doses.

POSSIBLE SIDE EFFECTS OF THIS MEDICINE

Side Effects That Usually Do Not Require Medical Attention

These possible side effects may go away during treatment; however, if they continue or are bothersome, check with your doctor, nurse, or pharmacist.

> *More common*—Yellowing of palms, hands, soles of feet, or face

> *Rare*—Diarrhea; dizziness; joint pain; unusual bleeding or bruising

Other side effects not listed above may also occur in some patients. If you notice any other effects, check with your doctor, nurse, or pharmacist.

BETHANECHOL Systemic

■ For the Pharmacist ■

In providing consultation, consider emphasizing the following selected information (» = major clinical significance):

Before using this medication
» Conditions affecting use, especially:
   Sensitivity to bethanechol
   Other medical problems, especially anastomosis, recent bladder surgery or gastrointestinal resection; asthma; pronounced bradycardia or hypotension; coronary artery disease; hyperthyroidism; peptic ulcer; peritonitis; or conditions in which the strength or integrity of the gastrointestinal or bladder wall is in question or in the presence of mechanical obstruction; or marked vagotonia

Proper use of this medication
» Taking medication on an empty stomach to minimize the possibility of nausea and vomiting, unless otherwise directed by physician
» Importance of not taking more medication than the amount prescribed
» Proper dosing
   Missed dose: Taking if remembered within an hour or so; not taking if remembered after 2 or more hours; not doubling doses
» Proper storage

Precautions while using this medication
   Caution when getting up suddenly from a lying or sitting position

Side/adverse effects
   Signs of potential side effects, especially shortness of breath, wheezing, or tightness in chest

▲ For the Patient ▲

913342

ABOUT YOUR MEDICINE

Bethanechol (be-THAN-e-kole) is taken to treat certain disorders of the urinary tract or bladder. It helps to cause urination and emptying of the bladder. Bethanechol may also be used for other conditions as determined by your doctor.

If any of the information in this leaflet causes you special concern or if you want additional information about your medicine and its use, check with your doctor, nurse, or pharmacist. **Remember, keep this and all other medicines out of the reach of children and never share your medicines with others.**

BEFORE USING THIS MEDICINE

Tell your doctor, nurse, and pharmacist if you . . .
   • are allergic to any medicine, either prescription or non-prescription (OTC);

- are pregnant or intend to become pregnant while using this medicine;
- are breast-feeding;
- are taking any other prescription or nonprescription (OTC) medicine;
- have any other medical problems, especially asthma, heart or blood vessel disease, intestinal blockage or other intestinal problems, overactive thyroid, recent bladder or intestinal surgery, or stomach ulcer or other stomach problems.

PROPER USE OF THIS MEDICINE

Take this medicine on an empty stomach (either 1 hour before or 2 hours after meals) to lessen the possibility of nausea and vomiting, unless otherwise directed by your doctor.

Take this medicine only as directed. Do not take more of it, do not take it more often, and do not take it for a longer time than your doctor ordered. To do so may increase the chance of side effects.

If you miss a dose of this medicine and you remember within an hour or so of the missed dose, take it right away. Then go back to your regular dosing schedule. However, if you do not remember until 2 or more hours after the missed dose, skip it and go back to your regular dosing schedule. Do not double doses.

PRECAUTIONS WHILE USING THIS MEDICINE

Dizziness, lightheadedness, or fainting may occur, especially when you get up from a lying or sitting position. Getting up slowly may help lessen this problem.

POSSIBLE SIDE EFFECTS OF THIS MEDICINE
Side Effects That Should Be Reported To Your Doctor

    Rare—Shortness of breath, wheezing, or tightness in chest

Other side effects not listed above may also occur in some patients. If you notice any other effects, check with your doctor, nurse, or pharmacist.

BROMOCRIPTINE   Systemic

■For the Pharmacist■

In providing consultation, consider emphasizing the following selected information (» = major clinical significance):

Before using this medication
» Conditions affecting use, especially:
   Sensitivity to bromocriptine or other ergot alkaloids
   Pregnancy—Use is not generally recommended
   Breast-feeding—Will prevent lactation in mothers who intend to breast-feed
   Use in the elderly—CNS effects may occur more frequently
   Dental—Reduced salivary flow caused by large doses may contribute to dental disorders
   Other medications, especially alcohol, oral contraceptives, estrogens, progestins, or other ergot alkaloids
   Other medical problems, especially history of hypertension or pregnancy-induced hypertension

Proper use of this medication
   Taking with meals or milk to reduce gastrointestinal irritation; taking dose at bedtime or first dose vaginally to better tolerate nausea
   Missed dose: Taking if remembered within 4 hours; otherwise not taking at all; not doubling doses
» Proper dosing
» Proper storage

Precautions while using this medication
   Regular visits to physician to check progress
» Caution when driving or doing jobs requiring alertness because of possible drowsiness or dizziness
   Dizziness may be more likely to occur after initial dose; taking first dose at bedtime or lying down; getting up slowly from sitting or lying position; taking first dose vaginally
» Possible dryness of mouth; using sugarless gum or candy, ice, or saliva substitute for relief; checking with physician or dentist if dry mouth continues for more than 2 weeks
   Checking with physician before reducing dosage or discontinuing medication
» Possibility of disulfiram-like reaction with alcohol
For treatment of amenorrhea, galactorrhea, acromegaly, or pituitary prolactinomas in females of child-bearing potential
   Advisability of using nonhormonal contraception during therapy; patients desiring pregnancy should discuss with physician proper time to discontinue use of contraception; telling physician immediately if pregnancy is suspected
» Telling physician right away if symptoms of enlargement of pituitary tumor (blurred vision, sudden headache, severe nausea and vomiting) occur
For treatment of female infertility
   Advisability of using nonhormonal contraception until normal menstrual cycle is established; discussing with physician proper time to discontinue use of contraception; telling physician immediately if pregnancy is suspected

» Telling physician right away if symptoms of enlargement of pituitary tumor (blurred vision, sudden headache, severe nausea and vomiting) occur

Side/adverse effects

Signs of potential side effects, especially CNS effects, fainting, myocardial infarction, seizures, gastrointestinal hemorrhage, peptic ulcer, retroperitoneal fibrosis, rhinorrhea, and strokes

---

▲ For the Patient ▲

913069

ABOUT YOUR MEDICINE

Bromocriptine (broe-moe-KRIP-teen) is a medicine used to treat several different types of medical problems. It is used to treat certain menstrual problems; as a fertility medicine in some women who are unable to become pregnant; to stop milk production in some women; to treat Parkinson's disease; to treat acromegaly (overproduction of growth hormone); or to treat pituitary prolactinomas (tumors of the pituitary gland). Bromocriptine may also be used for other conditions as determined by your doctor.

If any of the information in this leaflet causes you special concern or if you want additional information about your medicine and its use, check with your doctor, nurse, or pharmacist. **Remember, keep this and all other medicines out of the reach of children and never share your medicines with others.**

BEFORE USING THIS MEDICINE

Tell your doctor, nurse, and pharmacist if you . . .

- are allergic to any medicine, either prescription or non-prescription (OTC);
- are pregnant or intend to become pregnant while using this medicine;
- are breast-feeding;
- are taking any other prescription or nonprescription (OTC) medicine, especially birth control pills, ergot alkaloids, estrogens, or progestins;
- have any other medical problems, especially high blood pressure (history of or pregnancy-induced).

PROPER USE OF THIS MEDICINE

If bromocriptine upsets your stomach, it may be taken with meals or milk or at bedtime. If stomach upset continues, check with your doctor.

If you miss a dose of this medicine, take the missed dose if you remember it within 4 hours. However, if a longer time has passed, skip the missed dose and go back to your regular schedule. Do not double doses.

PRECAUTIONS WHILE USING THIS MEDICINE

This medicine may cause some people to become drowsy, dizzy, or less alert than they are normally. **Make sure you**

know how you react before you drive, use machines, or do other jobs that require you to be alert.

Dizziness is more likely to occur after the first dose of bromocriptine. It may be helpful if you get up slowly from a lying or sitting position. Taking the first dose vaginally or at bedtime or when you are able to lie down may also lessen problems.

It may take several weeks for bromocriptine to work. Do not stop taking it or reduce the amount you are taking without first checking with your doctor.

For females who are able to bear children:

- It is best to use some type of birth control while you are taking bromocriptine. However, do not use oral contraceptives (the "Pill") since they may prevent bromocriptine from working. If you wish to become pregnant, you and your doctor should decide on the best time for you to stop using birth control.
- Tell your doctor right away if you think you have become pregnant. You and your doctor should discuss whether you should continue to take bromocriptine during pregnancy. **Check with your doctor right away** if you have blurred vision, a sudden headache, or severe nausea and vomiting.

Drinking alcohol while you are taking bromocriptine may cause you to have a certain reaction. **Avoid alcohol until you have discussed this with your doctor.**

POSSIBLE SIDE EFFECTS OF THIS MEDICINE

Some serious side effects have occurred during the use of bromocriptine to stop milk flow after pregnancy or abortion. These side effects have included strokes, seizures (convulsions), and heart attacks. Some deaths have also occurred. You should discuss with your doctor the good that this medicine will do as well as the risks of using it.

Side Effects That Should Be Reported To Your Doctor Immediately

Rare—Black, tarry stools; bloody vomit; chest pain (severe); convulsions (seizures); fainting; fast heartbeat; headache (unusual); increased sweating; nausea and vomiting (severe); nervousness; shortness of breath (unexplained); vision changes (such as blurred vision or temporary blindness); weakness (sudden)

Other Side Effects That Should Be Reported To Your Doctor

Less common (reported more often in patients with Parkinson's disease)—Confusion; hallucinations; uncontrolled movements of the body

Rare—Abdominal or stomach pain (continuing or severe); increased frequency of urination; loss of appetite (continuing); lower back pain; runny nose (continuing); weakness

Side Effects That Usually Do Not Require Medical Attention

These possible side effects may go away during treatment; however, if they continue or are bothersome, check with your doctor, nurse, or pharmacist.

More common—Dizziness or lightheadedness; nausea

Other side effects not listed above may also occur in some patients. If you notice any other effects, check with your doctor, nurse, or pharmacist.

BRONCHODILATORS, ADRENERGIC   Systemic

Including Albuterol; Bitolterol; Ephedrine; Epinephrine; Ethylnorepinephrine; Fenoterol; Isoetharine; Isoproterenol; Metaproterenol; Pirbuterol; Procaterol; Racepinephrine; Terbutaline.

■ For the Pharmacist ■

In providing consultation, consider emphasizing the following selected information (» = major clinical significance):

Before using this medication
» Conditions affecting use, especially:
    Sensitivity to sympathomimetics
    Allergies to sulfites present in some preparations of ephedrine, epinephrine, ethylnorepinephrine, fenoterol, isoetharine, and isoproterenol
    Pregnancy—
        For albuterol, bitolterol, and metaproterenol
            Studies in animals have shown albuterol, bitolterol, and metaproterenol to cause teratogenic effects when medication given in doses many times human dose
        For epinephrine
            Studies in animals have shown epinephrine to cause teratogenic effects when medication given in doses many times human dose
            Use of epinephrine during pregnancy may cause anoxia in fetus
        For pirbuterol
            Studies in animals have shown pirbuterol at high doses to cause abortions and fetal mortality
        For terbutaline
            Parenteral administration of terbutaline during pregnancy reported to cause fetal tachycardia
    Labor and/or delivery—
        For albuterol
            Albuterol given intravenously or orally reportedly inhibits uterine contractions
        For epinephrine
            Epinephrine is not recommended for use during labor because it may delay second stage; also may cause prolonged uterine atony with hemorrhage when given in sufficient dosage to reduce uterine contractions
        For terbutaline
            Terbutaline inhibits uterine activity during second and third trimesters of pregnancy and may inhibit labor; when administered during labor, terbutaline reported to cause serious adverse reactions (e.g., transient hypokalemia, pulmonary edema, hypoglycemia) in mother and hypoglycemia in neonates of mothers treated with parenteral terbutaline
    Breast-feeding—
        For albuterol
            Not known if albuterol is distributed into breast milk; however, some animal studies have shown albuterol to be potentially tumorigenic

For epinephrine

Epinephrine distributed into breast milk; use by nursing mothers may cause serious adverse reactions in infant

For terbutaline

Terbutaline distributed into breast milk; some animal studies have shown terbutaline to be potentially tumorigenic

Use in children—

For epinephrine

Epinephrine should be used with caution in infants and children, since syncope has occurred following administration of epinephrine in asthmatic children

Dental—

For epinephrine

Epinephrine present in gingival retraction cords; systemic absorption of epinephrine from retraction cords may occur; epinephrine retraction cords should be used with caution in patients with cardiovascular problems

Other medications, especially—

For all adrenergic bronchodilators

Beta-adrenergic blocking agents; cocaine, mucosal-local; digitalis glycosides

For albuterol, metaproterenol, pirbuterol, procaterol, and terbutaline only

Maprotiline, monoamine oxidase (MAO) inhibitors, tricyclic antidepressants

For ephedrine only

Ergoloid mesylates, ergotamine, monoamine oxidase (MAO) inhibitors

For epinephrine only

Ergoloid mesylates, ergotamine, maprotiline, tricyclic antidepressants

For fenoterol only

Monoamine oxidase (MAO) inhibitors

For isoproterenol only

Maprotiline, tricyclic antidepressants

Other medical problems, especially—

For all adrenergic bronchodilators

Cardiovascular disease

For epinephrine only

Brain damage, organic

Proper use of this medication

For all adrenergic bronchodilators

» Importance of not using more medication than the amount recommended

» Proper dosing

» Proper storage

For all adrenergic bronchodilators, except ethylnorepinephrine

Missed dose: If on scheduled dosing regimen, using as soon as possible; using any remaining doses for the day at regularly spaced intervals; not doubling doses

For ephedrine only

» Taking the medication a few hours before bedtime to minimize the possibility of insomnia

For epinephrine only

Not using if solution or suspension is pinkish to brownish in color or if solution contains a precipitate

» Not using inhalation dosage form of epinephrine without a physician's prescription unless medical problem is diagnosed as asthma

For isoetharine and isoproterenol only
> Not using if solution is pinkish to brownish in color or if solution contains a precipitate

For all inhalation dosage forms
> Proper administration:
>> Reading patient instructions carefully before using
>> Knowing correct administration technique if using in a nebulizer or a combination nebulizer and respirator; checking with physician, nurse, or pharmacist if necessary

For all inhalation aerosols
» Avoiding contact with the eyes
» Taking no more than 2 inhalations at one time with interval of 1 to 2 minutes between inhalations
> Saving applicator; refill units may be available

For albuterol extended-release tablet dosage form only
> Swallowing tablet whole; not crushing, breaking, or chewing

For epinephrine and ethylnorepinephrine injection dosage forms only
» Using only for conditions as prescribed by physician
> Keeping ready for use at all times; also keeping telephone numbers for physician and nearest hospital emergency room readily available
> Checking expiration date routinely; replacing medication before it expires
> Knowing correct administration technique for self-administration; checking with physician if necessary

For emergency use of epinephrine injection in allergic reaction—
» Using medication immediately
> Notifying physician immediately or going to nearest hospital emergency room
> If stung by an insect, removing insect's stinger; applying ice packs or sodium bicarbonate soaks, if available, to area stung
> For auto-injector use:
>> Importance of not removing safety cap on auto-injector before ready to use
>> Reading patient instructions carefully before need to use medication
>> Procedures for using—
>>> Removing gray safety cap
>>> Placing black tip on thigh at right angle to leg
>>> Pressing hard into thigh until auto-injector functions; holding in place several seconds; removing and properly discarding
>>> Massaging injection area for 10 seconds

For isoproterenol sublingual tablet dosage form only
> Not chewing or swallowing tablet whole, but dissolving slowly under tongue; not swallowing until tablet completely dissolved

Precautions while using this medication
For albuterol, bitolterol, epinephrine inhalation, metaproterenol, pirbuterol, procaterol, and terbutaline
» Checking with physician immediately if difficulty in breathing persists after use of medication or if condition becomes worse

For ephedrine and ethylnorepinephrine
» Possibility of allergic reaction to sulfites contained in some preparations; checking with physician immediately if signs of allergic reaction occur

For epinephrine only
> Diabetics: May increase blood glucose concentrations

»   Possibility of allergic reaction to sulfites contained in some preparations; checking with physician immediately if signs of allergic reaction occur

For fenoterol, isoetharine, and isoproterenol

»   Checking with physician immediately if difficulty in breathing persists after use of medication or if condition becomes worse

»   Possibility of allergic reaction to sulfites contained in some preparations; checking with physician immediately if signs of allergic reaction occur

For inhalation dosage forms only

Possible dryness of mouth and throat; rinsing mouth with water after each dose to help prevent dryness

For inhalation aerosol dosage forms

»   For patients also using a corticosteroid or ipratropium inhalation aerosol: Using adrenergic bronchodilator inhalation aerosol 5 minutes prior to the corticosteroid or ipratropium inhalation aerosol, unless otherwise directed by physician

Checking with physician if contents of one canister of albuterol inhalation aerosol is used in less than 2 weeks

Side/adverse effects

Signs of potential side effects, especially:

For all adrenergic bronchodilators

Paradoxical bronchospasm

For albuterol

Chest discomfort or pain, unusual or bad taste

In some animal studies, albuterol caused increased incidence of benign leiomyomas of mesovarium when administered at doses many times the maximum human inhalation or oral dose

For bitolterol

Chest discomfort or pain, irregular heartbeat

For ephedrine

Chest discomfort or pain, irregular heartbeat, allergic reaction to sulfites present in some preparations, hallucinations (with high doses), mood or mental changes

For epinephrine

Chest discomfort or pain, irregular heartbeat, allergic reaction to sulfites present in some preparations, hallucinations (with high doses)

For ethylnorepinephrine

Allergic reaction to sulfites present in some preparations

For fenoterol

Allergic reaction to sulfites present in some preparations, unusual or bad taste

For isoetharine

Allergic reaction to sulfites present in some preparations

For isoproterenol

Chest discomfort or pain, irregular heartbeat, allergic reaction to sulfites present in some preparations

Pinkish to red coloration of saliva caused by oxidation of isoproterenol in mouth may be alarming to patient although medically insignificant

For metaproterenol

Unusual or bad taste

For pirbuterol

Chest discomfort or pain, irregular heartbeat, mood or mental changes, changes in smell or taste, numbness in feet or hands, unusual bruising

For procaterol

Chest discomfort or pain

For terbutaline
> Chest discomfort or pain, irregular heartbeat, unusual or bad taste
>
> Some studies in animals have shown that terbutaline caused increased incidence of leiomyomas of mesovarium, ovarian cysts, and hyperplasia of mesovarium when administered at oral doses many times the recommended daily adult dose

---

▲ For the Patient ▲

912769

ADRENERGIC BRONCHODILATORS (Inhalation):
Including Albuterol; Bitolterol; Epinephrine; Fenoterol; Isoetharine; Isoproterenol; Metaproterenol; Pirbuterol; Procaterol; Racepinephrine; Terbutaline.

ABOUT YOUR MEDICINE

Adrenergic bronchodilators are taken by oral inhalation to treat the symptoms of bronchial asthma, chronic bronchitis, emphysema, and other lung diseases. These medicines relieve cough, wheezing, shortness of breath, and troubled breathing.

If any of the information in this leaflet causes you special concern or if you want additional information about your medicine and its use, check with your doctor, nurse, or pharmacist. **Remember, keep this and all other medicines out of the reach of children and never share your medicines with others.**

BEFORE USING THIS MEDICINE

If you are taking this medicine without a prescription, carefully read and follow any precautions on the label. You should be especially careful if you . . .
- are allergic to any medicine, either prescription or nonprescription (OTC);
- are pregnant, intend to become pregnant, or are breast-feeding;
- are taking **any** other prescription or nonprescription (OTC) medicine;
- have **any** other medical problems;
- are now using or have used cocaine.

If you have any questions, check with your doctor, nurse, or pharmacist.

PROPER USE OF THIS MEDICINE

For patients using epinephrine, isoetharine, isoproterenol, or racepinephrine:
- Do not use if the solution becomes cloudy or turns pinkish to brownish in color.

Some epinephrine preparations are available without a doctor's prescription. However, **do not use this medicine without** a doctor's prescription, unless your medical problem has been diagnosed as asthma by a doctor.

Some of these preparations may come with patient directions. Read them carefully before using this medicine.

Use this medicine only as directed. Do not use more of it and do not use it more often than recommended.

For patients using the inhalation aerosol form of this medicine:

- **Keep spray away from the eyes because it may cause irritation.**
- **Do not take more than 2 inhalations of this medicine at any one time,** unless otherwise directed by your doctor. Allow 1 to 2 minutes after the first inhalation to make certain that a second inhalation is necessary.
- Save your applicator. Refill units may be available.
- Store away from heat and direct sunlight. Do not puncture, break, or burn container, even if it is empty.

If you are using this medicine regularly and you miss a dose, use it as soon as possible. Then use any remaining doses for that day at regularly spaced intervals. Do not double doses.

PRECAUTIONS WHILE USING THIS MEDICINE

If you still have trouble breathing after using this medicine, or if your condition becomes worse, check with your doctor at once.

If you are using the inhalation aerosol form of this medicine and you are also using an adrenocorticoid or ipratropium inhaler to help you breathe better, allow 5 minutes between using this medicine and the adrenocorticoid or ipratropium, unless otherwise directed.

POSSIBLE SIDE EFFECTS OF THIS MEDICINE

Side Effects That Should Be Reported To Your Doctor Immediately

Bluish coloration of skin; dizziness (severe) or feeling faint; flushing or redness of face or skin (continuing); increased wheezing or difficulty in breathing; skin rash, hives, or itching; swelling of face, lips, or eyelids

Other Side Effects That Should Be Reported To Your Doctor

Rare—Chest discomfort or pain; irregular heartbeat; numbness in hands or feet; unusual bruising

With high doses—Hallucinations

Possible signs of overdose—Dizziness (severe); fast, slow, irregular, or pounding heartbeat (continuing); headache (continuing or severe); increase or decrease in blood pressure (severe); nausea or vomiting (continuing or severe); weakness (severe)

Side Effects That Usually Do Not Require Medical Attention

These possible side effects may go away during treatment; however, if they continue or are bothersome, check with your doctor, nurse, or pharmacist.

> *More common*—Nervousness or restlessness; trembling

> *Less common*—Coughing or other bronchial irritation; dizziness or lightheadedness; dryness or irritation of mouth or throat; headache; increased sweating; nausea or vomiting; trouble in sleeping; weakness

While you are using some of these medicines, you may notice an unusual or unpleasant taste. Also, pirbuterol may cause changes in smell or taste and isoproterenol may cause the saliva to turn pinkish to red. These effects may be expected and will go away when you stop using the medicine.

Other side effects not listed above may also occur in some patients. If you notice any other effects, check with your doctor, nurse, or pharmacist.

▲ For the Patient ▲

912770

ADRENERGIC BRONCHODILATORS (Oral/ Injection): *Including Albuterol; Ephedrine; Epinephrine; Ethylnorepinephrine; Fenoterol; Isoproterenol; Metaproterenol; Terbutaline.*

ABOUT YOUR MEDICINE

Adrenergic bronchodilators are used to treat the symptoms of bronchial asthma, chronic bronchitis, emphysema, and other lung diseases. These medicines relieve cough, wheezing, shortness of breath, and troubled breathing. Adrenergic bronchodilators may also be used for other conditions as determined by your doctor.

If any of the information in this leaflet causes you special concern or if you want additional information about your medicine and its use, check with your doctor, nurse, or pharmacist. **Remember, keep this and all other medicines out of the reach of children and never share your medicines with others.**

BEFORE USING THIS MEDICINE

If you are taking this medicine without a prescription, carefully read and follow any precautions on the label. You should be especially careful if you . . .

- are allergic to any medicine, either prescription or non-prescription (OTC);
- are pregnant, intend to become pregnant, or are breast-feeding;
- are taking **any** other prescription or nonprescription (OTC) medicine;

- have **any** other medical problems;
- are now using or have used cocaine.

If you have any questions, check with your doctor, nurse, or pharmacist.

PROPER USE OF THIS MEDICINE

Use this medicine only as directed. Do not use more of it and do not use it more often than ordered. To do so may increase the chance of side effects.

Adrenergic bronchodilators, especially ephedrine, may cause some people to have trouble in sleeping. To help prevent this, **take the last dose for each day a few hours before bedtime.**

For patients taking **albuterol extended-release tablets:**
- Swallow the tablet whole.
- Do not crush, break, or chew before swallowing.

For patients using **epinephrine injection:**
- Do not use if the solution or suspension turns pinkish to brownish in color or if the solution becomes cloudy.
- **Use this medicine only for the conditions for which it was prescribed by your doctor.**
- If you are using this medicine **for an allergic reaction emergency** and an allergic reaction as described by your doctor occurs, **use the epinephrine injection immediately**.

If you are using this medicine regularly and you miss a dose, use it as soon as possible. Then use any remaining doses for that day at regularly spaced intervals. Do not double doses.

PRECAUTIONS WHILE USING THIS MEDICINE

If you still have trouble breathing after using this medicine, or if your condition becomes worse, check with your doctor at once.

POSSIBLE SIDE EFFECTS OF THIS MEDICINE

Side Effects That Should Be Reported To Your Doctor Immediately

Bluish coloration of skin; dizziness (severe) or feeling faint; flushing or redness of face or skin (continuing); increased wheezing or difficulty in breathing; skin rash, hives, or itching; swelling of face, lips, or eyelids

Other Side Effects That Should Be Reported To Your Doctor

Rare—Chest discomfort or pain; irregular heartbeat

With high doses—Hallucinations

Possible signs of overdose—Dizziness (severe); fast, slow, irregular, or pounding heartbeat (continuing); headache (continuing or severe); increase or decrease in blood pressure (severe); nausea or vomiting (continuing or severe); weakness (severe)

Side Effects That Usually Do Not Require Medical Attention

These possible side effects may go away during treatment; however, if they continue or are bothersome, check with your doctor, nurse, or pharmacist.

More common—Nervousness or restlessness; trembling

Less common—Dizziness or lightheadedness; fast or pounding heartbeat; headache; increase in blood pressure; increased sweating; nausea or vomiting; trouble in sleeping; weakness

While you are using albuterol, fenoterol, metaproterenol, or terbutaline, you may notice an unusual or unpleasant taste. This is to be expected and will go away when you stop using the medicine.

Other side effects not listed above may also occur in some patients. If you notice any other effects, check with your doctor, nurse, or pharmacist.

BRONCHODILATORS, XANTHINE-DERIVATIVE Systemic

Including Aminophylline; Dyphylline; Oxtriphylline; Theophylline.

■For the Pharmacist■

In providing consultation, consider emphasizing the following selected information (» = major clinical significance):

Before using this medication
» Conditions affecting use, especially:
   Sensitivity to xanthines or to ethylenediamine in aminophylline
   Mutagenicity—Theophylline reported to cause chromosomal breakage in human cells in culture at concentrations up to 50 times maximum therapeutic serum concentration
   Pregnancy—Studies in mice have shown theophylline to cause teratogenic effects when given in doses 30 times the human dose (FDA Pregnancy Category C); use during pregnancy may result in potentially dangerous serum theophylline and caffeine concentrations in neonates; tachycardia, jitteriness, irritability, gagging, and vomiting reported in some neonates; neonates of mothers taking theophylline during pregnancy should be monitored for signs of theophylline toxicity
   Breast-feeding—Theophylline and dyphylline distributed into breast milk; use of aminophylline, oxtriphylline, or theophylline by nursing mothers may cause irritability, fretfulness, or insomnia in infants
   Use in children—Possible decreased plasma clearance and increased serum concentrations and/or toxicity in neonates, especially premature neonates; repeated doses should not be given if heart rate greater than 180 beats per minute
   Use in the elderly—Possible decreased plasma clearance and increased potential for toxicity in patients over 55 years of age
   Other medications, especially beta-adrenergic blocking agents, cimetidine, ciprofloxacin, corticosteroids, erythromycin, phenytoin, nicotine chewing gum, norfloxacin, ranitidine, troleandomycin, or smoking tobacco or marijuana
   Other medical problems, especially active gastritis, active or history of peptic ulcer, congestive heart failure (for aminophylline and sodium chloride only), or renal function impairment (for aminophylline and sodium chloride and dyphylline only)

Proper use of this medication
» Importance of not using more medication than the amount prescribed
» Compliance with therapy; not missing any doses
» Proper dosing
   Missed dose: Taking as soon as possible; not taking if almost time for next dose; not doubling doses
» Proper storage
   Proper administration:
   For enteric-coated or delayed-release tablet dosage form
      Swallowing tablets whole
      Not breaking, crushing, or chewing

For extended-release dosage forms
   Swallowing capsules or tablets whole
   Not breaking (unless tablet dosage form is scored for breaking),
      crushing, or chewing
For oral liquid, immediate-release capsule or tablet, or extended-release (not including once-a-day) capsule or tablet dosage forms
» Taking on empty stomach with a glass of water for faster absorption
      or, if necessary, taking with meals or immediately after meals
      to lessen gastrointestinal irritation, unless otherwise directed
For once-a-day capsule or tablet dosage forms
» Taking once a day each morning after fasting overnight and at least
      1 hour before eating or taking each morning or evening with or
      without food, depending on product; trying to take at same time
      each day

Precautions while using this medication
   Regular visits to physician to check progress during initial period
      of therapy
» Not changing brands or dosage forms without first checking with
      physician
» Caution in eating or drinking large amounts of xanthine-containing
      foods or beverages during therapy with this medication
For aminophylline, oxtriphylline, and theophylline only
   Not eating charcoal-broiled foods daily because of possible decrease
      in effects of medication
» Notifying physician immediately if symptoms of influenza, a fever,
      or diarrhea occur because of possible need to alter dosage

Side/adverse effects
   Signs of potential side effects, especially gastroesophageal reflux,
      allergic reaction to ethylenediamine in aminophylline, and re-
      action to too-rapid intravenous administration or to solution or
      administration technique (parenteral dosage forms only)

▲ For the Patient ▲

912882

ABOUT YOUR MEDICINE

Xanthine bronchodilators are used to treat and/or prevent
the symptoms of bronchial asthma, chronic bronchitis, and
emphysema. These medicines relieve cough, wheezing,
shortness of breath, and troubled breathing. Aminophylline
and theophylline may also be used for other conditions as
determined by your doctor.

If any of the information in this leaflet causes you special
concern or if you want additional information about your
medicine and its use, check with your doctor, nurse, or pharmacist. **Remember, keep this and all other medicines out of
the reach of children and never share your medicines with
others.**

BEFORE USING THIS MEDICINE

Tell your doctor, nurse, and pharmacist if you . . .
   • are allergic to any medicine, either prescription or non-
      prescription (OTC);
   • are pregnant or intend to become pregnant while using
      this medicine;

- are breast-feeding;
- are taking any other prescription or nonprescription (OTC) medicine, especially adrenocorticoids (cortisone-like medicine), beta-blockers, cimetidine, ciprofloxacin, erythromycin, nicotine chewing gum, norfloxacin, phenytoin, ranitidine, or troleandomycin;
- smoke or have smoked (tobacco or marijuana) within the last 2 years;
- have any other medical problems, especially stomach ulcer (or history of) or other stomach problems.

PROPER USE OF THIS MEDICINE

For patients taking the capsule, tablet, liquid, or extended-release (not including the once-a-day capsule or tablet) form of this medicine:

- **This medicine works best when taken with a glass of water on an empty stomach** (either 30 minutes to 1 hour before or 2 hours after meals) since that way it will get into the blood sooner. However, in some cases your doctor may want you to take this medicine with or right after meals to lessen stomach upset.

For patients taking the once-a-day capsule or tablet form of this medicine:

- **Some products are to be taken each morning after fasting overnight and at least 1 hour before eating. However, other products are to be taken in the morning or evening with or without food. Be sure you understand exactly how to take the medicine prescribed for you.** Try to take the medicine at about the same time each day.

Use this medicine only as directed by your doctor. Do not use more of it, do not use it more often, and do not use it for a longer time than your doctor ordered. To do so may increase the chance of serious side effects.

In order for this medicine to help your medical problem, it must be taken every day in regularly spaced doses.

If you miss a dose of this medicine, take it as soon as possible. However, if it is almost time for your next dose, skip the missed dose and go back to your regular dosing schedule. Do not double doses.

PRECAUTIONS WHILE USING THIS MEDICINE

Your doctor should check your progress at regular visits, especially for the first few weeks after you begin using this medicine.

Do not change brands or dosage forms of this medicine without first checking with your doctor. Different products may not work the same way.

This medicine may add to the central nervous system (CNS) stimulant effects of caffeine-containing foods or beverages such as chocolate, cocoa, tea, coffee, and cola drinks. **Avoid eating or drinking large amounts of these foods or beverages while using this medicine.**

Check with your doctor at once if you develop symptoms of influenza (flu) or a fever since either of these may increase the chance of side effects with this medicine. Also, **check with your doctor if diarrhea occurs** because the dose of this medicine may need to be changed.

POSSIBLE SIDE EFFECTS OF THIS MEDICINE
Side Effects That Should Be Reported To Your Doctor

> *Less common*—Heartburn and/or vomiting

> *Rare*—Skin rash or hives

> *Signs of overdose*—Bloody or black tarry stools; confusion or change in behavior; convulsions (seizures); diarrhea; dizziness or lightheadedness; fast breathing; fast, pounding, or irregular heartbeat; flushing or redness of face; headache; increased urination; irritability; loss of appetite; muscle twitching; stomach cramps or pain; trembling; trouble in sleeping; unusual tiredness or weakness; vomiting of blood or material that looks like coffee grounds

Side Effects That Usually Do Not Require Medical Attention

These possible side effects may go away during treatment; however, if they continue or are bothersome, check with your doctor, nurse, or pharmacist.

> *More common*—Nausea; nervousness or restlessness

Other side effects not listed above may also occur in some patients. If you notice any other effects, check with your doctor, nurse, or pharmacist.

BUCLIZINE Systemic

∎For the Pharmacist∎

In providing consultation, consider emphasizing the following selected information (» = major clinical significance):

Before using this medication
» Conditions affecting use, especially:
    Sensitivity to buclizine
    Pregnancy—Animal studies have shown buclizine to be terato-genic at doses above therapeutic range
    Breast-feeding—May be distributed into breast milk; may inhibit lactation due to anticholinergic effects
    Use in children—Possible increased susceptibility to anticholinergic side effects
    Use in the elderly—Possible increased susceptibility to anticholinergic side effects
    Other medications, especially other CNS depressants

Proper use of this medication
    Taking with food, water, or milk to minimize gastric irritation
    Not taking more medication than the amount recommended
    For motion sickness, taking at least 30 minutes before traveling
» Proper dosing
    Missed dose (if on a regular dosing regimen): Taking as soon as possible; not taking if almost time for next dose; not doubling doses
» Proper storage

Precautions while using this medication
    Possible interference with skin tests using allergens; need to inform physician of using this medication
» Avoiding use of alcohol or other CNS depressants
» Caution if drowsiness occurs
    Possible dryness of mouth; using sugarless gum or candy, ice, or saliva substitute for relief

▲ For the Patient ▲

912394

MECLIZINE/BUCLIZINE/CYCLIZINE (Oral):
Including Meclizine; Buclizine; Cyclizine.

ABOUT YOUR MEDICINE

Meclizine (MEK-li-zeen), **buclizine** (BYOO-kli-zeen), and **cyclizine** (SYE-kli-zeen) are used to prevent and treat nausea, vomiting, and dizziness associated with motion sickness, and dizziness caused by other medical problems.

If any of the information in this leaflet causes you special concern or if you want additional information about your medicine and its use, check with your doctor, nurse, or pharmacist. **Remember, keep this and all other medicines out of the reach of children and never share your medicines with others.**

BEFORE USING THIS MEDICINE

If you are taking this medicine without a prescription, carefully read and follow any precautions on the label. You should be especially careful if you . . .

- are allergic to any medicine, either prescription or non-prescription (OTC);
- are pregnant, intend to become pregnant, or are breast-feeding;
- are taking any other prescription or nonprescription (OTC) medicine, especially other CNS depressants;
- have any other medical problems.

If you have any questions, check with your doctor, nurse, or pharmacist.

PROPER USE OF THIS MEDICINE

This medicine is used to relieve or prevent the symptoms of motion sickness or dizziness caused by other medical problems. Take it only as directed. Do not take more of it or take it more often than stated on the label or ordered by your doctor. To do so may increase the chance of side effects.

For patients taking this medicine for motion sickness:

—take buclizine or cyclizine at least 30 minutes before you begin to travel.
—take meclizine at least 1 hour before you begin to travel.

Take this medicine with food or a glass of water or milk to lessen stomach irritation, if necessary.

If you must take this medicine regularly and you miss a dose, take the missed dose as soon as possible. However, if it is almost time for your next dose, skip the missed dose and go back to your regular dosing schedule. Do not double doses.

PRECAUTIONS WHILE USING THIS MEDICINE

This medicine will add to the effects of alcohol and other CNS depressants (medicines that slow down the nervous system). **Check with your doctor before taking any such depressants while you are taking this medicine.**

This medicine may cause some people to become drowsy or less alert than they are normally. **Make sure you know how you react to this medicine before you drive, use machines, or do other jobs that require you to be alert.**

Buclizine, cyclizine, and meclizine may cause dryness of the mouth. For temporary relief use sugarless candy or gum, dissolve bits of ice in your mouth, or use a saliva substitute. However, if your mouth continues to feel dry for more than 2 weeks, check with your physician or dentist. Continuing dryness of the mouth may increase the chance of dental disease, including tooth decay, gum disease, and fungus infections.

POSSIBLE SIDE EFFECTS OF THIS MEDICINE
Side Effects That Usually Do Not Require Medical Attention

These possible side effects may go away during treatment; however, if they continue or are bothersome, check with your doctor, nurse, or pharmacist.

More common—Drowsiness

Less common or rare—Blurred vision; constipation; difficult or painful urination; dizziness; dryness of mouth, nose, and throat; fast heartbeat; headache; loss of appetite; nervousness, restlessness, or trouble in sleeping; skin rash; upset stomach

Other side effects not listed above may also occur in some patients. If you notice any other effects, check with your doctor, nurse, or pharmacist.

BUPROPION   Systemic

■ For the Pharmacist ■

In providing consultation, consider emphasizing the following selected information (» = major clinical significance):

Before using this medication
» Conditions affecting use, especially:
   Sensitivity to bupropion
   Pregnancy—Crosses placenta
   Breast-feeding—Distributed into breast milk; because of potential for serious adverse effects in the infant, use is not recommended
   Other medications, especially alcohol, antipsychotic medications, fluoxetine, lithium, MAO inhibitors, maprotiline, trazodone, or tricyclic antidepressants
   Other medical problems, especially anorexia nervosa, bulimia, CNS tumor, head trauma, hepatic or renal function impairment, recent myocardial infarction, or seizure disorders

Proper use of this medication
» Compliance with therapy; not taking more or less medication than prescribed
   Taking with food if needed to lessen gastrointestinal irritation
   May require up to 4 weeks or longer for optimal antidepressant effects
» Proper dosing
   Missed dose: Taking as soon as possible; taking any remaining doses for that day at regularly spaced intervals of no less than 4 hours; not doubling doses
» Proper storage

Precautions while using this medication
   Regular visits to physician to check progress during therapy
» Checking with physician before discontinuing medication; gradual dosage reduction may be necessary to prevent adverse effects
» Minimizing consumption of or avoiding use of alcoholic beverages to prevent possible seizures
» Possible dizziness, drowsiness, or euphoria; caution when driving, using machinery, or doing other things requiring alertness and judgment

Side/adverse effects
   Signs of potential side effects, especially CNS stimulation, fast or irregular heartbeat, severe headache, hallucinations, skin rash, fainting, or seizures

▲ For the Patient ▲

916952

ABOUT YOUR MEDICINE
Bupropion (byoo-PROE-pee-on) is an antidepressant or "mood elevator." It relieves mental depression.

If any of the information in this leaflet causes you special concern or if you want additional information about your medicine and its use, check with your doctor, nurse, or pharmacist. **Remember, keep this and all other medicines out of**

the reach of children and never share your medicines with others.

BEFORE USING THIS MEDICINE
Tell your doctor, nurse, and pharmacist if you . . .

- are allergic to any medicine, either prescription or non-prescription (OTC);
- are pregnant or intend to become pregnant while using this medicine;
- are breast-feeding;
- are taking any other prescription or nonprescription (OTC) medicine, especially antipsychotics (medicine for mental illness), fluoxetine, lithium, MAO inhibitors, maprotiline, trazodone, or tricyclic antidepressants;
- have any other medical problems, especially anorexia nervosa; brain tumor; bulimia; head injury (history of); heart attack (recent); kidney disease; liver disease; other nervous, mental, or emotional conditions; or seizure disorder.

PROPER USE OF THIS MEDICINE
Use bupropion only as directed by your doctor. Do not use more of it, do not use it more often, and do not use it for a longer time than your doctor ordered. To do so may increase the chance of side effects.

To lessen stomach upset, this medicine may be taken with food, unless your doctor has told you to take it on an empty stomach.

Usually this medicine must be taken for several weeks before you feel better. Your doctor should check your progress at regular visits.

If you miss a dose of this medicine, take it as soon as possible. However, if it is within 4 hours of your next dose, skip the missed dose and go back to your regular dosing schedule. Do not double doses.

PRECAUTIONS WHILE USING THIS MEDICINE
Your doctor should check your progress at regular visits, especially during the first few months of treatment with this medicine. The amount of bupropion you take may have to be changed often to meet the needs of your condition and to help avoid unwanted effects.

If you have been taking this medicine regularly, do not stop taking it without first checking with your doctor. Your doctor may want you to reduce gradually the amount you are taking before stopping completely. This will help reduce the chance of side effects.

Drinking of alcoholic beverages should be limited or avoided, if possible, while taking bupropion. This will help prevent unwanted effects.

This medicine may cause some people to feel a false sense of well-being, or to become drowsy, dizzy, or less alert than they are normally. **Make sure you know how you react to this medicine before you drive, use machines, or do other jobs that require you to be alert and clearheaded.**

POSSIBLE SIDE EFFECTS OF THIS MEDICINE
Side Effects That Should Be Reported To Your Doctor

> *More common*—Agitation or excitement; anxiety; confusion; fast or irregular heartbeat; headache (severe); restlessness; trouble in sleeping

> *Less common*—Hallucinations; skin rash

> *Rare*—Fainting; convulsions (seizures), especially with higher doses

Side Effects That Usually Do Not Require Medical Attention

These possible side effects may go away during treatment; however, if they continue or are bothersome, check with your doctor, nurse, or pharmacist.

> *More common*—Constipation; decrease in appetite; dizziness; dryness of mouth; increased sweating; nausea or vomiting; tremor; weight loss (unusual)

> *Less common*—Blurred vision; difficulty in concentration; drowsiness; fever or chills; hostility or anger; tiredness; unusual feeling of well-being

Other side effects not listed above may also occur in some patients. If you notice any other effects, check with your doctor, nurse, or pharmacist.

BUSPIRONE   Systemic

■For the Pharmacist■

In providing consultation, consider emphasizing the following selected information (» = major clinical significance):

Before using this medication
» Conditions affecting use, especially:
   Sensitivity to buspirone
   Other medications, especially monoamine oxidase (MAO) inhibitors

Proper use of this medication
» Importance of not using more medication than the amount prescribed
   One to two weeks of therapy may be required before antianxiety effect is noticeable
» Proper dosing
   Missed dose: If on scheduled dosing regimen—Taking as soon as possible; not taking if almost time for next dose; not doubling doses
» Proper storage

Precautions while using this medication
   Regular visits to physician to check progress during prolonged therapy
   Caution in taking alcohol or other CNS depressants during therapy
» Caution if dizziness or drowsiness occurs
» Suspected overdose: Getting emergency help at once

Side/adverse effects
   Signs of potential side effects, especially chest pain, confusion, fast or pounding heartbeat, mental depression, neurological effects, and sore throat or fever

▲ For the Patient ▲

915268

ABOUT YOUR MEDICINE

Buspirone (byoo-SPYE-rone) is used to treat certain anxiety disorders or to relieve the symptoms of anxiety. However, buspirone is usually not used for anxiety or tension caused by the stress of everyday life.

If any of the information in this leaflet causes you special concern or if you want additional information about your medicine and its use, check with your doctor, nurse, or pharmacist. **Remember, keep this and all other medicines out of the reach of children and never share your medicines with others.**

BEFORE USING THIS MEDICINE

Tell your doctor, nurse, and pharmacist if you . . .
 • are allergic to any medicine, either prescription or nonprescription (OTC);

- are pregnant or intend to become pregnant while using this medicine;
- are breast-feeding;
- are taking any other prescription or nonprescription (OTC) medicine, especially MAO inhibitors;
- have any other medical problems.

PROPER USE OF THIS MEDICINE

Take buspirone only as directed by your doctor. Do not take more of it, do not take it more often, and do not take it for a longer time than your doctor ordered. To do so may increase the chance of unwanted effects.

After you begin taking buspirone, 1 to 2 weeks may pass before you feel the full effects of the medicine.

If you are taking this medicine regularly and you miss a dose, take it as soon as possible. However, if it is almost time for your next dose, skip the missed dose and go back to your regular dosing schedule. Do not double doses.

PRECAUTIONS WHILE USING THIS MEDICINE

If you will be using buspirone regularly for a long time, your doctor should check your progress at regular visits to make sure the medicine does not cause unwanted effects.

Buspirone when taken with alcohol or other CNS depressants (medicines that slow down the nervous system) may increase the chance of drowsiness. Check with your doctor before taking any such depressants while you are taking this medicine.

Buspirone may cause some people to become dizzy, light-headed, drowsy, or less alert than they are normally. **Make sure you know how you react to this medicine before you drive, use machines, or do other jobs that require you to be alert.**

If you think you or someone else may have taken an overdose of buspirone, get emergency help at once. Some signs of an overdose are severe dizziness or drowsiness; severe stomach upset, including nausea or vomiting; or unusually small pupils.

POSSIBLE SIDE EFFECTS OF THIS MEDICINE

Side Effects That Should Be Reported To Your Doctor

> *Rare*—Chest pain; confusion or mental depression; fast or pounding heartbeat; muscle weakness; numbness, tingling, pain, or weakness in hands or feet; sore throat or fever; uncontrolled movements of the body

Side Effects That Usually Do Not Require Medical Attention

These possible side effects may go away during treatment; however, if they continue or are bothersome, check with your doctor, nurse, or pharmacist.

More common—Dizziness or lightheadedness; headache; nausea; restlessness, nervousness, or unusual excitement

Less common or rare—Blurred vision; decreased concentration; drowsiness; dryness of mouth; muscle pain, spasms, cramps, or stiffness; ringing in the ears; stomach upset; trouble in sleeping, nightmares, or vivid dreams; unusual tiredness or weakness

Other side effects not listed above may also occur in some patients. If you notice any other effects, check with your doctor, nurse, or pharmacist.

CALCIUM CHANNEL BLOCKING AGENTS   Systemic
Including Bepridil; Diltiazem; Felodipine; Flunarizine; Isradipine; Nicardipine; Nifedipine; Nimodipine; Verapamil.

■For the Pharmacist■

In providing consultation, consider emphasizing the following selected information (» = major clinical significance):

Before using this medication
» Conditions affecting use, especially:
　　Sensitivity to the calcium channel blocker prescribed
　　Pregnancy—High doses in animals cause birth defects, prolonged pregnancy, poor bone development, and stillbirth
　　Use in the elderly—Elderly patients may be more sensitive to effects
　　Other medications, especially parenteral amphotericin B (for bepridil), beta-blockers, carbamazepine, carbonic anhydrase inhibitors, corticosteroids (for bepridil), cyclosporine, digitalis glycosides, disopyramide, potassium-depleting diuretics (for bepridil), procainamide, or quinidine
　　Other medical problems, especially arrhythmias (for bepridil), other cardiovascular problems, or hypokalemia (for bepridil)

Proper use of this medication
» Compliance with therapy; importance of not taking more medication than amount prescribed
» Proper dosing
　　Missed dose: Taking as soon as possible; not taking if almost time for next scheduled dose; not doubling doses
» Proper storage
For bepridil
　　If nausea occurs, may be taken with meals or at bedtime
For extended-release diltiazem capsules
　　Swallowing capsules whole without crushing or chewing
» Caution if switching brands; one is for once-daily dosing and one is for twice-daily dosing
For extended-release nifedipine or verapamil capsules
　　Swallowing capsules whole without crushing or chewing
For regular nifedipine or extended-release felodipine or nifedipine tablets
　　Swallowing tablets whole, without breaking, crushing, or chewing
　　For *Procardia XL*—Patient may notice empty shell in stool left over after medication is absorbed
For extended-release verapamil tablets
　　Swallowing tablets whole, without crushing or chewing; may be broken in half on instructions from physician
　　Taking with food or milk
For use as an antihypertensive
　　Importance of diet; possible need for sodium restriction and/or weight reduction
» Patient may not experience symptoms of hypertension; importance of taking medication even if feeling well
» Does not cure, but helps control hypertension; possible need for lifelong therapy; serious consequences of untreated hypertension

Precautions while using this medication

Regular visits to physician to check progress during therapy

Checking with physician before discontinuing medication; gradual dosage reduction may be necessary

» Discussing exercise or physical exertion limits with physician; reduced occurrence of chest pain may tempt patient to be overactive

Possible headache; checking with physician if continuing or severe

» Maintaining good dental hygiene and seeing dentist frequently for teeth cleaning to prevent tenderness, bleeding, and gum enlargement

For use as an antihypertensive

» Not taking other medications, especially nonprescription sympathomimetics, unless discussed with physician

For patients taking bepridil, diltiazem, or verapamil

» Checking pulse as directed; checking with physician if less than 50 beats per minute

For patients taking flunarizine

Caution when driving or doing other things requiring alertness because of risk of drowsiness

Side/adverse effects

Signs of potential side effects, especially angina, congestive heart failure or pulmonary edema, extrapyramidal effects (for flunarizine), galactorrhea (for flunarizine), peripheral edema, tachycardia, bradycardia, excessive hypotension, gingival hyperplasia, allergic reaction, mental depression (for flunarizine), arthritis (for nifedipine), and transient blindness (for nifedipine)

▲ For the Patient ▲

912816

ABOUT YOUR MEDICINE

Calcium channel blockers are used to relieve and control angina (chest pain). Some are also used to treat high blood pressure (hypertension), prevent migraine headaches, or prevent and treat problems caused by a burst blood vessel in the head (also known as a ruptured aneurysm or subarachnoid hemorrhage). Channel blockers may also be used for other conditions as determined by your doctor.

If any of the information in this leaflet causes you special concern or if you want additional information about your medicine and its use, check with your doctor, nurse, or pharmacist. **Remember, keep this and all other medicines out of the reach of children and never share your medicines with others.**

BEFORE USING THIS MEDICINE

Tell your doctor, nurse, and pharmacist if you . . .

• are allergic to any medicine, either prescription or nonprescription (OTC);

• are pregnant or intend to become pregnant while using this medicine;

• are breast-feeding;

• are taking any other prescription or nonprescription (OTC) medicine, especially *any* other medicines for the

heart, carbamazepine, corticosteroids, cyclosporine, or diuretics (water pills);
- have any other medical problems, especially other heart disease.

PROPER USE OF THIS MEDICINE

For patients taking bepridil:
- If bepridil causes upset stomach, it may be taken with meals or at bedtime.

For patients taking extended-release capsules or tablets or regular nifedipine:
- Swallow whole, without breaking, crushing, or chewing.

For patients taking diltiazem extended-release capsules:
- **Do not change to another brand without first checking with your doctor.**

For patients taking *Procardia XL*:
- You may notice what looks like a tablet in your stool. That is just the empty shell that is left after the medicine has been absorbed into your body.

For patients taking verapamil extended-release tablets:
- Your doctor may tell you to break the tablet in half. Do this only if you are instructed to do so. Also, take the tablets with food or milk.

Take exactly as directed even if you feel well. Do not take more of this medicine and do not take it more often than your doctor ordered. Do not miss any doses.

If you do miss a dose of this medicine, take it as soon as possible. However, if it is almost time for your next dose, skip the missed dose and go back to your regular dosing schedule. Do not double doses.

PRECAUTIONS WHILE USING THIS MEDICINE

If you have been using this medicine regularly for several weeks, do not suddenly stop using it. Stopping suddenly may bring on your previous problem. Check with your doctor for the best way to reduce gradually the amount you are taking before stopping completely.

Chest pain resulting from exercise or exertion is usually reduced or prevented by this medicine. This may tempt you to be overly active. **Make sure you discuss with your doctor a safe amount of exercise for your medical problem.**

In some patients, tenderness, swelling, or bleeding of the gums may occur. Brushing and flossing your teeth carefully and regularly and massaging your gums may help prevent this. **See your dentist regularly to have your teeth cleaned. Check with your physician or dentist if you notice any tenderness, swelling, or bleeding of your gums.**

For patients taking bepridil, diltiazem, or verapamil:
- **Ask your doctor or pharmacist how to count your pulse rate. Then, while you are taking this medicine, check**

your pulse regularly. If it is much slower than your usual rate, or less than 50 beats per minute, check with your doctor.

For patients taking flunarizine:
* This medicine may cause some people to become drowsy or less alert than they are normally. **Make sure you know how you react before you drive, use machines, or do other jobs that require you to be alert.**

POSSIBLE SIDE EFFECTS OF THIS MEDICINE
Side Effects That Should Be Reported To Your Doctor

Less common—Breathing difficulty, coughing, or wheezing; dizziness; irregular or fast or slow heartbeat; skin rash; swelling of ankles, feet, or lower legs

Rare—Bleeding, tender, or swollen gums; chest pain; fainting; painful, swollen joints (nifedipine only); trouble in seeing (nifedipine only); unusual secretion of milk (flunarizine and verapamil only)

For flunarizine only: Less common (in addition to the above)—Loss of balance control; mask-like face; mental depression; shuffling walk; stiff arms or legs; trembling of hands and fingers; trouble in speaking or swallowing

Side Effects That Usually Do Not Require Medical Attention

These possible side effects may go away during treatment; however, if they continue or are bothersome, check with your doctor, nurse, or pharmacist.

For flunarizine: More common—Drowsiness; increased appetite or weight

For amlodipine, isradipine, and nifedipine: More common—Flushing

For amlodipine, felodipine, nicardipine, nifedipine: More common—Headache

Other side effects not listed above may also occur in some patients. If you notice any other effects, check with your doctor, nurse, or pharmacist.

CAPSAICIN   Topical

■For the Pharmacist■

In providing consultation, consider emphasizing the following selected
information (» = major clinical significance):

Before using this medication
» Conditions affecting use, especially:
    Sensitivity to capsaicin or to the fruits of capsicum plants (e.g.,
        hot peppers)
    Use in children—Not recommended in infants and children up
        to 2 years of age, except under the direction of a physician
    Other medical problems, especially broken or irritated skin on
        area to be treated

Proper use of this medication
    If using capsaicin for treatment of neuralgia due to herpes zoster,
        not applying medicine until after zoster sores have healed
    Washing areas to be treated will not cause harm, but is not necessary
    Rubbing cream into the affected area well so that little or no cream
        is left on surface of skin
    Washing hands with soap and water after applying capsaicin to avoid
        getting medicine in eyes or on other sensitive areas of body;
        however, if medication used on arthritic hands, not washing hands
        for at least 30 minutes after application
    If bandage is being used, not applying tightly
    Warm, stinging, or burning sensation may occur and is related to
        the action of capsaicin on the skin; usually disappears after first
        several days of treatment, however, may last 2 to 4 weeks or
        longer; heat, humidity, clothing, bathing in warm water, or sweat-
        ing may increase sensation; sensation usually lessens in frequency
        and intensity the longer medication is used; reducing number of
        daily doses of capsaicin will not lessen sensation, and may prolong
        period of time that sensation occurs; reducing number of doses
        also will reduce amount of pain relief obtained
    Relief from pain may not occur right away; also, time it takes for
        capsaicin to work differs depending on type of pain; with ar-
        thritis, pain relief usually begins within 1 or 2 weeks; with neur-
        algia, pain relief usually begins within 2 to 4 weeks; with head
        and neck neuralgias, pain relief may take 4 to 6 weeks
    Using capsaicin 3 or 4 times a day or as directed by doctor; pain
        relief will last only as long as capsaicin is used regularly; if
        medicine is discontinued and pain recurs, capsaicin treatment
        may be restarted
» Proper dosage
    Missed dose: Using as soon as possible; if almost time for next dose,
        skipping missed dose and returning to regular dosing schedule;
        not doubling doses
» Proper storage

Precautions while using this medication
    If capsaicin gets into eyes, flushing with water; if capsaicin gets on
        other sensitive areas of body, washing with warm (not hot) soapy
        water
    If condition worsens, or does not improve after 1 month, discontin-
        uing use and checking with physician

▲ For the Patient ▲

918550

ABOUT YOUR MEDICINE

Capsaicin (cap-SAY-sin) is used to help relieve a certain type of pain known as neuralgia (new-RAL-ja). Capsaicin is also used to temporarily help relieve the pain from osteoarthritis (OS-te-o-ar-THRI-tis) or rheumatoid arthritis (ROO-ma-toid ar-THRI-tis). This medicine will not cure any of these conditions. Capsaicin may also be used for neuralgias caused by other conditions as determined by your doctor.

If any of the information in this leaflet causes you special concern or if you want additional information about your medicine and its use, check with your doctor, nurse, or pharmacist. **Remember, keep this and all other medicines out of the reach of children and never share your medicines with others.**

BEFORE USING THIS MEDICINE

If you are taking this medicine without a prescription, carefully read and follow any precautions on the label. You should be especially careful if you . . .

- are allergic to any medicine, either prescription or nonprescription (OTC);
- are pregnant, intend to become pregnant, or are breast-feeding;
- are taking any other prescription or nonprescription (OTC) medicine;
- have any other medical problems, especially broken or irritated skin on area to be treated with capsaicin.

If you have any questions, check with your doctor, nurse, or pharmacist.

PROPER USE OF THIS MEDICINE

If you are using capsaicin for the treatment of neuralgia caused by herpes zoster, do not apply the medicine until the zoster sores have healed.

You do not need to wash the areas to be treated before you apply capsaicin, but doing so will not cause harm.

Apply a small amount of cream and use your fingers to rub it well into the affected area so that little or no cream is left on the surface of the skin afterwards.

Wash your hands with soap and water after applying capsaicin to avoid getting the medicine in your eyes or on other sensitive areas of the body. However, if you are using capsaicin for arthritis in your hands, do not wash your hands for at least 30 minutes after applying the cream.

If a bandage is being used on the treated area, it should not be applied tightly.

When you first begin to use capsaicin, a warm, stinging, or burning sensation (feeling) may occur. This is to be expected.

Although this sensation usually disappears after the first several days of treatment, it may last 2 to 4 weeks or longer. Heat, humidity, clothing, bathing in warm water, or sweating may increase the sensation. However, the sensation usually occurs less often and is less severe the longer you use the medicine. Reducing the number of doses of capsaicin that you use each day will not lessen the sensation, and may lengthen the period of time that you get the sensation. Also, reducing the number of doses you use may reduce the amount of pain relief that you get.

Capsaicin must be used regularly every day as directed if it is to work properly. Even then, it may not relieve your pain right away. The length of time it takes to work depends on the type of pain you have. In persons with arthritis, pain relief usually begins within 1 to 2 weeks. In most persons with neuralgia, relief usually begins within 2 to 4 weeks, although with head and neck neuralgias, relief may take as long as 4 to 6 weeks.

Once capsaicin has begun to relieve pain, you must continue to use it regularly 3 or 4 times a day to keep the pain from returning. If you stop using capsaicin and your pain returns, you can begin using it again.

If you miss a dose of this medicine, use it as soon as possible. However, if it is almost time for your next dose, skip the missed dose and go back to your regular dosing schedule. Do not double doses.

PRECAUTIONS WHILE USING THIS MEDICINE

If capsaicin gets into your eyes or on other sensitive areas of the body, it will cause a burning sensation. If capsaicin gets into your eyes, flush your eyes with water. If capsaicin gets on other sensitive areas of your body, wash the areas with warm (not hot) soapy water.

If your condition gets worse, or does not improve after 1 month, stop using this medicine and check with your doctor.

POSSIBLE SIDE EFFECTS OF THIS MEDICINE
Side Effects That Usually Do Not Require Medical Attention

These possible side effects may go away during treatment; however, if they continue or are bothersome, check with your doctor, nurse, or pharmacist.

>   *More common*—Warm, stinging, or burning feeling at the place of treatment

Other side effects not listed above may also occur in some patients. If you notice any other effects, check with your doctor, nurse, or pharmacist.

CARBACHOL   Ophthalmic

■For the Pharmacist■

In providing consultation, consider emphasizing the following selected information (» = major clinical significance):

Before using this medication
» Conditions affecting use, especially:
   Sensitivity to carbachol
   Other medical problems, especially acute iritis or other conditions in which pupillary constriction is undesirable

Proper use of this medication
For the ophthalmic solution
» Importance of not using more medication than the amount prescribed
   Proper administration technique
   Washing hands immediately after applying eye drops
   Preventing contamination: Not touching applicator tip to any surface; keeping container tightly closed
» Proper dosing
   Missed dose: Applying as soon as possible; not applying if almost time for next dose; applying next dose at regularly scheduled time
» Proper storage

Precautions while using this medication
For the ophthalmic solution
   Regular visits to physician to check eye pressure during therapy
» Caution if driving or doing anything else at night or in dim light
» Caution if blurred vision or change in near or distance vision occurs

Side/adverse effects
   Signs of potential side effects, especially retinal detachment or symptoms of systemic absorption

▲ For the Patient ▲

912849

GLAUCOMA EYE MEDICINE—SHORT-ACTING CHOLINERGIC: *Including Carbachol; Physostigmine; Pilocarpine.*

ABOUT YOUR MEDICINE

Short-acting cholinergic (ko-lin-ER-jik) **glaucoma eye medicines** are used in the eye to treat certain kinds of glaucoma and other eye conditions.

If any of the information in this leaflet causes you special concern or if you want additional information about your medicine and its use, check with your doctor, nurse, or pharmacist. **Remember, keep this and all other medicines out of the reach of children and never share your medicines with others.**

BEFORE USING THIS MEDICINE

Tell your doctor, nurse, and pharmacist if you . . .
- are allergic to any medicine, either prescription or non-prescription (OTC);
- are pregnant or intend to become pregnant while using this medicine;
- are breast-feeding;
- are taking **any** other prescription or nonprescription (OTC) medicine;
- have any other medical problems, especially other eye disease or problems.

PROPER USE OF THIS MEDICINE

Use this medicine only as directed. Do not use more of it and do not use it more often than your doctor ordered. To do so may increase the chance of too much medicine being absorbed into the body and the chance of side effects.

To use the ophthalmic solution (eye drops) form of this medicine:
- First, wash your hands. Tilt the head back and, pressing your finger gently on the skin just beneath the lower eyelid, pull the lower eyelid away from the eye to make a space. Drop the medicine into this space. Let go of the eyelid and gently close the eyes. Do not blink. Keep the eyes closed and apply pressure to the inner corner of the eye with your finger for 1 or 2 minutes to allow the medicine to be absorbed by the eye.
- Wash hands to remove any medicine that may be on them.
- Do not use solution if it is discolored.

To use the ophthalmic ointment (eye ointment) or the eye gel form of this medicine:
- First, wash your hands. Pull lower eyelid away from eye to form a pouch. Squeeze a thin strip of ointment or gel into the pouch. A 1-cm (approximately 1/3-inch) strip of ointment or a 1 and 1/2-cm (approximately 1/2-inch) strip of gel is usually enough unless otherwise directed by your doctor. Close eyes and keep them closed for 1 or 2 minutes.
- Wash hands to remove any medicine that may be on them.
- Wipe the tip of the tube with a clean tissue.

To use the eye system form of this medicine:
- This medicine usually comes with patient directions. Read them carefully.
- If you think a medicine unit may be damaged, do not use it.
- If the unit seems to be releasing too much medicine into your eye, remove it and replace with a new unit.
- Insert the unit at bedtime, unless otherwise directed by your doctor.

To keep the medicine as germ-free as possible, do not touch the applicator tip to any surface (including the eye) and keep the container tightly closed.

If you miss a dose of this medicine, apply the missed dose as soon as possible. However, if it is almost time for your next dose, skip the missed dose and go back to your regular dosing schedule. Do not double doses.

PRECAUTIONS WHILE USING THIS MEDICINE
Your doctor should check your eye pressure at regular visits.

For a short time after you apply this medicine, your vision may be blurred or there may be a change in your near or distant vision, especially at night. **Make sure your vision is clear before you drive, use machines, or do other jobs that require you to see well.**

POSSIBLE SIDE EFFECTS OF THIS MEDICINE
Side Effects That Should Be Reported To Your Doctor

> *Signs of too much medicine being absorbed into the body*—Flushing or redness of face; frequent urge to urinate; increased sweating; loss of bladder control; muscle tremors or weakness; nausea, vomiting, or diarrhea; shortness of breath, troubled breathing, wheezing, or tightness in chest; slow or irregular heartbeat; stomach cramps or pain; unusual tiredness or weakness; watering of mouth

Side Effects That Usually Do Not Require Medical Attention

These possible side effects may go away during treatment; however, if they continue or are bothersome, check with your doctor, nurse, or pharmacist.

> *More common*—Blurred vision; change in near or distant vision; eye pain

> *Less common*—Burning, redness, stinging, watering, or other eye irritation; headache or browache; twitching of eyelids

Other side effects not listed above may also occur in some patients. If you notice any other effects, check with your doctor, nurse, or pharmacist.

CARBAMAZEPINE   Systemic

■ For the Pharmacist ■

In providing consultation, consider emphasizing the following selected information (» = major clinical significance):

Before using this medication
» Conditions affecting use, especially:

Sensitivity to tricyclic antidepressants or carbamazepine

Pregnancy—Crosses placenta; babies reportedly born with small head circumference, low birth weight, craniofacial defects, fingernail hypoplasia, developmental delays, and spina bifida; animal studies have shown rib anomalies, cleft palate, foot deformities, or anophthalmos with doses 10 to 25 times the human dose

Breast-feeding—Distributed into breast milk; animal studies have shown lack of weight gain and unkempt appearance of young at high doses

Use in children—Appropriate studies have not been done in children up to 6 years of age; behavior changes more likely to occur in children

Use in elderly—Elderly more likely to have confusion or agitation, AV heart block, SIADH, or bradycardia than are younger people

Dental—Increased incidence of blood dyscrasias that cause infection, delayed healing, or gingival bleeding; proper oral hygiene necessary

Other medications, especially anticoagulants, other anticonvulsants, tricyclic antidepressants, barbiturates, benzodiazepines metabolized via hepatic microsomal enzymes (especially clonazepam), cimetidine, clarithromycin, oral estrogen-containing contraceptives, corticosteroids, diltiazem, erythromycin, estrogens, isoniazid, MAO inhibitors, propoxyphene, quinidine, or verapamil

Other medical problems, especially absence, atonic, or myoclonic seizures; AV heart block; blood disorders; or bone marrow depression

Proper use of this medication
» Taking with food to lessen gastrointestinal irritation
» Not using medication for minor aches and pains
» Compliance with therapy; not taking more or less medication than prescribed
» Proper dosing

Missed dose: Taking as soon as possible; not taking if almost time for next dose; not doubling doses; calling physician if more than one dose a day is missed

» Proper storage; not storing tablet dosage forms in bathroom or other high-moisture areas due to loss of potency and effectiveness

For use in epilepsy
» Checking with physician before discontinuing medication; gradual dosage reduction may be necessary to prevent seizures or status epilepticus

Precautions while using this medication
» Regular visits to physician to check progress of therapy
» Avoiding the use of alcoholic beverages and other CNS depressants while taking this medicine

» Possible drowsiness, dizziness, lightheadedness, blurred or double vision, weakness, or muscular incoordination; caution when driving or using machinery, or doing jobs requiring alertness and coordination

» Possible skin photosensitivity; avoiding unprotected exposure to sun; using protective clothing; using a sun block product that includes protection against both UVA-caused photosensitivity reactions and UVB-caused sunburn reactions; avoiding use of sunlamp, tanning bed, or tanning booth

Diabetic patients: May increase urine sugar concentrations

Caution if any laboratory tests required; possible interference with results of metyrapone or pregnancy tests

» Caution if any kind of surgery, dental treatment, or emergency treatment is needed

Carrying medical identification card or bracelet during therapy

Side/adverse effects

Signs of potential side effects, especially CNS toxicity, allergic reaction, Stevens-Johnson syndrome, toxic epidermal necrolysis, behavioral changes, severe diarrhea, dilutional hyponatremia or water intoxication (SIADH), SLE-like syndrome, adenopathy or lymphadenopathy, blood dyscrasias, bone marrow depression, cardiovascular effects, hypersensitivity hepatitis, hypocalcemia, renal toxicity or failure, paresthesias or peripheral neuritis, porphyria, pulmonary hypersensitivity, or thrombophlebitis

---

▲ For the Patient ▲

912168

ABOUT YOUR MEDICINE

Carbamazepine (kar-ba-MAZ-e-peen) is used to control some types of seizures in the treatment of epilepsy. It is also used to relieve pain due to trigeminal neuralgia (tic douloureux). Carbamazepine may also be used for other conditions as determined by your doctor.

If any of the information in this leaflet causes you special concern or if you want additional information about your medicine and its use, check with your doctor, nurse, or pharmacist. **Remember, keep this and all other medicines out of the reach of children and never share your medicines with others.**

BEFORE USING THIS MEDICINE

Tell your doctor, nurse, and pharmacist if you . . .

- are allergic to any medicine, either prescription or nonprescription (OTC);
- are pregnant or intend to become pregnant while using this medicine;
- are breast-feeding;
- are taking any other prescription or nonprescription (OTC) medicine, especially adrenocorticoids; anticoagulants (blood thinners); antidepressants; cimetidine; diltiazem; erythromycin; estrogens; isoniazid; MAO inhibitors; oral contraceptives (birth control pills) containing estrogen; other anticonvulsants (seizure medicine); propoxyphene; quinidine; or verapamil;

- have any other medical problems, especially anemia or other blood problems, or heart or blood vessel disease.

PROPER USE OF THIS MEDICINE

Take carbamazepine exactly as directed. It should be taken with meals to lessen the chance of stomach upset.

For patients taking this medicine for epilepsy: Do not suddenly stop taking it without first checking with your doctor.

If you miss a dose of this medicine, take it as soon as possible. However, if it is almost time for your next dose, skip the missed dose and go back to your regular dosing schedule. Do not double doses.

PRECAUTIONS WHILE USING THIS MEDICINE

It is very important that your doctor check your progress at regular visits. Your doctor may want to do certain tests to see if you are receiving the right amount of medicine or if certain side effects are occurring.

This medicine will add to the effects of alcohol and other CNS depressants (medicines that slow down the nervous system). **Check with your doctor before taking any such depressants while you are using this medicine.**

Some people who take carbamazepine may become more sensitive to sunlight than they are normally. **Avoid too much sun and do not use a sunlamp until you see how you react to the sun,** especially if you tend to burn easily. **If you have a severe reaction, check with your doctor.**

Before having any kind of surgery or dental or emergency treatment, tell the physician or dentist in charge that you are taking carbamazepine.

This medicine may cause some people to become drowsy, dizzy, lightheaded, or less alert than they are normally especially when starting treatment or increasing the dose. It may also cause blurred or double vision, weakness, or loss of muscle control. **Make sure you know how you react before you drive or do jobs that require you to be alert and well-coordinated or able to see well.**

POSSIBLE SIDE EFFECTS OF THIS MEDICINE
Side Effects That Should Be Reported To Your Doctor Immediately

Check with your doctor immediately if you notice black, tarry stools; blood in urine or stools; bone or joint pain; cough or hoarseness; darkening of urine; lower back or side pain; nosebleeds or other unusual bleeding or bruising; painful or difficult urination; pain, tenderness, swelling, or bluish color in leg or foot; pale stools; pinpoint red spots on skin; shortness of breath; sores, ulcers, or white spots on lips or in the mouth; sore throat, chills, and fever; swollen or painful glands; unusual tiredness or weakness; wheezing, tightness in chest, or troubled breathing; or yellow eyes or skin.

Other Side Effects That Should Be Reported To Your Doctor

More common—Blurred or double vision; continuous back-and-forth eye movements

Less common—Behavioral changes (especially in children); confusion, agitation, or hostility (especially in the elderly); diarrhea (severe); headache (continuing); increase in seizures; nausea and vomiting (severe); skin rash, hives, or itching; unusual drowsiness

Rare—Buzzing or ringing in ears; chest pain; difficulty in speaking or slurred speech; fainting; frequent urination; irregular, pounding, or slow heartbeat; mental depression with restlessness; numbness, tingling, pain, or weakness in hands and feet; rapid weight gain; rigidity; sudden decrease in amount of urine; swelling of face, hands, feet or lower legs; trembling; uncontrolled body movements; visual hallucinations

Side Effects That Usually Do Not Require Medical Attention

These possible side effects may go away during treatment; however, if they continue or are bothersome, check with your doctor, nurse, or pharmacist.

More common—Clumsiness or unsteadiness; dizziness or lightheadedness (mild); drowsiness (slight); nausea or vomiting (mild)

Other side effects not listed above may also occur in some patients. If you notice any other effects, check with your doctor, nurse, or pharmacist.

CARBIDOPA AND LEVODOPA   Systemic

■ For the Pharmacist ■

In providing consultation, consider emphasizing the following selected information (» = major clinical significance):

Before using this medication
» Conditions affecting use, especially:

Sensitivity to carbidopa and/or levodopa

Pregnancy—No studies in humans; depressed growth and malformations in animal studies

Breast-feeding—Levodopa is distributed into breast milk; may inhibit lactation

Use in the elderly—Reduced tolerance to effects of levodopa; caution in resuming normal activity, especially in patients with osteoporosis; psychic effects more common with concurrent use of anticholinergics

Dental—Possible difficulty in retention of full dentures

Other medications, especially haloperidol, hydantoin anticonvulsants, hydrocarbon inhalation anesthetics, phenothiazines, cocaine, MAO inhibitors, and selegiline

Other medical problems, especially severe cardiovascular disease, severe pulmonary diseases, glaucoma, melanoma (history of or suspected), peptic ulcer (history of), psychosis, renal function impairment, or urinary retention

Proper use of this medication
» Taking food shortly after taking medication to relieve gastric irritation; taking food before or concurrently may retard levodopa's effect

» Compliance with therapy; taking medication only as directed; not stopping medication unless ordered by physician

» Maximum effectiveness of medication may not occur for several weeks or months after therapy is initiated

Missed dose: Taking as soon as possible; skipping dose if next scheduled dose is within 2 hours; not doubling doses

» Proper storage

Precautions while using this medication
Caution if any kind of surgery (including dental surgery) or emergency treatment is required

For diabetic patients—May interfere with urine tests for sugar and ketones

» Caution if drowsiness occurs

» Caution when getting up suddenly from lying or sitting position; dizziness and fainting may occur

Possibility of "on-off" phenomenon

Side/adverse effects
Occasional darkening of urine or sweat may be alarming to patient although medically insignificant

Signs of potential side effects, especially difficult urination, duodenal ulcer, hemolytic anemia, hypertension, irregular heartbeat, mental depression, mood or mental changes, severe nausea or vomiting, orthostatic hypotension, spasm or closing of eyelids, or uncontrolled movements of body

▲ For the Patient ▲

912383

LEVODOPA/CARBIDOPA WITH LEVODOPA

(Oral): *Including Carbidopa with Levodopa; Levodopa.*

ABOUT YOUR MEDICINE

Levodopa (LEE-voe-doe-pa) is a medicine used alone or in combination with **carbidopa** (KAR-bi-doe-pa) to treat Parkinson's disease, sometimes referred to as shaking palsy or paralysis agitans.

If any of the information in this leaflet causes you special concern or if you want additional information about your medicine and its use, check with your doctor, nurse, or pharmacist. **Remember, keep this and all other medicines out of the reach of children and never share your medicines with others.**

BEFORE USING THIS MEDICINE

Tell your doctor, nurse, and pharmacist if you . . .

- are allergic to any medicine, either prescription or nonprescription (OTC);
- are pregnant or intend to become pregnant while using this medicine;
- are breast-feeding;
- are taking any other prescription or nonprescription (OTC) medicine, especially anticonvulsants, haloperidol, MAO inhibitors, phenothiazines, pyridoxine (vitamin B_6), or selegiline;
- have any other medical problems, especially asthma, bronchitis, emphysema, or other chronic lung disease; glaucoma; heart or blood vessel disease; kidney disease or difficult urination; mental illness; skin cancer; or stomach ulcer;
- use cocaine.

PROPER USE OF THIS MEDICINE

Take this medicine only as directed. Do not take more or less of it, do not take it more often, and do not stop taking it unless ordered by your doctor. Some people must take this medicine for several weeks before full benefit is received.

Your doctor may want you to take food shortly after taking this medicine (about 15 minutes after) to lessen possible stomach upset. If stomach upset is severe or continues, check with your doctor.

For patients taking carbidopa and levodopa extended-release tablets:

- Swallow the tablet whole without crushing or chewing, unless your doctor tells you not to. If your doctor tells you to, you may break the tablet in half.

If you miss a dose of this medicine, take it as soon as possible. However, if your next scheduled dose is within 2 hours, skip the missed dose and go back to your regular dosing schedule. Do not double doses.

PRECAUTIONS WHILE USING THIS MEDICINE
This medicine may cause some people to become drowsy or less alert than they are normally. **Make sure you know how you react to this medicine before you drive, use machines, or do other jobs that require you to be alert.**

Dizziness, lightheadedness, or fainting may occur, especially when you get up from a lying or sitting position. Getting up slowly may help.

Pyridoxine (vitamin B_6) has been found to reduce the effects of levodopa when taken alone (not in combination with carbidopa). If you are taking levodopa, do not take vitamin products containing vitamin B_6 unless prescribed. Also remember that certain foods contain large amounts of vitamin B_6.

As your condition improves and your body movements become easier, **be careful not to overdo physical activities. Injuries resulting from falls may occur.**

POSSIBLE SIDE EFFECTS OF THIS MEDICINE
Side Effects That Should Be Reported To Your Doctor

More common—Mental depression; mood changes; unusual and uncontrolled movements of the upper body (such as the tongue, arms, head)

Less common (more common when levodopa is used alone)—Difficult urination; dizziness or lightheadedness; irregular heartbeat; nausea and vomiting (severe or continuing); spasm or closing of eyelids

Rare—High blood pressure; stomach pain; unusual tiredness or weakness

After taking this medicine for long periods of time, such as one to several years, some patients suddenly lose the ability to move. This may last from a few minutes to hours. The patient is then able to move as before until the condition unexpectedly occurs again. If you should have this problem, check with your doctor.

Side Effects That Usually Do Not Require Medical Attention

These possible side effects may go away during treatment; however, if they continue or are bothersome, check with your doctor, nurse, or pharmacist.

More common—Anxiety

Less common—Constipation or diarrhea; dryness of mouth

This medicine sometimes causes the urine and sweat to be darker than usual. The urine may at first be reddish, then turn to nearly black after being exposed to air. This effect is not important and is to be expected.

Other side effects not listed above may also occur in some patients. If you notice any other effects, check with your doctor, nurse, or pharmacist.

CEPHALOSPORINS Systemic

Including Cefaclor; Cefadroxil; Cefamandole; Cefaxolin; Cefixime; Cefmetazole; Cefonicid; Cefoperazone; Cefotaxime; Cefotetan; Cefoxitin; Cefpodoxime; Cefprozil; Ceftazidime; Ceftizoxime; Ceftriaxone; Cefuroxime; Cephalexin; Cephalothin; Cephapirin; Cephradine.

■For the Pharmacist■

In providing consultation, consider emphasizing the following selected information (» = major clinical significance):

Before using this medication
» Conditions affecting use, especially:
  Allergies to penicillins, penicillin derivatives, penicillamine, or cephalosporins
  Pregnancy—Cephalosporins cross the placenta
  Breast-feeding—Most cephalosporins are distributed into breast-milk; however, it is not known if cefixime is distributed into breast-milk; no problems in humans have been documented
  Use in children—Accumulation of cephalosporins, with resulting prolonged half-life, has been reported in newborn infants. Cefoxitin and ceftizoxime have been associated with an increased incidence of eosinophilia and elevated aspartate aminotransferase (AST [SGOT]). Ceftizoxime has also been associated with elevated alanine aminotransferase (ALT [SGPT]) and creatine kinase (CK). Ceftriaxone should be used with caution in hyperbilirubinemic neonates since it may be more likely than other cephalosporins to displace bilirubin from serum albumin
  Other medications, especially alcohol, anticoagulants, heparin, thrombolytic agents, platelet aggregation inhibitors, or probenecid
  Other medical problems, especially a history of bleeding disorders; a history of gastrointestinal disease, such as colitis; hepatic function impairment; or renal function impairment

Proper use of this medication
  Taking on a full or empty stomach, or with food if gastrointestinal irritation occurs; absorption of cefuroxime axetil and cefpodoxime proxetil is enhanced when they are administered with food
  Proper administration technique for oral liquids and/or pediatric drops; not using after expiration date
» Compliance with full course of therapy, especially in streptococcal infections
» Importance of not missing doses and taking at evenly spaced times
» Proper dosing
  Missed dose: Taking as soon as possible; not taking if almost time for next dose; not doubling doses
» Proper storage
For patients unable to swallow cefuroxime axetil tablets whole
  Crushing tablets and mixing with food to mask the strong, persistent bitter taste

Precautions while using this medication
  Checking with physician if no improvement within a few days
» Diabetics: False-positive reactions with copper sulfate urine glucose tests may occur

» For severe diarrhea, checking with physician before taking any antidiarrheals; for mild diarrhea, kaolin- or attapulgite-containing,
but not other, antidiarrheals may be tried; checking with physician or pharmacist if mild diarrhea continues or worsens

» Avoiding alcoholic beverages or other alcohol-containing preparations while receiving, and for several days after discontinuing,
cefamandole, cefmetazole, cefoperazone, or cefotetan

Side/adverse effects
Signs of potential side effects, especially hypoprothrombinemia,
pseudomembranous colitis, allergic reactions, hemolytic anemia,
renal dysfunction, serum sickness–like reactions, hypersensitivity
reactions, seizures, thrombophlebitis, or biliary "sludge" or pseu-
dolithiasis

▲ For the Patient ▲

912179

ABOUT YOUR MEDICINE

Cephalosporins (sef-a-loe-SPOR-ins) are used to treat infections caused by bacteria. They will not work for colds, flu,
or other virus infections.

If any of the information in this leaflet causes you special
concern or if you want additional information about your
medicine and its use, check with your doctor, nurse, or pharmacist. **Remember, keep this and all other medicines out of
the reach of children and never share your medicines with
others.**

BEFORE USING THIS MEDICINE

Tell your doctor, nurse, and pharmacist if you . . .
* are allergic to any medicine, either prescription or nonprescription (OTC);
* are pregnant or intend to become pregnant while using
this medicine;
* are breast-feeding;
* are taking any other prescription or nonprescription
(OTC) medicine, especially probenecid or thrombolytic
agents (blood thinners);
* have any other medical problems, especially history of
stomach or intestinal disease, such as colitis, including
colitis caused by antibiotics, or enteritis.

PROPER USE OF THIS MEDICINE

Cephalosporins may be taken on a full or empty stomach.
If this medicine upsets your stomach, it may be taken with
food. Cefuroxime axetil tablets and cefpodoxime should be
taken with food to increase absorption of the medicine.

For patients taking the oral liquid form of this medicine:
* This medicine is to be taken by mouth even if it comes
in a dropper bottle. If this medicine does not come in
a dropper bottle, use a specially marked measuring spoon
or other device to measure each dose accurately. The
average household teaspoon may not hold the right
amount of liquid.

For patients unable to swallow cefuroxime tablets whole:
- Cefuroxime tablets may be crushed and mixed with food (e.g., applesauce, ice cream) or drinks (apple, orange, or grape juice, or chocolate milk) to cover up the strong, lasting, bitter taste.

To help clear up your infection completely, **keep taking this medicine for the full time of treatment** even if you begin to feel better after a few days; **do not miss any doses**.

If you do miss a dose of this medicine, take it as soon as possible. This will help to keep a constant amount of medicine in the blood or urine. However, if it is almost time for your next dose, skip the missed dose and go back to your regular dosing schedule. Do not double doses.

PRECAUTIONS WHILE USING THIS MEDICINE

If your symptoms do not improve within a few days, or if they become worse, check with your doctor.

Diabetics—This medicine may cause false test results with some urine sugar tests. Check with your doctor before changing your diet or the dosage of your diabetes medicine.

For patients with phenylketonuria (PKU):
- Cefprozil oral suspension contains phenylalanine. Check with your doctor before taking this medicine.

If diarrhea occurs, do not take any diarrhea medicine without first checking with your doctor or pharmacist. Diarrhea medicines may make your diarrhea worse or make it last longer.

This medicine must not be given to other people or used for other infections unless you are otherwise directed by your doctor.

POSSIBLE SIDE EFFECTS OF THIS MEDICINE

Side Effects That Should Be Reported To Your Doctor Immediately

Less common or rare—Abdominal or stomach cramps and pain (severe); diarrhea (watery and severe), which may also be bloody; fever

The above side effects may also occur up to several weeks after you stop taking this medicine.

Rare—Convulsions (seizures); decrease in urine output; dizziness or lightheadedness; joint pain; loss of appetite; skin rash, itching, redness, or swelling; trouble in breathing

Side Effects That Usually Do Not Require Medical Attention

These possible side effects may go away during treatment; however, if they continue or are bothersome, check with your doctor, nurse, or pharmacist.

More common (less common with some cephalosporins)—Diarrhea (mild); nausea and vomiting; sore mouth or tongue; stomach cramps (mild)

Other side effects not listed above may also occur in some patients. If you notice any other effects, check with your doctor, nurse, or pharmacist.

CHLORAL HYDRATE   Systemic

■For the Pharmacist■

In providing consultation, consider emphasizing the following selected information (» = major clinical significance):

Before using this medication
» Conditions affecting use, especially:
    Sensitivity to chloral hydrate
    Pregnancy—Chloral hydrate crosses placenta; chronic use during pregnancy may cause withdrawal symptoms in neonate
    Breast-feeding—Chloral hydrate is distributed into breast milk; use by nursing mothers may cause sedation in the infant
    Other medications, especially alcohol or other CNS depression–producing medications or coumarin- or indandione-derivative anticoagulants
    Other medical problems, especially esophagitis, gastritis, gastric or duodenal ulcers, hepatic function impairment, or renal function impairment

Proper use of this medication
» Importance of not using more medication than the amount prescribed because of habit-forming potential
    Proper administration:
    For capsule dosage form
        Swallowing capsule whole; not chewing because of unpleasant taste
        Taking with a full glass (240 mL) of water, fruit juice, or ginger ale to reduce gastric irritation
    For syrup dosage form
        Taking each dose mixed with up to ½ glass (120 mL) of clear liquid (e.g., water, apple juice, ginger ale) to improve flavor and reduce gastric irritation
    For suppository dosage form
        Proper administration technique
        Chilling in refrigerator for 30 minutes or running cold water over suppository before removing foil wrapper if too soft for insertion
» Proper dosing
    Missed dose: Not taking missed dose; not doubling doses
» Proper storage

Precautions while using this medication
    Regular visits to physician to check progress during prolonged therapy
    Checking with physician before discontinuing medication after prolonged use; gradual dosage reduction may be necessary to avoid the possibility of withdrawal symptoms
» Avoiding use of alcohol or other CNS depressants
» Suspected overdose: Getting emergency help at once
» Caution if dizziness, lightheadedness, or drowsiness occurs

Side/adverse effects
    Signs of potential side effects, especially allergic reaction, confusion, and paradoxical reaction

▲ For the Patient ▲

913444

ABOUT YOUR MEDICINE

Chloral hydrate (KLOR-al HYE-drate) belongs to the group of medicines called sedatives and hypnotics. It is sometimes used before surgery or certain procedures to relieve anxiety or tension or to produce sleep. In addition, chloral hydrate may be used with analgesics (pain medicine) for control of pain following surgery.

Chloral hydrate has been used in the treatment of insomnia (trouble in sleeping) and to help calm or relax patients who are nervous or tense. However, this medicine has generally been replaced by other medicines for the treatment of insomnia and nervousness or tension.

If any of the information in this leaflet causes you special concern or if you want additional information about your medicine and its use, check with your doctor, nurse, or pharmacist. **Remember, keep this and all other medicines out of the reach of children and never share your medicines with others.**

BEFORE USING THIS MEDICINE

Tell your doctor, nurse, and pharmacist if you . . .
- are allergic to any medicine, either prescription or non-prescription (OTC);
- are pregnant or intend to become pregnant while using this medicine;
- are breast-feeding;
- are taking any other prescription or nonprescription (OTC) medicine, especially anticoagulants (blood thinners), other CNS depressants, or tricyclic antidepressants;
- have any other medical problems, especially esophagitis or inflammation of the esophagus, gastritis or inflammation of the stomach, kidney disease, liver disease, or stomach ulcers.

PROPER USE OF THIS MEDICINE

For patients taking chloral hydrate capsules:
- Swallow the capsule whole. Do not chew since the medicine may cause an unpleasant taste.
- Take this medicine with a full glass (8 ounces) of water, fruit juice, or ginger ale to lessen stomach upset.

For patients taking chloral hydrate syrup:
- Take each dose of medicine mixed with 1/2 glass (4 ounces) of water, fruit juice, or ginger ale to improve flavor and lessen stomach upset.

Use this medicine only as directed by your doctor. Do not use more of it, do not use it more often, and do not use it for a longer time than your doctor ordered. If too much is used, it may become habit-forming.

If you miss a dose of this medicine, skip the missed dose and go back to your regular dosing schedule. Do not double doses.

PRECAUTIONS WHILE USING THIS MEDICINE

Chloral hydrate comes in different strengths. Serious problems, including deaths, have occurred when children were given the wrong strength. **Make sure your doctor has told your pharmacist how many milligrams (mg), not just the number of capsules or teaspoonfuls, should be used**.

This medicine will add to the effects of alcohol and other CNS depressants (medicines that slow down the nervous system). **Check with your doctor before taking any such depressants while you are using this medicine.**

If you think you or someone else may have taken an overdose, get emergency help at once. Taking an overdose of chloral hydrate or taking alcohol or other CNS depressants with chloral hydrate may lead to unconsciousness and possibly death. Some signs of an overdose are continuing confusion, convulsions (seizures), difficulty in swallowing, severe drowsiness, severe weakness, shortness of breath or troubled breathing, staggering, and slow or irregular heartbeat.

This medicine may cause some people to become dizzy, lightheaded, drowsy, or less alert than they are normally. Even if taken at bedtime, it may cause some people to feel drowsy or less alert on arising. **Make sure you know how you react to this medicine before you drive, use machines, or do other jobs that require you to be alert.**

POSSIBLE SIDE EFFECTS OF THIS MEDICINE
Side Effects That Should Be Reported To Your Doctor

 Less common—Skin rash or hives

 Rare—Confusion; hallucinations; unusual excitement

Side Effects That Usually Do Not Require Medical Attention

These possible side effects may go away during treatment; however, if they continue or are bothersome, check with your doctor, nurse, or pharmacist.

 More common—Nausea; stomach pain; vomiting

Other side effects not listed above may also occur in some patients. If you notice any other effects, check with your doctor, nurse, or pharmacist.

After you stop using this medicine, your body may need time to adjust. The length of time this takes depends on the amount of medicine you were using and how long you used it. During this time check with your doctor if you notice any unusual effects, especially confusion, hallucinations, nausea or vomiting, nervousness, restlessness, stomach pain, trembling, or unusual excitement.

CHLORAMPHENICOL   Systemic

■ For the Pharmacist ■

In providing consultation, consider emphasizing the following selected information (» = major clinical significance):

Before using this medication
»   Conditions affecting use, especially:
       Allergies or toxic reactions to chloramphenicol
       Pregnancy—Chloramphenicol crosses the placenta; use at term or during labor may cause "gray syndrome" in infants
       Breast feeding—Chloramphenicol is excreted in breast milk; may cause bone marrow depression in the infant
       Use in children—Because of possible accumulation and toxic reactions, serum concentrations must be measured in premature and newborn infants
       Dental—May result in an increased incidence of infection, delayed healing, and gingival bleeding
       Other medications, especially alfentanil, hydantoin anticonvulsants, bone marrow depressants, radiation therapy, oral antidiabetic agents, erythromycins, lincomycins, phenobarbital, phenytoin, warfarin, or other medicines metabolized by mixed-function oxidase system
       Other medical problems, especially bone marrow depression, liver dysfunction, previous cytotoxic drug therapy, or radiation therapy

Proper use of this medication
       Taking on an empty stomach
       Proper administration technique for oral liquids
»   Compliance with full course of therapy
»   Proper dosing
       Missed dose: Taking as soon as possible; not taking if almost time for next dose; not doubling doses
»   Proper storage

Precautions while using this medication
       Checking with physician if no improvement within a few days
»   Regular visits to physician to check for blood problems
       Using caution in use of regular toothbrushes, dental floss, and toothpicks; completing dental work prior to initiation of therapy or deferring dental work until blood counts have returned to normal; checking with physician or dentist concerning proper oral hygiene
»   Diabetics: False-positive reactions with copper sulfate urine glucose tests may occur

Side/adverse effects
       May also cause bone marrow aplasia and "gray syndrome"
       Signs of potential side effects, especially blood dyscrasias, gray syndrome, optic neuritis, peripheral neuritis, neurotoxic reactions, or hypersensitivity reactions

▲ For the Patient ▲

913466

ABOUT YOUR MEDICINE

Chloramphenicol (klor-am-FEN-i-kole) is used to treat serious infections in different parts of the body. It is sometimes given with other antibiotics. However, chloramphenicol should not be used for colds, flu, other virus infections, sore throats or other minor infections, or to prevent infections.

If any of the information in this leaflet causes you special concern or if you want additional information about your medicine and its use, check with your doctor, nurse, or pharmacist. **Remember, keep this and all other medicines out of the reach of children and never share your medicines with others.**

BEFORE USING THIS MEDICINE

Chloramphenicol should only be used for serious infections in which other medicines do not work. This medicine may cause some serious side effects, including blood problems and eye problems. **You and your doctor should talk about the good this medicine will do as well as the risks of taking it.**

Tell your doctor, nurse, and pharmacist if you . . .
- are allergic to any medicine, either prescription or non-prescription (OTC);
- are pregnant or intend to become pregnant while using this medicine;
- are breast-feeding;
- are taking **any** other prescription or nonprescription (OTC) medicine;
- have any other medical problems, especially anemia, bleeding, or other blood problems;
- have ever been treated with x-rays or cancer medicine.

PROPER USE OF THIS MEDICINE

Chloramphenicol is best taken with a full glass (8 ounces) of water on an empty stomach (either 1 hour before or 2 hours after meals), unless otherwise directed by your doctor.

To help clear up your infection completely, **keep taking this medicine for the full time of treatment** even if you begin to feel better after a few days; **do not miss any doses.**

If you do miss a dose of this medicine, take it as soon as possible. However, if it is almost time for your next dose, skip the missed dose and go back to your regular dosing schedule. Do not double doses.

PRECAUTIONS WHILE USING THIS MEDICINE

If your symptoms do not improve within a few days, or if they become worse, check with your doctor.

It is very important that your doctor check you at regular visits for any blood problems that may be caused by this medicine. These problems may result in a greater chance of infection, slow healing, and bleeding of the gums. Be careful when using regular toothbrushes, dental floss, and toothpicks. Dental work should be done before you begin taking this medicine or delayed until your blood counts have returned to normal. Check with your medical doctor or dentist if you have any questions.

Diabetics—This medicine may cause false test results with urine sugar tests. Check with your doctor before changing your diet or the dosage of your diabetes medicine.

This medicine must not be given to other people or used for other infections unless otherwise directed by your doctor.

POSSIBLE SIDE EFFECTS OF THIS MEDICINE
Side Effects That Should Be Reported To Your Doctor Immediately

Stop taking this medicine and get emergency help immediately if you notice:

> *In babies only*
>> *Rare*—Bloated stomach; drowsiness; gray skin color; low body temperature; uneven breathing

Other Side Effects That Should Be Reported To Your Doctor Immediately

> *Less common*—Pale skin; sore throat and fever; unusual bleeding or bruising; unusual tiredness or weakness

> *Rare*—Confusion, delirium, or headache; eye pain, blurred vision, or loss of vision; numbness, tingling, burning pain, or weakness in the hands or feet; skin rash, fever, or difficulty in breathing

Some of the above side effects may also occur up to weeks or months after you stop taking this medicine.

Other side effects not listed above may also occur in some patients. If you notice any other effects, check with your doctor, nurse, or pharmacist.

CHLORDIAZEPOXIDE AND CLIDINIUM   Systemic

■For the Pharmacist■

In providing consultation, consider emphasizing the following selected information (» = major clinical significance):

Before using this medication
» Conditions affecting use, especially:
   Sensitivity to clidinium and chlordiazepoxide or to other benzodiazepines or any of the belladonna alkaloids
   Pregnancy—Use is not recommended; chronic use of chlordiazepoxide may cause physical dependence and withdrawal symptoms in the neonate; chlordiazepoxide increases risk of congenital malformations in first trimester
   Breast-feeding—Chlordiazepoxide distributed into breast milk; clidinium may cause inhibition of lactation
   Use in children—Increased susceptibility to anticholinergic effects of clidinium and to CNS effects of chlordiazepoxide
   Use in the elderly—Increased susceptibility to mental and other anticholinergic effects of clidinium and to CNS effects of chlordiazepoxide; danger of precipitating undiagnosed glaucoma; possible impairment of memory
   Dental—Possible development of dental problems because of decreased salivary flow
   Other medications, especially other anticholinergics, antacids, antidiarrheals, CNS depressants, ketoconazole, or potassium chloride
   Other medical problems, especially cardiac disease, glaucoma, hepatic disease, hiatal hernia with reflux esophagitis, intestinal atony, myasthenia gravis, obstruction in gastrointestinal or urinary tract, ulcerative colitis, or urinary retention

Proper use of this medication
   Taking dose 30 to 60 minutes before meals unless told otherwise by physician
» Taking medication only as directed
» Proper dosing
   Missed dose: Taking as soon as possible; not taking if almost time for next dose; not doubling doses
» Proper storage

Precautions while using this medication
   Regular visits to physician to check progress of therapy if used for extended period of time
   Avoiding medicine for diarrhea within 1 to 2 hours of taking this medication
» Caution if dizziness, lightheadedness, drowsiness, or blurred vision occurs
» Avoiding use of alcohol or other CNS depressants during and for a few days following therapy
» Caution during exercise and hot weather; overheating may result in heat stroke
   Possible dryness of mouth, nose, and throat; using sugarless gum or candy, ice, or saliva substitute for relief; checking with dentist if mouth continues to feel dry for more than 2 weeks
» Checking with physician if constipation occurs

Checking with physician before discontinuing medication after prolonged use; gradual dosage reduction may be necessary to avoid the possibility of withdrawal symptoms

Side/adverse effects

Signs of potential side effects, especially agranulocytosis, granulocytopenia, or leukopenia; allergic reaction; CNS depression; increased intraocular pressure; jaundice; and paradoxical reaction

---

▲ For the Patient ▲

912180

ABOUT YOUR MEDICINE

Chlordiazepoxide (klor-dye-az-e-POX-ide) and **clidinium** (kli-DI-nee-um) is a combination of medicines used to relax the digestive system and to reduce stomach acid. It is used to treat stomach and intestinal problems such as ulcers and colitis.

If any of the information in this leaflet causes you special concern or if you want additional information about your medicine and its use, check with your doctor, nurse, or pharmacist. **Remember, keep this and all other medicines out of the reach of children and never share your medicines with others.**

BEFORE USING THIS MEDICINE

Tell your doctor, nurse, and pharmacist if you . . .

- are allergic to any medicine, either prescription or non-prescription (OTC);
- are pregnant or intend to become pregnant while using this medicine;
- are breast-feeding;
- are taking any other prescription or nonprescription (OTC) medicine, especially CNS depressants, ketoconazole, medicine for diarrhea, other medicine for abdominal or stomach spasms or cramps, or potassium chloride;
- have any other medical problems, especially difficult urination, glaucoma, hiatal hernia, intestinal blockage, liver disease, myasthenia gravis, or severe ulcerative colitis.

PROPER USE OF THIS MEDICINE

Take this medicine only as directed. If too much is taken, it may become habit-forming.

Take this medicine about 1/2 to 1 hour before meals unless otherwise directed by your doctor.

If you miss a dose of this medicine, take it as soon as possible. However, if it is almost time for your next dose, skip the missed dose and go back to your regular dosing schedule. Do not double doses.

PRECAUTIONS WHILE USING THIS MEDICINE

If you will be taking this medicine regularly for a long period of time, your doctor should check your progress at regular visits.

Chlordiazepoxide and clidinium may cause some people to have blurred vision or to become dizzy, lightheaded, drowsy, or less alert than they are normally. **Make sure you know how you react to this medicine before you drive, use machines, or do other jobs that require you to be alert or able to see well.**

This medicine will add to the effects of alcohol and other CNS depressants (medicines that slow down the nervous system). **Check with your doctor before taking any such depressants while you are using this medicine.**

This medicine will often make you sweat less, causing your body temperature to increase. **Use extra care not to become overheated during exercise or hot weather while you are taking this medicine** as this could result in heat stroke. Also, hot baths or saunas may make you feel dizzy or faint while you are taking this medicine.

Check with your doctor if you develop intestinal problems such as constipation. This is especially important if you are taking other medicine while you are taking chlordiazepoxide and clidinium. If not corrected, complications may result.

POSSIBLE SIDE EFFECTS OF THIS MEDICINE
Side Effects That Should Be Reported To Your Doctor

> *Less common or rare*—Constipation; eye pain; mental depression; shortness of breath; skin rash or hives; slow heartbeat; sore throat and fever; troubled breathing; trouble in sleeping; unusual excitement; yellow eyes or skin

Side Effects That Usually Do Not Require Medical Attention

These possible side effects may go away during treatment; however, if they continue or are bothersome, check with your doctor, nurse, or pharmacist.

> *More common*—Bloated feeling; decreased sweating; dizziness; drowsiness; dryness of mouth; headache

Other side effects not listed above may also occur in some patients. If you notice any other effects, check with your doctor, nurse, or pharmacist.

After you stop using this medicine, your body may need time to adjust. The length of time this takes depends on the amount of medicine you were using and how long you used it. **During this time check with your doctor** if you have muscle cramps, nausea or vomiting, seizures, stomach cramps, or trembling.

CHLORHEXIDINE   Mucosal-Local

■ For the Pharmacist ■

In providing consultation, consider emphasizing the following selected information (» = major clinical significance):

Before using this medication
» Conditions affecting use, especially:
  Allergy to chlorhexidine or to disinfectant skin cleansers containing chlorhexidine

Proper use of this medication
  Using medication after brushing and flossing; rinsing toothpaste completely from mouth with water before using oral rinse; not eating or drinking for several hours after using oral rinse
  Using the cap of the original container to measure the dose or acquiring another measuring device to use; asking your pharmacist for help
» Swishing medication around in mouth for 30 seconds and spitting out; using full strength; not swallowing
» Proper dosing
  Missed dose: Using as soon as possible; not using if almost time for next dose; not doubling doses
» Proper storage

Precautions while using this medication
  Not rinsing mouth with water immediately after using medication, since doing so will increase medication's bitter aftertaste and may decrease medication's effect
  Medication causes change in taste; change may last up to 4 hours after dose; change in taste should be less noticeable as medication is continued; after medication is discontinued, taste should return to normal
  Staining and increase in tartar (calculus) may occur; brushing with tartar-control toothpaste and flossing teeth daily to help reduce tartar build-up; visiting dentist at least every 6 months for teeth cleaning and gum examination
» Getting emergency help at once if a child weighing 22 pounds (10 kg) or less drinks more than 4 ounces of dental rinse or if any child experiences symptoms of alcohol intoxication, such as slurred speech, sleepiness, or staggering or stumbling walk, after drinking the dental rinse

Side/adverse effects
  Signs of potential side effects, especially allergic reaction

▲ For the Patient ▲

915610
ABOUT YOUR MEDICINE

Chlorhexidine (klor-HEX-i-deen) is used to treat gingivitis. It helps to reduce the inflammation (redness) and swelling of your gums and to reduce gum bleeding.

If any of the information in this leaflet causes you special concern or if you want additional information about your medicine and its use, check with your dentist, physician, nurse, or pharmacist. **Remember, keep this and all other medicines out of the reach of children and never share your medicines with others.**

BEFORE USING THIS MEDICINE

Tell your dentist, physician, nurse, and pharmacist if you . . .
- are allergic to any medicine, either prescription or nonprescription (OTC);
- are pregnant or intend to become pregnant while using this medicine;
- are breast-feeding;
- are taking any other prescription or nonprescription (OTC) medicine;
- have any other gum problems;
- have any front-tooth fillings.

PROPER USE OF THIS MEDICINE

Chlorhexidine oral rinse should be used after you have brushed and flossed your teeth. Rinse the toothpaste completely from your mouth with water before using the oral rinse. Do not eat or drink for several hours after using the oral rinse.

The cap on the original container of chlorhexidine can be used to measure the 15 mL (1/2 fluid ounce) dose of this medicine. Fill the cap to the "fill line." If you do not receive the dental rinse in its original container, make sure you have a measuring device to measure out the correct dose. Your pharmacist can help you with this.

Swish chlorhexidine around in the mouth for 30 seconds. Then spit out. **Use the medicine full strength**. Do not mix with water before using. **Do not swallow the medicine**.

If you miss a dose of this medicine, use it as soon as possible. However, if it is almost time for your next dose, skip the missed dose and go back to your regular dosing schedule. Do not double doses.

PRECAUTIONS WHILE USING THIS MEDICINE

Chlorhexidine may have a bitter aftertaste. Do not rinse your mouth with water immediately after using chlorhexidine, since doing so will increase the bitterness. Rinsing may also decrease the effect of the medicine.

Chlorhexidine may change the way foods taste to you. Sometimes this effect may last up to 4 hours after you use the oral rinse. In most cases, this effect will become less noticeable as you continue to use the medicine. When you stop using chlorhexidine, your taste should return to normal.

Chlorhexidine may cause staining and an increase in tartar (calculus) on your teeth. Brushing with a tartar-control toothpaste and flossing your teeth daily may help reduce this tartar build-up and stain. In addition, you should visit your dentist at least every 6 months to have your teeth cleaned and your gums examined.

If you think that a child weighing 22 pounds (10 kilograms) or less has swallowed more than 4 ounces of the dental rinse, **get emergency help at once.** In addition, if a child of any age drinks the dental rinse and has symptoms of alcohol intoxication, such as slurred speech, sleepiness, or a staggering or stumbling walk, **get emergency help at once.**

POSSIBLE SIDE EFFECTS OF THIS MEDICINE

Side Effects That Should Be Reported To Your Doctor Immediately

> *Rare*—Signs of allergic reactions, such as nasal congestion; shortness of breath or troubled breathing; skin rash, hives, or itching; or swelling of face

Side Effects That Usually Do Not Require Medical Attention

These possible side effects may go away during treatment; however, if they continue or are bothersome, check with your dentist, physician, nurse, or pharmacist.

> *More common*—Change in taste; increase in tartar (calculus) on teeth; staining of teeth, mouth, tooth fillings, and dentures or other mouth appliances

> *Less common or rare*—Mouth irritation; swollen glands on side of face or neck; tongue tip irritation

Other side effects not listed above may also occur in some patients. If you notice any other effects, check with your dentist, physician, nurse, or pharmacist.

CHLOROQUINE   Systemic

∎For the Pharmacist∎

In providing consultation, consider emphasizing the following selected
information (» = major clinical significance):

Before using this medication
» Conditions affecting use, especially:
>   Hypersensitivity to chloroquine or hydroxychloroquine
>   Pregnancy—May cause toxicity to the fetus when given to mother
>   in therapeutic doses; however, chloroquine has not been shown
>   to cause adverse effects in the fetus when used as a prophy-
>   lactic agent against malaria
>   Use in children—Infants and children are especially sensitive to
>   effects of chloroquine
>   Other medical problems, especially impaired hepatic function,
>   severe blood disorders, severe neurologic disorders, or pres-
>   ence of retinal or visual field changes

Proper use of this medication
» Taking with meals or milk to minimize possible gastrointestinal ir-
>   ritation
» Keeping medication out of reach of children; fatalities reported with
>   as little as 300 mg of chloroquine base (1 tablet) in a 12 month
>   old
» Importance of not taking more medication than the amount pre-
>   scribed
» Compliance with full course of therapy
» Importance of not missing doses and taking medication on regular
>   schedule
» Proper dosing
>   Missed dose: If dosing schedule is—
>   Every 7 days: Taking as soon as possible
>   Once a day: Taking as soon as possible; not taking if not re-
>   membered until next day; not doubling doses
>   More than once a day: Taking right away if remembered within
>   an hour or so; not taking if not remembered until later; not
>   doubling doses
» Proper storage
For prevention of malaria
>   Starting medication 1 to 2 weeks before entering malarious area to
>   ascertain patient response and allow time to substitute another
>   medication if reactions occur
» Continuing medication while staying in area and for 4 weeks after
>   leaving area; checking with physician immediately if fever de-
>   velops while traveling or within 2 months after departure from
>   endemic area
For arthritis and lupus erythematosus
>   Importance of taking medication on regular schedule
>   May require up to 6 months for full benefit

Precautions while using this medication
» Regular visits to physician to check for blood problems, muscle
>   weakness, and ophthalmologic examinations during or after long-
>   term therapy
>   Checking with physician if no improvement within a few days (or
>   a few weeks or months for arthritis)

» Caution if blurred vision, difficulty in reading, or other change in
vision occurs
Mosquito-control measures to reduce the chance of getting malaria:
Sleeping under mosquito netting
Wearing long-sleeved shirts or blouses and long trousers to pro-
tect arms and legs between dusk and dawn
Applying mosquito repellent to uncovered areas of skin between
dusk and dawn

Side/adverse effects
Signs of potential side effects, especially ocular toxicity, cardiovascular toxicity, neuromyopathy, emotional or psychological
changes, ototoxicity, seizures, and blood dyscrasias

▲ For the Patient ▲

913229
ABOUT YOUR MEDICINE

Chloroquine (KLOR–oh–kwin) is a medicine used to prevent
and treat malaria and to treat some conditions such as liver
disease caused by protozoa. It is also used in the treatment
of arthritis to help relieve inflammation, swelling, stiffness,
and joint pain, and to help control the symptoms of lupus
erythematosus (lupus; SLE). Chloroquine may also be used
for other conditions as determined by your doctor.

If any of the information in this leaflet causes you special
concern or if you want additional information about your
medicine and its use, check with your doctor, nurse, or pharmacist. **Remember, keep this and all other medicines out of
the reach of children and never share your medicines with
others.**

BEFORE USING THIS MEDICINE
Tell your doctor, nurse, and pharmacist if you . . .
- are allergic to any medicine, either prescription or nonprescription (OTC);
- are pregnant or intend to become pregnant while using
this medicine;
- are breast-feeding;
- are taking **any** other prescription or nonprescription
(OTC) medicine;
- have any other medical problems, especially blood disease, eye or vision problems, liver disease, or nerve or
brain disease, including convulsions (seizures).

PROPER USE OF THIS MEDICINE
Take this medicine with meals or milk to lessen possible
stomach upset, unless otherwise directed by your doctor.

Keep this medicine out of the reach of children. Overdose is
especially dangerous in children.

Take this medicine only as directed. If you are taking this
medicine to treat or prevent malaria, **keep taking it for the
full time of treatment.**

If you miss a dose of this medicine, take it as soon as possible. However, if it is almost time for your next dose, skip the missed dose and go back to your regular dosing schedule. Do not double doses.

For patients taking this medicine to prevent malaria: Your doctor may want you to start taking this medicine 1 to 2 weeks before you travel to an area where there is a chance of getting malaria and for 6 weeks after you leave the area. If fever develops during your travels or within 2 months after you leave the area, **check with your doctor immediately.**

For patients taking this medicine for arthritis or lupus: It may take up to several weeks before you begin to feel better and up to 6 months before you feel the full benefit of this medicine.

PRECAUTIONS WHILE USING THIS MEDICINE

This medicine may cause blurred vision, difficulty in reading, or other changes in vision. It may also cause some people to become lightheaded. **Make sure you know how you react to this medicine before you drive, use machines, or do other jobs that require you to be alert or to see well.**

POSSIBLE SIDE EFFECTS OF THIS MEDICINE

Side Effects That Should Be Reported To Your Doctor Immediately

> *Less common*—Blurred vision or any other change in vision

> *Rare*—Convulsions (seizures); fatigue; feeling faint or lightheaded; increased muscle weakness; mood or other mental changes; ringing or buzzing in ears or any loss of hearing; sore throat and fever; unusual bleeding or bruising; weakness

Side Effects That Usually Do Not Require Medical Attention

These possible side effects may go away during treatment; however, if they continue or are bothersome, check with your doctor, nurse, or pharmacist.

> *More common*—Diarrhea; difficulty in seeing to read; headache; itching (more common in black patients); loss of appetite; nausea or vomiting; stomach cramps or pain

> *Less common*—Bleaching of hair or increased hair loss; blue-black discoloration of skin, fingernails, or inside of mouth; skin rash

Other side effects not listed above may also occur in some patients. If you notice any other effects, check with your doctor, nurse, or pharmacist.

CHOLESTYRAMINE Oral-Local

■For the Pharmacist■

In providing consultation, consider emphasizing the following selected information (» = major clinical significance):

Before using this medication
» Conditions affecting use, especially:
> Sensitivity to cholestyramine
> Use in children—Caution with use in children less than 10 years of age since cholesterol is required for normal development
> Use in the elderly—Increased incidence of gastrointestinal side effects and potentially adverse nutritional effects in patients over 60 years of age
> Other oral medications, especially anticoagulants, digitalis glycosides, thiazide diuretics, penicillin G, phenylbutazone, propranolol, tetracyclines, thyroid hormones, or vancomycin
> Other medical problems, especially complete biliary obstruction or complete atresia, constipation, or phenylketonuria

Proper use of this medication
» Importance of not taking more or less medication than the amount prescribed
» Proper dosing
> Missed dose: Taking as soon as possible; not taking if almost time for next dose; not doubling doses
» Proper storage
» Importance of mixing with fluids before taking; instructions for measuring and mixing—Placing in 2 ounces of any beverage and stirring vigorously, then adding 2 to 4 ounces of beverage and shaking vigorously (does not dissolve); rinsing glass and drinking to make sure all medication is taken; may also be mixed with milk in cereals, thin soups, or pulpy fruits
For use as an antihyperlipidemic
» Diet as preferred therapy; importance of following prescribed diet
> This medication does not cure the condition but rather helps control it

Precautions while using this medication
» Importance of close monitoring by the physician
» Not taking any other medication unless discussed with physician
For use as an antihyperlipidemic
» Checking with physician before discontinuing medication; blood lipid concentrations may increase significantly

Side/adverse effects
> Signs of potential side effects, especially constipation, gallstones, pancreatitis, gastrointestinal bleeding, peptic ulcer, and steatorrhea or malabsorption syndrome

---

▲ For the Patient ▲

916125

CHOLESTEROL-LOWERING RESINS (Oral):
Including Cholestyramine; Colestipol.

ABOUT YOUR MEDICINE

Cholesterol-lowering resins are used to lower levels of cholesterol (a fat-like substance) in the blood. This may help prevent medical problems caused by cholesterol clogging the blood vessels. These medicines may also be used for other conditions as determined by your doctor.

If any of the information in this leaflet causes you special concern or if you want additional information about your medicine and its use, check with your doctor, nurse, or pharmacist. **Remember, keep this and all other medicines out of the reach of children and never share your medicines with others.**

BEFORE USING THIS MEDICINE

Importance of diet—Before prescribing medicine for your condition, your doctor will probably try to control your condition by prescribing a personal diet for you. Such a diet may be low in fats, sugars, and/or cholesterol. Many people are able to control their condition by carefully following their doctor's orders for proper diet and exercise. Medicine is prescribed only when additional help is needed and is effective only when a schedule of diet and exercise is properly followed.

Also, this medicine is less effective if you are greatly overweight. It may be very important for you to go on a reducing diet. However, check with your doctor before going on any diet.

Tell your doctor, nurse, and pharmacist if you . . .
- are allergic to any medicine, either prescription or nonprescription (OTC);
- are pregnant or intend to become pregnant while using this medicine;
- are breast-feeding;
- are taking any other prescription or nonprescription (OTC) medicine, especially anticoagulants (blood thinners), digitalis glycosides (heart medicine), diuretics (water pills), phenylbutazone, penicillins, propranolol, tetracyclines, thyroid hormones, or vancomycin;
- have any other medical problems, especially constipation or stomach problems;
- have phenylketonuria, since some brands of cholestyramine may contain aspartame.

PROPER USE OF THIS MEDICINE

For patients taking the powder form of this medicine:

- **This medicine should never be taken in its dry form, since it could cause you to choke.** Instead, always mix as follows:
  - —For cholestyramine: Place the medicine in 2 ounces of any beverage and mix thoroughly. Then add an additional 2 to 4 ounces of beverage and again mix thoroughly (it will **not** dissolve) before drinking.
  - —For colestipol: Add this medicine to 3 ounces or more of water, milk, flavored drink, or your favorite juice or carbonated drink. If you use a carbonated drink, slowly mix in the powder in a large glass to prevent too much foaming.
  - —Stir until the medicine is completely mixed (it will **not** dissolve) before drinking. After drinking all the liquid, rinse the glass with a little more liquid and drink that also, to make sure you get the full dose.
  - —You may also mix this medicine with milk in hot or regular breakfast cereals, or in thin soups such as tomato or chicken noodle. Or you may add it to some pulpy fruits such as crushed pineapple, pears, peaches, or fruit cocktail.

For patients taking the chewable bar form of cholestyramine:

- Chew each bite well before swallowing.

Take this medicine exactly as directed by your doctor. Try not to miss any doses and do not take more medicine than your doctor ordered.

If you miss a dose of this medicine, take it as soon as possible. However, if it is almost time for your next dose, skip the missed dose and go back to your regular dosing schedule. Do not double doses.

PRECAUTIONS WHILE USING THIS MEDICINE

It is very important that your doctor check your progress at regular visits.

Do not take any other medicine unless prescribed by your doctor since cholesterol-lowering resins may change the effect of other medicines.

Do not stop taking this medicine without first checking with your doctor. When you stop taking this medicine, your blood cholesterol levels may increase again. Your doctor may want you to follow a special diet to help prevent this.

POSSIBLE SIDE EFFECTS OF THIS MEDICINE

Side Effects That Should Be Reported To Your Doctor Immediately

> *Rare*—Black, tarry stools; stomach pain (severe) with nausea and vomiting

Other Side Effects That Should Be Reported To Your Doctor

    More common—Constipation

    Rare—Loss of weight (sudden)

Side Effects That Usually Do Not Require Medical Attention

These possible side effects may go away during treatment; however, if they continue or are bothersome, check with your doctor, nurse, or pharmacist.

    More common (less common for colestipol)—Heartburn or indigestion; nausea or vomiting; stomach pain

Other side effects not listed above may also occur in some patients. If you notice any other effects, check with your doctor, nurse, or pharmacist.

CIPROFLOXACIN   Ophthalmic

■For the Pharmacist■

In providing consultation, consider emphasizing the following selected information (» = major clinical significance):

Before using this medication
» Conditions affecting use, especially:
   Sensitivity to ciprofloxacin or other quinolones
   Breast-feeding—Oral ciprofloxacin is distributed into breast milk; it is not known whether ophthalmic ciprofloxacin is distributed into breast milk
   Use in children—Safety and efficacy have not been established in children up to 12 years of age

Proper use of this medication
   Proper administration technique
» Compliance with full course of therapy
» Proper dosing
   Missed dose: Applying as soon as possible; not applying if almost time for next dose
» Proper storage

Precautions while using this medication
   Checking with physician if no improvement within a few days
   Possible photophobic reactions; wearing sunglasses and avoiding prolonged exposure to bright light

Side/adverse effects
   Signs of potential side effects, especially corneal infiltrates, corneal staining, decreased vision, keratopathy, keratitis, nausea, or skin rash

▲ For the Patient ▲

919859

ABOUT YOUR MEDICINE

Ophthalmic **ciprofloxacin** (sip-roe-FLOX-a-sin) is used in the eye to treat bacterial infections of the eye and corneal ulcers of the eye.

If any of the information in this leaflet causes you special concern or if you want additional information about your medicine and its use, check with your doctor, nurse, or pharmacist. **Remember, keep this and all other medicines out of the reach of children and never share your medicines with others.**

BEFORE USING THIS MEDICINE

Tell your doctor, nurse, and pharmacist if you . . .
   • are allergic to any medicine, either prescription or non-prescription (OTC);
   • are pregnant or intend to become pregnant while using this medicine;
   • are breast-feeding;

- are taking any other prescription or nonprescription (OTC) medicine;
- have any other medical problems.

PROPER USE OF THIS MEDICINE
To use:

- First, wash your hands. Tilt the head back and, pressing your finger gently on the skin just beneath the lower eyelid, pull the lower eyelid away from the eye to make a space. Drop the medicine into the space. Let go of the eyelid and gently close the eyes. Do not blink. Keep the eyes closed for 1 or 2 minutes to allow the medicine to come into contact with the infection.
- If you think you did not get the drop of medicine into your eye properly, use another drop.
- To keep the medicine as germ-free as possible, do not touch the applicator tip to any surface (including the eye). Also, keep the container tightly closed.

To help clear up your infection completely, **keep using this medicine for the full time of treatment,** even if your symptoms begin to clear up after a few days. If you stop using this medicine too soon, your symptoms may return. **Do not miss any doses.**

If you do miss a dose of this medicine, use it as soon as possible. However, if it is almost time for your next dose, skip the missed dose and go back to your regular dosing schedule.

PRECAUTIONS WHILE USING THIS MEDICINE
If your symptoms do not improve within a few days, or if they become worse, check with your doctor.

This medicine may cause your eyes to become more sensitive to light than they are normally. Wearing sunglasses and avoiding too much exposure to bright light may help lessen the discomfort.

POSSIBLE SIDE EFFECTS OF THIS MEDICINE
Side Effects That Should Be Reported To Your Doctor Immediately

  Rare—Blurred vision or other change in vision; irritation (severe) or redness of eye; nausea; skin rash

Side Effects That Usually Do Not Require Medical Attention

These possible side effects may go away during treatment; however, if they continue or are bothersome, check with your doctor, nurse, or pharmacist.

  More common—Burning or other discomfort of eye; crusting or crystals in corner of eye

  Less common—Bad taste following use in the eye; feeling of something in eye; itching of eye; redness of the lining of the eyelid

Rare—Increased sensitivity of eyes to light; swelling of eyelid; tearing of eye

Other side effects not listed above may also occur in some patients. If you notice any other effects, check with your doctor, nurse, or pharmacist.

CISAPRIDE   Systemic

■ For the Pharmacist ■

In providing consultation, consider emphasizing the following selected information (» = major clinical significance):

Before using this medication
» Conditions affecting use, especially:
   Sensitivity to cisapride
   Breast-feeding—Distributed into breast milk in small amounts
   Other medical problems, especially gastrointestinal bleeding, mechanical obstruction, or perforation

Proper use of this medication
» Taking 15 minutes before meals and at bedtime with a beverage
» Proper dosing
   Missed dose: Using as soon as possible; not using if almost time for next dose
» Proper storage

Precautions while using this medication
» Checking with physician before using alcohol
» Caution if drowsiness occurs

Side/adverse effects
   Seizures

▲ For the Patient ▲

919677

ABOUT YOUR MEDICINE

Cisapride (SIS-a-pride) is used to treat symptoms such as heartburn caused by a backward flow of gastric acid into the esophagus. Cisapride may also be used for other conditions as determined by your doctor.

If any of the information in this leaflet causes you special concern or if you want additional information about your medicine and its use, check with your doctor, nurse, or pharmacist. **Remember, keep this and all other medicines out of the reach of children and never share your medicines with others.**

BEFORE USING THIS MEDICINE

Tell your doctor, nurse, and pharmacist if you . . .
- are allergic to any medicine, either prescription or nonprescription (OTC);
- are pregnant or intend to become pregnant while using this medicine;
- are breast-feeding;
- are taking any other prescription or nonprescription (OTC) medicine, especially anticholinergics (medicines for abdominal or stomach spasms or cramps);
- have any other medical problems, especially abdominal or stomach bleeding, or intestinal blockage.

PROPER USE OF THIS MEDICINE

Take this medicine 15 minutes before meals and at bedtime with a beverage, unless otherwise directed by your doctor.

If you miss a dose of this medicine, take it as soon as possible. However, if it is almost time for your next dose, skip the missed dose and go back to your regular dosing schedule. Do not double doses.

PRECAUTIONS WHILE USING THIS MEDICINE

This medicine may cause your body to absorb alcohol more quickly than you normally would. Therefore, you may notice the effects sooner. **Check with your doctor before drinking alcohol while you are using this medicine.**

This medicine may cause some people to become drowsy or less alert than they are normally. **Make sure you know how you react to this medicine before you drive, use machines, or do other jobs that require you to be alert.**

POSSIBLE SIDE EFFECTS OF THIS MEDICINE

Side Effects That Should Be Reported To Your Doctor Immediately

   Rare—Convulsions (seizures)

Side Effects That Usually Do Not Require Medical Attention

These possible side effects may go away during treatment; however, if they continue or are bothersome, check with your doctor, nurse, or pharmacist.

   Less common—Abdominal cramping; constipation; diarrhea; drowsiness; headache; nausea; unusual tiredness or weakness

Other side effects not listed above may also occur in some patients. If you notice any other effects, check with your doctor, nurse, or pharmacist.

CLARITHROMYCIN Systemic

■ For the Pharmacist ■

In providing consultation, consider emphasizing the following selected information (» = major clinical significance):

Before using this medication
» Conditions affecting use, especially:
    Hypersensitivity to erythromycins or other macrolides
    Pregnancy—Clarithromycin has produced embryotoxicity and fetal toxicity in animals
    Other medications, especially carbamazepine, rifabutin, terfenadine, theophylline, and zidovudine

Proper use of this medication
    May be taken with food or milk or on an empty stomach
    Compliance with full course of therapy
    Proper administration technique for oral liquids
» Proper dosing
    Missed dose: Taking as soon as possible; not taking if almost time for next dose; not doubling doses
» Proper storage

Precautions while using this medication
    Checking with physician if no improvement within a few days

Side/adverse effects
    Signs of potential side effects, especially thrombocytopenia

▲ For the Patient ▲

918313

ABOUT YOUR MEDICINE

Clarithromycin (kla-RITH-roe-mye-sin) is used to treat bacterial infections in many different parts of the body. It is also used to treat *Mycobacterium avium* complex (MAC) infection. However, this medicine will not work for colds, flu, or other virus infections. Clarithromycin may be used for other problems as determined by your doctor.

If any of the information in this leaflet causes you special concern or if you want additional information about your medicine and its use, check with your doctor, nurse, or pharmacist. **Remember, keep this and all other medicines out of the reach of children and never share your medicines with others.**

BEFORE USING THIS MEDICINE

Tell your doctor, nurse, and pharmacist if you . . .
- are allergic to any medicine, either prescription or nonprescription (OTC);
- are pregnant or intend to become pregnant while using this medicine;
- are breast-feeding;

- are taking any other prescription or nonprescription (OTC) medicine, especially carbamazepine, rifabutin, terfenadine, theophylline, or zidovudine;
- have any other medical problems.

PROPER USE OF THIS MEDICINE

Clarithromycin may be taken with meals or milk or on an empty stomach.

To help clear up your infection completely, **keep taking clarithromycin for the full time of treatment,** even if you begin to feel better after a few days. If you stop taking this medicine too soon, your symptoms may return.

If you are using clarithromycin oral suspension, use a specially marked measuring spoon or other device to measure each dose accurately. The average household teaspoon may not hold the right amount of liquid.

If you miss a dose of this medicine, take it as soon as possible. However, if it is almost time for your next dose, skip the missed dose and go back to your regular dosing schedule. Do not double doses.

PRECAUTIONS WHILE USING THIS MEDICINE

If your symptoms do not improve within a few days, or if they become worse, check with your doctor.

POSSIBLE SIDE EFFECTS OF THIS MEDICINE

Side Effects That Should Be Reported To Your Doctor

   Rare—Unusual bleeding or bruising

Side Effects That Usually Do Not Require Medical Attention

These possible side effects may go away during treatment; however, if they continue or are bothersome, check with your doctor, nurse, or pharmacist.

   Less common—Abnormal taste; diarrhea; headache; nausea; stomach pain or discomfort; vomiting

Other side effects not listed above may also occur in some patients. If you notice any other effects, check with your doctor, nurse, or pharmacist.

CLINDAMYCIN   Systemic

■For the Pharmacist■

In providing consultation, consider emphasizing the following selected information (» = major clinical significance):

Before using this medication
» Conditions affecting use, especially:
>> Hypersensitivity to clindamycin, lincomycin, or doxorubicin
>> Pregnancy—Clindamycin crosses the placenta
>> Breast-feeding—Clindamycin is excreted in breast milk
>> Use in children—Clindamycin should be used cautiously in infants up to 1 month of age; clindamycin injection contains benzyl alcohol, which has been associated with a fatal gasping syndrome in infants
>> Other medications, especially hydrocarbon inhalation anesthetics, neuromuscular blocking agents, adsorbent antidiarrheals, chloramphenicol, or erythromycins
>> Other medical problems, especially a history of gastrointestinal disease, particularly ulcerative colitis, or severe hepatic function impairment

Proper use of this medication
» Taking clindamycin capsules with a full glass of water or with meals to avoid esophageal ulceration
>> Proper administration technique for clindamycin oral solution; not using after expiration date
» Compliance with full course of therapy, especially in streptococcal infections
» Importance of not missing doses and taking at evenly spaced times
» Proper dosing
>> Missed dose: Taking as soon as possible; not taking if almost time for next dose; not doubling doses
» Proper storage

Precautions while using this medication
>> Regular visits to physician to check progress
>> Checking with physician if no improvement within a few days
» For severe diarrhea, checking with physician before taking any antidiarrheals; for mild diarrhea, taking attapulgite-containing antidiarrheals at least 2 hours before or 3 to 4 hours after taking oral clindamycin; other antidiarrheals may worsen or prolong the diarrhea; checking with physician or pharmacist if mild diarrhea continues or worsens
>> Caution if surgery with general anesthesia is required

Side/adverse effects
>> Signs of potential side effects, especially pseudomembranous colitis, hypersensitivity, neutropenia, and thrombocytopenia

---

▲ For the Patient ▲

914210

LINCOMYCINS (Oral): *Including Clindamycin;*
Lincomycin.

ABOUT YOUR MEDICINE

Lincomycins (lin-koe-MYE-sins) belong to the general family of medicines called antibiotics. These medicines are used to treat infections. They will not work for colds, flu, or other virus infections.

If any of the information in this leaflet causes you special concern or if you want additional information about your medicine and its use, check with your doctor, nurse, or pharmacist. **Remember, keep this and all other medicines out of the reach of children and never share your medicines with others.**

BEFORE USING THIS MEDICINE

Tell your doctor, nurse, and pharmacist if you . . .
- are allergic to any medicine, either prescription or non-prescription (OTC);
- are pregnant or intend to become pregnant while using this medicine;
- are breast-feeding;
- are taking any other prescription or nonprescription (OTC) medicine, especially chloramphenicol, diarrhea medicine, or erythromycins;
- have any other medical problems, especially liver disease, or stomach or intestinal disease (history of) (especially colitis, including colitis caused by antibiotics, or enteritis).

PROPER USE OF THIS MEDICINE

If you are taking the capsule form of clindamycin, it should be taken with a full glass (8 ounces) of water or with meals to prevent irritation of the esophagus.

For patients taking lincomycin:
- Lincomycin is best taken with a full glass (8 ounces) of water on an empty stomach (either 1 hour before or 2 hours after meals).

To help clear up your infection completely, **keep taking this medicine for the full time of treatment** even if you begin to feel better after a few days. **If you have a "strep" infection, you should keep taking this medicine for at least 10 days. This is especially important in "strep" infections. Serious heart problems could develop later** if your infection is not cleared up completely. Also, if you stop taking this medicine too soon, your symptoms may return.

This medicine works best when there is a constant amount in the blood. **To help keep this amount constant, do not miss** any doses. Also, it is best to take each dose at evenly spaced times day and night.

If you do miss a dose of this medicine, take it as soon as possible. This will help to keep a constant amount of medicine in the blood. However, if it is almost time for your next dose, skip the missed dose and go back to your regular dosing schedule. Do not double doses.

PRECAUTIONS WHILE USING THIS MEDICINE

If your symptoms do not improve within a few days, or if they become worse, check with your doctor.

In some patients, lincomycins may cause diarrhea.
- Severe diarrhea may be a sign of a serious side effect. **Do not take any diarrhea medicine without first checking with your doctor.**
- For mild diarrhea, diarrhea medicine containing attapulgite (e.g., Kaopectate tablets, Diasorb) may be taken. However, attapulgite may keep lincomycins from being absorbed into the body. Therefore, these diarrhea medicines should be taken at least 2 hours before or 3 to 4 hours after you take lincomycins by mouth.

If you have any questions about this or if mild diarrhea continues or gets worse, check with your doctor, nurse, or pharmacist.

This medicine must not be given to other people or used for other infections unless you are otherwise directed by your doctor.

POSSIBLE SIDE EFFECTS OF THIS MEDICINE

Side Effects That Should Be Reported To Your Doctor Immediately

 More common—Abdominal or stomach cramps and pain (severe); abdominal tenderness; diarrhea (watery and severe), which may also be bloody; fever

The above side effects may also occur up to several weeks after you stop taking this medicine.

 Less common—Skin rash, redness, and itching; sore throat and fever; unusual bleeding or bruising

Side Effects That Usually Do Not Require Medical Attention

These possible side effects may go away during treatment; however, if they continue or are bothersome, check with your doctor, nurse, or pharmacist.

 More common—Diarrhea (mild); nausea and vomiting; stomach pain

Other side effects not listed above may also occur in some patients. If you notice any other effects, check with your doctor, nurse, or pharmacist.

CLINDAMYCIN   Topical

■ For the Pharmacist ■

In providing consultation, consider emphasizing the following selected information (» = major clinical significance):

Before using this medication
» Conditions affecting use, especially:
> Sensitivity to clindamycin or lincomycin
> Breast feeding—May be distributed into breast milk in small quantities since systemic clindamycin is distributed into breast milk
> Other medical problems, especially a history of antibiotic-associated colitis, ulcerative colitis, or regional enteritis

Proper use of this medication
> Before applying, washing affected areas with warm water and soap, rinsing, and patting dry
» Importance of applying medication to entire affected area
> Avoiding too frequent washing of affected areas
» Compliance with full course of therapy, which may take months or longer
» Proper dosing
> Missed dose: Applying as soon as possible; not applying if almost time for next dose
» Proper storage
For topical solution only
> Waiting 30 minutes after washing or shaving before applying
» Not using near heat, near open flame, or while smoking
> Proper administration technique for applicator-tip bottle:
» Avoiding contact with eyes, nose, mouth, or other mucous membranes
> Not using more often than prescribed
For topical suspension only
» Shaking well before using

Precautions while using this medication
> Checking with physician or pharmacist if no improvement within about 6 weeks
> Applying other medications at different times
> Checking with physician if treated skin becomes excessively dry (for topical solution only)
» For severe diarrhea, checking with physician before taking any antidiarrheals; for mild diarrhea, taking attapulgite-containing, but not other, antidiarrheals; checking with physician or pharmacist if mild diarrhea continues or worsens
> Using only "water-base" cosmetics; not applying too heavily or too often

Side/adverse effects
> Signs of potential side effects, especially hypersensitivity reactions and pseudomembranous colitis

▲ For the Patient ▲

913524

ABOUT YOUR MEDICINE

Clindamycin (klin-da-MYE-sin) belongs to the family of medicines called antibiotics. Topical clindamycin is used to help control acne. This medicine may also be used for other problems as determined by your doctor.

If any of the information in this leaflet causes you special concern or if you want additional information about your medicine and its use, check with your doctor, nurse, or pharmacist. **Remember, keep this and all other medicines out of the reach of children and never share your medicines with others.**

BEFORE USING THIS MEDICINE

Tell your doctor, nurse, and pharmacist if you . . .
- are allergic to any medicine, either prescription or non-prescription (OTC);
- are pregnant or intend to become pregnant while using this medicine;
- are breast-feeding;
- are taking any other prescription or nonprescription (OTC) medicine;
- have any other medical problems.

PROPER USE OF THIS MEDICINE

When applying this medicine, use enough to cover the affected area lightly. **You should apply the medicine to the whole area usually affected by acne, not just to the pimples themselves.**

For patients using the gel form of clindamycin:
- Apply a thin film to the affected areas.

For patients using the topical suspension (lotion) form of clindamycin:
- **Shake well** before applying.

For patients using the topical solution form of clindamycin:
- This medicine contains alcohol and is flammable. **Do not use near heat, near open flame, or while smoking.**
- **To apply this medicine:**
  —This medicine comes in a bottle with an applicator tip. Use the applicator with a dabbing motion instead of a rolling motion (not like a roll-on deodorant, for example). Tilt the bottle and press the tip firmly against your skin. If the applicator tip becomes dry, turn the bottle upside down and press the tip several times to moisten it.
  —Since this medicine contains alcohol, it will sting or burn. Also, it has an unpleasant taste if it gets on the mouth or lips. Therefore, **do not get this medicine in the eyes, nose, mouth, or on other mucous membranes.**

This medicine will not cure your acne. However, to help keep your acne under control, **keep using this medicine for the full time of treatment,** even if your symptoms begin to clear up after a few days. You may have to continue using this medicine every day for months or even longer. If you stop using this medicine too soon, your symptoms may return. **Do not miss any doses.**

If you do miss a dose of this medicine, apply it as soon as possible. However, if it is almost time for your next dose, skip the missed dose and go back to your regular dosing schedule.

PRECAUTIONS WHILE USING THIS MEDICINE

If there is no improvement in your acne after you have used this medicine for about 6 weeks, or if it becomes worse, check with your doctor or pharmacist.

In some patients, clindamycin may cause diarrhea.
- Severe diarrhea may be a sign of a serious side effect. **Do not take any diarrhea medicine without first checking with your doctor.** Diarrhea medicines may make your diarrhea worse or make it last longer.
- For mild diarrhea, only diarrhea medicine containing attapulgite may be taken.
- If you have any questions about this or if mild diarrhea continues or gets worse, check with your doctor or pharmacist.

You may continue to use cosmetics (make-up) while using this medicine for acne. However, it is best to use only "water-base" cosmetics. Also, it is best not to use cosmetics too heavily or too often. They may make your acne worse.

POSSIBLE SIDE EFFECTS OF THIS MEDICINE

Side Effects That Should Be Reported To Your Doctor Immediately

Rare—Abdominal or stomach cramps, pain, and bloating (severe); diarrhea (watery and severe) which may also be bloody; fever; increased thirst; nausea or vomiting; unusual tiredness or weakness; weight loss (unusual)

The above side effects may also occur up to several weeks after you stop using this medicine.

Other Side Effects That Should Be Reported To Your Doctor

Less common—Skin rash, itching, redness, swelling, or other sign of irritation not present before use of this medicine

Side Effects That Usually Do Not Require Medical Attention

These possible side effects may go away during treatment; however, if they continue or are bothersome, check with your doctor, nurse, or pharmacist.

More common—Dryness, scaliness, or peeling of skin (for topical solution)

Other side effects not listed above may also occur in some patients. If you notice any other effects, check with your doctor, nurse, or pharmacist.

CLOFIBRATE   Systemic

■ For the Pharmacist ■

In providing consultation, consider emphasizing the following selected
   information (» = major clinical significance):

Before using this medication
   Potential serious toxicity; WHO study controversy
   Diet as preferred therapy
» Conditions affecting use, especially:
      Sensitivity to clofibrate
      Pregnancy—May cross placenta; enzyme system required for
         excretion may not be developed in fetus; withdrawal of clo-
         fibrate therapy several months before conception is recom-
         mended if pregnancy is planned
      Breast-feeding—Use not recommended while nursing because of
         potentially serious adverse effects on nursing infants
      Use in children—Not recommended in children less than 2 years
         of age since cholesterol is required for normal development
      Other medications, especially anticoagulants
      Other medical problems, especially primary biliary cirrhosis, he-
         patic function impairment, or renal function impairment

Proper use of this medication
» Importance of not taking more or less medication than the amount
      prescribed
» Compliance with prescribed diet
      Taking with meals to prevent possible gastric irritation
» Proper dosing
      Missed dose: Taking as soon as possible; not taking if almost time
         for next dose; not doubling doses
» Proper storage

Precautions while using this medication
» Importance of close monitoring by the physician
» Checking with physician before discontinuing medication; blood lipid
      concentrations may increase significantly

Side/adverse effects
      Signs of potential side effects, especially angina, cardiac arrhyth-
         mias, leukopenia, anemia, pancreatitis, gallstones, and renal tox-
         icity

▲ For the Patient ▲

913535

ABOUT YOUR MEDICINE

Clofibrate (kloe-FYE-brate) is used to lower cholesterol and
triglyceride (fat-like substances) levels in the blood. This
may help prevent medical problems caused by such substances clogging the blood vessels. Clofibrate may also be
used for other conditions as determined by your doctor.

If any of the information in this leaflet causes you special
concern or if you want additional information about your
medicine and its use, check with your doctor, nurse, or pharmacist. **Remember, keep this and all other medicines out of**

**the reach of children and never share your medicines with
others.**

BEFORE USING THIS MEDICINE

In addition to its helpful effects in treating your medical
problem, this medicine may have some harmful effects.

You may have read or heard about a study called the WHO
Study. This study compared the effects in patients who used
clofibrate with effects in those who used a placebo (sugar
pill). The results of this study suggested that clofibrate might
increase the patient's risk of cancer, liver disease, and pancreatitis (inflammation of the pancreas), although it might
also decrease the risk of heart attack. It may also increase
the risk of gallstones and problems from gallbladder surgery.
Other studies have not found all of these effects. Be sure
you have discussed this with your doctor before taking this
medicine.

Importance of diet—Before prescribing medicine for your
condition, your doctor will probably try to control your condition by prescribing a personal diet for you. Such a diet
may be low in fats, sugars, and/or cholesterol. Many people
are able to control their condition by carefully following their
doctor's orders for proper diet and exercise. **Medicine is prescribed only when additional help is needed** and is effective
only when a schedule of diet and exercise is properly followed.

Also, this medicine is less effective if you are greatly overweight. It may be very important for you to go on a reducing diet. However, check with your doctor before going
on any diet.

Tell your doctor, nurse, and pharmacist if you . . .
- are allergic to any medicine, either prescription or nonprescription (OTC);
- are pregnant or intend to become pregnant while using
  this medicine;
- are breast-feeding;
- are taking any other prescription or nonprescription
  (OTC) medicine, especially anticoagulants (blood thinners);
- have any other medical problems, especially kidney disease or liver disease.

PROPER USE OF THIS MEDICINE

Use this medicine only as directed by your doctor. Do not
use more or less of it, and do not use it more often or for a
longer time than your doctor ordered.

Stomach upset may occur but usually lessens after a few
doses. Take this medicine with food or immediately after
meals to lessen possible stomach upset.

If you miss a dose of this medicine, take it as soon as possible.
However, if it is almost time for your next dose, skip the

missed dose and go back to your regular dosing schedule. Do not double doses.

PRECAUTIONS WHILE USING THIS MEDICINE

It is very important that your doctor check your progress at regular visits. This will allow your doctor to see if the medicine is working properly to lower your cholesterol and triglyceride levels and if you should continue to take it.

Do not stop taking this medicine without first checking with your doctor. When you stop taking this medicine, your blood fat levels may increase again. Your doctor may want you to follow a special diet to help prevent that.

POSSIBLE SIDE EFFECTS OF THIS MEDICINE

Side Effects That Should Be Reported To Your Doctor Immediately

> *Rare*—Chest pain; irregular heartbeat; shortness of breath; stomach pain (severe) with nausea and vomiting

Other Side Effects That Should Be Reported To Your Doctor

> *Rare*—Blood in urine; cough or hoarseness; decrease in urination; fever or chills; lower back or side pain; painful or difficult urination; swelling of feet or lower legs

Side Effects That Usually Do Not Require Medical Attention

These possible side effects may go away during treatment; however, if they continue or are bothersome, check with your doctor, nurse, or pharmacist.

> *More common*—Diarrhea; nausea

Other side effects not listed above may also occur in some patients. If you notice any other effects, check with your doctor, nurse, or pharmacist.

CLOMIPHENE   Systemic

■ For the Pharmacist ■

In providing consultation, consider emphasizing the following selected
    information (» = major clinical significance):

Before using this medication
» Conditions affecting use, especially:
    Sensitivity to clomiphene
    Carcinogenicity—Bilateral female breast cancer and testicular
        cancer have occurred very rarely during use of clomiphene
    Pregnancy—Use during pregnancy is not recommended since
        animal studies have shown teratogenicity
    Other medical problems, especially hepatic function impairment,
        mental depression, ovarian cyst, thrombophlebitis, undi-
        agnosed abnormal vaginal bleeding, endometriosis, uterine
        fibroids, and polycystic ovary syndrome

Proper use of this medication
» Compliance with therapy; clarification of schedule; taking at same
    time every day to aid in remembering each dose
» Proper dosing
    Missed dose: Taking as soon as possible; doubling dose if not re-
        membered until time of next dose; checking with physician if
        more than one dose missed
» Proper storage

Precautions while using this medication
» Importance of close monitoring by physician
» Importance of following physician's instructions for timing of in-
    tercourse
» Telling physician immediately if pregnancy is suspected; importance
    of not taking medication while pregnant
» Caution when driving or doing jobs requiring alertness because of
    visual disturbances, dizziness, or lightheadedness

Side/adverse effects
    Signs of potential side effects, especially ovarian enlargement, ovar-
        ian cyst formation, uterine fibroid enlargement, premenstrual
        syndrome, hepatotoxicity, thromboembolism, or vision changes

▲ For the Patient ▲

913546

ABOUT YOUR MEDICINE

Clomiphene (KLOE-mi-feen) is used as a fertility medicine
in some women who are unable to become pregnant. It may
also be used for other conditions in both females and males,
as determined by your doctor. The following information
applies only to female patients taking clomiphene. Check
with your doctor if you are a male and have any questions
about the use of clomiphene.

If any of the information in this leaflet causes you special
concern or if you want additional information about your
medicine and its use, check with your doctor, nurse, or pharmacist. **Remember, keep this and all other medicines out of**

the reach of children and never share your medicines with others.

BEFORE USING THIS MEDICINE

If you become pregnant as a result of using this medicine, there is a chance of a multiple birth (for example, twins, triplets) occurring.

Tell your doctor, nurse, and pharmacist if you . . .
- are allergic to any medicine, either prescription or non-prescription (OTC);
- are taking any other prescription or nonprescription (OTC) medicine;
- have any other medical problems, especially cysts on the ovaries, endometriosis, fibroid tumors of the uterus, inflamed veins due to blood clots, liver disease (or history of), mental depression, or unusual vaginal bleeding.

PROPER USE OF THIS MEDICINE

Take this medicine only as directed by your doctor. If you are to begin on Day 5, count the first day of your menstrual period as Day 1. Beginning on Day 5, take the correct dose every day for as many days as your doctor ordered. To help you remember to take your dose of medicine, take it at the same time every day.

If you miss a dose of this medicine, take it as soon as possible. If you do not remember until it is time for the next dose, take both doses together. If you miss more than one dose, check with your doctor.

PRECAUTIONS WHILE USING THIS MEDICINE

It is very important that your doctor check your progress at regular visits to make sure this medicine is working and to check for unwanted effects.

If your doctor has asked you to record your temperature daily, make sure that you do this every day as soon as you awaken and before getting up. This will help you know if you have begun to ovulate. It is important that intercourse take place at the correct time to give you the best chance of becoming pregnant. **Follow your doctor's instructions carefully.**

There is a chance that clomiphene may cause birth defects if it is taken after you become pregnant. **Stop taking this medicine and tell your doctor immediately if you think you have become pregnant** while still taking clomiphene.

This medicine may cause blurred vision, difficulty in reading, or other changes in vision. It may also cause some people to become dizzy or lightheaded. **Make sure you know how you react to this medicine before you drive, use machines, or do other jobs that require you to see well or be clear-headed.**

POSSIBLE SIDE EFFECTS OF THIS MEDICINE

Side Effects That Should Be Reported To Your Doctor Immediately

> *More common*—Bloating; stomach or pelvic pain

> *Less common or rare*—Shortness of breath (sudden)

Other Side Effects That Should Be Reported To Your Doctor

> *Less common or rare*—Blurred vision; decreased or double vision or other vision problems; sensitivity of eyes to light; yellow eyes or skin

Side Effects That Usually Do Not Require Medical Attention

These possible side effects may go away during treatment; however, if they continue or are bothersome, check with your doctor, nurse, or pharmacist.

> *More common*—Hot flashes

Other side effects not listed above may also occur in some patients. If you notice any other effects, check with your doctor, nurse, or pharmacist.

CLONIDINE Systemic
Including Clonidine (Oral); Clonidine (Transdermal).

■For the Pharmacist■

In providing consultation, consider emphasizing the following selected information (» = major clinical significance):

Before using this medication
» Conditions affecting use, especially:
    Sensitivity to clonidine or to ophthalmic apraclonidine
    Pregnancy—Increased resorptions in rats and mice
    Breast-feeding—Distributed into breast milk
    Use in children—Caution recommended in children because accidental overdoses have been reported
    Use in the elderly—Hypotensive effects may be more likely
    Other medications, especially tricyclic antidepressants or beta-adrenergic blocking agents

Proper use of this medication
    Proper administration of the transdermal dosage form:
»   Compliance with therapy; reading patient instructions carefully
    Not trimming or cutting patch
    Applying to clean, dry skin area on upper arm or torso; area should be free of hair, scars, cuts, or irritation
    Should remain in place even during showering, bathing, or swimming; applying adhesive overlay to loose systems; replacing systems that have loosened excessively or fallen off
    Alternating application sites
    Folding used patches in half with adhesive sides together; disposing of patch carefully, out of reach of children
    Getting into the habit of taking or using at same time each day or week to help increase compliance
» Proper dosing
» Missed dose: Taking or using as soon as possible; checking with physician if miss two or more oral doses in a row or if are late in changing the transdermal system by 3 or more days; possible severe reaction if stopped abruptly
» Proper storage
For use as an antihypertensive
    Possible need for control of weight and diet, especially sodium intake
» Patient may not experience symptoms of hypertension; importance of taking medication even if feeling well
» Does not cure, but helps control hypertension; possible need for lifelong therapy; serious consequences of untreated hypertension

Precautions while using this medication
    Regular visits to physician to check progress
» Checking with physician before discontinuing medication; gradual dosage reduction may be necessary to avoid serious rebound hypertension
» Having enough medication on hand to get through weekends, holidays, and vacations; possibly carrying second prescription for emergency use
» Caution in taking alcohol or other CNS depressants
» Caution when driving or doing things requiring alertness, because of possible drowsiness
» Caution if any kind of surgery or emergency treatment is required
    Caution when getting up suddenly from a lying or sitting position

      Caution in using alcohol, while standing for long periods or exercising, and during hot weather, because of enhanced orthostatic hypotensive effects

      Possible dryness of mouth; using sugarless candy or gum, ice, or saliva substitute for relief; checking with physician or dentist if dry mouth continues for more than 2 weeks

For use as an antihypertensive

» Not taking other medications, especially nonprescription sympathomimetics, unless discussed with physician

Side/adverse effects

      Signs of potential side effects, especially itching or redness of skin (transdermal), mental depression, sodium and water retention, edema, Raynaud's phenomenon, vivid dreams or nightmares, and withdrawal reaction

---

▲ For the Patient ▲

912215

CLONIDINE (Oral)

ABOUT YOUR MEDICINE

Clonidine (KLOE-ni-deen) belongs to the general class of medicines called antihypertensives. It is used to treat high blood pressure (hypertension). Clonidine also may be prescribed for other conditions as determined by your doctor.

If any of the information in this leaflet causes you special concern or if you want additional information about your medicine and its use, check with your doctor, nurse, or pharmacist. **Remember, keep this and all other medicines out of the reach of children and never share your medicines with others.**

BEFORE USING THIS MEDICINE

Tell your doctor, nurse, and pharmacist if you . . .

- are allergic to any medicine, either prescription or nonprescription (OTC);
- are pregnant or intend to become pregnant while using this medicine;
- are breast-feeding;
- are taking any other prescription or nonprescription (OTC) medicine, especially beta-blockers or tricyclic antidepressants (medicine for depression);
- have any other medical problems.

PROPER USE OF THIS MEDICINE

For patients taking this medicine for high blood pressure:

- This medicine will not cure your high blood pressure but it does help control it. You must continue to take it—even if you feel well—if you expect to keep your blood pressure down. **You may have to take high blood pressure medicine for the rest of your life.**

If you miss a dose of this medicine, take it as soon as possible. Then go back to your regular dosing schedule. **If you miss 2 or more doses in a row, check with your doctor right away.**

If your body goes without this medicine for too long, your blood pressure may go up to a dangerously high level and some unpleasant effects may occur.

PRECAUTIONS WHILE USING THIS MEDICINE

Check with your doctor before you stop taking this medicine. Your doctor may want you to reduce your dose gradually before stopping completely.

Make sure that you have enough medicine on hand to last through weekends, holidays, or vacations. You should not miss taking any doses. You may want to ask your doctor for another written prescription for clonidine to carry in your wallet or purse. You can then have it filled if you run out of medicine when you are away from home.

Clonidine will add to the depressant effects of alcohol and other CNS depressants (medicines that slow down the nervous system). **Check with your doctor before taking any such depressants while you are taking this medicine.**

Since clonidine may cause some people to become drowsy, **make sure you know how you react to it before you drive, use machines, or do other jobs that require you to be alert.**

Before having any kind of surgery or dental or emergency treatment, tell the physician or dentist in charge that you are using this medicine.

Dizziness, lightheadedness, or fainting may occur after you take this medicine, especially when you get up from a lying or sitting position. Getting up slowly may help. These effects are also more likely to occur if you drink alcohol, stand for long periods of time, exercise, or if the weather is hot.

POSSIBLE SIDE EFFECTS OF THIS MEDICINE
Side Effects That Should Be Reported To Your Doctor

> *Less common*—Mental depression; swelling of feet and lower legs
>
> *Rare*—Cold feeling or paleness in fingertips and toes; vivid dreams or nightmares

Side Effects That Usually Do Not Require Medical Attention

These possible side effects may go away during treatment; however, if they continue or are bothersome, check with your doctor, nurse, or pharmacist.

> *More common*—Constipation; dizziness; drowsiness; dryness of mouth; unusual tiredness or weakness
>
> *Less common*—Decreased sexual ability; nausea or vomiting

Other side effects not listed above may also occur in some patients. If you notice any other effects, check with your doctor, nurse, or pharmacist.

After you stop taking clonidine, check with your doctor immediately if you notice anxiety or tenseness, chest pain, fast
or pounding heartbeat, headache, increase in saliva, nausea
or vomiting, nervousness, restlessness, shaking or trembling
of hands and fingers, stomach cramps, sweating, or trouble
in sleeping.

▲ For the Patient ▲

917140

CLONIDINE (Transdermal)

ABOUT YOUR MEDICINE

Clonidine (KLOE-ni-deen) belongs to the general class of
medicines called antihypertensives. It is used to treat high
blood pressure (hypertension). Clonidine may also be used
for other conditions as determined by your doctor.

If any of the information in this leaflet causes you special
concern or if you want additional information about your
medicine and its use, check with your doctor, nurse, or pharmacist. Remember, keep this and all other medicines out of
the reach of children and never share your medicines with
others.

BEFORE USING THIS MEDICINE

Tell your doctor, nurse, and pharmacist if you . . .
- are allergic to any medicine, either prescription or nonprescription (OTC);
- are pregnant or intend to become pregnant while using
  this medicine;
- are breast-feeding;
- are taking any other prescription or nonprescription
  (OTC) medicine, especially beta-blockers; tricyclic antidepressants (medicine for depression); or medicines for
  appetite control, asthma, colds, cough, hay fever, or sinus;
- have any other medical problems.

PROPER USE OF THIS MEDICINE

For patients using this medicine for high blood pressure:
- This medicine will not cure your high blood pressure
  but it does help control it. You must continue to use it
  as directed—even if you feel well—if you expect to
  lower your blood pressure and keep it down. You may
  have to take high blood pressure medicine for the rest
  of your life.

This medicine usually comes with patient instructions. Read
them carefully before using this medicine.

Wash and dry your hands before and after handling the
patch.

Do not trim or cut the patch to change the dose. Check with
your doctor, instead.

Put the patch on a clean, dry area on your upper arm or chest that has little hair. Do not put it on scars, cuts, or irritation. Press the patch firmly in place. Put each patch on a different area of skin to prevent skin problems.

The patch will stay in place, even during showering, bathing, or swimming. If the patch becomes loose, cover it with the extra adhesive overlay provided. Apply a new patch if the first one becomes too loose or falls off.

After taking off a used patch, fold it in half with sticky sides together. Discard it carefully out of the reach of children.

If you forget to apply a new patch when you are supposed to, apply it as soon as possible. **If you miss changing the patch for three or more days, check with your doctor right away.**

PRECAUTIONS WHILE USING THIS MEDICINE
Check with your doctor before you stop using this medicine. Your doctor may want you to reduce your dose gradually before stopping completely.

Make sure you have enough clonidine on hand to last through weekends, holidays, or vacations. Ask your doctor for another prescription for clonidine that you can have filled if you run out of medicine when you are away from home.

Clonidine will add to the depressant effects of alcohol and other CNS depressants (medicines that slow down the nervous system). **Check with your doctor before taking any such depressants while you are using this medicine.**

Since clonidine may cause some people to become drowsy, **make sure you know how you react to it before you drive, use machines, or do other jobs that require you to be alert.**

Dizziness, lightheadedness, or fainting may occur, especially when you get up from a lying or sitting position. Getting up slowly may help. These effects are also more likely to occur if you drink alcohol, stand for long periods of time, exercise, or if the weather is hot.

POSSIBLE SIDE EFFECTS OF THIS MEDICINE
Side Effects That Should Be Reported To Your Doctor

> *More common*—Itching or redness of skin
>
> *Less common*—Mental depression; swelling of feet and lower legs
>
> *Rare*—Paleness or cold feeling in fingertips and toes; vivid dreams or nightmares

Side Effects That Usually Do Not Require Medical Attention

These possible side effects may go away during treatment; however, if they continue or are bothersome, check with your doctor, nurse, or pharmacist.

More common—Constipation; dizziness; drowsiness; dry mouth; unusual tiredness or weakness

Other side effects not listed above may also occur in some patients. If you notice any other effects, check with your doctor, nurse, or pharmacist.

After you stop using clonidine, check with your doctor immediately if you notice anxiety or tenseness, chest pain, fast or irregular heartbeat, headache, increased salivation, nausea or vomiting, nervousness, restlessness, shaking or trembling of hands and fingers, stomach cramps, sweating, or trouble in sleeping.

CLOZAPINE   Systemic

■For the Pharmacist■

In providing consultation, consider emphasizing the following selected
information (» = major clinical significance):

Before using this medication
» Conditions affecting use, especially:
    Pregnancy—Crosses the placenta
    Breast-feeding—May cause sedation, decreased suckling, and
      restlessness or irritability in nursing infant
    Use in elderly—Greater risk of orthostatic hypotension and an-
      ticholinergic side effects in these patients
    Dental—Clozapine-induced blood dyscrasias may result in in-
      fections, delayed healing, and bleeding; dry mouth may cause
      caries and candidiasis; hypersalivation occurs frequently
    Other medications, especially alcohol, other CNS depression-
      producing medications, other bone marrow depressants, or
      lithium
    Other medical problems, especially severe CNS depression, mye-
      loproliferative disorders, cardiovascular disorders, gastroin-
      testinal disorders, predisposition to narrow-angle glaucoma,
      impairment of hepatic or renal function, prostatic hypertro-
      phy, and seizure disorders

Proper use of this medication
    Compliance with therapy; not taking more or less medication than
      prescribed
» Proper dosing
    Missed dose: Taking as soon as possible; not taking if almost time
      for next dose; not doubling doses
» Proper storage

Precautions while using this medication
    Regular visits to physician to check progress of therapy and to
      laboratory for blood tests
    Checking with physician before discontinuing medication; gradual
      dosage reduction may be needed
    Avoiding use of alcoholic beverages or other CNS depressants dur-
      ing therapy
    Possible drowsiness, blurred vision, or seizures; not driving, swim-
      ming, climbing, operating machinery, or doing other things that
      require alertness or accurate vision
    Possible orthostatic hypotension; caution when getting up from a
      lying or sitting position
    Possible dryness of mouth; using sugarless gum or candy, ice, or
      saliva substitute for relief; checking with physician or dentist if
      dryness of mouth continues for more than 2 weeks

Side/adverse effects
    Signs of potential side effects, especially cardiovascular effects, fe-
      ver, difficulty in accommodation, agitation, akathisia, confusion,
      ECG changes, extrapyramidal effects, insomnia, mental depres-
      sion, syncope, blood dyscrasias, difficulty in urinating, impo-
      tence, neuroleptic malignant syndrome, tardive dyskinesia, and
      seizures

▲ For the Patient ▲

916883

ABOUT YOUR MEDICINE

Clozapine (KLOE-za-peen) is used to treat schizophrenia in patients who have not been helped by or are unable to take other medicines.

Clozapine is only available from pharmacies that agree to participate with your doctor in a plan to test your blood. **You will need to have blood tests done every week,** and you will receive a 7-day supply of clozapine only if your blood tests show that it is safe for you to take this medicine.

If any of the information in this leaflet causes you special concern or if you want additional information about your medicine and its use, check with your doctor, nurse, or pharmacist. **Remember, keep this and all other medicines out of the reach of children and never share your medicines with others.**

BEFORE USING THIS MEDICINE

Tell your doctor, nurse, and pharmacist if you . . .

- are allergic to any medicine, either prescription or non-prescription (OTC);
- are pregnant or intend to become pregnant while using this medicine;
- are breast-feeding;
- are taking **any** other prescription or nonprescription (OTC) medicine;
- have any other medical problems, especially blood diseases, enlarged prostate or difficult urination, or epilepsy or other seizure disorder.

PROPER USE OF THIS MEDICINE

Take this medicine exactly as directed. Do not take more of this medicine and do not take it more often than your doctor ordered. Do not miss any doses.

This medicine has been prescribed for your current medical problem only. It must not be given to other people or used for other problems.

If you miss a dose of this medicine, take it as soon as possible. However, if it is almost time for your next dose, skip the missed dose and go back to your regular dosing schedule. Do not double doses.

PRECAUTIONS WHILE USING THIS MEDICINE

It is important that you have your blood tests done weekly and that your doctor check your progress at regular visits. This will allow your doctor to make sure the medicine is working properly and to change the dosage if needed.

If you have been using this medicine regularly, do not stop taking it without first checking with your doctor. Your doctor may want you to reduce gradually the amount you are taking before stopping completely.

This medicine will add to the effects of alcohol and other CNS depressants (medicines that slow down the nervous system). **Check with your doctor before taking any such depressants while you are using this medicine.**

Clozapine may cause drowsiness, blurred vision, or convulsions (seizures). **Do not drive, climb, swim, operate machines, or do anything else that could be dangerous** while you are taking this medicine.

Dizziness, lightheadedness, or fainting may occur, especially when you get up from a lying or sitting position. Getting up slowly may help. If this problem continues or gets worse, check with your doctor.

POSSIBLE SIDE EFFECTS OF THIS MEDICINE
Side Effects That Should Be Reported To Your Doctor Immediately

> *More common*—Fast or irregular heartbeat; fever; low blood pressure
>
> *Less common*—High blood pressure
>
> *Rare*—Chills; convulsions (seizures); difficult or fast breathing; increased sweating; loss of bladder control; muscle stiffness (severe); sore throat; sores, ulcers, or white spots on lips or in mouth; unusual bleeding or bruising; unusual tiredness or weakness; unusually pale skin

Other Side Effects That Should Be Reported To Your Doctor

> *More common*—Dizziness or fainting
>
> *Less common*—Blurred vision; confusion; restlessness or need to keep moving; trembling; unusual anxiety, nervousness, or irritability
>
> *Rare*—Absence of or decrease in movement; decreased sexual ability; difficulty in sleeping; difficulty in urinating; headache (severe or continuing); lip smacking or puckering; mental depression; puffing of cheeks; rapid or worm-like movements of tongue; uncontrolled chewing movements; uncontrolled movements of arms and legs

Side Effects That Usually Do Not Require Medical Attention

These possible side effects may go away during treatment; however, if they continue or are bothersome, check with your doctor, nurse, or pharmacist.

> *More common*—Constipation; dizziness or lightheadedness (mild); drowsiness; headache (mild); increased

watering of mouth; nausea or vomiting; unusual weight gain

Other side effects not listed above may also occur in some patients. If you notice any other effects, check with your doctor, nurse, or pharmacist.

COLCHICINE   Systemic

■ For the Pharmacist ■

In providing consultation, consider emphasizing the following selected
information (» = major clinical significance):

Before using this medication
» Conditions affecting use, especially:
Sensitivity to colchicine
Use in the elderly—Increased susceptibility to cumulative tox-
icity
Other medications, especially other bone marrow depressants or
radiation therapy
Other medical problems, especially blood dyscrasias, severe car-
diac disorders, gastrointestinal disorders, renal function im-
pairment, or hepatic function impairment

Proper use of this medication
» Importance of not taking more medication than prescribed
For prophylactic use
Compliance with therapy
Not using additional colchicine to relieve an acute gout attack
that occurs during prophylactic therapy, unless otherwise di-
rected by physician; using alternative treatment as prescribed
For intermittent use to relieve acute attack
Starting medication at earliest sign of attack
» Stopping medication when pain relieved; at first sign of diarrhea,
nausea or vomiting, or stomach pain; or when maximum dos-
age reached (even if symptoms not relieved)
Noting total quantity of colchicine taken before gastrointestinal
symptoms occur and, in subsequent attacks, stopping treatment before this cumulative dose has been reached
» Not taking additional colchicine for 3 days after using therapeutic oral doses to relieve an acute attack or for 7 days after
receiving intravenous colchicine
» Continuing other gout medication (if applicable) while taking
colchicine
» Proper dosing
Missed dose: If on fixed-dosage chronic therapy—Taking as soon
as possible; not taking if almost time for next dose; not doubling
doses
» Proper storage

Precautions while using this medication
Regular visits to physician to check progress and possibly to be tested
for adverse effects during long-term therapy
» Possibility that large quantities of alcohol may increase the risk of
gastrointestinal toxicity; also, alcohol may increase uric acid concentrations and thereby decrease the effectiveness of medication
when used for gout
Not discontinuing prophylactic treatment without first consulting
physician if acute attacks continue to occur

Side/adverse effects
» Checking with physician if diarrhea, nausea, vomiting, or stomach
pain occurs and continues for more than 3 hours after medication
is discontinued
» Checking with physician immediately if symptoms of angioedema,
bone marrow depression, or overdose occur

Signs and symptoms of other potential side effects, especially skin rash or hives, localized reactions to extravasation after intravenous administration, myopathy, and neuropathy

---

▲ For the Patient ▲

913590

Colchicine (Oral)

ABOUT YOUR MEDICINE

Colchicine (KOL-chi-seen) is used to prevent or relieve the pain and inflammation that occur with attacks of gout. Most people take small amounts of colchicine regularly for a long time (months or even years) to prevent attacks or other problems caused by inflammation. Other people take large amounts of it for a short time (several hours) only when an attack is occurring. Colchicine may also be used for other conditions as determined by your doctor.

If any of the information in this leaflet causes you special concern or if you want additional information about your medicine and its use, check with your doctor, nurse, or pharmacist. **Remember, keep this and all other medicines out of the reach of children and never share your medicines with others.**

BEFORE USING THIS MEDICINE

Tell your doctor, nurse, and pharmacist if you . . .
- are allergic to any medicine, either prescription or nonprescription (OTC);
- are pregnant or intend to become pregnant while using this medicine;
- are breast-feeding;
- are taking **any** other prescription or nonprescription (OTC) medicine;
- have any other medical problems, especially heart, intestine, kidney, or liver disease, low white blood cell or platelet count, or stomach ulcer.

PROPER USE OF THIS MEDICINE

Do not take more of this medicine or take it more often than directed by your doctor. This is especially important for elderly patients. Also, stop taking colchicine when you have taken the largest amount that your doctor ordered for each attack, even if the pain is not relieved.

For patients taking small amounts regularly (preventive treatment):
- Take this medicine regularly as directed by your doctor, even if you feel well. If you stop taking it too soon, your gout attacks may return or get worse.
- Most people with gout who take preventive amounts of colchicine should not take extra colchicine to relieve an attack. Ask your doctor to recommend other medicine for an attack. If you do need to take colchicine for an

attack, ask your doctor to tell you the largest amount of colchicine you should take and how long you should wait before starting to take the smaller preventive amounts again. Be sure to follow these directions carefully.

For patients taking colchicine only to relieve an attack:
- Start taking this medicine at the first sign of the attack for best results.
- **Stop taking this medicine as soon as the pain is relieved or at the first sign of nausea, vomiting, stomach pain, or diarrhea.**
- The first few times you take colchicine, keep a record of each dose as you take it. If nausea, vomiting, stomach pain, or diarrhea occurs, count the number of doses you have taken. For the next attack, take fewer doses. If stomach upset occurs again, check with your doctor.
- After taking colchicine tablets to treat an attack, **do not take any more colchicine for at least 3 days. Also, after receiving the medicine by injection, do not take any more colchicine for at least 7 days.** Elderly patients may have to wait even longer between treatments.
- If you are also taking other medicine to reduce the amount of uric acid in your body, **do not stop taking the other medicine.**

If you are taking colchicine regularly (for example, every day) and you miss a dose, take it as soon as possible. However, if it is almost time for your next dose, skip the missed dose. Do not double doses.

PRECAUTIONS WHILE USING THIS MEDICINE

Stomach problems may be more likely to occur if you drink large amounts of alcohol while taking colchicine. Also, too much alcohol may lessen the effects of colchicine in patients with gout. Therefore, people who take colchicine should be careful to limit the amount of alcohol they drink.

For patients taking small amounts regularly (preventive treatment):
- Attacks of gout should occur less often, and should not be as severe as they were before you started taking colchicine. However, if you think the colchicine is not working, **do not stop taking it and do not increase the dose.** Check with your doctor instead.

POSSIBLE SIDE EFFECTS OF THIS MEDICINE

Side Effects That Should Be Reported To Your Doctor Immediately

Stop taking this medicine immediately if diarrhea, nausea, stomach pain, or vomiting occurs. **If any of these continue for 3 hours or longer after you have stopped taking colchicine, check with your doctor.**

> *Rare*—Black, tarry stools; blood in urine or stools; difficult breathing with exercise; fever; headache; large,

hive-like swellings on face, eyelids, mouth, lips, or tongue; pinpoint red spots on skin; sores, ulcers, or white spots on lips or in mouth; sore throat; unusual bleeding or bruising; unusual tiredness or weakness

Signs of overdose—Burning feeling in the stomach, throat, or skin; diarrhea (severe or bloody); nausea, stomach pain, or vomiting (severe)

Other Side Effects That Should Be Reported To Your Doctor

Rare—Hives; muscle weakness; numbness in fingers or toes; skin rash

Other side effects not listed above may also occur in some patients. If you notice any other effects, check with your doctor, nurse, or pharmacist.

COLESTIPOL   Oral-Local

■ For the Pharmacist ■

In providing consultation, consider emphasizing the following selected information (» = major clinical significance):

Before using this medication
Diet as preferred therapy; importance of following prescribed diet
This medication does not cure the condition but rather helps control it
» Conditions affecting use, especially:
Sensitivity to colestipol
Use in children—Not recommended in children under 2 years of age since cholesterol is required for normal development
Use in the elderly—Increased incidence of gastrointestinal side effects and adverse nutritional effects in patients over 60 years of age
Other medications, especially anticoagulants, digitalis glycosides, oral penicillin G, oral tetracyclines, oral propranolol, thyroid hormones, thiazide diuretics, or oral vancomycin
Other medical problems, especially primary biliary cirrhosis, complete biliary obstruction or complete atresia, or constipation

Proper use of this medication
» Importance of not taking more or less medication than the amount prescribed
» Compliance with prescribed diet
» Importance of mixing with fluids before taking; instructions for mixing: Stirring until completely mixed (does not dissolve); rinsing glass and drinking to make sure all medication is taken; may also be mixed with milk in cereals, thin soups, or pulpy fruits
» Proper dosing
Missed dose: Taking as soon as possible; not taking if almost time for next dose; not doubling doses
» Proper storage

Precautions while using this medication
» Importance of close monitoring by the physician
» Checking with physician before discontinuing medication; blood lipid concentrations may increase significantly
» Not taking any other medication unless discussed with physician

Side/adverse effects
Signs of potential side effects, especially constipation, gallstones, gastrointestinal bleeding, peptic ulcer, and steatorrhea or malabsorption syndrome

▲ For the Patient ▲

916125

CHOLESTEROL-LOWERING RESINS (Oral):
Including Cholestyramine; Colestipol.

ABOUT YOUR MEDICINE

Cholesterol-lowering resins are used to lower levels of cholesterol (a fat-like substance) in the blood. This may help prevent medical problems caused by cholesterol clogging the blood vessels. These medicines may also be used for other conditions as determined by your doctor.

If any of the information in this leaflet causes you special concern or if you want additional information about your medicine and its use, check with your doctor, nurse, or pharmacist. **Remember, keep this and all other medicines out of the reach of children and never share your medicines with others.**

BEFORE USING THIS MEDICINE

Importance of diet—Before prescribing medicine for your condition, your doctor will probably try to control your condition by prescribing a personal diet for you. Such a diet may be low in fats, sugars, and/or cholesterol. Many people are able to control their condition by carefully following their doctor's orders for proper diet and exercise. Medicine is prescribed only when additional help is needed and is effective only when a schedule of diet and exercise is properly followed.

Also, this medicine is less effective if you are greatly overweight. It may be very important for you to go on a reducing diet. However, check with your doctor before going on any diet.

Tell your doctor, nurse, and pharmacist if you . . .
- are allergic to any medicine, either prescription or nonprescription (OTC);
- are pregnant or intend to become pregnant while using this medicine;
- are breast-feeding;
- are taking any other prescription or nonprescription (OTC) medicine, especially anticoagulants (blood thinners), digitalis glycosides (heart medicine), diuretics (water pills), phenylbutazone, penicillins, propranolol, tetracyclines, thyroid hormones, or vancomycin;
- have any other medical problems, especially constipation or stomach problems;
- have phenylketonuria, since some brands of cholestyramine may contain aspartame.

PROPER USE OF THIS MEDICINE

For patients taking the powder form of this medicine:
- **This medicine should never be taken in its dry form, since it could cause you to choke.** Instead, always mix as follows:
  —For cholestyramine: Place the medicine in 2 ounces of any beverage and mix thoroughly. Then add an additional 2 to 4 ounces of beverage and again mix thoroughly (it will **not** dissolve) before drinking.
  —For colestipol: Add this medicine to 3 ounces or more of water, milk, flavored drink, or your favorite juice or carbonated drink. If you use a carbonated drink,

slowly mix in the powder in a large glass to prevent too much foaming.

—Stir until the medicine is completely mixed (it will **not** dissolve) before drinking. After drinking all the liquid, rinse the glass with a little more liquid and drink that also, to make sure you get the full dose.

—You may also mix this medicine with milk in hot or regular breakfast cereals, or in thin soups such as tomato or chicken noodle. Or you may add it to some pulpy fruits such as crushed pineapple, pears, peaches, or fruit cocktail.

For patients taking the chewable bar form of cholestyramine:
• Chew each bite well before swallowing.

Take this medicine exactly as directed by your doctor. Try not to miss any doses and do not take more medicine than your doctor ordered.

If you miss a dose of this medicine, take it as soon as possible. However, if it is almost time for your next dose, skip the missed dose and go back to your regular dosing schedule. Do not double doses.

PRECAUTIONS WHILE USING THIS MEDICINE

It is very important that your doctor check your progress at regular visits.

Do not take any other medicine unless prescribed by your doctor since cholesterol-lowering resins may change the effect of other medicines.

Do not stop taking this medicine without first checking with your doctor. When you stop taking this medicine, your blood cholesterol levels may increase again. Your doctor may want you to follow a special diet to help prevent this.

POSSIBLE SIDE EFFECTS OF THIS MEDICINE
Side Effects That Should Be Reported To Your Doctor Immediately

Rare—Black, tarry stools; stomach pain (severe) with nausea and vomiting

Other Side Effects That Should Be Reported To Your Doctor

More common—Constipation

Rare—Loss of weight (sudden)

Side Effects That Usually Do Not Require Medical Attention

These possible side effects may go away during treatment; however, if they continue or are bothersome, check with your doctor, nurse, or pharmacist.

More common (less common for colestipol)—Heartburn or indigestion; nausea or vomiting; stomach pain

Other side effects not listed above may also occur in some patients. If you notice any other effects, check with your doctor, nurse, or pharmacist.

CORTICOSTEROIDS   Inhalation-Local
*Including Beclomethasone; Budesonide; Dexamethasone;
Flunisolide; Triamcinolone.*

■For the Pharmacist■

In providing consultation, consider emphasizing the following selected
information (» = major clinical significance):

Before using this medication
» Conditions affecting use, especially:
  Sensitivity to corticosteroids
  Use in children—Higher doses may result in retarded growth
    rate and reduced cortisol secretion; monitoring of growth and
    development and adrenal function is important with pro-
    longed or high-dose therapy. The use of a spacer is necessary
    for better compliance and improved airway delivery. Expo-
    sure to chickenpox or measles should be avoided

Proper use of this medication
» Not using to relieve acute asthma attack; continuing use even if
    using other medication for asthma attack
» Importance of not using more medication than the amount pre-
    scribed
» Compliance with therapy by using every day in regularly spaced
    doses; patients who are not taking systemic corticosteroids when
    inhalation therapy started may require up to 4 weeks for initial
    improvement and several months for full benefits
  Gargling and rinsing mouth with water after each dose; not swal-
    lowing rinse water
» Reading patient instructions carefully; checking frequently with
    health care professional for proper use of inhaler
» Proper dosing
  Missed dose: Using as soon as possible; using any remaining doses
    for that day at regularly spaced intervals
  Checking with pharmacist to determine availability of refills for
    aerosol inhalers; saving inhaler if refills available
» Proper storage
  Proper dose may not be delivered if aerosol canister is cold
*For beclomethasone, flunisolide, or triamcinolone inhalation aerosol
dosage form*
  Testing inhaler before using first time
  Proper administration technique
  Proper administration technique with use of spacer device
  Proper cleaning procedure for inhaler
For beclomethasone capsule for inhalation dosage form
» Not swallowing capsules; medication not effective if swallowed
  Proper loading technique for inhaler
  Proper administration technique
  Proper cleaning procedure for inhaler
For beclomethasone powder for inhalation dosage form
  Proper loading technique for inhaler
  Proper administration technique
  Proper cleaning procedure for inhaler
For budesonide powder for inhalation dosage form
  Proper loading technique for inhaler
  Proper administration technique

For budesonide suspension for inhalation dosage form
   Using in a power-operated nebulizer with an adequate flow rate and
      equipped with face mask or mouthpiece
   Preparation of medication for use in nebulizer
   Proper administration technique
   Proper cleaning procedure for nebulizer

Precautions while using this medication
» Checking with physician if:
      Unusual physical stress occurs, such as surgery, injury, or in-
         fections
      Asthma attack is not responsive to bronchodilator
      Any sign indicating possible mouth, throat, or lung infection
         occurs
      Symptoms do not improve or condition becomes worse
   Carrying medical identification card stating that supplemental sys-
      temic corticosteroid therapy may be required in emergency sit-
      uations, periods of unusual stress, or acute asthma attack
» Caution if any kind of surgery or emergency treatment is required;
   informing physician or dentist in charge that inhalation corticosteroid is being used
For patients receiving systemic corticosteroid therapy
» Importance of not discontinuing systemic corticosteroid therapy
   without physician's advice; carefully reducing dose or discontinuing treatment if so directed
» Importance of regular visits to physician during time that systemic
   corticosteroid therapy is being withdrawn; obtaining physician's
   instructions to follow if severe asthma attack occurs, medical or
   surgical treatment is needed, or symptoms of corticosteroid withdrawal occur

Side/adverse effects
   Signs of potential side effects, especially increased bronchospasm,
      oropharyngeal or esophageal candidiasis, and, with budesonide,
      psychic changes

▲ For the Patient ▲

912780

ABOUT YOUR MEDICINE

Inhalation corticosteroids (kor-ti-koe-STER-oids) are used to
help prevent asthma attacks. They will not relieve an attack
that has already started. They are cortisone-like medicines.
Corticosteroids also belong to the general family of medicines called steroids.

If any of the information in this leaflet causes you special
concern or if you want additional information about your
medicine and its use, check with your doctor, nurse, or pharmacist. **Remember, keep this and all other medicines out of
the reach of children and never share your medicines with
others.**

BEFORE USING THIS MEDICINE
Tell your doctor, nurse, and pharmacist if you . . .
   • are allergic to any medicine, either prescription or non-
      prescription (OTC);
   • are pregnant or intend to become pregnant while using
      this medicine;

- are breast-feeding;
- are taking any other prescription or nonprescription (OTC) medicine, especially oral antidiabetics (diabetes medicine you take by mouth), or insulin;
- have any other medical problems, especially certain types of lung disease, diabetes mellitus (sugar diabetes), fungus infection, heart disease or recent heart attack, herpes simplex of the eye, myasthenia gravis, or stomach ulcer or other stomach problems.

PROPER USE OF THIS MEDICINE

In order for this medicine to help you, it must be used every day in regularly spaced doses as ordered by your doctor. Up to four weeks may pass before you feel its full effects.

Do not use this medicine more often than ordered. To do so may increase the chance of absorption into the body and the chance of unwanted effects.

This medicine is used with a special inhaler and usually comes with patient directions. **Read the directions carefully before using.**

If you miss a dose of this medicine, use it as soon as possible. However, if it is almost time for your next dose, skip the missed dose and go back to your regular dosing schedule. Do not double doses.

PRECAUTIONS WHILE USING THIS MEDICINE

If you are also taking another corticosteroid (for example, cortisone or prednisone) for your asthma along with this medicine, do not stop taking the other one without your doctor's advice, even if your asthma seems better. If your doctor tells you to reduce or stop taking your other corticosteroid, check with him or her if you notice abdominal or back pain; dizziness or fainting; fever; muscle or joint pain; nausea or vomiting; prolonged loss of appetite; shortness of breath; unusual tiredness or weakness; unusual weight loss.

Also check with your doctor if you go through a period of unusual stress or have an asthma attack that does not improve with a bronchodilator.

If you are also using a bronchodilator inhaler, use it first, then wait about 5 minutes before using this medicine, unless otherwise directed by your doctor.

Check with your doctor if signs of mouth, throat, or lung infection occur; if you do not get better within four weeks; or if you get worse.

For patients who have used corticosteroids in the past:
- Your doctor may want you to carry a medical identification card stating that you are using this medicine.
- **Tell the doctor in charge that you are using this medicine before having any kind of surgery (including dental surgery) or emergency treatment.**

POSSIBLE SIDE EFFECTS OF THIS MEDICINE

Side Effects That Should Be Reported To Your Doctor Immediately

   Rare—Increased shortness of breath, troubled breathing, tightness in chest, or wheezing

Other Side Effects That Should Be Reported To Your Doctor

   More common—Creamy white, curd-like patches in mouth; fast or pounding heartbeat; increased susceptibility to infection; skin rash

   Less common or rare—Decreased or blurred vision; filling out of face; mood or mental changes; swelling of feet or lower legs; unusual weight gain

   With long-term use—Acne or other skin problems; back or rib pain; bloody or black, tarry stools; frequent urination; increased thirst; irregular heartbeats; menstrual problems; muscle weakness, cramps, or pains; stomach pain or burning (severe and continuing); unusual tiredness or weakness; wounds that will not heal

Side Effects That Usually Do Not Require Medical Attention

These possible side effects may go away during treatment; however, if they continue or are bothersome, check with your doctor, nurse, or pharmacist.

   More common—Cough; headache; hoarseness

   Less common or rare—Nosebleeds; nose, mouth, tongue or throat irritation or dryness

Other side effects not listed above may also occur in some patients. If you notice any other effects, check with your doctor, nurse, or pharmacist.

CORTICOSTEROIDS Nasal

Including Beclomethasone; Budesonide; Dexamethasone;
Flunisolide; Triamcinolone.

■For the Pharmacist■

In providing consultation, consider emphasizing the following selected
information (» = major clinical significance):

Before using this medication
» Conditions affecting use, especially:
>
> Intolerance to corticosteroids
>
> Pregnancy—Risk-benefit must be considered, since systemic cor-
> ticosteroids cross the placenta and have demonstrated em-
> bryotoxicity, fetotoxicity, and teratogenicity in animals; bec-
> lomethasone oral inhalation study in humans has shown no
> adverse effects on fetus; infants born to mothers who received
> substantial doses of corticosteroids during pregnancy should
> be observed for hypoadrenalism
>
> Breast-feeding—Use of dexamethasone is not recommended, since
> dexamethasone is distributed into breast milk
>
> Use in children—Significant effect on growth by beclometha-
> sone or flunisolide has not been documented; importance of
> monitoring growth and development with prolonged or high-
> dose therapy
>
> Other medical problems, especially fungal, bacterial, or systemic
> viral infections, ocular herpes simplex, or latent or active
> tuberculosis of respiratory tract

Proper use of this medication
» Proper administration technique; reading patient directions carefully
before use

> Blowing nose to clear nasal passages before administration; aiming
> spray away from nasal septum (aiming towards the inner corner
> of eye)

» Compliance with therapy; may require up to 3 weeks for full benefit
» Importance of not using more medication than the amount prescribed, because of potential enhanced absorption and increased
severity of side effects
» Checking with physician before using medication for other nasal
problems

> Saving special inhaler used for beclomethasone or dexamethasone;
> refills may be available

» Proper dosing

> Missed dose: Using as soon as possible if remembered within an
> hour or so; if remembered later, not using at all; not doubling
> doses

» Proper storage; not storing budesonide powder in damp places, especially if cap has not been tightly screwed on; decreased efficacy if aerosol canister is cold; not puncturing, breaking, or burning aerosol container; discarding unused portion of beclomethasone
solution or flunisolide solution 3 months after opening package

Precautions while using this medication
> Regular visits to physician to check progress during prolonged ther-
> apy

» Checking with physician if:
>
> —signs of infection of nose, throat, or sinuses occur
> —no improvement within 7 days (for dexamethasone)

—no improvement within 3 weeks (for beclomethasone, budesonide, flunisolide, or triamcinolone)
—condition becomes worse

Side/adverse effects

Signs of potential side effects, especially headache, crusting inside nose or epistaxis, sore throat, ulceration of nasal mucosa, allergic reaction or bronchial asthma, cough, dizziness or lightheadedness, hoarseness, lethargy, loss of sense of taste or smell, nausea or vomiting, continuing rhinorrhea, continuing stuffy nose, continuing watery eyes, stomach pains, nasal candidiasis, nasal septal perforation, ocular hypertension, pharyngeal candidiasis, delayed or immediate hypersensitivity reaction, atrophic rhinitis, dermatitis, urticaria, continuing burning or stinging after use of spray, or irritation inside nose

---

▲ For the Patient ▲

913182

ABOUT YOUR MEDICINE

Nasal corticosteroids (kor-ti-koh-STER-oids) are cortisone-like medicines. They belong to the family of medicines called steroids. These medicines are sprayed or inhaled into the nose to help relieve the stuffy nose, irritation, and discomfort of hay fever, other allergies, and other nasal problems. These medicines are also used to prevent nasal polyps from growing back after they have been removed by surgery.

If any of the information in this leaflet causes you special concern or if you want additional information about your medicine and its use, check with your doctor, nurse, or pharmacist. **Remember, keep this and all other medicines out of the reach of children and never share your medicines with others.**

BEFORE USING THIS MEDICINE

Children using this medicine should have their progress checked by their doctor at regular visits. Also, if used in high doses or too often, this medicine may get into the bloodstream through the lining of the nose and may affect growth. It is important to follow your doctor's directions carefully.

Tell your doctor, nurse, and pharmacist if you . . .
- are allergic to any medicine, either prescription or nonprescription (OTC);
- are pregnant or intend to become pregnant while using this medicine;
- are breast-feeding;
- have **any** other medical problems.

PROPER USE OF THIS MEDICINE

This medicine usually comes with patient directions. **Read them carefully before using the medicine.** Beclomethasone, budesonide, dexamethasone and triamcinolone are used with a special inhaler. If you do not understand the directions, or if you are not sure how to use the inhaler, check with your doctor, nurse, or pharmacist.

Before using this medicine, clear the nasal passages by blowing your nose. Then, with the nosepiece inserted into the nostril, aim the spray towards the inner corner of the eye.

In order for this medicine to help you, it must be used regularly as ordered by your doctor. This medicine usually begins to work in about 1 week, but up to 3 weeks may pass before you feel its full effects.

Use this medicine only as directed. Do not use more of it and do not use it more often than your doctor ordered. To do so may increase the chance of unwanted effects.

Check with your doctor before using this medicine for nasal problems other than the one for which it was prescribed, since it should not be used on many types of nasal infections.

Save the inhaler that comes with beclomethasone or dexamethasone, since refill units may be available at lower cost.

If you miss a dose of this medicine and remember within an hour or so, use it right away. However, if you do not remember until later, skip the missed dose and go back to your regular dosing schedule. Do not double doses.

PRECAUTIONS WHILE USING THIS MEDICINE

If you will be using this medicine for more than a few weeks, your doctor should check your progress at regular visits.

Check with your doctor:
   —**if signs of a nose, sinus, or throat infection occur.**
   —**if your symptoms do not improve within 7 days (for dexamethasone) or within 3 weeks (for beclomethasone, budesonide, flunisolide, or triamcinolone).**
   —**if your condition gets worse.**

POSSIBLE SIDE EFFECTS OF THIS MEDICINE
Side Effects That Should Be Reported To Your Doctor

   Less common or rare—Bad smell; bloody mucus or unexplained nosebleeds; burning or stinging after use of spray or irritation inside nose (continuing); crusting, white patches, or sores inside nose; eye pain; gradual loss of vision; headache; hives; lightheadedness or dizziness; loss of sense of taste or smell; nausea or vomiting; shortness of breath, troubled breathing, tightness in chest, or wheezing; skin rash; sore throat, cough, or hoarseness; stomach pains; stuffy, dry, or runny nose or watery eyes (continuing); swelling of eyelids, face, or lips; unusual tiredness or weakness; white patches in throat

Side Effects That Usually Do Not Require Medical Attention

These possible side effects may go away during treatment; however, if they continue or are bothersome, check with your doctor, nurse, or pharmacist.

More common—Burning, dryness, or other irritation inside the nose (mild, lasting only a short time); increase in sneezing; irritation of throat

Other side effects not listed above may also occur in some patients. If you notice any other effects, check with your doctor, nurse, or pharmacist.

CORTICOSTEROIDS/CORTICOTROPIN—
Glucocorticoid Effects Systemic

Including Betamethasone; Corticotropin; Cortisone;
Dexamethasone; Hydrocortisone; Methylprednisolone;
Paramethasone; Prednisolone; Prednisone; Triamcinolone.

■ For the Pharmacist ■

In providing consultation, consider emphasizing the following selected
information (» = major clinical significance):

Before using this medication
» Conditions affecting use, especially:
  Allergies to cosyntropin, corticotropin, or corticosteroids
  Pregnancy—Pharmacologic doses in animals show some evi-
    dence of increased risk of placental insufficiency, decreased
    birthweight, or stillbirths; other animal studies show in-
    creased incidence of cleft palate, placental insufficiency,
    spontaneous abortions, or intrauterine growth retardation.
    Hypoadrenalism may occur in infants if mothers received
    substantial doses of corticosteroids prenatally
  Breast-feeding—Breast-feeding is not recommended during use
    of higher doses
  Use in children—Close monitoring required since chronic ther-
    apy may result in suppression of growth and development;
    possible increased severity of chickenpox or measles in chil-
    dren receiving immunosuppressant doses; discussing possible
    effects with physician
  Use in the elderly—Increased risk of osteoporosis (especially in
    postmenopausal females) or hypertension
  Other medications, especially aminoglutethimide, parenteral
    amphotericin B, antacids, oral antidiabetic agents, insulin,
    digitalis glycosides, diuretics, hepatic enzyme–inducing agents,
    mitotane, potassium supplements, ritodrine, sodium-contain-
    ing medications, human growth hormone, or immunizations
  Other medical problems, especially:
    For all uses—AIDS, systemic or local infections, gastroin-
      testinal disorders, cardiac disease, chickenpox, congestive
      heart failure, renal diseases, diabetes, measles, or myas-
      thenia gravis
    For intra-articular injection only—Arthroplasty, clotting dis-
      orders, fracture, osteoporosis, or unstable joint
    For rectal use only—Recent ileocolostomy
    For neonatal respiratory distress syndrome prophylaxis only—
      Amnionitis, uterine bleeding, febrile illness, placental in-
      sufficiency, or premature membrane rupture
    For corticotropin only—Adrenocortical hyperfunction,
      congestive heart failure, hypertension, ocular herpes sim-
      plex, osteoporosis, scleroderma, porcine protein sensitiv-
      ity, or recent surgery

Proper use of this medication
  For oral dosage forms:
» Taking with food to minimize gastrointestinal irritation
  Possibility that alcohol may enhance ulcerogenic effects of med-
    ication

For rectal dosage forms:
    Proper administration technique; reading patient directions carefully
    Saving applicator for methylprednisolone acetate for enema; refill units may be available

» Importance of not using more medication than the amount prescribed
» Proper dosing
    Missed dose: If dosing schedule is—
        Every other day: Taking as soon as possible if remembered same morning; if remembered later, not taking until next morning, then skipping a day
        Once a day: Taking as soon as possible; not taking if almost time for next dose; not doubling doses
        Several times a day: Taking as soon as possible; doubling if time for next dose
» Proper storage

Precautions while using this medication
» Regular visits to physician to check progress during and following therapy
» Checking with physician before discontinuing medication; gradual dosage reduction may be necessary
    Checking with physician if symptoms recur or worsen when dose decreased or therapy discontinued
» Possible need for calorie and/or sodium restriction or potassium supplementation during long-term therapy
    Possible need for increased protein intake during long-term therapy
    Ophthalmologic examinations during long-term therapy
    Carrying medical identification card indicating use of medication during long-term therapy
» Caution in receiving skin tests
» Caution if any kind of surgery or emergency treatment is required
» Avoiding exposure to chickenpox or measles (especially for children); telling physician right away if exposure occurs
» Caution in receiving vaccinations or other immunizations or coming in contact with persons receiving oral poliovirus vaccine
» Caution if serious infections or injuries occur
    Diabetics: May increase blood sugar concentrations
For parenteral dosage forms
    Restricting use of joint following intra-articular injection
    Checking with physician if redness or swelling occurs, and continues or becomes worse, following local injection
For rectal dosage forms
    Checking with physician if signs of rectal irritation or infection occur

Side/adverse effects
    Signs of potential side effects, especially visual disturbances, diabetes mellitus, local irritation, allergic reactions, local or systemic infection, psychic disturbances, seizures, hypertension, tachycardia, musculoskeletal disorders, Cushing's syndrome, edema, endocrine imbalance, hypokalemic syndrome, gastrointestinal effects, myopathy, striae, tissue atrophy, scarring at injection site, bruising, or delayed wound healing

▲ For the Patient ▲

912011

ABOUT YOUR MEDICINE

Corticosteroids (kor-ti-koh-STER-oids) are produced naturally by the body and are necessary for good health. If your
body does not make enough, your doctor may prescribe this
medicine to help make up the difference. These medicines
are used also to relieve inflamed areas of the body or for
severe allergies or skin problems, asthma, or arthritis. Corticosteroids may also be used for other conditions as determined by your doctor.

If any of the information in this leaflet causes you special
concern or if you want additional information about your
medicine and its use, check with your doctor, nurse, or pharmacist. **Remember, keep this and all other medicines out of
the reach of children and never share your medicines with
others.**

BEFORE USING THIS MEDICINE

Tell your doctor, nurse, and pharmacist if you . . .
  • are allergic to any medicine, either prescription or non-
    prescription (OTC);
  • are pregnant or intend to become pregnant while using
    this medicine;
  • are breast-feeding;
  • are taking **any** other prescription or nonprescription
    (OTC) medicine;
  • have **any** other medical problems;

PROPER USE OF THIS MEDICINE

Take this medicine with food to help prevent upset stomach.

Use this medicine only as directed.

If you miss a dose of this medicine, and your dosing schedule
is:
  • One dose every other day—Take the missed dose as
    soon as possible if you remember it the same morning,
    then go back to your regular schedule. If you do not
    remember until later, wait and take it the following
    morning. Then skip a day and start your regular dosing
    schedule again.
  • One dose a day—Take the missed dose as soon as pos-
    sible, then go back to your regular dosing schedule. If
    you do not remember until the next day, skip the missed
    dose and do not double the next one.
  • Several doses a day—Take the missed dose as soon as
    possible, then go back to your regular dosing schedule.
    If you do not remember until your next dose is due,
    double the next dose.

PRECAUTIONS WHILE USING THIS MEDICINE

Do not stop using this medicine without first checking with your doctor.

Your doctor may want you to follow a low-salt or potassium-rich diet.

Tell the doctor in charge that you are using this medicine before having skin tests, before having any kind of surgery (including dental surgery) or emergency treatment, or if you get a serious infection or injury.

While you are being treated with this medicine, and after you stop taking it, **do not have any immunizations without your doctor's approval.**

Diabetic patients: Check with your doctor if you notice a change in your blood sugar levels.

Children should avoid close contact with anyone who has chickenpox or measles. Tell the doctor right away if you think the child has been exposed to chickenpox or measles.

POSSIBLE SIDE EFFECTS OF THIS MEDICINE
Side Effects That Should Be Reported To Your Doctor

> *Less common*—Decreased or blurred vision; frequent urination; increased thirst

> *Rare*—Confusion; excitement; false sense of well-being; hallucinations; mental depression; mistaken feelings of self-importance or being mistreated; mood swings; restlessness

> *With long-term use*—Abdominal or stomach pain or burning (continuing); acne or other skin problems; bloody or black, tarry stools; filling or rounding out of face; irregular heartbeat; menstrual problems; muscle cramps, pain, or weakness; nausea; pain in back, hips, ribs, arms, shoulders, or legs; reddish purple lines on skin; swelling of feet or lower legs; thin, shiny skin; unusual bruising; unusual tiredness or weakness; vomiting; weight gain (rapid); wounds that will not heal

Side Effects That Usually Do Not Require Medical Attention

These possible side effects may go away during treatment; however, if they continue or are bothersome, check with your doctor, nurse, or pharmacist.

> *More common*—Increased appetite; indigestion; loss of appetite (triamcinolone only); nervousness or restlessness; trouble in sleeping

After you stop using this medicine, your body may need time to adjust. During this time, **check with your doctor immediately if any of the following side effects occur:** Abdominal, stomach, or back pain; dizziness; fainting; fever; loss of appetite (continuing); muscle or joint pain; nausea; reappearance of disease symptoms; shortness of breath; unexplained headaches (frequent or continuing); unusual tiredness or weakness; vomiting; weight loss (rapid).

Other side effects not listed above may also occur in some patients. If you notice any other effects, check with your doctor, nurse, or pharmacist.

COUGH/COLD COMBINATIONS   Systemic

■For the Pharmacist■

In providing consultation, consider emphasizing the following selected information (**»** = major clinical significance):

Before using this medication
» Conditions affecting use, especially:
   Sensitivity to any of the medications in the combination being taken
   Pregnancy—
      For all combinations
      Concern for the fetus or newborn infant, especially with high-dose and/or long-term usage
      In addition to the above, the following specific information may apply:
         For decongestant-containing
         Psychiatric disorders more likely with use of phenylpropanolamine in postpartum women
         For iodine/iodide-containing
         Use not recommended during pregnancy; may induce fetal goiter
         For opioid (narcotic) antitussive–containing
         Physical dependence in the neonate possible with regular use by mother during pregnancy
   Breast-feeding—
      For antihistamine-containing
      Antihistamines may cause excitement or irritability in nursing infant
      For decongestant-containing
      High risk for infants from sympathomimetic amines
      For iodine/iodide-containing
      Use not recommended during breast-feeding, because may induce skin rash and thyroid suppression in nursing infant
      For salicylate-containing
      Caution with high doses and chronic use because of high salicylate intake by infant
   Use in children—
      For anticholinergic-containing
      Increased susceptibility to anticholinergic effects
      Paradoxical reaction (hyperexcitability) possible
      For antihistamine-containing
      Increased susceptibility to anticholinergic effects
      Paradoxical reaction (hyperexcitability) possible
      For decongestant-containing
      Increased susceptibility to vasopressor effects of sympathomimetic amines
      Psychiatric disorders more likely with use of phenylpropanolamine in children up to 6 years of age
      For iodine/iodide-containing
      Increased susceptibility to goitrogenic effects of iodides
      For opioid (narcotic) antitussive–containing
      Paradoxical reaction (hyperexcitability) possible
      Increased susceptibility to respiratory depressant effects in children up to 2 years of age

For salicylate-containing
Increased susceptibility to toxic effects of salicylates, especially
if fever and dehydration present
Possible association between aspirin usage and Reye's syndrome
Use in the elderly—
For anticholinergic-containing
Anticholinergic effects more likely to occur
For antihistamine-containing
Anticholinergic effects more likely to occur
For decongestant-containing
Increased sensitivity to CNS and vasopressor effects of sym-
pathomimetic amines
For opioid (narcotic) antitussive–containing
Increased susceptibility to respiratory depressant effects
For salicylate-containing
Increased susceptibility to toxic effects of salicylates
Other medications, especially—
For acetaminophen-containing
Zidovudine
For anticholinergic-containing
Anticholinergics, other, or monoamine oxidase (MAO) inhib-
itors
For antihistamine-containing
Alcohol; anticholinergics; antidepressants, tricyclic; CNS de-
pressants; or monoamine oxidase (MAO) inhibitors
For decongestant-containing
Antidepressants, tricyclic; antihypertensives; beta-adrenergic
blocking agents, oral; CNS stimulants; monoamine oxidase
(MAO) inhibitors; or rauwolfia alkaloids
For dextromethorphan-containing
Alcohol or other CNS depressants, or monoamine oxidase
(MAO) inhibitors
For iodine/iodide-containing
Antithyroid agents or lithium
For opioid (narcotic) antitussive-containing
Alcohol or other CNS depressants
For salicylate-containing, especially aspirin
Alcohol; alkalizers, urinary; anticoagulants; antidiabetic agents,
oral; anti-inflammatory drugs, nonsteroidal; heparin; meth-
otrexate; platelet aggregation inhibitors; probenecid; sulfin-
pyrazone; thrombolytic agents; vancomycin; or zidovudine
Other medical problems, especially—
For all combinations (alcohol-containing only)
Alcohol abuse or history of
In addition to the above, the following specific information may
apply:
For anticholinergic-containing
Glaucoma or prostatic hypertrophy
For antihistamine-containing
Glaucoma or prostatic hypertrophy
For decongestant-containing
Cardiovascular disease, diabetes, hypertension, or thyroid
disease
For dextromethorphan-containing
Asthma
For iodine/iodide-containing
Thyroid disease
For opioid (narcotic) antitussive–containing
Asthma, diarrhea, or inflammatory bowel disease

For salicylate-containing, especially aspirin
Asthma, bleeding problems, gastritis, or peptic ulcer

Proper use of this medication

For all combinations

» Importance of drinking a glass of water after each dose of medication to help loosen mucus in lungs

» Importance of not taking more medication than the amount recommended (for all products; danger of overdose of acetaminophen, salicylates, or opioid [narcotic] antitussives; also, acetaminophen may cause liver damage with long-term or high-dose use)

Swallowing extended-release dosage form whole

Missed dose: If on scheduled dosing regimen—Taking as soon as possible; not taking if almost time for next dose; not doubling doses (for all products)

» Proper storage

In addition to the above, the following specific information may apply:

For antihistamine-containing

Taking with food, water, or milk to minimize gastric irritation

For salicylate-containing, especially aspirin

Taking with food, water, or milk to minimize gastric irritation

» Not taking combinations containing aspirin if a strong vinegar-like odor is present

Precautions while using this medication

For all combinations

» Checking with physician if symptoms persist after medication has been used for 7 days or if high fever, skin rash, or continuing headache is present with cough

In addition to the above, the following specific information may apply:

For analgesic-containing

» Caution if other medications containing acetaminophen, aspirin, or other salicylates (including diflunisal) are used

Diabetics: Aspirin or sodium salicylate present in some of these combinations may cause false urine sugar test results with prolonged use of 8 or more 325-mg doses per day

Not taking products containing aspirin for 5 days prior to any kind of surgery, unless otherwise directed by physician

For anticholinergic-containing

Possible dryness of mouth; using sugarless candy or gum, ice, or saliva substitute for relief; checking with physician or dentist if dry mouth continues for more than 2 weeks

» Caution during exercise and hot weather; overheating may result in heat stroke

For antihistamine-containing

Possible interference with skin tests using allergens; need to inform physician of use of antihistamine-containing medication

» Avoiding use of alcohol or other CNS depressants

» Caution if drowsiness or dizziness occurs

Possible dryness of mouth; using sugarless candy or gum, ice, or saliva substitute for relief; checking with physician or dentist if dry mouth continues for more than 2 weeks

May mask ototoxic effects of large doses of salicylates

For decongestant-containing

» Caution if taking phenylpropanolamine-containing appetite suppressants

» Possible insomnia; taking the medication a few hours before bedtime; however, the possibility of insomnia may be minimized with preparations that also contain an antihistamine or an opioid (narcotic) antitussive

Need to inform physician or dentist of use of medication if any kind of surgery (including dental surgery) or emergency treatment is required
For iodine/iodide-containing
Possible interference with thyroid tests
For opioid (narcotic) antitussive–containing
» Avoiding use of alcohol or other CNS depressants
» Caution if drowsiness or dizziness occurs; also, in addition to drowsiness and dizziness, a false sense of well-being may also occur
Lying down if nausea occurs
Caution when getting up suddenly from a lying or sitting position
Need to inform physician or dentist of use of medication if any kind of surgery (including dental surgery) or emergency treatment is required

Side/adverse effects
Signs of potential side effects, especially:
For all combinations
Allergic reactions
In addition to the above, the following specific information may apply:
For analgesic-containing
Anemia, gastrointestinal irritation or bleeding (for salicylates, particularly aspirin), and jaundice (for acetaminophen-containing)
For anticholinergic-containing only
Anticholinergic effects
For antihistamine-containing only
Anticholinergic effects and blood dyscrasias
For iodine/iodide-containing
Parotitis, acute

▲ For the Patient ▲

915315

ABOUT YOUR MEDICINE

Cough/cold combinations are used mainly to relieve the cough due to colds, influenza, or hay fever.

Cough/cold combination products contain more than one ingredient. For example, some products may contain an antihistamine, a decongestant, and an analgesic, in addition to a medicine for coughing. If you are treating yourself, it is important to choose a product that is best for your symptoms. Also, in general, it is best to buy a product that includes only those medicines you really need. If you have questions about which product to buy, check with your pharmacist.

If any of the information in this leaflet causes you special concern or if you want additional information about your medicine and its use, check with your doctor, nurse, or pharmacist. **Remember, keep this and all other medicines out of the reach of children and never share your medicines with others.**

BEFORE USING THIS MEDICINE

Do not give medicine containing aspirin or other salicylates to a child or a teenager with a fever or other symptoms of

a virus infection, especially flu or chickenpox, without first discussing its use with your child's doctor.

If you are taking this medicine without a prescription, carefully read and follow any precautions on the label. You should be especially careful if you . . .

- are allergic to any medicine, either prescription or nonprescription (OTC);
- are pregnant, intend to become pregnant, or are breastfeeding;
- are taking **any** other prescription or nonprescription (OTC) medicine;
- have **any** other medical problems.

If you have any questions, check with your doctor, nurse, or pharmacist.

PROPER USE OF THIS MEDICINE

To help loosen mucus or phlegm in the lungs, **drink a glass of water after each dose of this medicine**, unless otherwise directed by your doctor.

Take this medicine only as directed. Do not take more of it and do not take it more often than recommended on the label, unless otherwise directed by your doctor. To do so may increase the chance of side effects. Also, if you are taking an extended-release form of this medicine, swallow the capsule or tablet whole without breaking it or chewing it.

If you must take this medicine regularly and you miss a dose, take it as soon as possible. However, if it is almost time for your next dose, skip the missed dose and go back to your regular dosing schedule. Do not double doses.

PRECAUTIONS WHILE USING THIS MEDICINE

For patients taking an antihistamine- or narcotic-containing combination:

- This medicine will add to the effects of alcohol and other CNS depressants. **Check with your doctor before taking any other CNS depressants while you are taking this medicine.**
- This medicine may cause some people to become drowsy, dizzy, or less alert than they are normally. **Make sure you know how you react to this medicine before you drive, use machines, or do other jobs that require you to be alert and clearheaded.**

For patients taking an analgesic-containing combination:

- **Check the labels of all over-the-counter (OTC) and prescription medicines you now take.** Avoid any that contain acetaminophen or aspirin or other salicylates, since taking them while taking a cough/cold combination medicine that already contains them may lead to overdose.

For patients taking a decongestant-containing combination:
- This medicine may add to the central nervous system (CNS) stimulant and other effects of phenylpropanolamine (PPA)-containing diet aids. **Do not use medicines for diet or appetite control while taking this medicine unless you have checked with your doctor.**
- **This medicine may cause some people to be nervous or restless or to have trouble in sleeping. If you have trouble in sleeping, take the last dose of this medicine for each day a few hours before bedtime.**

POSSIBLE SIDE EFFECTS OF THIS MEDICINE
Side Effects That Should Be Reported To Your Doctor

The side effects that may occur with cough/cold combinations will differ, depending on the ingredients. **Ask your doctor, nurse, or pharmacist if there are any serious side effects that may occur with the medicine you are taking.**

CROMOLYN   Inhalation-Local

■ For the Pharmacist ■

In providing consultation, consider emphasizing the following selected information (» = major clinical significance):

Before using this medication
» Conditions affecting use, especially:
    Sensitivity to cromolyn

Proper use of this medication
» Helps prevent, but does not relieve, acute attacks of asthma or bronchospasm
» Importance of not using more medication than the amount prescribed
    Reading patient instructions carefully before using
    Checking periodically with physician, nurse, or pharmacist for proper use of inhaler to prevent incorrect dosage
» Proper dosing
    Missed dose: If used regularly, using as soon as possible; using any remaining doses for that day at regularly spaced intervals
» Proper storage
For inhalation aerosol dosage form
    Keeping record of number of sprays used, if possible; not floating canister in water to test fullness
    Testing inhaler before using first time or if not used for a while
    Proper administration technique
    Proper administration technique with spacer device
    Proper cleaning procedure for inhaler
For inhalation capsule dosage form
» Not swallowing capsules; medication not effective if swallowed
    Using with Spinhaler or Halermatic inhaler
    Proper loading technique for inhaler
    Proper administration technique
    Proper cleaning procedure for inhaler
For inhalation solution dosage form
    Not using if solution cloudy or contains particles
    Proper breaking of ampul
    Using in a power-operated nebulizer with an adequate flow rate and equipped with face mask or mouthpiece; not using hand-squeezed bulb nebulizers
For patients on scheduled dosing regimen
» Compliance with therapy; may require up to 4 weeks for full benefit

Precautions while using this medication
» Checking with physician if symptoms do not improve within first 4 weeks; checking with physician immediately if condition becomes worse
» Importance of not discontinuing concurrent systemic corticosteroid or bronchodilator therapy without physician's advice
    Possible dryness of mouth or throat, throat irritation, and hoarseness; gargling and rinsing mouth or taking drink of water after each dose to help prevent these effects

Side/adverse effects
    Signs of potential side effects, especially bronchospasm (increased); anaphylactic reaction; angioedema; dizziness; problems with urination; eosinophilic pneumonia; headache, severe or continuing;

joint pain or swelling; laryngeal edema; muscle pain or weakness; and skin rash, hives, or itching

Cromolyn inhalation aerosol may cause an unpleasant taste

▲ For the Patient ▲

912791

ABOUT YOUR MEDICINE

Cromolyn (KROE-moe-lin) is taken by oral inhalation to prevent asthma attacks. It is also used before and during exposure to substances that cause allergic reactions to prevent bronchospasm (wheezing or difficulty in breathing). In addition, this medicine is used to prevent bronchospasm caused by exercise.

If any of the information in this leaflet causes you special concern or if you want additional information about your medicine and its use, check with your doctor, nurse, or pharmacist. **Remember, keep this and all other medicines out of the reach of children and never share your medicines with others.**

BEFORE USING THIS MEDICINE

Tell your doctor, nurse, and pharmacist if you . . .
- are allergic to any medicine, either prescription or non-prescription (OTC);
- are using the capsule form of cromolyn and are allergic to lactose, milk, or milk products;
- are pregnant or intend to become pregnant while using this medicine;
- are breast-feeding;
- are taking any other prescription or nonprescription (OTC) medicine;
- have any other medical problems.

PROPER USE OF THIS MEDICINE

Cromolyn oral inhalation is used to prevent asthma or bronchospasm attacks. It will not relieve an attack that has already started. If this medicine is used during a severe attack, it may cause irritation and make the attack worse.

For patients using cromolyn aerosol:
- This medicine usually comes with patient directions. Read them carefully before using this medicine.
- Keep the spray away from the eyes because it may cause irritation.

For patients using cromolyn capsules for inhalation:
- This medicine is used with a special inhaler. Follow directions for use.
- **Do not swallow the capsules. The medicine will not work this way.**

For patients using cromolyn solution for inhalation:
- Use this medicine only in a power-operated nebulizer with an adequate flow rate and equipped with a face

mask or mouthpiece. Make sure you understand exactly how to use it. Hand-operated nebulizers are not suitable.

Use cromolyn oral inhalation only as directed. Do not use more of it and do not use it more often than your doctor ordered. To do so may increase the chance of side effects.

In order for cromolyn to work properly, it must be inhaled every day in regularly spaced doses as ordered by your doctor. Up to 4 weeks may pass before you feel the full effects of the medicine.

If you miss a dose of this medicine, use it as soon as possible. Then use any remaining doses for that day at regularly spaced intervals. Do not double doses.

PRECAUTIONS WHILE USING THIS MEDICINE

If your symptoms do not improve or if your condition becomes worse, check with your doctor.

If you are also using an adrenocorticoid (cortisone-like medicine) for your asthma along with this medicine, do not stop using the adrenocorticoid even if your asthma seems better, unless told to do so by your doctor.

If you are also using a bronchodilator inhaler, use the bronchodilator first. Then wait about 5 minutes before using cromolyn, unless otherwise directed.

Dryness of the mouth or throat, throat irritation, and hoarseness may occur after using this medicine. Gargling and rinsing the mouth after each dose may help prevent these effects.

POSSIBLE SIDE EFFECTS OF THIS MEDICINE

Side Effects That Should Be Reported To Your Doctor

> *Less common*—Difficult or painful urination; dizziness; frequent urge to urinate; headache (severe or continuing); increased wheezing; joint pain or swelling; muscle pain or weakness; nausea or vomiting; skin rash, hives, or itching; swelling of the lips and eyes; tightness in chest; troubled breathing; trouble in swallowing

> *Rare*—Chest pain; chills; sweating

Side Effects That Usually Do Not Require Medical Attention

These possible side effects may go away during treatment; however, if they continue or are bothersome, check with your doctor, nurse, or pharmacist.

> *More common*—Cough; hoarseness

Other side effects not listed above may also occur in some patients. If you notice any other effects, check with your doctor, nurse, or pharmacist.

CROMOLYN   Nasal

■ For the Pharmacist ■

In providing consultation, consider emphasizing the following selected information (» = major clinical significance):

Before using this medication
» Conditions affecting use, especially:
    Sensitivity to cromolyn
    Use in children—Safety and efficacy have not been established in the U.S. in children up to 6 years of age (in Canada, up to 5 years of age)

Proper use of this medication
    Reading patient directions carefully
    Clearing nasal passages before use
    For *cromolyn nasal solution:* Using with a special spray device; wiping nosepiece with a clean tissue and replacing dust cap after use to keep unit clean
    For *cromolyn for nasal insufflation:* Using with a special inhaler; understanding exactly how to use inhaler; wiping nosepiece with a clean tissue and replacing dust cap after use; washing only nosepiece in warm water, drying thoroughly; not washing bulb or dampening bulb interior
» Importance of not using more medication than the amount prescribed
» Using every day in regularly spaced doses in order for medication to work properly; results are usually noticeable in approximately 1 week; however in perennial allergic rhinitis, up to 4 weeks may be required for full benefit
» Proper dosing
    Missed dose: Using as soon as possible; using any remaining doses for that day at regularly spaced intervals; not doubling doses
» Proper storage

Precautions while using this medication
» Checking with physician if symptoms do not improve or if condition becomes worse

Side/adverse effects
    Signs of potential side effects, especially anaphylactic reaction, epistaxis, and skin rash

▲ For the Patient ▲

913626

ABOUT YOUR MEDICINE

Cromolyn (KROE-moe-lin) nasal solution is used to help prevent or treat the symptoms (sneezing, wheezing, runny nose, itching) of seasonal (short-term) or chronic (long-term) allergic rhinitis. Cromolyn powder for nasal inhalation is used to help prevent seasonal (short-term) allergic rhinitis.

When cromolyn is used to treat chronic (long-term) allergic rhinitis, an antihistamine and/or a nasal decongestant may be used with this medicine, especially during the first few weeks of treatment.

If any of the information in this leaflet causes you special concern or if you want additional information about your medicine and its use, check with your doctor, nurse, or pharmacist. **Remember, keep this and all other medicines out of the reach of children and never share your medicines with others.**

BEFORE USING THIS MEDICINE

Tell your doctor, nurse, and pharmacist if you . . .
- are allergic to any medicine, either prescription or non-prescription (OTC);
- are pregnant or intend to become pregnant while using this medicine;
- are breast-feeding;
- are taking any other prescription or nonprescription (OTC) medicine;
- have any other medical problems.

PROPER USE OF THIS MEDICINE

This medicine usually comes with patient directions. Read them carefully before using the medicine.

Before using this medicine, clear the nasal passages by blowing your nose.

For patients using cromolyn nasal solution:
- Cromolyn nasal solution is used with a special spray device.
- To keep clean, wipe the nosepiece with a clean tissue and replace the dust cap after use.

For patients using cromolyn powder for nasal inhalation:
- This medicine is used with a special inhaler. Be sure you understand exactly how to use it.
- To keep clean, wipe the nosepiece with a clean tissue and replace the dust cap after use. Only the nosepiece may be washed in warm water, but must be dried thoroughly. **Do not wash the bulb unit or let it get wet.**

Use this medicine only as directed. Do not use more of it and do not use it more often than your doctor ordered. To do so may increase the chance of side effects.

In order for this medicine to work properly, it must be used every day in regularly spaced doses as ordered by your doctor:
- For patients using cromolyn for seasonal (short-term) allergic rhinitis, up to 1 week may pass before you begin to feel better.
- For patients using cromolyn for chronic (long-term) allergic rhinitis, up to 4 weeks may pass before you feel the full effects of this medicine, although you may begin to feel better after 1 week.

If you miss a dose of this medicine, use it as soon as possible. Then use any remaining doses for that day at regularly spaced intervals. Do not double doses.

PRECAUTIONS WHILE USING THIS MEDICINE
If your symptoms do not improve or if your condition becomes worse, check with your doctor.

POSSIBLE SIDE EFFECTS OF THIS MEDICINE
Side Effects That Should Be Reported To Your Doctor

  Rare—Allergic reaction (coughing; difficulty in swallowing; hives or itching; swelling of face, lips, or eyelids; wheezing or difficulty in breathing); nosebleeds; skin rash

Side Effects That Usually Do Not Require Medical Attention

  More common—Burning, stinging, or irritation inside of nose; increase in sneezing

  Less common—Cough; headache; postnasal drip; unpleasant taste

Other side effects not listed above may also occur in some patients. If you notice any other effects, check with your doctor, nurse, or pharmacist.

CYCLIZINE   Systemic

■ For the Pharmacist ■

In providing consultation, consider emphasizing the following selected information (» = major clinical significance):

Before using this medication
» Conditions affecting use, especially:
   Sensitivity to cyclizine
   Pregnancy—Animal studies have shown cyclizine to be terato-genic at doses above therapeutic range
   Breast-feeding—May be distributed into breast milk; may inhibit lactation due to anticholinergic effects
   Use in children—Possible increased susceptibility to anticholinergic side effects
   Use in the elderly—Possible increased susceptibility to anticholinergic side effects
   Other medications, especially other CNS depressants

Proper use of this medication
   Taking with food, water, or milk to minimize gastric irritation
   Not taking more medication than the amount prescribed
   For motion sickness, taking at least 30 minutes before traveling
» Proper dosing
   Missed dose (if on a regular dosing schedule): Taking as soon as possible; not taking if almost time for next dose; not doubling doses
» Proper storage

Precautions while using this medication
   Possible interference with skin tests using allergens; need to inform physician of using this medication
» Avoiding use of alcohol or other CNS depressants
» Caution if drowsiness occurs
   Possible dryness of mouth; using sugarless gum or candy, ice, or saliva substitute for relief

▲ For the Patient ▲

912394

MECLIZINE/BUCLIZINE/CYCLIZINE (Oral):
Including Meclizine; Buclizine; Cyclizine.

ABOUT YOUR MEDICINE

Meclizine (MEK-li-zeen), **buclizine** (BYOO-kli-zeen), and **cyclizine** (SYE-kli-zeen) are used to prevent and treat nausea, vomiting, and dizziness associated with motion sickness, and dizziness caused by other medical problems.

If any of the information in this leaflet causes you special concern or if you want additional information about your medicine and its use, check with your doctor, nurse, or pharmacist. **Remember, keep this and all other medicines out of the reach of children and never share your medicines with others.**

BEFORE USING THIS MEDICINE

If you are taking this medicine without a prescription, carefully read and follow any precautions on the label. You should be especially careful if you . . .

- are allergic to any medicine, either prescription or nonprescription (OTC);
- are pregnant, intend to become pregnant, or are breastfeeding;
- are taking any other prescription or nonprescription (OTC) medicine, especially other CNS depressants;
- have any other medical problems.

If you have any questions, check with your doctor, nurse, or pharmacist.

PROPER USE OF THIS MEDICINE

This medicine is used to relieve or prevent the symptoms of motion sickness or dizziness caused by other medical problems. Take it only as directed. Do not take more of it or take it more often than stated on the label or ordered by your doctor. To do so may increase the chance of side effects.

For patients taking this medicine for motion sickness:

—take buclizine or cyclizine at least 30 minutes before you begin to travel.

—take meclizine at least 1 hour before you begin to travel.

Take this medicine with food or a glass of water or milk to lessen stomach irritation, if necessary.

If you must take this medicine regularly and you miss a dose, take the missed dose as soon as possible. However, if it is almost time for your next dose, skip the missed dose and go back to your regular dosing schedule. Do not double doses.

PRECAUTIONS WHILE USING THIS MEDICINE

This medicine will add to the effects of alcohol and other CNS depressants (medicines that slow down the nervous system). **Check with your doctor before taking any such depressants while you are taking this medicine.**

This medicine may cause some people to become drowsy or less alert than they are normally. **Make sure you know how you react to this medicine before you drive, use machines, or do other jobs that require you to be alert.**

Buclizine, cyclizine, and meclizine may cause dryness of the mouth. For temporary relief use sugarless candy or gum, dissolve bits of ice in your mouth, or use a saliva substitute. However, if your mouth continues to feel dry for more than 2 weeks, check with your physician or dentist. Continuing dryness of the mouth may increase the chance of dental disease, including tooth decay, gum disease, and fungus infections.

POSSIBLE SIDE EFFECTS OF THIS MEDICINE
Side Effects That Usually Do Not Require Medical Attention

These possible side effects may go away during treatment; however, if they continue or are bothersome, check with your doctor, nurse, or pharmacist.

> *More common*—Drowsiness

> *Less common or rare*—Blurred vision; constipation; difficult or painful urination; dizziness; dryness of mouth, nose, and throat; fast heartbeat; headache; loss of appetite; nervousness, restlessness, or trouble in sleeping; skin rash; upset stomach

Other side effects not listed above may also occur in some patients. If you notice any other effects, check with your doctor, nurse, or pharmacist.

CYCLOBENZAPRINE   Systemic

■ For the Pharmacist ■

In providing consultation, consider emphasizing the following selected information (» = major clinical significance):

Before using this medication
» Conditions affecting use, especially:
  Sensitivity to cyclobenzaprine
  Other medications, especially other CNS depression–producing medications, monoamine oxidase inhibitors, and tricyclic antidepressants
  Other medical problems, especially cardiac arrhythmias, congestive heart failure, heart block or other conduction disturbances, hyperthyroidism, and myocardial infarction (acute recovery phase)

Proper use of this medication
  Not taking more medication than the amount prescribed, to minimize possibility of side effects
» Proper dosing
  Missed dose: Taking if remembered within an hour; not taking if not remembered until later; not doubling doses
» Proper storage

Precautions while using this medication
» Avoiding alcohol or other CNS depressants unless prescribed or otherwise approved by physician
» Caution if blurred vision, drowsiness, or dizziness occurs
  Possible dryness of mouth; using sugarless gum or candy, ice, or saliva substitute for relief; checking with dentist if dry mouth continues for more than 2 weeks

Side/adverse effects
  Signs and symptoms of potential side effects, especially anaphylaxis, angioedema, allergic dermatitis, hepatitis, and syncope

▲ For the Patient ▲

913648

ABOUT YOUR MEDICINE

Cyclobenzaprine (sye-kloe-BEN-za-preen) is a medicine that is used to help relax certain muscles in your body. It is used to relieve the pain, stiffness, and discomfort caused by strains, sprains, or injuries to your muscles. However, this medicine does not take the place of rest, excercise or physical therapy, or other treatment that your doctor may recommend for your medical problem. Cyclobenzaprine may also be used for other conditions as determined by your doctor.

If any of the information in this leaflet causes you special concern or if you want additional information about your medicine and its use, check with your doctor, nurse, or pharmacist. **Remember, keep this and all other medicines out of the reach of children and never share your medicines with others.**

BEFORE USING THIS MEDICINE

Tell your doctor, nurse, and pharmacist if you . . .

- are allergic to any medicine, either prescription or non-prescription (OTC);
- are pregnant or intend to become pregnant while using this medicine;
- are breast-feeding;
- compete in athletics;
- are taking any other prescription or nonprescription (OTC) medicine, especially CNS depressants, MAO inhibitors, or tricyclic antidepressants;
- have any other medical problems, especially heart or blood vessel disease or overactive thyroid.

PROPER USE OF THIS MEDICINE

Take this medicine only as directed by your doctor. Do not take more of it and do not take it more often than your doctor ordered. To do so may increase the chance of serious side effects.

If you miss a dose of this medicine and remember within an hour or so of the missed dose, take it right away. Then go back to your regular dosing schedule. However, if you do not remember until later, skip the missed dose and go back to your regular dosing schedule. Do not double doses.

PRECAUTIONS WHILE USING THIS MEDICINE

Cyclobenzaprine will add to the effects of alcohol and other CNS depressants (medicines that slow down the nervous system). **Check with your doctor before taking any such depressants while you are taking this medicine.**

Cyclobenzaprine may cause some people to have blurred vision or to become drowsy, dizzy, or less alert than they are normally. **Make sure you know how you react to this medicine before you drive, use machines, or do other jobs that require you to be alert and see well.**

Cyclobenzaprine may cause dryness of the mouth. For temporary relief, use sugarless candy or gum, melt bits of ice in your mouth, or use a saliva substitute. However, if your mouth continues to feel dry for more than 2 weeks, check with your medical doctor or dentist. Continuing dryness of the mouth may increase the chance of dental disease, including tooth decay, gum disease, and fungal infections.

POSSIBLE SIDE EFFECTS OF THIS MEDICINE

Side Effects That Should Be Reported To Your Doctor Immediately

   Rare—Fainting; swelling of face, lips, or tongue

   Signs of overdose—Convulsions (seizures); hallucinations; troubled breathing

Other Side Effects That Should Be Reported To Your Doctor

> *Rare*—Clumsiness or unsteadiness; confusion; mental depression or other mood or mental changes; problems in urinating; ringing or buzzing in ears; skin rash, hives, or itching; unusual thoughts or dreams; yellow eyes or skin

Side Effects That Usually Do Not Require Medical Attention

These possible side effects may go away during treatment; however, if they continue or are bothersome, check with your doctor, nurse, or pharmacist.

> *More common*—Dizziness or lightheadedness; drowsiness; dryness of mouth

Other side effects not listed above may also occur in some patients. If you notice any other effects, check with your doctor, nurse, or pharmacist.

CYCLOPHOSPHAMIDE   Systemic

■For the Pharmacist■

In providing consultation, consider emphasizing the following selected information (» = major clinical significance):

Before using this medication
» Conditions affecting use, especially:
   Sensitivity to cyclophosphamide
   Pregnancy—Use not recommended because of mutagenic, teratogenic, and carcinogenic potential; advisability of using contraception; telling physician immediately if pregnancy is suspected
   Breast-feeding—Not recommended because of risk of serious side effects
   Other medications, especially probenecid, sulfinpyrazone, other bone marrow depressants, other immunosuppressants, or cytotoxic drug or radiation therapy
   Other medical problems, especially chickenpox, herpes zoster, hepatic function impairment, infection, or renal function impairment

Proper use of this medication
» Importance of not taking more or less medication than the amount prescribed
   Caution in taking combination therapy; taking each medication at the right time
» Importance of ample fluid intake and subsequent increase in urine output, as well as frequent voiding (including at least once during night), to prevent hemorrhagic cystitis and aid in excretion of uric acid; following physician instructions for recommended fluid intake; some patients may require up to 3000 mL (3 quarts) per day
   Usually best if taken in the morning to reduce risk of hemorrhagic cystitis; however, physician may recommend taking in small doses throughout day to lessen stomach upset; following physician's instructions for timing of doses
» Probability of nausea, vomiting, and loss of appetite; importance of continuing medication despite stomach upset; checking with physician before discontinuing medication
   Checking with physician if vomiting occurs shortly after dose is taken
» Proper dosing
   Missed dose: Not taking at all; not doubling doses; checking with physician
» Proper storage

Precautions while using this medication
» Importance of close monitoring by physician
» Avoiding immunizations unless approved by physician; other persons in patient's household should avoid immunizations with oral poliovirus vaccine; avoiding persons who have taken oral poliovirus vaccine or wearing a protective mask that covers nose and mouth
   Caution if any kind of surgery, including dental surgery, or emergency treatment with general anesthesia is required within 10 days of treatment

Caution if bone marrow depression occurs:

» Avoiding exposure to persons with bacterial infections, especially during periods of low blood counts; checking with physician immediately if fever or chills, cough or hoarseness, lower back or side pain, or painful or difficult urination occur

» Checking with physician immediately if unusual bleeding or bruising; black, tarry stools; blood in urine; or pinpoint red spots on skin occur

Caution in use of regular toothbrush, dental floss, or toothpick; physician, dentist, or nurse may suggest alternatives; checking with physician before having dental work done

Not touching eyes or inside of nose unless hands washed immediately before

Using caution to avoid accidental cuts with use of sharp objects such as safety razor or fingernail or toenail cutters

Avoiding contact sports or other situations where bruising or injury could occur

Caution if any laboratory tests required; possible interference with test results

Side/adverse effects

May cause adverse effects such as blood problems; loss of hair; toxicity to lungs, heart, or bladder; and cancer; importance of discussing possible effects with physician

Signs of potential side effects, especially gonadal suppression, leukopenia, infection, cardiotoxicity, hemorrhagic cystitis, hyperuricemia, uric acid nephropathy, nonhemorrhagic cystitis, nephrotoxicity, pneumonitis, interstitial pulmonary fibrosis, SIADH secretion, anemia, thrombocytopenia, anaphylactic reaction, hemorrhagic colitis, hepatitis, hyperglycemia, redness or swelling or pain at site of injecton, and stomatitis

Physician or nurse can help in dealing with side effects

Possibility of hair loss; normal hair growth should return after treatment has ended; new hair may be slightly different in color or texture

---

▲ For the Patient ▲

916249

ABOUT YOUR MEDICINE

Cyclophosphamide (sye-kloe-FOSS-fa-mide) is used to treat some kinds of cancer as well as some noncancer conditions, including some kinds of kidney disease.

If any of the information in this leaflet causes you special concern or if you want additional information about your medicine and its use, check with your doctor, nurse, or pharmacist. **Remember, keep this and all other medicines out of the reach of children and never share your medicines with others.**

BEFORE USING THIS MEDICINE

Discuss with your doctor the possible side effects that may be caused by this medicine. Some of them may be serious and/or long-term.

Tell your doctor, nurse, and pharmacist if you . . .

- are allergic to any medicine, either prescription or non-prescription (OTC);

- are pregnant or intend to have children;
- are breast-feeding;
- are taking **any** other prescription or nonprescription (OTC) medicine;
- have any other medical problems, especially chickenpox (including recent exposure), herpes zoster (shingles), infection, kidney disease, or liver disease;
- have ever been treated with x-rays or cancer medicines.

PROPER USE OF THIS MEDICINE

Take this medicine only as directed by your doctor. Do not take more or less and do not take it more often than ordered.

While you are using cyclophosphamide, it is important that you drink extra fluids so that you will pass more urine. Also, empty your bladder frequently.

Cyclophosphamide often causes nausea, vomiting, and loss of appetite. Ask your doctor, nurse, or pharmacist for ways to lessen these effects.

If you vomit shortly after a dose, check with your doctor.

If you miss a dose of this medicine, do not take the missed dose at all and do not double the next one. Instead, go back to your regular dosing schedule and check with your doctor.

PRECAUTIONS WHILE USING THIS MEDICINE

It is very important that your doctor check your progress at regular visits to make sure this medicine is working properly and to check for unwanted effects.

While you are being treated with cyclophosphamide, and after you stop treatment, **do not have any immunizations (vaccinations) without your doctor's approval.**

Cyclophosphamide can lower the number of white blood cells in your blood, increasing the chance of getting an infection. It can also lower the number of platelets, which are necessary for proper blood clotting. If this occurs:
- Avoid people with infections.
- Be careful when using a regular toothbrush, dental floss, or toothpick.
- Do not touch your eyes or the inside of your nose unless you have just washed your hands and have not touched anything else in the meantime.
- Be careful not to cut, bruise, or injure yourself.

POSSIBLE SIDE EFFECTS OF THIS MEDICINE

Side Effects That Should Be Reported To Your Doctor Immediately

Less common—Cough or hoarseness; fever or chills; lower back or side pain; painful or difficult urination

Rare—Black, tarry stools; blood in urine or stools; pinpoint red spots on skin; shortness of breath (sudden); unusual bleeding or bruising

With high doses or long-term treatment—Blood in urine; painful urination

Other Side Effects That Should Be Reported To Your Doctor

More common—Dizziness, confusion, or agitation; missing periods; unusual tiredness or weakness

Less common—Fast heartbeat; joint pain; shortness of breath; swelling of feet or lower legs

Rare—Frequent urination; redness, pain, or swelling at place of injection; sores in mouth and on lips; unusual thirst; yellow eyes or skin

Side Effects That Usually Do Not Require Medical Attention

These possible side effects may go away during treatment; however, if they continue or are bothersome, check with your doctor, nurse, or pharmacist.

More common—Darkening of skin and fingernails; loss of appetite; nausea or vomiting

Cyclophosphamide may cause a temporary loss of hair. After treatment has ended, hair growth should return.

Other side effects not listed above may also occur in some patients. If you notice any other effects, check with your doctor, nurse, or pharmacist.

After you stop using cyclophosphamide, it may still produce some side effects that need attention. Check with your doctor immediately if you notice blood in your urine.

CYCLOSERINE   Systemic

■For the Pharmacist■

In providing consultation, consider emphasizing the following selected
information (» = major clinical significance):

Before using this medication
» Conditions affecting use, especially:
Pregnancy—Cycloserine crosses the placenta and fetal serum
concentrations may approach maternal serum concentrations
Breast-feeding—Cycloserine is distributed into breast milk. Concentrations may approach or exceed maternal serum concentrations
Other medications, especially alcohol and ethionamide
Other medical problems, especially alcoholism (active or in remission), a history of seizure disorders, or renal function impairment

Proper use of this medication
Taking this medication after meals if gastrointestinal irritation oc-
curs
» Compliance with full course of therapy; in tuberculosis, therapy may
take months or years
» Importance of not missing doses and taking at evenly spaced times
» Proper dosing
Missed dose: Taking as soon as possible; not taking if almost time
for next dose; not doubling doses
» Proper storage

Precautions while using this medication
Regular visits to physician to check progress
Checking with physician if no improvement within 2 to 3 weeks
» Checking with physician immediately if thoughts of suicide occur
» Caution if dizziness or drowsiness occurs
» Avoiding alcoholic beverages while taking this medication

Side/adverse effects
Signs of potential side effects, especially CNS toxicity, hypersensitivity reactions, peripheral neuropathy, and seizures

▲ For the Patient ▲

913659

ABOUT YOUR MEDICINE

Cycloserine (sye-kloe-SER-een) belongs to the family of
medicines called antibiotics. It is used to treat tuberculosis
(TB). When cycloserine is used for TB, it is given with other
medicines for TB. Cycloserine may also be used for other
conditions as determined by your doctor.

**To help clear up your tuberculosis (TB) completely, you must
keep taking this medicine for the full time of treatment, even
if you begin to feel better. This is very important. It is also
very important that you do not miss any doses.**

If any of the information in this leaflet causes you special
concern or if you want additional information about your

medicine and its use, check with your doctor, nurse, or pharmacist. **Remember, keep this and all other medicines out of the reach of children and never share your medicines with others.**

BEFORE USING THIS MEDICINE

Tell your doctor, nurse, and pharmacist if you . . .

- are allergic to any medicine, either prescription or non-prescription (OTC);
- are pregnant or intend to become pregnant while using this medicine;
- are breast-feeding;
- are taking any other prescription or nonprescription (OTC) medicine, especially ethionamide;
- have any other medical problems, especially alcohol abuse (or history of), convulsive disorders such as seizures or epilepsy, or severe kidney disease.

PROPER USE OF THIS MEDICINE

Cycloserine may be taken after meals if it upsets your stomach.

To help clear up your infection completely, **it is very important that you keep taking this medicine for the full time of treatment** even if you begin to feel better after a few weeks. If you are taking this medicine for TB, you may have to take it every day for as long as 1 to 2 years or more. If you stop taking this medicine too soon, your symptoms may return.

This medicine works best when there is a constant amount in the blood or urine. **To help keep this amount constant, do not miss any doses. Also, it is best to take each dose at evenly spaced times day and night.** If this interferes with your sleep or other daily activities, check with your doctor, nurse, or pharmacist.

If you do miss a dose of this medicine, take it as soon as possible. This will help to keep a constant amount of medicine in the blood or urine. However, if it is almost time for your next dose, skip the missed dose and go back to your regular dosing schedule. Do not double doses.

PRECAUTIONS WHILE USING THIS MEDICINE

If your symptoms do not improve within 2 to 3 weeks, or if they become worse, check with your doctor.

If cycloserine causes you to feel very depressed or to have thoughts of suicide, check with your doctor immediately.

This medicine may cause some people to become dizzy, drowsy, or less alert than they are normally. **Make sure you know how you react to this medicine before you drive, use machines, or do other jobs that require you to be alert.** If these reactions are especially bothersome, check with your doctor.

Some of cycloserine's side effects may be more likely to occur if you drink alcoholic beverages regularly while you are taking this medicine. Therefore, **you should not drink alcoholic beverages while you are taking this medicine.**

This medicine must not be given to other people or used for other infections unless you are otherwise directed by your doctor.

POSSIBLE SIDE EFFECTS OF THIS MEDICINE

Side Effects That Should Be Reported To Your Doctor Immediately

More common—Anxiety; confusion; dizziness; drowsiness; increased irritability; increased restlessness; mental depression; muscle twitching or trembling; nervousness; nightmares; other mood or mental changes; speech problems; thoughts of suicide

Less common—Convulsions (seizures); numbness, tingling, burning pain, or weakness in the hands or feet; skin rash

Side Effects That Usually Do Not Require Medical Attention

These possible side effects may go away during treatment; however, if they continue or are bothersome, check with your doctor, nurse, or pharmacist.

More common—Headache

Other side effects not listed above may also occur in some patients. If you notice any other effects, check with your doctor, nurse, or pharmacist.

CYCLOSPORINE Systemic

■ For the Pharmacist ■

In providing consultation, consider emphasizing the following selected information (» = major clinical significance):

Before using this medication
» Conditions affecting use, especially:
 Sensitivity to cyclosporine
 Pregnancy—Causes birth defects or fetal death in animals
 Breast-feeding—Distributed into breast milk; breast-feeding not recommended because of risk of serious side effects
 Other medications, especially androgens, cimetidine, danazol, diltiazem, potassium-sparing diuretics, erythromycin, estrogens, ketoconazole, other immunosuppressants, or lovastatin
 Other medical problems, especially chickenpox, herpes zoster, hepatic function impairment, infection, or renal function impairment

Proper use of this medication
» Importance of not taking more or less medication than the amount prescribed
 Getting into the habit of taking at the same time each day to help increase compliance and maintain steady blood concentrations
 Taking solution orally; special dropper to be used for accurate measuring; making sure dropper is properly dried after cleaning before using
 Mixing oral solution with milk, chocolate milk, or orange juice (preferably at room temperature) in a glass (not wax-lined or plastic disposable) container to improve palatability; stirring well and drinking immediately, then rinsing glass and drinking to make sure all medication is taken; wiping pipette dry but not rinsing with water (to prevent cloudiness)
 Taking with meals to reduce gastrointestinal irritation
» Checking with physician before discontinuing medication; possible need for lifelong therapy
» Proper dosing
 Missed dose: Taking as soon as possible if remembered within 12 hours; not taking if almost time for next dose; not doubling doses
» Proper storage

Precautions while using this medication
» Importance of close monitoring by physician
» Avoiding immunizations unless approved by physician; other persons in patient's household should avoid immunizations with oral poliovirus vaccine; avoiding persons who have taken oral poliovirus vaccine or wearing a protective mask that covers nose and mouth
» Maintaining good dental hygiene and seeing dentist frequently for teeth cleaning to prevent tenderness, bleeding, and gum enlargement

Side/adverse effects
 Importance of discussing possible effects, including cancer, with physician
 Signs of potential side effects, especially gingival hyperplasia, convulsions, infection, anaphylaxis, hyperkalemia, pancreatitis, and renal toxicity

Asymptomatic side effects, including hypertension, nephrotoxicity, and hepatotoxicity

▲ For the Patient ▲

916511

ABOUT YOUR MEDICINE

Cyclosporine (SYE-kloe-spor-een) belongs to the group of medicines known as immunosuppressive agents. It is used to help prevent the body from rejecting an organ (for example, kidney, liver, and heart) transplant. Cyclosporine may also be used for other conditions as determined by your doctor.

If any of the information in this leaflet causes you special concern or if you want additional information about your medicine and its use, check with your doctor, nurse, or pharmacist. **Remember, keep this and all other medicines out of the reach of children and never share your medicines with others.**

BEFORE USING THIS MEDICINE

Discuss with your doctor the possible side effects that may be caused by this medicine. Some of them may be serious and/or long-term.

Tell your doctor, nurse, and pharmacist if you . . .
- are allergic to any medicine, either prescription or non-prescription (OTC);
- are pregnant or intend to become pregnant while using this medicine;
- are breast-feeding;
- are taking **any** other prescription or nonprescription (OTC) medicine;
- have any other medical problems, especially chickenpox (including recent exposure); herpes zoster (shingles); infection; or kidney or liver disease.

PROPER USE OF THIS MEDICINE

Take this medicine only as directed by your doctor. Do not take more or less of it and do not take it more often than your doctor ordered.

To help you remember to take your medicine, try to get into the habit of taking it at the same time each day. This will also help cyclosporine work better by keeping a constant amount in the blood.

To make cyclosporine taste better, mix it in a glass container with milk, chocolate milk, or orange juice (preferably at room temperature). Do not use a wax-lined or plastic disposable container. Stir it well, then drink it immediately. After drinking all the liquid containing the medicine, rinse the glass with a little more liquid and drink that also, to make sure you get all the medicine. Dry the dropper used to measure the cyclosporine, but do not rinse it with water.

If this medicine upsets your stomach, your doctor may recommend that you take it with meals. However, check with your doctor first.

Do not stop taking this medicine without first checking with your doctor. You may have to take medicine for the rest of your life to prevent your body from rejecting the transplant.

If you miss a dose of cyclosporine and remember it within 12 hours, take the missed dose as soon as you remember. However, if it is almost time for the next dose, skip the missed dose, go back to your regular dosing schedule, and check with your doctor. Do not double doses.

PRECAUTIONS WHILE USING THIS MEDICINE

It is very important that your doctor check your progress at regular visits. Your doctor will want to do laboratory tests to make sure that cyclosporine is working properly and to check for unwanted effects.

While you are being treated with cyclosporine, and after you stop treatment with it, **do not have any immunizations (vaccinations) without your doctor's approval.**

In some patients (usually younger patients), tenderness, swelling, or bleeding of the gums may appear soon after treatment with cyclosporine is started. Brushing and flossing your teeth carefully and regularly and massaging your gums may help prevent this. **See your dentist regularly to have your teeth cleaned. Check with your physician or dentist if you have any questions about how to take care of your teeth and gums, or if you notice any tenderness, swelling, or bleeding of your gums.**

POSSIBLE SIDE EFFECTS OF THIS MEDICINE

Side Effects That Should Be Reported To Your Doctor Immediately

> *Less common*—Fever or chills; frequent urge to urinate

> *Rare*—Blood in urine

Other Side Effects That Should Be Reported To Your Doctor

> *More common*—Bleeding, tender, or enlarged gums

> *Less common*—Convulsions (seizures)

> *Rare*—Confusion; irregular heartbeat; numbness or tingling in hands, feet, or lips; shortness of breath or difficult breathing; stomach pain (severe) with nausea and vomiting; unexplained nervousness; unusual tiredness or weakness; weakness or heaviness of legs

Side Effects That Usually Do Not Require Medical Attention

These possible side effects may go away during treatment; however, if they continue or are bothersome, check with your doctor, nurse, or pharmacist.

More common—Increase in hair growth; trembling and
   shaking of hands

Less common—Acne or oily skin; headache; leg cramps;
   nausea or vomiting

Other side effects not listed above may also occur in some
patients. If you notice any other effects, check with your
doctor, nurse, or pharmacist.

DANAZOL   Systemic

■ For the Pharmacist ■

In providing consultation, consider emphasizing the following selected information (» = major clinical significance):

Before using this medication
»   Conditions affecting use, especially:
Sensitivity to anabolic steroids, androgens, or danazol
Pregnancy—Use is not recommended during pregnancy because of possible androgenic effects on female fetus
Breast-feeding—Use is usually not recommended because of possible androgenic effects in the infant
Use in children—Caution is recommended because of possible androgenic effects
Other medications, especially coumarin- or indandione-derivative anticoagulants
Other medical problems, especially severe cardiac function impairment, undiagnosed abnormal vaginal bleeding, severe hepatic function impairment, or severe renal function impairment

Proper use of this medication
»   Taking for full time of therapy
»   Proper dosing
Missed dose: Taking as soon as possible; not taking if almost time for next dose; not doubling doses
»   Proper storage

Precautions while using this medication
Regular visits to physician to check progress during therapy
Diabetics: May alter blood sugar levels
»   Possible photosensitivity reactions: caution during exposure to sun or when using sunlamps, tanning booths or beds
For treatment of endometriosis or fibrocystic breast disease
Possibility of amenorrhea or irregular menstrual periods; checking with physician if regular menstruation does not occur within 60 to 90 days after discontinuation of medication
Advisability of using nonhormonal forms of contraception during therapy; not using oral contraceptives
»   Stopping medication and checking with physician if pregnancy is suspected

Side/adverse effects
Signs of potential side effects, especially edema, virilism in females, liver dysfunction, peliosis hepatis, polyneuritis, pancreatitis, carpal tunnel syndrome, hematologic disorders, Stevens-Johnson syndrome, cataracts, intracranial hypertension, bladder telangiectasia, testicular atrophy, and irregular menstrual periods

▲ For the Patient ▲

913660

ABOUT YOUR MEDICINE

Danazol (DA-na-zole) may be used for a number of different medical problems. These include treatment of:
• pain and/or infertility due to endometriosis;

- a tendency for females to develop cysts in the breasts (fibrocystic breast disease);
- hereditary angioedema, which causes swelling of the face, arms, legs, throat, windpipe, bowels, or sexual organs.

Danazol may also be used for other conditions as determined by your doctor.

If any of the information in this leaflet causes you special concern or if you want additional information about your medicine and its use, check with your doctor, nurse, or pharmacist. **Remember, keep this and all other medicines out of the reach of children and never share your medicines with others.**

BEFORE USING THIS MEDICINE

Tell your doctor, nurse, and pharmacist if you . . .

- are allergic to any medicine, either prescription or non-prescription (OTC);
- are pregnant or intend to become pregnant while using this medicine;
- are breast-feeding;
- are taking any other prescription or nonprescription (OTC) medicine, especially anticoagulants (blood thinners);
- have any other medical problems, especially diabetes mellitus (sugar diabetes); epilepsy; heart, kidney, or liver disease; or migraine headaches.

PROPER USE OF THIS MEDICINE

In order for danazol to help you, **it must be taken regularly for the full time of treatment** as ordered by your doctor.

If you miss a dose of this medicine, take it as soon as possible. Then go back to your regular dosing schedule. However, if it is almost time for your next dose, skip the missed dose and go back to your regular dosing schedule. Do not double doses.

PRECAUTIONS WHILE USING THIS MEDICINE

For patients taking danazol for endometriosis or fibrocystic breast disease:

- During the time you are taking danazol, you should use birth control methods that do not contain hormones. **If you suspect that you may have become pregnant, stop taking this medicine and check with your doctor.** Continued use may cause male-like changes in female babies.

Some people who take danazol may become more sensitive to sunlight than they are normally. **When you first begin taking this medicine, avoid too much sun and do not use a sunlamp until you see how you react to the sun. If you have a severe reaction, check with your doctor.**

POSSIBLE SIDE EFFECTS OF THIS MEDICINE
Side Effects That Should Be Reported To Your Doctor

For both males and females
    Less common—Acne or increased oiliness of skin or hair;
        muscle cramps or spasms; rapid weight gain; swelling
        of feet or lower legs; unusual tiredness or weakness

    Rare—Bleeding gums; bloating, pain, or tenderness of
        abdomen or stomach; blood in urine; changes in vision;
        chest pain; chills; cough; dark-colored urine; diarrhea;
        discharge from nipple; eye pain; fast heartbeat; fever;
        headache; hives or other skin rashes; joint pain; light-
        colored stools; loss of appetite (continuing); more fre-
        quent nosebleeds; muscle aches; nausea; pain, numb-
        ness, tingling, or burning in all fingers except the
        smallest finger; purple- or red-colored, or other spots
        on body or inside the mouth or nose; sore throat; tin-
        gling, numbness, or weakness in legs, which may move
        upward to arms, trunk or face; unusual bruising or
        bleeding; unusual tiredness, weakness, or general feel-
        ing of illness; vomiting; yellow eyes or skin

For females only
    More common—Decrease in breast size; irregular men-
        strual periods; weight gain

    Rare—Enlarged clitoris; hoarseness or deepening of voice;
        unnatural hair growth

For males only
    Rare—Decrease in size of testicles

Side Effects That Usually Do Not Require Medical Attention

These possible side effects may go away during treatment;
however, if they continue or are bothersome, check with your
doctor, nurse, or pharmacist.

For both males and females
    Less common—Flushing or redness of skin; mood or men-
        tal changes; nervousness; sweating

    Rare—Increased sensitivity of skin to sunlight

For females only
    Less common—Burning, dryness, or itching of vagina or
        vaginal bleeding

Other side effects not listed above may also occur in some
patients. If you notice any other effects, check with your
doctor, nurse, or pharmacist.

DANTROLENE   Systemic

■ For the Pharmacist ■

In providing consultation, consider emphasizing the following selected information (» = major clinical significance):

Before using this medication
» Conditions affecting use, especially:
    Other medications, especially CNS depression–producing medications and other hepatotoxic medications
    Other medical problems, especially active hepatic disease

Proper use of this medication
    Mixing contents of capsule with fruit juice or other liquid if unable to swallow capsule; drinking immediately after mixing
» Not taking more medication than the amount prescribed, to minimize risk of hepatotoxicity or other adverse effects
» Proper dosing
    Missed dose: Taking if remembered within an hour or so; not taking if not remembered within an hour; not doubling doses
» Proper storage

Precautions while using this medication
    Regular visits to physician to check progress during long-term therapy; possibility of blood tests to check for side effects
» Avoiding alcohol or other CNS depressants during therapy unless prescribed or otherwise approved by physician
» Caution if drowsiness, dizziness or lightheadedness, vision disturbances, or muscle weakness occurs

Side/adverse effects
    Signs of potential side effects, especially bloody or dark urine; confusion; constipation, severe; convulsions; allergic dermatitis; diarrhea, severe; difficult urination; hepatitis; mental depression; phlebitis; pleural effusion with pericarditis; and respiratory depression

▲ For the Patient ▲

913670

ABOUT YOUR MEDICINE

Dantrolene (DAN-troe-leen) is a medicine used to help relax certain muscles in your body. It relieves the spasms, cramping, and tightness of muscles caused by certain medical problems such as multiple sclerosis (MS), cerebral palsy, stroke, or injury to the spine. Dantrolene does not cure these problems, but it may allow other treatment, such as physical therapy, to be more helpful in improving your condition.

Dantrolene is also used to prevent or treat a medical problem called malignant hyperthermia that may occur in some people during or following surgery or anesthesia.

If any of the information in this leaflet causes you special concern or if you want additional information about your medicine and its use, check with your doctor, nurse, or pharmacist. **Remember, keep this and all other medicines out of**

the reach of children and never share your medicines with others.

BEFORE USING THIS MEDICINE

Tell your doctor, nurse, and pharmacist if you . . .

- are allergic to any medicine, either prescription or non-prescription (OTC);
- are pregnant or intend to become pregnant while using this medicine;
- are breast-feeding;
- are taking **any** other prescription or nonprescription (OTC) medicine;
- have any other medical problems, especially liver disease (or history of).

PROPER USE OF THIS MEDICINE

If you are unable to swallow the capsules, you may empty the number of capsules needed for one dose into a small amount of fruit juice or other liquid. Stir gently to mix the powder with the liquid before drinking. Drink the medicine right away. Rinse the glass with a little more liquid, and drink that also to make sure that you have taken all of the medicine.

This medicine may be taken with or without food. Take it as directed.

Take this medicine only as directed by your doctor. Do not take more of it and do not take it more often than your doctor ordered. Dantrolene may cause liver damage or other unwanted effects if too much is taken.

If you miss a dose of this medicine and remember within an hour or so of the missed dose, take it right away. Then go back to your regular dosing schedule. But if you do not remember until later, skip the missed dose and go back to your regular dosing schedule. Do not double doses.

PRECAUTIONS WHILE USING THIS MEDICINE

If you will be taking dantrolene for a long period of time (for example, for several months at a time), your doctor should check your progress at regular visits. It may be necessary to have certain blood tests to check for unwanted effects while you are taking dantrolene.

This medicine will add to the effects of alcohol and other CNS depressants (medicines that slow down the nervous system). **Check with your doctor before taking any such depressants while you are using this medicine.**

This medicine may cause dizziness or lightheadedness, drowsiness, muscle weakness, or vision problems in some people. **Make sure you know how you react to this medicine before you drive, use machines, or do other jobs that require you to be alert, well-coordinated, and able to see well.**

POSSIBLE SIDE EFFECTS OF THIS MEDICINE

Side Effects That Should Be Reported To Your Doctor Immediately

> *Less common*—Convulsions (seizures); pain, tenderness, changes in skin color, or swelling of foot or leg; shortness of breath or slow or troubled breathing

Other Side Effects That Should Be Reported To Your Doctor

> *Less common*—Bloody or dark urine; chest pain; confusion; constipation (severe); diarrhea (severe); difficult urination; mental depression; skin rash, hives, or itching; yellow eyes or skin

Side Effects That Usually Do Not Require Medical Attention

These possible side effects may go away during treatment; however, if they continue or are bothersome, check with your doctor, nurse, or pharmacist.

> *More common*—Diarrhea (mild); dizziness or lightheadedness; drowsiness; general feeling of discomfort or illness; muscle weakness; nausea or vomiting; unusual tiredness

Other side effects not listed above may also occur in some patients. If you notice any other effects, check with your doctor, nurse, or pharmacist.

DAPSONE   Systemic

■ For the Pharmacist ■

In providing consultation, consider emphasizing the following selected information (» = major clinical significance):

Before using this medication
» Conditions affecting use, especially:
    Allergy to sulfonamides
    Pregnancy—Dapsone crosses the placenta
    Breast-feeding—Dapsone is distributed into breast milk; it may cause hemolytic anemia in G6PD-deficient neonates
    Other medications, especially other hemolytics and dideoxyinosine
    Other medical problems, especially severe anemia, G6PD deficiency, or methemoglobin reductase deficiency

Proper use of this medication
» Proper dosing
    Missed dose: Taking as soon as possible; not taking if almost time for next dose; not doubling doses
» Proper storage
For leprosy
» Compliance with full course of therapy, which may take years
» Importance of not missing doses and taking at same time every day
For dermatitis herpetiformis
    Possible need for gluten-free diet
For Pneumocystis carinii pneumonia
» Compliance with full course of therapy

Precautions while using this medication
    Regular visits to physician to check progress
    Checking with physician if no improvement within 2 to 3 months (leprosy), within 1 week (PCP), or within a few days (dermatitis herpetiformis)

Side/adverse effects
    Signs of potential side effects, especially hemolytic anemia, blood dyscrasias, hypersensitivity reactions, methemoglobinemia, exfoliative dermatitis, peripheral neuropathy, hepatic damage, "sulfone syndrome," and mood and other mental changes

▲ For the Patient ▲

913681

ABOUT YOUR MEDICINE

Dapsone (DAP-sone), a sulfone, belongs to the family of medicines called anti-infectives. It is used to treat leprosy (Hansen's disease) and to help control dermatitis herpetiformis, a skin problem. When it is used to control leprosy, dapsone may be given with one or more other medicines. Dapsone may also be used for other conditions as determined by your doctor.

If any of the information in this leaflet causes you special concern or if you want additional information about your

medicine and its use, check with your doctor, nurse, or pharmacist. **Remember, keep this and all other medicines out of the reach of children and never share your medicines with others.**

BEFORE USING THIS MEDICINE
Tell your doctor, nurse, and pharmacist if you . . .
- are allergic to any medicine, either prescription or non-prescription (OTC);
- are pregnant or intend to become pregnant while using this medicine;
- are breast-feeding;
- are taking **any** other prescription or nonprescription (OTC) medicine;
- have any other medical problems, especially glucose-6-phosphate dehydrogenase (G6PD) deficiency, methemoglobin reductase deficiency, or severe anemia.

PROPER USE OF THIS MEDICINE
For patients taking this medicine for leprosy:
- To help clear up your leprosy completely or to keep it from coming back, **it is very important that you keep taking this medicine for the full time of treatment** even if you begin to feel better after a few weeks or months. You may have to take it every day for as long as 3 years or more, or for life. If you stop taking this medicine too soon, your symptoms may return.
- This medicine works best when there is a constant amount in the blood. **To help keep the amount constant, do not miss any doses. Also, it is best to take each dose at the same time every day.** If you need help in planning the best time to take your medicine, check with your doctor, nurse, or pharmacist.

For patients taking this medicine for dermatitis herpetiformis:
- Your doctor may want you to follow a gluten-free diet. If you have any questions about this, check with your doctor.

You may skip a missed dose if it does not make your symptoms come back or get worse. If your symptoms do come back or get worse, take the missed dose as soon as possible. Then go back to your regular dosing schedule.

PRECAUTIONS WHILE USING THIS MEDICINE
It is very important that your doctor check your progress at regular visits.

If your symptoms do not improve within 2 to 3 months (for leprosy) or within a few days (for dermatitis herpetiformis), or if your condition becomes worse, check with your doctor.

POSSIBLE SIDE EFFECTS OF THIS MEDICINE
Side Effects That Should Be Reported To Your Doctor Immediately

More common—Back, leg, or stomach pains; bluish fingernails, lips, or skin; fever; loss of appetite; pale skin; skin rash; unusual tiredness or weakness

Rare—Difficult breathing; itching, dryness, redness, scaling, or peeling of the skin, or loss of hair; mood or other mental changes; numbness, tingling, pain, burning, or weakness in hands or feet; sore throat; unusual bleeding or bruising; yellow eyes or skin

Other side effects not listed above may also occur in some patients. If you notice any other effects, check with your doctor, nurse, or pharmacist.

DECONGESTANTS AND ANALGESICS Systemic

*Including Phenylephrine and Acetaminophen;
Phenylpropanolamine and Acetaminophen;
Phenylpropanolamine, Acetaminophen, and Aspirin;
Phenylpropanolamine, Acetaminophen, Aspirin, and
Caffeine; Phenylpropanolamine, Acetaminophen, and
Caffeine; Phenylpropanolamine, Acetaminophen,
Salicylamide, and Caffeine; Phenylpropanolamine and
Aspirin; Pseudoephedrine and Acetaminophen;
Pseudoephedrine, Acetaminophen, and Caffeine;
Pseudoephedrine and Aspirin; Pseudoephedrine, Aspirin, and
Caffeine; Pseudoephedrine and Ibuprofen.*

■For the Pharmacist■

In providing consultation, consider emphasizing the following selected information (» = major clinical significance):

Before using this medication
» Conditions affecting use, especially:

Sensitivity to other sympathomimetic amines, salicylates or other nonsteroidal anti-inflammatory drugs

Pregnancy—Concern with high doses and long-term therapy because of salicylate effects; use of aspirin-containing combinations not recommended during third trimester; use of ibuprofen-containing combinations during second half of pregnancy not recommended because of potential adverse effect on fetal blood flow

Breast-feeding—High risk for infants from sympathomimetic amines; also, concern with high doses and chronic use because of high salicylate intake by infant

Use in children—Increased sensitivity to vasopressor and psychiatric effects of sympathomimetic amines; also, increased susceptibility to toxic effects of salicylates, especially if fever and dehydration present; possible association between aspirin usage and Reye's syndrome

Use in adolescents—Possible association between aspirin usage and Reye's syndrome

Use in the elderly—Increased susceptibility to effects of sympathomimetic amines and toxic effects of salicylates; increased risk of toxicity with ibuprofen

Other medications, especially for high blood pressure or depression, CNS depressants or stimulants, and others that may interact with acetaminophen, ibuprofen, and/or salicylates depending on specific ingredients of combination

Other medical problems, especially hypertension (for all combinations); alcoholism or hepatitis (for acetaminophen-containing combinations); hemophilia or other bleeding problems (for aspirin-containing combinations); asthma, gastritis, or peptic ulcer (with salicylate-containing combinations); clotting defects, peptic ulcer or other gastrointestinal tract disease, or stomatitis (for ibuprofen-containing combinations)

Proper use of this medication
» Importance of not taking more medication than the amount recommended

» Proper dosing
　　Missed dose: If on scheduled dosing regimen—Taking as soon as possible; not taking if almost time for next dose; not doubling doses
» Proper storage

For salicylate-containing combinations
　　Taking with food or a full glass (240 mL) of water to minimize gastrointestinal irritation
» Not taking combinations containing aspirin if a strong vinegar-like odor is present

For ibuprofen-containing combinations
　　Taking with food or antacids (a magnesium- and aluminum-containing antacid may be preferred) to reduce gastrointestinal irritation; not lying down for 15 to 30 minutes after taking

Precautions while using this medication
　　Checking with physician if symptoms persist or become worse, or if high fever is present
» Caution if taking phenylpropanolamine-containing appetite suppressants
» Possible insomnia; taking the medication a few hours before bedtime
　　Need to inform physician or dentist of use of medication if any kind of surgery (including dental surgery or emergency treatment is required)
» Caution if other medications containing acetaminophen, aspirin, or other salicylates (including diflunisal) are used
» Avoiding use of alcoholic beverages while taking these medications; alcohol consumption may increase risk of ibuprofen- or salicylate-induced gastrointestinal toxicity and acetaminophen-induced liver toxicity
» Suspected overdose: Getting emergency help at once
　　Not taking products containing aspirin for 5 days prior to any kind of surgery, unless otherwise directed by physician
　　Diabetics: Aspirin present in some combination formulations may cause false urine sugar test results with prolonged use of 8 or more 325-mg (5-grain) doses per day

For ibuprofen-containing combinations
» Caution if drowsiness or dizziness occurs

Side/adverse effects
　　Signs of potential side effects, especially allergic reactions, anemia, cardiac effects, CNS stimulation, psychotic episodes, severe dizziness, severe nervousness or restlessness (for all combinations); blood dyscrasias, hepatitis, hepatotoxicity (for acetaminophen-containing); signs of gastrointestinal irritation or bleeding (for ibuprofen- or salicylate-containing); and cutaneous adverse effects, hepatitis, renal impairment (for ibuprofen-containing)

▲ For the Patient ▲

916715

ABOUT YOUR MEDICINE

Decongestant and **analgesic** combinations are taken by mouth to relieve sinus and nasal congestion (stuffy nose) and headache of colds, allergy, and hay fever.

If any of the information in this leaflet causes you special concern or if you want additional information about your medicine and its use, check with your doctor, nurse, or pharmacist. **Remember, keep this and all other medicines out of**

the reach of children and never share your medicines with others.

BEFORE USING THIS MEDICINE

If you are taking this medicine without a prescription, carefully read and follow any precautions on the label. You should be especially careful if you . . .

- are allergic to any medicine, either prescription or nonprescription (OTC);
- are pregnant, intend to become pregnant, or are breast-feeding;
- are taking **any** other prescription or nonprescription (OTC) medicine;
- have **any** other medical problems.

If you have any questions, check with your doctor, nurse, or pharmacist.

PROPER USE OF THIS MEDICINE

For aspirin or salicylate-containing products:

- Use of aspirin in children or teenagers with fever due to a virus infection (especially flu or chickenpox) has been associated with a serious illness called Reye's syndrome. **Do not give medicines containing aspirin or other salicylates to a child or a teenager with symptoms of flu or chickenpox** unless you have first discussed this with your child's doctor.

Take this medicine only as directed. Do not take more of it or take it more often than recommended on the label, unless otherwise directed by your doctor.

If this medicine irritates your stomach, you may take it with food or a glass of water or milk to lessen the irritation.

If you must take this medicine regularly and you miss a dose, take it as soon as possible. However, if it is almost time for your next dose, skip the missed dose and go back to your regular dosing schedule. Do not double doses.

PRECAUTIONS WHILE USING THIS MEDICINE

Check with your doctor if your symptoms do not improve or become worse, or if you have a high fever.

This medicine may cause some people to become nervous or restless or to have trouble in sleeping. If you have trouble in sleeping, **take the last dose of this medicine for each day a few hours before bedtime**.

Do not drink alcoholic beverages while taking this medicine.

If you think that you or anyone else may have taken an overdose of this medicine, get emergency help at once.

For patients taking **ibuprofen-containing medicine:**

- This medicine may cause some people to become confused, drowsy, dizzy, lightheaded, or less alert than they are normally. It may also cause blurred vision or other vision problems in some people. **Make sure you know how you react to this medicine before you drive, use machines, or do other jobs that require you to be alert and clearheaded.**

POSSIBLE SIDE EFFECTS OF THIS MEDICINE

Side Effects That Should Be Reported To Your Doctor

> *More common*—Nausea, vomiting, or stomach pain (mild—for combinations containing aspirin or ibuprofen)

> *Less common or rare*—Bloody, or black, tarry stools; bloody or cloudy urine; blurred vision or any changes in vision or eyes; changes in facial skin color; changes in hearing; difficult or painful urination; fever; headache (severe), with fever and stiff neck; increased blood pressure; muscle cramps or pain; skin rash, hives, or itching; sores, ulcers, or white spots on lips or in mouth; swelling of face, fingers, feet, or lower legs; swollen or painful glands; unexplained sore throat and fever; unusual bleeding or bruising; unusual tiredness or weakness; vomiting of blood or material that looks like coffee grounds; weight gain (unusual); yellow eyes or skin

Side Effects That Usually Do Not Require Medical Attention

These possible side effects may go away during treatment; however, if they continue or are bothersome, check with your doctor, nurse, or pharmacist.

> *More common*—Heartburn or indigestion (for medicines containing salicylates or ibuprofen); nervousness or restlessness

Other side effects not listed above may also occur in some patients. If you notice any other effects, check with your doctor, nurse, or pharmacist.

DIDANOSINE   Systemic

■ For the Pharmacist ■

In providing consultation, consider emphasizing the following selected information (» = major clinical significance):

Before using this medication
» Conditions affecting use, especially:
   Use in children—May cause retinal depigmentation, which is more likely to occur in children receiving doses above 300 mg/m^2 per day
   Other medications, especially other drugs associated with pancreatitis and peripheral neuropathy, dapsone or medications that require an acidic environment for absorption, tetracyclines, or fluoroquinolone antibiotics
   Other medical problems, especially alcoholism, hypertriglyceridemia, pancreatitis or a history of pancreatitis, conditions requiring sodium-restriction, or peripheral neuropathy

Proper use of this medication
» Importance of not taking more medication than prescribed; importance of not discontinuing medication without checking with physician; discontinuing medication and calling physician at first signs and symptoms of pancreatitis
» Importance of not missing doses and of taking at evenly spaced times
» Proper administration:
   For buffered didanosine for oral solution
   Preparing by opening the packet and dissolving its contents in 1/2 glass (4 ounces) of water. The powder should not be mixed with fruit juice or other acid-containing liquid
   Stirring the mixture for approximately 2 to 3 minutes until the powder is completely dissolved
   Swallowing the entire solution immediately
   For tablets
   Patients older than 1 year of age must take 2 tablets at each dose to provide adequate buffering and to prevent gastric acid degradation of didanosine
   Children under 1 year of age should receive a 1-tablet dose. The recommended dose for children is based on body surface area and, for adults, on body weight
   Thoroughly chewing, manually crushing, or dispersing in at least 1 ounce of water prior to consumption. Because the tablets are hard, they may be difficult to chew for some patients; manually crushing or dispersing the tablets may be preferable. To disperse tablets, 2 tablets should be added to at least 1 ounce of drinking water. The mixture should be stirred until a uniform dispersion forms and consumed immediately
» Proper dosing
   Missed dose: Taking as soon as possible; not taking if almost time for next dose; not doubling doses
» Proper storage

Precautions while using this medication
» Regular visits to physician for blood tests
» Importance of not taking other medications concurrently without checking with physician

» Using a condom to help prevent transmission of the AIDS virus to others; not sharing needles or injectable equipment with anyone

Side/adverse effects

Signs of potential side effects, especially peripheral neuropathy, pancreatitis, cardiomyopathy, hematologic toxicities, hepatitis, hypersensitivity, retinal depigmentation, and seizures

---

▲ For the Patient ▲

918153

ABOUT YOUR MEDICINE

Didanosine (di-DAN-oe-seen), also called ddI, is used to treat patients who are infected with the human immunodeficiency virus (HIV). HIV is the virus that causes acquired immune deficiency syndrome (AIDS). HIV attacks the immune system. This medicine appears to slow down the destruction of the immune system caused by HIV. This may help slow down the progress of HIV disease and the serious infections that occur with AIDS. However, didanosine will not cure or prevent HIV infection, and it will not keep you from spreading the virus to other people. Patients who are taking this medicine may continue to have the problems usually related to AIDS or HIV disease.

If any of the information in this leaflet causes you special concern or if you want additional information about your medicine and its use, check with your doctor, nurse, or pharmacist. **Remember, keep this and all other medicines out of the reach of children and never share your medicines with others.**

BEFORE USING THIS MEDICINE

Tell your doctor, nurse, and pharmacist if you . . .
- are allergic to any medicine, either prescription or non-prescription (OTC);
- are pregnant or intend to become pregnant while using this medicine;
- are breast-feeding;
- are taking **any** other prescription or nonprescription (OTC) medicine;
- have any other medical problems, especially alcoholism, edema, heart disease, high blood pressure, kidney disease, liver disease, pancreatitis, or peripheral neuropathy.

PROPER USE OF THIS MEDICINE

Take this medicine exactly as directed by your doctor. Do not take more of it, do not take it more often, and do not take it for a longer time than your doctor ordered. Also, do not stop taking this medicine without checking with your doctor first. However, stop taking didanosine and call your doctor right away if you have severe nausea, vomiting, and stomach pain. **Otherwise, keep taking didanosine for the full time of treatment,** even if you begin to feel better.

There are different instructions for preparing didanosine, depending on the dosage form you are taking. Make sure you have received and understand these instructions. If you have any questions about this, check with your doctor or pharmacist.

Didanosine should be taken on an empty stomach since food may decrease the absorption in the stomach and keep the medicine from working properly. Didanosine should be taken at least 2 hours before or 2 hours after you eat.

This medicine works best when there is a constant amount in the blood. **To help keep the amount constant, do not miss any doses.** If you need help in planning the best times to take your medicine, check with your doctor, nurse, or pharmacist.

If you do miss a dose of this medicine, take it as soon as possible. However, if it is almost time for your next dose, skip the missed dose and go back to your regular dosing schedule. Do not double doses.

Only take medicine that your doctor has prescribed specifically for you. Do not share your medicine with others.

PRECAUTIONS WHILE USING THIS MEDICINE

It is very important that your doctor check your progress at regular visits.

Do not take any other medicines without checking with your doctor first.

HIV is spread to other people through infected body fluids, such as blood, vaginal fluid, or semen. **If you are infected with HIV, it is best not to have sex** or do anything that involves an exchange of body fluids with other people.

If you do have sex, always wear (or have your partner wear) a condom ("rubber"). Only use condoms made of latex, and **use them every time you have vaginal, anal, or oral sex.** Using a spermicide (such as nonoxynol-9) may also help keep you from spreading HIV, as long as the spermicide does not irritate the vagina, rectum, or mouth. Do not use oil-based jelly, cold cream, baby oil, or shortening as a lubricant—these products can cause the condom (rubber) to break. Lubricants without oil, such as *K-Y Jelly,* are recommended. **If you inject drugs,** get help to stop. **Do not share needles with anyone.** If you have any questions about this, check with your doctor, nurse, or pharmacist.

POSSIBLE SIDE EFFECTS OF THIS MEDICINE
Side Effects That Should Be Reported To Your Doctor Immediately

   Less common—Nausea and vomiting; stomach pain; tingling, burning, numbness, and pain in the hands or feet

   Rare—Convulsions (seizures); fever and chills; shortness of breath; skin rash and itching; sore throat; swelling of feet or lower legs; unusual bleeding and bruising; unusual tiredness and weakness; yellow eyes and skin

Side Effects That Usually Do Not Require Medical Attention

These possible side effects may go away during treatment; however, if they continue or are bothersome, check with your doctor, nurse, or pharmacist.

More common—Anxiety; diarrhea; difficulty in sleeping; dryness of mouth; headache; irritability; restlessness

Other side effects not listed above may also occur in some patients. If you notice any other effects, check with your doctor, nurse, or pharmacist.

DIFENOXIN AND ATROPINE   Systemic

■ For the Pharmacist ■

In providing consultation, consider emphasizing the following selected information (» = major clinical significance):

Before using this medication
» Conditions affecting use, especially:
   Sensitivity to atropine or difenoxin
   Pregnancy—Studies in rats show increased delivery time and stillbirth at doses 20 times maximum human dose
   Breast-feeding—Difenoxin and atropine distributed into breast milk; potential for serious adverse effects in nursing infant
   Use in children—Not recommended for use in children; increased susceptibility to toxic effects of atropine and respiratory depressant effects of difenoxin; risk of dehydration
   Use in the elderly—Increased risk of respiratory depression; risk of dehydration
   Other medications, especially other anticholinergics, CNS depressants, MAO inhibitors, or naltrexone
   Other medical problems, especially acute dysentery; dehydration; diarrhea caused by antibiotics or poisoning; gastrointestinal tract obstruction; hepatic function impairment or jaundice; or severe colitis

Proper use of this medication
   Taking with food or meals if gastric irritation occurs
» Importance of not taking more medication than the amount prescribed because of habit-forming potential
» Importance of maintaining adequate hydration and proper diet
» Proper dosing
   Missed dose: If on scheduled dosing regimen—Taking as soon as possible; not taking if almost time for next dose; not doubling doses
» Proper storage

Precautions while using this medication
   Regular visits to physician to check progress during prolonged therapy
» Consulting physician if diarrhea is not controlled within 48 hours and/or fever develops
» Avoiding use of alcohol or other CNS depressants during therapy
» Suspected overdose: Getting emergency help at once
   Need to inform physician or dentist of use of medication if any kind of surgery (including dental surgery) or emergency treatment is required
» Caution if dizziness or drowsiness occurs

Side/adverse effects
   Signs of potential side effects, especially paralytic ileus or toxic megacolon

▲ For the Patient ▲

913739

ABOUT YOUR MEDICINE

Difenoxin (dye-fen-OX-in) and **atropine** (A-troe-peen) is a combination medicine used along with other measures to treat severe diarrhea.

Do not give antidiarrheals to young children (under 3 years of age) without first checking with their doctor. In older children and elderly persons with diarrhea, antidiarrheals may be used, but it is also very important that liquids be taken to replace the fluids lost by the body. If you have any questions about this, check with your doctor, nurse, or pharmacist.

If any of the information in this leaflet causes you special concern or if you want additional information about your medicine and its use, check with your doctor, nurse, or pharmacist. **Remember, keep this and all other medicines out of the reach of children and never share your medicines with others.**

BEFORE USING THIS MEDICINE

Tell your doctor, nurse, and pharmacist if you . . .
- are allergic to any medicine, either prescription or non-prescription (OTC);
- are pregnant or intend to become pregnant while using this medicine;
- are breast-feeding;
- are taking any other prescription or nonprescription (OTC) medicine, especially antibiotics, other medicine for abdominal or stomach spasms or cramps, other CNS depressants, or naltrexone;
- have any other medical problems, especially colitis (severe), dysentery, or liver disease.

PROPER USE OF THIS MEDICINE

Take this medicine only as directed by your doctor. Do not take more of it, do not take it more often, and do not take it for a longer time than ordered.

Importance of diet and fluid intake:
- **In addition to using medicine for diarrhea, it is very important that you replace the fluid lost by the body and follow a proper diet.** For the first 24 hours, you should drink plenty of clear liquids, such as ginger ale, decaffeinated cola, decaffeinated tea, broth, and gelatin. During the next 24 hours you may eat bland foods, such as cooked cereals, bread, crackers, and applesauce.
- Check with your doctor as soon as possible if any of the following signs of too much fluid loss occur: decreased urination; dizziness and lightheadedness; dryness of mouth; increased thirst; wrinkled skin.

If you must take this medicine regularly and you miss a dose, take it as soon as possible. However, if it is almost time for your next dose, skip the missed dose and go back to your regular dosing schedule. Do not double doses.

PRECAUTIONS WHILE USING THIS MEDICINE
Check with your doctor if your diarrhea does not stop after two days or if you develop a fever.

This medicine will add to the effects of alcohol and other CNS depressants (medicines that slow down the nervous system). **Check with your doctor before taking any such depressants while you are taking this medicine.**

This medicine may cause some people to become dizzy, drowsy, or less alert than they are normally. Even if taken at bedtime, it may cause some people to feel drowsy or less alert on arising. **Make sure you know how you react to this medicine before you drive, use machines, or do other jobs that require you to be alert.**

If you think you or someone else in your home may have taken an overdose, get emergency help at once. Taking an overdose of this medicine may lead to unconsciousness and possibly death. Signs of overdose include severe drowsiness; shortness of breath or troubled breathing; unusually fast heartbeat; and unusual warmth, dryness, and flushing of skin.

Before having any kind of surgery or dental or emergency treatment, tell the physician or dentist in charge that you are using this medicine.

POSSIBLE SIDE EFFECTS OF THIS MEDICINE
Side Effects That Should Be Reported To Your Doctor Immediately

Check with your doctor immediately if any of the following side effects are severe and occur suddenly, since they may indicate a more severe and dangerous problem with your bowels:

> Bloating; constipation; loss of appetite; stomach pain (severe) with nausea and vomiting

Side Effects That Usually Do Not Require Medical Attention

These possible side effects may go away during treatment; however, if they continue or are bothersome, check with your doctor, nurse, or pharmacist.

> *Less common or rare*—Blurred vision; confusion; difficult urination; dizziness or drowsiness; dry skin and mouth; fever; headache; trouble in sleeping; unusual tiredness or weakness

Other side effects not listed above may also occur in some patients. If you notice any other effects, check with your doctor, nurse, or pharmacist.

After you stop using this medicine, your body may need time to adjust. The length of time this takes depends on the amount of medicine you were using and how long you used it. During this time check with your doctor if you notice increased sweating; muscle cramps; nausea or vomiting; shivering or trembling; or stomach cramps.

DIGITALIS GLYCOSIDES Systemic

Including Digitoxin; Digoxin.

■ For the Pharmacist ■

In providing consultation, consider emphasizing the following selected information (» = major clinical significance):

Before using this medication
» Conditions affecting use, especially:

Sensitivity to the digitalis glycoside prescribed

Pregnancy—Cross placenta

Use in children—Infant responses vary; careful dosage adjustment required

Use in the elderly—Increased sensitivity to effects

Other medications, especially potassium-depleting diuretics or other hypokalemia-causing medications, amiodarone, other antiarrhythmics, sympathomimetics, antidiarrheal adsorbents, calcium channel blocking agents, cholestyramine, colestipol, potassium-containing medications or supplements, quinidine, spironolactone, or sucralfate

Other medical problems, especially severe pulmonary disease, conduction disturbance, ventricular arrhythmias, ischemic heart disease, recent myocardial infarction, or myocarditis

Proper use of this medication
» Compliance with therapy; taking exactly as directed, not taking more or less

Proper administration of elixir: Taking orally; special dropper to be used for accurate measuring

Taking medication at the same time each day to help increase compliance

Checking apical pulse as directed (checking with physician if less than 60 beats per minute)

» Proper dosing

Missed dose: Taking as soon as remembered if within 12 hours of scheduled dose; not taking if remembered later; not doubling doses; checking with doctor if dose missed for 2 days or more

» Proper storage

Precautions while using this medication
Regular visits to physician to check progress

» Checking with physician before discontinuing medication

» Keeping medication out of reach of children

» Reporting to physician any nausea, vomiting, diarrhea, loss of appetite, or extremely slow pulse as possible signs of overdose

» Caution if medical or dental surgery or emergency treatment is required

Carrying medical identification card

» Avoiding other medications unless prescribed by physician

Caution in using medications of similar appearance

Side/adverse effects
Signs of potential side effects, especially allergic reaction, and signs and symptoms of overdose

▲ For the Patient ▲

912248

ABOUT YOUR MEDICINE

Digitalis (di-ji-TAL-iss) **medicines** are used to improve the strength and efficiency of the heart or to control the rate and rhythm of the heartbeat. This leads to better blood circulation and reduced swelling of hands and ankles in patients with heart problems.

If any of the information in this leaflet causes you special concern or if you want additional information about your medicine and its use, check with your doctor, nurse, or pharmacist. **Remember, keep this and all other medicines out of the reach of children and never share your medicines with others.**

BEFORE USING THIS MEDICINE

Tell your doctor, nurse, and pharmacist if you . . .
- are allergic to any medicine, either prescription or nonprescription (OTC);
- are pregnant or intend to become pregnant while using this medicine;
- are breast-feeding;
- are taking any other prescription or nonprescription (OTC) medicine, especially any other heart medicines, calcium channel blockers, cholestyramine, colestipol, cortisone-like medicines, diarrhea medicine, diuretics (water pills), ephedrine, epinephrine, medicine for colds or sinus, potassium-containing medicines or supplements, propafenone, quinidine, reducing or diet medicine, or sucralfate;
- have any other medical problems, especially heart disease, heart rhythm problems, severe lung disease, or if you have had a recent heart attack.

PROPER USE OF THIS MEDICINE

To keep your heart working properly, **take this medicine exactly as directed even though you may feel well.** Do not miss taking any of the doses and do not take more medicine than ordered.

Ask your doctor about checking your pulse rate. Then, while you are taking this medicine, check your pulse regularly. If it is much slower, or faster, than usual (or less than 60 beats per minute), or if it changes in rhythm or force, check with your doctor. Such changes may mean that side effects are developing.

After you begin taking digitalis medicine, your doctor may sometimes check your blood level of digitalis medicine to find out if your dose needs to be changed. **Do not change your dose** unless your doctor tells you to do so.

If you miss a dose of this medicine, and you remember it within 12 hours, take it as soon as you remember. However, if you do not remember until later, do not take the missed dose at all and do not double the next one. Instead, go back to your regular dosing schedule. If you have any questions about this or if you miss doses for 2 or more days in a row, check with your doctor.

PRECAUTIONS WHILE USING THIS MEDICINE

Do not suddenly stop taking this medicine without first checking with your doctor.

Watch for signs of overdose (too much medicine) while you are taking digitalis medicine. The amount of medicine needed to help most people is very close to the amount that could cause serious problems from overdose. Follow directions carefully and watch for the early warning signs of overdose.

Before having any kind of surgery or dental or emergency treatment, tell the physician or dentist in charge that you are using this medicine.

Do not take any other medicine unless ordered by your doctor. Many nonprescription medicines contain ingredients which may interfere with digitalis medicines or which may make your condition worse. They include antacids; asthma remedies; cold, cough, or sinus preparations; laxatives; medicine for diarrhea; and reducing or diet medicines.

POSSIBLE SIDE EFFECTS OF THIS MEDICINE

Side Effects That Should Be Reported To Your Doctor

   Rare—Skin rash or hives

   Possible signs of overdose (in the order in which they may occur)—Loss of appetite; nausea or vomiting; lower stomach pain; diarrhea; unusual tiredness or weakness (extreme); slow or uneven heartbeat (may be fast in children); blurred vision or "yellow, green, or white vision" (a yellow, green, or white halo seen around objects); drowsiness; confusion or mental depression; headache; fainting

Other side effects not listed above may also occur in some patients. If you notice any other effects, check with your doctor, nurse, or pharmacist.

DIPHENIDOL   Systemic

■ For the Pharmacist ■

In providing consultation, consider emphasizing the following selected information (» = major clinical significance):

Before using this medication
» Conditions affecting use, especially:
  Sensitivity to diphenidol
  Use in children—Not recommended for prophylaxis or treatment of nausea and vomiting in children weighing less than 22.8 kg
  Other medications, especially CNS depressants
  Other medical problems, especially anuria, hypotension, renal function impairment

Proper use of this medication
  Taking with food, water, or milk to minimize gastric irritation
» Importance of not taking more medication than the amount prescribed
» Proper dosing
  Missed dose: If on a regular dosing schedule—using as soon as possible; if almost time for next dose, not using at all; not doubling doses
» Proper storage

Precautions while using this medication
» Avoiding use of alcohol or other CNS depressants
» Caution if drowsiness or blurred vision occurs

Side/adverse effects
  Signs of potential side effects, especially confusion and hallucinations

▲ For the Patient ▲

913761

ABOUT YOUR MEDICINE

Diphenidol (dye-FEN-i-dole) is used to relieve or prevent nausea, vomiting, and dizziness caused by certain medical problems.

If any of the information in this leaflet causes you special concern or if you want additional information about your medicine and its use, check with your doctor, nurse, or pharmacist. **Remember, keep this and all other medicines out of the reach of children and never share your medicines with others.**

BEFORE USING THIS MEDICINE

Tell your doctor, nurse, and pharmacist if you . . .
  • are allergic to any medicine, either prescription or non-prescription (OTC);
  • are pregnant or intend to become pregnant while using this medicine;
  • are breast-feeding;

- are taking any other prescription or nonprescription (OTC) medicine, especially CNS depressants;
- have any other medical problems, especially kidney disease, or low blood pressure.

PROPER USE OF THIS MEDICINE

If you are taking diphenidol to prevent nausea and vomiting, it may be taken with food or a glass of water or milk to lessen stomach irritation, unless otherwise directed by your doctor. However, if you are already suffering from nausea and vomiting, it is best to keep the stomach empty, and this medicine should be taken only with a small amount of water.

Take this medicine only as directed. Do not take more of it and do not take it more often than directed by your doctor. To do so may increase the chance of side effects.

If you must take this medicine regularly and you miss a dose, take the missed dose as soon as possible. However, if it is almost time for your next dose, skip the missed dose and go back to your regular dosing schedule. Do not double doses.

PRECAUTIONS WHILE USING THIS MEDICINE

This medicine will add to the effects of alcohol and other CNS depressants (medicines that slow down the nervous system). **Check with your doctor before taking any such depressants while you are using this medicine.**

This medicine may cause some people to have blurred vision or to become drowsy or less alert than they are normally. **Make sure you know how you react to this medicine before you drive, use machines, or do other jobs that require you to be alert.**

POSSIBLE SIDE EFFECTS OF THIS MEDICINE

Side Effects That Should Be Reported To Your Doctor

   Rare—Confusion; hallucinations

Side Effects That Usually Do Not Require Medical Attention

These possible side effects may go away during treatment; however, if they continue or are bothersome, check with your doctor, nurse, or pharmacist.

   More common—Drowsiness

   Less common or rare—Blurred vision; dizziness; dryness of mouth; headache; heartburn; nervousness, restlessness, or trouble in sleeping; skin rash; stomach upset or pain; unusual tiredness or weakness

Other side effects not listed above may also occur in some patients. If you notice any other effects, check with your doctor, nurse, or pharmacist.

DIPHENOXYLATE AND
ATROPINE   Systemic

■ For the Pharmacist ■

In providing consultation, consider emphasizing the following selected information (» = major clinical significance):

Before using this medication
» Conditions affecting use, especially:
    Sensitivity to atropine or diphenoxylate
    Pregnancy—Studies in rats show decreased fertility and decreased maternal weight gain
    Breast-feeding—Diphenoxylate and atropine distributed into breast milk; potential for serious adverse effects in nursing infant
    Use in children—Not recommended for use in children; increased susceptibility to toxic effects of atropine and respiratory depressant effects of diphenoxylate; risk of dehydration
    Use in the elderly—Increased risk of respiratory depression, anticholinergic effects, and confusion; risk of dehydration
    Other medications, especially other anticholinergics, CNS depressants, MAO inhibitors, or naltrexone
    Other medical problems, especially acute dysentery; dehydration; diarrhea caused by antibiotics or poisoning; gastrointestinal tract obstruction; hepatic function impairment or jaundice; or severe colitis

Proper use of this medication
    Taking with food or meals if gastric irritation occurs
» Importance of not taking more medication than the amount prescribed because of habit-forming potential
» Importance of maintaining adequate hydration and proper diet
» Proper dosing
    Missed dose: If on a scheduled dosing regimen—Taking as soon as possible; not taking if almost time for next dose; not doubling doses
» Proper storage
For liquid dosage form
    Proper administration technique: Measuring amount with dropper and taking by mouth

Precautions while using this medication
    Regular visits to physician to check progress during prolonged therapy
» Consulting physician if diarrhea is not controlled within 48 hours and/or fever develops
» Avoiding use of alcohol or other CNS depressants during therapy
» Suspected overdose: Getting emergency help at once
    Need to inform physician or dentist of use of medication if any kind of surgery (including dental surgery) or emergency treatment is required
» Caution if dizziness or drowsiness occurs

Side/adverse effects
    Signs of potential side effects, especially paralytic ileus or toxic megacolon

▲ For the Patient ▲

912259

ABOUT YOUR MEDICINE

Diphenoxylate (dye-fen-OX-i-late) and **atropine** (AT-troepeen) is a combination medicine used along with other measures to treat severe diarrhea.

Do not give antidiarrheals to young children (under 3 years of age) without first checking with their doctor. In older children and elderly persons with diarrhea, antidiarrheals may be used, but it is also very important that liquids be taken to replace the fluids lost by the body. If you have any questions about this, check with your doctor, nurse, or pharmacist.

If any of the information in this leaflet causes you special concern or if you want additional information about your medicine and its use, check with your doctor, nurse, or pharmacist. **Remember, keep this and all other medicines out of the reach of children and never share your medicines with others.**

BEFORE USING THIS MEDICINE

Tell your doctor, nurse, and pharmacist if you . . .
- are allergic to any medicine, either prescription or non-prescription (OTC);
- are pregnant or intend to become pregnant while using this medicine;
- are breast-feeding;
- are taking any other prescription or nonprescription (OTC) medicine, especially antibiotics, other CNS depressants, other medicine for abdominal or stomach spasms or cramps, monoamine oxidase (MAO) inhibitors, naltrexone, or tricyclic antidepressants;
- have any other medical problems, especially colitis (severe), dysentery, or liver disease.

PROPER USE OF THIS MEDICINE

Take diphenoxylate and atropine only as directed. Do not take more of it, do not take it more often, and do not take it for a longer time than ordered.

Importance of diet and fluid intake:
- **In addition to using medicine for diarrhea, it is very important that you replace the fluid lost by the body and follow a proper diet.** For the first 24 hours, you should drink plenty of clear liquids, such as ginger ale, decaffeinated cola, decaffeinated tea, broth, and gelatin. During the next 24 hours you may eat bland foods, such as cooked cereals, bread, crackers, and applesauce.
- Check with your doctor as soon as possible if any of the following signs of too much fluid loss occur: decreased urination; dizziness and lightheadedness; dryness of mouth; increased thirst; wrinkled skin.

Keep this medicine out of the reach of children since overdose is especially dangerous in children.

If you must take this medicine regularly and you miss a dose, take it as soon as possible. However, if it is almost time for your next dose, skip the missed dose and go back to your regular dosing schedule. Do not double doses.

PRECAUTIONS WHILE USING THIS MEDICINE
Check with your doctor if your diarrhea does not stop after two days or if you develop a fever.

This medicine will add to the effects of alcohol and other CNS depressants (medicines that slow down the nervous system). **Check with your doctor before taking any such depressants while you are using this medicine.**

Since this medicine may cause some people to become drowsy, **make sure you know how you react to it before you drive, use machines, or do other jobs that require you to be alert.**

If you think you or someone in your household may have taken an overdose, get emergency help at once. Some signs of overdose are severe drowsiness; shortness of breath or troubled breathing; unusually fast heartbeat; and unusual warmth, dryness, and flushing of skin.

POSSIBLE SIDE EFFECTS OF THIS MEDICINE
Side Effects That Should Be Reported To Your Doctor Immediately

Check with your doctor immediately if any of the following side effects are severe and occur suddenly, since they may be signs of a more severe and dangerous problem with your bowels: bloating; constipation; loss of appetite; stomach pain (severe) with nausea and vomiting.

Side Effects That Usually Do Not Require Medical Attention

These possible side effects may go away during treatment; however, if they continue or are bothersome, check with your doctor, nurse, or pharmacist.

> *Less common or rare*—Blurred vision; difficult urination; dizziness or drowsiness; dry skin and mouth; fever; headache; mental depression; numbness of hands or feet; skin rash or itching; swelling of the gums

Other side effects not listed above may also occur in some patients. If you notice any other effects, check with your doctor, nurse, or pharmacist.

After you stop using this medicine, your body may need time to adjust. The length of time this takes depends on the amount of medicine you were using and how long you used it. **During this time check with your doctor** if you notice muscle cramps, nausea and vomiting, shivering or trembling, stomach cramps, or increased sweating.

DIPIVEFRIN   Ophthalmic

■ For the Pharmacist ■

In providing consultation, consider emphasizing the following selected information (》 = major clinical significance):

Before using this medication
》 Conditions affecting use, especially:
    Sensitivity to dipivefrin or epinephrine
    Other medical problems, especially predisposition to angle-closure glaucoma

Proper use of this medication
》 Importance of not using more medication than the amount prescribed
    Proper administration technique
    Washing hands immediately after applying eye drops
    Preventing contamination: Not touching applicator tip to any surface; keeping container tightly closed
》 Proper dosing
    Missed dose: Applying as soon as possible; if almost time for next dose, skipping missed dose and going back to regular dosing schedule; not doubling doses
》 Proper storage

Precautions while using this medication
    Regular visits to physician to check eye pressure during therapy

Side/adverse effects
    Signs of potential side effects, especially fast or irregular heartbeat or increase in blood pressure

▲ For the Patient ▲

913080

GLAUCOMA EYE MEDICINE—EPINEPHRINE-TYPE: *Including Dipivefrin; Epinephrine; Epinephryl Borate.*

ABOUT YOUR MEDICINE

Epinephrine-type (ep-i-NEF-rin) **glaucoma eye medicines** are used in the eye to treat certain types of glaucoma. Epinephrine and epinephryl borate may also be used in eye surgery.

If any of the information in this leaflet causes you special concern or if you want additional information about your medicine and its use, check with your doctor, nurse, or pharmacist. **Remember, keep this and all other medicines out of the reach of children and never share your medicines with others.**

BEFORE USING THIS MEDICINE
Tell your doctor, nurse, and pharmacist if you . . .
- are allergic to any medicine, either prescription or nonprescription (OTC);

- are pregnant or intend to become pregnant while using this medicine;
- are breast-feeding;
- are taking any other prescription or nonprescription (OTC) medicine;
- have any other medical problems, especially heart or blood vessel disease, or other eye disease.

PROPER USE OF THIS MEDICINE

Use this medicine only as directed. Do not use more of it and do not use it more often than your doctor ordered. To do so may increase the chance of too much medicine being absorbed into the body and the chance of side effects.

To use:
- First, wash your hands. Tilt the head back and, pressing your finger gently on the skin just beneath the lower eyelid, pull the lower eyelid away from the eye to make a space. Drop the medicine into this space. Let go of the eyelid and gently close the eyes. Do not blink. Keep the eyes closed and apply pressure to the inner corner of the eye with your finger for 1 or 2 minutes to allow the medicine to be absorbed by the eye.
- Immediately after using the eye drops, wash your hands to remove any medicine that may be on them.
- To keep the medicine as germ-free as possible, do not touch the applicator tip to any surface (including the eye) and keep the container tightly closed.

For patients using dipivefrin with the compliance cap (C Cap):
- Before using the eye drops for the first time, make sure the number 1 or the correct day of the week appears in the window of the cap.
- Remove the cap and use the eye drops as directed.
- Replace the cap. Holding the cap between your thumb and forefinger, rotate the bottle until the cap clicks to the next position. This will tell you your next dose.
- After every dose, rotate the bottle until the cap clicks to the position that tells you your next dose.

For patients using epinephrine ophthalmic solution:
- Do not use if the solution turns pinkish or brownish in color, or if it becomes cloudy.

For patients using epinephryl borate ophthalmic solution:
- The color of this solution may vary from colorless to amber yellow. Do not use if the solution turns dark brown or becomes cloudy.

If you miss a dose of this medicine, apply the missed dose as soon as possible. However, if it is almost time for your next dose, skip the missed dose and go back to your regular dosing schedule. Do not double doses.

PRECAUTIONS WHILE USING THIS MEDICINE

Your doctor should check your eye pressure at regular visits.

Dipivefrin may cause blurred vision or other vision problems for a short time after each dose is applied. If any of these occur, **do not drive, use machines, or do other jobs that require you to see well.**

POSSIBLE SIDE EFFECTS OF THIS MEDICINE
Side Effects That Should Be Reported To Your Doctor

> *Less common*—Blurred or decreased vision

> *Possible signs of too much medicine being absorbed into the body*—Fast, irregular, or pounding heartbeat; feeling faint; increase in blood pressure; increased sweating; paleness; trembling

Side Effects That Usually Do Not Require Medical Attention

These possible side effects may go away during treatment; however, if they continue or are bothersome, check with your doctor, nurse, or pharmacist.

> *More common*—Headache or browache; stinging, burning, redness, or other eye irritation; watering of eyes

> *Less common*—Eye pain or ache; increased sensitivity of eyes to light

Other side effects not listed above may also occur in some patients. If you notice any other effects, check with your doctor, nurse, or pharmacist.

DIPYRIDAMOLE Systemic

Including Dipyridamole (Diagnostic—Oral); Dipyridamole (Therapeutic—Oral).

■ For the Pharmacist ■

In providing consultation, consider emphasizing the following selected information (» = major clinical significance):

Before using this medication
» Conditions affecting use, especially:
Sensitivity to dipyridamole
Other medications, especially other platelet aggregation inhibitors, those cephalosporins that may cause hypoprothrombinemia, plicamycin, and valproic acid, and, for myocardial perfusion studies, caffeine and xanthine bronchodilators
Other medical problems, especially asthma (or history of)—for intravenous use in myocardial perfusion studies

Proper use of this medication
» Importance of taking at evenly spaced times
Taking medication with water at least 1 hour before or 2 hours after meals for faster absorption; may be taken with meals or milk if gastrointestinal irritation occurs
» Proper dosing
Missed dose: Taking as soon as possible unless next scheduled dose is within 4 hours; returning to regular dosing schedule; not doubling doses
» Proper storage

Precautions while using this medication
Possibility that concurrent use with an anticoagulant or with aspirin may increase the risk of bleeding
» Not taking aspirin concurrently unless specifically prescribed for concurrent use
» If taking aspirin concurrently, taking only the amount of aspirin prescribed; checking with physician about proper medication to use for relief of pain, fever
If taking aspirin concurrently, need for regular visits to physician to check progress during therapy
» Informing all physicians and dentists of use of dipyridamole and whether taking concurrently with an anticoagulant or aspirin
» Caution when getting up suddenly from lying or sitting position

Side/adverse effects
Signs of potential side effects, especially angina pectoris and, for diagnostic use only, bronchospasm, dyspnea, and migraine

▲ For the Patient ▲

918277

DIPYRIDAMOLE (Diagnostic—Oral)

ABOUT YOUR MEDICINE

Dipyridamole (dye-peer-ID-a-mole) is used as part of a medical test that shows how well blood is flowing to your heart. The test can show your doctor whether any of the blood vessels that bring blood to the heart are blocked or in danger of becoming blocked. Your doctor can then decide on the best treatment for you. Exercise (for example, walking on a treadmill) is usually used to give your doctor this information. Dipyridamole is used instead of exercise for people who are not able to exercise at all, or cannot exercise hard enough. Dipyridamole may also be used for other conditions as determined by your doctor. If you need information about other uses of dipyridamole, check with your doctor.

If any of the information in this leaflet causes you special concern or if you want additional information about your medicine and its use, check with your doctor, nurse, or pharmacist.

BEFORE HAVING THIS TEST

Tell your doctor, nurse, and pharmacist if you . . .
- are allergic to any medicine, either prescription or non-prescription (OTC);
- are pregnant;
- are breast-feeding;
- are taking any other prescription or nonprescription (OTC) medicine, especially aminophylline, anticoagulants (blood thinners), aspirin or other salicylates, caffeine, cefamandole, cefoperazone, cefotetan, diphylline, moxalactam, oxtriphylline, pentoxifylline, plicamycin, sulfinpyrazone, theophylline, ticarcillin, ticlopidine, or valproic acid;
- have any other medical problems.

POSSIBLE SIDE EFFECTS OF THIS MEDICINE

Side Effects That Should Be Reported To Your Doctor Immediately

> *More common*—Chest pain

> *Less common or rare*—Headache (severe and throbbing); shortness of breath, troubled breathing, tightness in chest, or wheezing; skin rash or itching

Side Effects That Usually Do Not Require Medical Attention

These possible side effects may go away during treatment; however, if they continue or are bothersome, check with your doctor, nurse, or pharmacist.

> *More common*—Dizziness or lightheadedness

> *Less common*—Flushing; headache; nausea or vomiting; skin rash

Other side effects not listed above may also occur in some patients. If you notice any other effects, check with your doctor, nurse, or pharmacist.

▲ For the Patient ▲

912260

DIPYRIDAMOLE (Therapeutic—Oral)

ABOUT YOUR MEDICINE

Dipyridamole (dye-peer-ID-a-mole) is used to lessen the chance of stroke or other serious medical problems that may occur when a blood vessel is blocked by blood clots. It is given only when there is a larger-than-usual chance that these problems may occur. For example, it is given to people who have had diseased heart valves replaced by mechanical valves, because dangerous blood clots are especially likely to occur in these patients. Dipyridamole may also be used for other conditions as determined by your doctor.

If any of the information in this leaflet causes you special concern or if you want additional information about your medicine and its use, check with your doctor, nurse, or pharmacist. **Remember, keep this and all other medicines out of the reach of children and never share your medicines with others.**

BEFORE USING THIS MEDICINE

Tell your doctor, nurse, and pharmacist if you . . .
- are allergic to any medicine, either prescription or non-prescription (OTC);
- are pregnant or intend to become pregnant while using this medicine;
- are breast-feeding;
- are taking any other prescription or nonprescription (OTC) medicine, especially anticoagulants (blood thinners), aspirin or other salicylates, cefamandole, cefoperazone, cefotetan, moxalactam, pentoxifylline, plicamycin, sulfinpyrazone, ticarcillin, ticlopidine, or valproic acid;
- have any other medical problems.

PROPER USE OF THIS MEDICINE

This medicine works best when taken with a full glass (8 ounces) of water at least 1 hour before or 2 hours after meals. However, to lessen stomach upset, your doctor may want you to take the medicine with food or milk.

Dipyridamole must be taken in regularly spaced doses, as ordered by your doctor.

If you miss a dose of this medicine, take it as soon as possible. However, if your next scheduled dose is within 4 hours, skip the missed dose and go back to your regular dosing schedule. Do not double doses.

PRECAUTIONS WHILE USING THIS MEDICINE

Dizziness, lightheadedness, or fainting may occur, especially when you get up from a lying or sitting position. Getting up

slowly may help. If this problem continues or gets worse, check with your doctor.

Do not take aspirin, or any combination medicine containing aspirin, unless the same doctor who directed you to take dipyridamole also directs you to take aspirin. This is especially important if you are taking an anticoagulant together with dipyridamole.

If you have been directed to take aspirin together with dipyridamole, **take only the amount of aspirin ordered by your doctor.**

Tell all physicians and dentists you go to that you are taking dipyridamole, and whether or not you are taking an anticoagulant (blood thinner) or aspirin together with it.

POSSIBLE SIDE EFFECTS OF THIS MEDICINE
Side Effects That Should Be Reported To Your Doctor

   Less common—Skin rash or itching

   Rare—Chest pain or tightness in chest

Side Effects That Usually Do Not Require Medical Attention

These possible side effects may go away during treatment; however, if they continue or are bothersome, check with your doctor, nurse, or pharmacist.

   More common—Dizziness

   Less common—Flushing; headache; nausea or vomiting; stomach cramping; weakness

Other side effects not listed above may also occur in some patients. If you notice any other effects, check with your doctor, nurse, or pharmacist.

DISOPYRAMIDE   Systemic

■ For the Pharmacist ■

In providing consultation, consider emphasizing the following selected
information (» = major clinical significance):

Before using this medication
» Conditions affecting use, especially:
   Sensitivity to disopyramide
   Pregnancy—May initiate uterine contractions
   Breast-feeding—Passes into breast milk
   Use in the elderly—Increased sensitivity to anticholinergic ef-
      fects
   Other medications, especially other antiarrhythmics or pimozide
   Other medical problems, especially second or third degree atrio-
      ventricular (AV) block, cardiogenic shock, cardiac conduc-
      tion abnormalities, cardiomyopathies, uncompensated or
      poorly compensated congestive heart failure, diabetes mel-
      litus, history of closed-angle glaucoma, hepatic function im-
      pairment, hyperkalemia or hypokalemia, myasthenia gravis,
      prostatic enlargement, or renal function impairment

Proper use of this medication
» Compliance with therapy; not taking more medication than directed
   Proper administration of extended-release capsules: Swallowing cap-
      sule whole, without breaking, crushing, or chewing
   Proper administration of extended-release tablets: Not crushing or
      chewing
» Importance of not missing doses and taking at evenly spaced inter-
      vals
» Proper dosing
» Missed dose: Taking as soon as possible, unless within 4 hours of
      next dose; not doubling doses
» Proper storage

Precautions while using this medication
» Regular visits to physician to check progress
» Checking with physician before stopping medication because of ad-
      verse cardiac effects with sudden withdrawal
» Caution when driving or doing things requiring alertness because of
      possible dizziness, lightheadedness, or fainting, especially when
      getting up suddenly from lying or sitting position
» Avoiding alcoholic beverages
» Notifying physician and taking sugar if symptoms of hypoglycemia
      occur
» Possible blurred vision; avoiding driving, using machines, or doing
      other things requiring clear vision if blurred vision occurs
   Possible dryness of eyes, mouth, and nose; using sugarless candy or
      gum, ice, or saliva substitute for relief of dry mouth; checking
      with physician or dentist if dry mouth continues for more than
      2 weeks
» Caution during exercise or hot weather because of possible reduced
      sweating and impaired heat tolerance

Side/adverse effects
  Signs of potential side effects, especially difficult urination, chest
    pains, confusion, congestive heart failure, fluid retention, hy-
    potension, muscle weakness, aggravation of glaucoma, agranu-
    locytosis, cholestatic jaundice, mental depression, and hypogly-
    cemia

▲ For the Patient ▲

913036

ANTIARRHYTHMICS, TYPE I (Oral): *Including*
Disopyramide; Encainide; Flecainide; Mexiletine;
Moricizine; Procainamide; Propafenone; Quinidine;
Tocainide.

ABOUT YOUR MEDICINE

Type I antiarrhythmics are used to correct irregular heartbeats to a normal rhythm and to slow an overactive heart.

There is a chance that these medicines may cause new heart
rhythm problems when they are used. Usually this effect is
rare and mild. However, some of these medicines are more
likely than others to cause this effect. For example, encainide
and flecainide have been shown to cause severe problems in
some patients, and so they are only used to treat serious
heart rhythm problems. Discuss this possible effect with
your doctor.

If any of the information in this leaflet causes you special
concern or if you want additional information about your
medicine and its use, check with your doctor, nurse, or pharmacist. **Remember, keep this and all other medicines out of
the reach of children and never share your medicines with
others.**

BEFORE USING THIS MEDICINE

Tell your doctor, nurse, and pharmacist if you . . .
  • are allergic to any medicine, either prescription or non-
    prescription (OTC);
  • are pregnant or intend to become pregnant while using
    this medicine;
  • are breast-feeding;
  • are taking **any** other prescription or nonprescription
    (OTC) medicine;
  • have **any** other medical problems.

PROPER USE OF THIS MEDICINE

Take this medicine exactly as directed by your doctor, even
though you may feel well. Do not take more medicine than
ordered.

For patients taking the extended-release capsules or tablets:
  • Swallow whole without breaking, crushing, or chewing.

**It is best to take each dose at evenly spaced times day and
night.**

For patients taking mexiletine:
- To lessen the possibility of stomach upset, this medicine should be taken with food or immediately after meals or with milk or an antacid.

If you miss a dose of this medicine, take it as soon as possible. However, if you do not remember until it is almost time for the next dose, skip the missed dose and go back to your regular dosing schedule. Do not double doses.

PRECAUTIONS WHILE USING THIS MEDICINE

It is important that your doctor check your progress at regular visits to make sure the medicine is working properly to help your heart.

Do not suddenly stop taking this medicine without first checking with your doctor. Stopping it suddenly may cause a serious change in heart activity.

Dizziness or lightheadedness or blurred vision may occur. **Make sure you know how you react to this medicine before you drive, use machines, or do other jobs that require you to be alert and able to see well.**

For patients taking disopyramide:
- **If signs of hypoglycemia (low blood sugar) such as chills, hunger, nausea, nervousness, or sweating appear, eat or drink a food containing sugar and call your doctor right away.**
- **Use extra care not to become overheated during exercise or hot weather,** since this medicine will often make you sweat less and could possibly result in heatstroke.

POSSIBLE SIDE EFFECTS OF THIS MEDICINE

Side Effects That Should Be Reported To Your Doctor Immediately

For quinidine only, especially after the first dose or first few doses—Breathing difficulty; changes in vision; dizziness, lightheadedness, or fainting; fever; severe headache; ringing in ears; skin rash

Other Side Effects That Should Be Reported To Your Doctor

For all antiarrhythmics—Chest pain; fast or irregular heartbeat; fever or chills; shortness of breath or painful breathing; skin rash or itching; unusual bleeding or bruising

For disopyramide (in addition to above)—Difficult urination; swelling of feet or lower legs

For encainide, flecainide, moricizine, and propafenone (in addition to above)—Swelling of feet or lower legs; trembling or shaking

Side Effects That Usually Do Not Require Medical Attention

These possible side effects may go away during treatment; however, if they continue or are bothersome, check with your doctor, nurse, or pharmacist.

For all antiarrhythmics—Blurred or double vision; dizziness or lightheadedness

For disopyramide (in addition to above)—Dry mouth and throat

For flecainide (in addition to above)—Seeing spots

For mexiletine (in addition to above)—Heartburn; nausea and vomiting; nervousness; trembling or shaking of hands; unsteadiness or trouble walking

For procainamide (in addition to above)—Diarrhea; loss of appetite

For propafenone (in addition to above)—Change in taste

For quinidine (in addition to above)—Bitter taste; diarrhea; flushing of skin with itching; loss of appetite; nausea or vomiting; stomach pain or cramps

For tocainide (in addition to above)—Loss of appetite; nausea

Other side effects not listed above may also occur in some patients. If you notice any other effects, check with your doctor, nurse, or pharmacist.

DISULFIRAM   Systemic

■ For the Pharmacist ■

In providing consultation, consider emphasizing the following selected information (» = major clinical significance):

Before using this medication
» Conditions affecting use, especially:
   Sensitivity to disulfiram, rubber, pesticides, or fungicides
   Other medications, especially alcohol; alfentanil; coumarin- or indandione-derivative anticoagulants; organic solvents; hydantoin anticonvulsants, especially phenytoin; isoniazid; metronidazole; or paraldehyde

Proper use of this medication
» Not taking this medication within 12 hours of using any alcohol-containing preparation or medication, or if the blood alcohol level is not zero
» Compliance with therapy
» Proper dosing
» Proper storage

Precautions while using this medication
» Not drinking or using any alcohol-containing products or medications while taking this medication and for 14 days after discontinuing this medication
   Symptoms of disulfiram-alcohol reaction:
   Blurred vision
   Chest pain
   Confusion
   Dizziness or fainting
   Fast or pounding heartbeat
   Flushing or redness of face
   Increased sweating
   Nausea and vomiting
   Throbbing headache
   Troubled breathing
   Weakness, severe
   Rarely, seizures, heart attack, unconsciousness, or death if reaction is severe
   Carrying medical identification card during therapy
   Regular visits to physician to check progress during long-term therapy
» Checking all liquid medications for presence of alcohol
» Caution if drowsiness occurs
» Checking with physician before using other CNS depressants

Side/adverse effects
   Signs of potential side effects, especially optic neuritis, peripheral neuritis, polyneuritis, or psychotic reaction

▲ For the Patient ▲

913772

ABOUT YOUR MEDICINE

Disulfiram (dye-SUL-fi-ram) is used to help overcome your drinking problem. It is not a cure for alcoholism, but rather will discourage you from drinking.

If any of the information in this leaflet causes you special concern or if you want additional information about your medicine and its use, check with your doctor, nurse, or pharmacist. **Remember, keep this and all other medicines out of the reach of children and never share your medicines with others.**

BEFORE USING THIS MEDICINE

Tell your doctor, nurse, and pharmacist if you . . .
- are allergic to any medicine, either prescription or non-prescription (OTC);
- are pregnant or intend to become pregnant while using this medicine;
- are breast-feeding;
- are taking any other prescription or nonprescription (OTC) medicine, especially anticoagulants (blood thinners), isoniazid, or phenytoin;
- are now taking or have taken within the past several days metronidazole or paraldehyde;
- have any other medical problems.

PROPER USE OF THIS MEDICINE

Before you take the first dose of this medicine, **make sure you have not taken any alcoholic beverage or alcohol-containing product or medicine** (for example, tonics, elixirs, and cough syrups) **during the past 12 hours.**

Take this medicine every day as directed by your doctor. The medicine is usually taken each morning. However, if it makes you drowsy, ask your doctor if you may take it at bedtime instead.

PRECAUTIONS WHILE USING THIS MEDICINE

Do not drink any alcohol, even small amounts, while you are taking this medicine and for 14 days after you stop taking it, because the alcohol may make you very sick. In addition to beverages, alcohol is found in many other products. Reading the list of ingredients on foods and other products before using them will help you to avoid alcohol. You can also avoid alcohol if you:
- Do not use alcohol-containing foods, products, or medicines, such as elixirs, tonics, sauces, vinegars, cough syrups, mouth washes, or gargles.
- **Do not come in contact with or breathe in the fumes of chemicals that may contain alcohol, acetaldehyde, paraldehyde, or other related chemicals**, such as paint thinner, paint, varnish, or shellac.
- **Use caution when using alcohol-containing products that are applied to the skin**, such as some transdermal (stick-on patch) medicines, rubbing alcohol, back rubs, after-shave lotions, colognes, perfumes, toilet waters, or after-bath preparations. Before using alcohol-containing products on your skin, first test the product by applying some to a small area of your skin. Allow the product to remain

on your skin for 1 to 2 hours. If no redness, itching, or other unwanted effects occur, you should be able to use the product.

- **Do not use any alcohol-containing products on raw skin or open wounds.**

Before buying or using any liquid prescription or nonprescription medicine, check with your pharmacist to see if it contains any alcohol.

Some of the symptoms you may experience if you use any alcohol while taking this medicine are throbbing headache, nausea and vomiting, confusion, fast or pounding heartbeat, dizziness or fainting, flushing or redness of face, increased sweating, troubled breathing, chest pain, weakness, or blurred vision. These symptoms will last as long as there is any alcohol left in your system, from 30 minutes to several hours. On rare occasions, if you have a severe reaction or have taken a large enough amount of alcohol, heart attack, unconsciousness, convulsions (seizures), or death may occur.

Your doctor may want you to carry an identification card stating that you are taking this medicine. This card should list the symptoms likely to occur if alcohol is taken, and the doctor or hospital to be contacted in case of emergency.

This medicine may cause some people to become drowsy or less alert than they are normally. **Make sure you know how you react to this medicine before you drive, use machines, or do other jobs that require you to be alert.**

Disulfiram will add to the effects of other CNS depressants (medicines that slow down the nervous system). **Check with your doctor before taking any such depressants while you are using this medicine.**

POSSIBLE SIDE EFFECTS OF THIS MEDICINE
Side Effects That Should Be Reported To Your Doctor

> *Less common*—Eye pain or tenderness or any change in vision; mood or mental changes; numbness, tingling, pain, or weakness in hands or feet
>
> *Rare*—Darkening of urine; light gray–colored stools; severe stomach pain; yellow eyes or skin

Side Effects That Usually Do Not Require Medical Attention

These possible side effects may go away during treatment; however, if they continue or are bothersome, check with your doctor, nurse, or pharmacist.

> *More common*—Drowsiness

Other side effects not listed above may also occur in some patients. If you notice any other effects, check with your doctor, nurse, or pharmacist.

DIURETICS, LOOP   Systemic
Including Bumetanide; Ethacrynic Acid; Furosemide.

■For the Pharmacist■

In providing consultation, consider emphasizing the following selected information (» = major clinical significance):

Before using this medication
» Conditions affecting use, especially:
   Sensitivity to the loop diuretic prescribed, or to sulfonamides (for bumetanide and furosemide)
   Pregnancy—Not recommended for routine use; reported to cause harmful effects, including birth defects, in animals
   Breast-feeding—Furosemide distributed into breast milk
   Use in the elderly—Elderly patients may be more sensitive to hypotensive and electrolyte effects, and may be at greater risk of developing circulatory collapse and thromboembolic episodes
   Other medications, especially parenteral amphotericin B, oral anticoagulants, other hypokalemia-causing medications, lithium, or other nephrotoxic medications
   Other medical problems, especially anuria or severe renal function impairment

Proper use of this medication
   Diuretic effects of the medication and timing of doses to minimize inconvenience of diuresis
   Getting into habit of taking at same time each day to help increase compliance
   Taking with food or milk to reduce gastrointestinal irritation
» Proper dosing
   Missed dose: Taking as soon as possible; not taking if almost time for next dose; not doubling doses
» Proper storage
For use as an antihypertensive
   Possible need for control of weight and diet, especially sodium intake
» Patient may not experience symptoms of hypertension; importance of taking medication even if feeling well
» Does not cure, but controls hypertension; possible need for lifelong therapy; serious consequences of untreated hypertension
For oral solution dosage form of furosemide (in addition to the above)
   Taking orally, even if in dropper bottle; importance of accurate measurement

Precautions while using this medication
   Regular visits to physician to check progress
» Possibility of hypokalemia; possible need for additional potassium in diet; not changing diet without first checking with physician
   To prevent dehydration, notifying physician if severe nausea, vomiting, or diarrhea occurs and continues
   Caution if any kind of surgery (including dental surgery) is required
» Caution when getting up suddenly from a lying or sitting position
» Caution in using alcohol, while standing for long periods or exercising, and during hot weather because of enhanced orthostatic hypotensive effects
   Diabetics: May increase blood sugar levels

For use as an antihypertensive
» Not taking other medications, especially nonprescription sympatho-
    mimetics, unless discussed with physician
For furosemide (in addition to the above)
» Possible skin photosensitivity; avoiding unprotected exposure to sun;
    using protective clothing; using a sun block product that includes
    protection against both UVA-caused photosensitivity reactions
    and UVB-caused sunburn reactions; avoiding use of sunlamp,
    tanning bed, or tanning booth

Side/adverse effects
Signs of potential side effects, especially allergic reaction, blood in
    urine, electrolyte imbalance, gastrointestinal bleeding, gout, he-
    patic dysfunction, leukopenia, agranulocytosis, ototoxicity, pan-
    creatitis, thrombocytopenia, and xanthopsia

▲ For the Patient ▲

912850

ABOUT YOUR MEDICINE

Loop diuretics help reduce the amount of water in the body
by increasing the flow of urine. Furosemide is also used to
treat high blood pressure (hypertension) in certain patients.
These medicines may also be used for other conditions as
determined by your doctor.

If any of the information in this leaflet causes you special
concern or if you want additional information about your
medicine and its use, check with your doctor, nurse, or pharmacist. **Remember, keep this and all other medicines out of
the reach of children and never share your medicines with
others.**

BEFORE USING THIS MEDICINE

Tell your doctor, nurse, and pharmacist if you . . .
  • are allergic to any medicine, either prescription or non-
    prescription (OTC);
  • are pregnant or intend to become pregnant while using
    this medicine;
  • are breast-feeding;
  • are taking **any** other prescription or nonprescription
    (OTC) medicine;
  • have any other medical problems, especially inflam-
    mation of the pancreas or severe kidney disease.

PROPER USE OF THIS MEDICINE

This medicine may cause an unusual feeling of tiredness
when you begin to take it. You may also notice an increase
in urine or in your frequency of urination. To keep this from
affecting sleep:
  • if you are to take a single dose a day, take it in the
    morning after breakfast.
  • if you are to take more than one dose, take the last one
    no later than 6 p.m.

For patients taking this medicine for high blood pressure:
- This medicine will not cure your high blood pressure but it does help control it. You must continue to take it—even if you feel well—if you expect to keep your blood pressure down. **You may have to take high blood pressure medicine for the rest of your life.**

If you miss a dose of this medicine, take it as soon as possible. However, if it is almost time for your next dose, skip the missed dose and go back to your regular dosing schedule. Do not double doses.

PRECAUTIONS WHILE USING THIS MEDICINE

This medicine may cause a loss of potassium from your body. To help prevent this, your doctor **may** want you to eat or drink foods that have a high potassium content, take a potassium supplement, or take another medicine to help prevent loss of potassium in the first place. It is very important to follow these directions. Also, it is important not to change your diet on your own and to check with your doctor if you become sick and have severe or continuing vomiting or diarrhea.

Dizziness, lightheadedness, or fainting may occur, especially when you get up from a lying or sitting position. Getting up slowly may help. **Also, drinking alcohol may make these effects worse and may cause a serious drop in blood pressure.** Check with your doctor before drinking alcohol.

POSSIBLE SIDE EFFECTS OF THIS MEDICINE
Side Effects That Should Be Reported To Your Doctor

Rare—Black, tarry stools; blood in urine or stools; cough or hoarseness; fever or chills; joint pain; lower back or side pain; painful or difficult urination; pinpoint red spots on skin; ringing or buzzing in ears or any loss of hearing; skin rash or hives; stomach pain (severe) with nausea and vomiting; unusual bleeding or bruising; yellow eyes or skin; yellow vision (furosemide only)

Signs of too much potassium loss—Dryness of mouth; increased thirst; irregular heartbeat; mood or mental changes; muscle cramps or pain; nausea or vomiting; unusual tiredness or weakness; weak pulse

Side Effects That Usually Do Not Require Medical Attention

These possible side effects may go away during treatment; however, if they continue or are bothersome, check with your doctor, nurse, or pharmacist.

More common—Dizziness or lightheadedness when getting up from a lying or sitting position

Other side effects not listed above may also occur in some patients. If you notice any other effects, check with your doctor, nurse, or pharmacist.

DIURETICS, POTASSIUM-SPARING, AND HYDROCHLOROTHIAZIDE   Systemic
*Including Amiloride and Hydrochlorothiazide;
Spironolactone and Hydrochlorothiazide; Triamterene and
Hydrochlorothiazide.*

■ For the Pharmacist ■

In providing consultation, consider emphasizing the following selected
information (» = major clinical significance):

Before using this medication
» Conditions affecting use, especially:
   Sensitivity to the potassium-sparing diuretic prescribed, hydro-
      chlorothiazide or other thiazide diuretics, other sulfonamide-
      type medications, bumetanide, furosemide, or carbonic an-
      hydrase inhibitors
   Pregnancy—Diuretics not recommended for routine use
   Breast-feeding—Hydrochlorothiazide distributed into breast milk;
      spironolactone may be distributed into breast milk
   Use in the elderly—Elderly patients may be more sensitive to
      hypotensive and electrolyte-depleting effects
   Other medications, especially angiotensin-converting enzyme in-
      hibitors, cholestyramine, colestipol, coumarin or indandione
      anticoagulants, cyclosporine, digitalis glycosides, heparin,
      lithium, low-salt milk, other potassium-sparing diuretics, po-
      tassium-containing medications or supplements, or stored blood
      from a blood bank
   Other medical problems, especially, diabetic nephropathy, he-
      patic function impairment, renal function impairment or an-
      uria

Proper use of this medication
   Diuretic effects of the medication and timing of doses to minimize
      inconvenience of diuresis
   Getting into habit of taking at same time each day to help increase
      compliance
   Taking with meals or milk to reduce stomach upset
» Proper dosing
   Missed dose: Taking as soon as possible; not taking if almost time
      for next dose; not doubling doses
» Proper storage
For use an an antihypertensive
   Possible need for control of weight and diet, especially sodium intake
» Patient may not experience symptoms of hypertension; importance
      of taking medication even if feeling well
» Does not cure, but helps control hypertension; possible need for
      lifelong therapy; checking with physician before discontinuing
      medication; serious consequences of untreated hypertension

Precautions while using this medication
   Regular visits to physician to check progress
» Possibility of hypokalemia or hyperkalemia; possible need for mon-
      itoring potassium in diet; not changing diet without first checking
      with physician
   To prevent dehydration, checking with physician if severe nausea,
      vomiting, or diarrhea occurs and continues
   Diabetics: May increase blood sugar levels

Possible photosensitivity; avoiding too much sun; using protective
clothing and sun block product; avoiding use of sunlamp, tanning
bed, or tanning booth

Caution if any kind of surgery or emergency treatment is required

Caution if any laboratory tests required; possible interference with
test results

For triamterene and hydrochlorothiazide combination

Not changing brands of triamterene and hydrochlorothiazide combination without checking with physician

For use an an antihypertensive

» Not taking other medications, especially nonprescription sympathomimetics, unless discussed with physician

Side/adverse effects

Signs of potential side effects, especially electrolyte imbalance,
agranulocytosis, allergic reaction, cholecystitis or pancreatitis,
gout or hyperuricemia, hepatic function impairment, thrombocytopenia, megaloblastosis (for triamterene)

For spironolactone

Possibility of enlargement of breasts in males and irregular menstrual periods in females; usually reversible within several months

---

▲ For the Patient ▲

913149

ABOUT YOUR MEDICINE

Potassium-sparing diuretics and **hydrochlorothiazide** combinations are used to treat high blood pressure (hypertension). They are used also to help reduce water in the body
by increasing the flow of urine. This combination is also
used to treat problems caused by too little potassium in the
body.

If any of the information in this leaflet causes you special
concern or if you want additional information about your
medicine and its use, check with your doctor, nurse, or pharmacist. **Remember, keep this and all other medicines out of
the reach of children and never share your medicines with
others.**

BEFORE USING THIS MEDICINE

Tell your doctor, nurse, and pharmacist if you . . .

- are allergic to any medicine, either prescription or nonprescription (OTC);
- are pregnant or intend to become pregnant while using
this medicine;
- are breast-feeding;
- are taking any other prescription or nonprescription
(OTC) medicine, especially captopril; cortisone-like
medicines; cyclosporine; digitalis; enalapril; lisinopril;
lithium; methenamine; other diuretics or antihypertensives; potassium-containing medicines or supplements;
or medicines for appetite control, asthma, colds, cough,
hay fever, or sinus;
- have any other medical problems, especially kidney or
liver disease.

PROPER USE OF THIS MEDICINE

This medicine may cause an unusual feeling of tiredness when you begin to take it. You may also notice an increase in urine or in frequency of urination. To keep this from affecting sleep:

- if you are to take a single dose a day, take it in the morning after breakfast.
- if you are to take more than one dose, take the last one no later than 6 p.m.

If this medicine upsets your stomach, it may be taken with meals or milk. If stomach upset continues, check with your doctor.

For patients taking this medicine for high blood pressure:

- This medicine will not cure your high blood pressure but it does help control it. You must continue to take it—even if you feel well—if you expect to keep your blood pressure down. **You may have to take high blood pressure medicine for the rest of your life.**

If you miss a dose of this medicine, take it as soon as possible. However, if it is almost time for your next dose, skip the missed dose and go back to your regular dosing schedule. Do not double doses.

PRECAUTIONS WHILE USING THIS MEDICINE

This medicine may cause either a loss or increase of potassium. Your doctor may have special instructions about eating or drinking foods or beverages that have a high potassium content, taking a potassium supplement, or using salt substitutes. Follow your doctor's directions and do not change your diet on your own. Check with your doctor if you become sick and have severe or continuing vomiting or diarrhea, as you may lose additional water and potassium.

POSSIBLE SIDE EFFECTS OF THIS MEDICINE

Side Effects That Should Be Reported To Your Doctor

Rare—Black, tarry stools; blood in urine or stools; cough or hoarseness; fever or chills; joint pain; lower back or side pain; painful or difficult urination; pinpoint red spots on skin; skin rash or hives; stomach pain (severe) with nausea and vomiting; unusual bleeding or bruising; yellow eyes or skin

Rare (for triamterene only)—Bright red tongue; burning, inflamed feeling in tongue; cracked corners of mouth

Signs of changes in potassium—Confusion; dryness of mouth; increased thirst; mood changes; muscle cramps or pain; numbness or tingling in hands, feet, or lips; shortness of breath or difficult breathing; unusual tiredness or weakness; weak or irregular heartbeat; weakness or heaviness of legs

Side Effects That Usually Do Not Require Medical Attention

These possible side effects may go away during treatment; however, if they continue or are bothersome, check with your doctor, nurse, or pharmacist.

> *More common (less common with triamterene)*—Loss of appetite; nausea and vomiting; stomach cramps and diarrhea; upset stomach

> *Less common*—Decreased sexual ability; headache; increased sensitivity of skin to sunlight; lightheadedness or dizziness when standing up

> *Less common (for amiloride only)*—Constipation

> *Less common (for spironolactone only)*—Breast tenderness, deepening of the voice, increased hair growth, and irregular menstrual periods in women; clumsiness; enlarged breasts in men; unusual sweating

Other side effects not listed above may also occur in some patients. If you notice any other effects, check with your doctor, nurse, or pharmacist.

DIURETICS, THIAZIDE   Systemic

*Including Bendroflumethiazide; Benzthiazide;
Chlorothiazide; Chlorthalidone; Cyclothiazide;
Hydrochlorothiazide; Hydroflumethiazide; Methyclothiazide;
Metolazone; Polythiazide; Quinethazone;
Trichlormethiazide.*

■For the Pharmacist■

In providing consultation, consider emphasizing the following selected
information (» = major clinical significance):

Before using this medication
» Conditions affecting use, especially:
   Sensitivity to thiazide diuretics, other sulfonamide-type medi-
      cations, bumetanide, furosemide, or carbonic anhydrase in-
      hibitors
   Pregnancy—Not recommended for routine use; may cause jaun-
      dice, thrombocytopenia, hypokalemia in infant
   Breast-feeding—Distributed into breast milk; recommended that
      nursing mothers avoid thiazides during first month of breast-
      feeding because of reports of suppression of lactation
   Pediatrics—Caution if giving to infants with jaundice
   Use in the elderly—Elderly patients may be more sensitive to
      hypotensive and electrolyte effects
   Other medications, especially cholestyramine, colestipol, digi-
      talis glycosides, or lithium
   Other medical problems, especially anuria or severe renal func-
      tion impairment or infants with jaundice

Proper use of this medication
   Diuretic effects of the medication and timing of doses to minimize
      inconvenience of diuresis (except in diabetes insipidus)
   Getting into habit of taking at same time each day to help increase
      compliance
   Proper administration of concentrated oral hydrochlorothiazide so-
      lution: Taking orally; special dropper to be used for accurate
      measuring
» Proper dosing
   Missed dose: Taking as soon as possible; not taking if almost time
      for next dose; not doubling doses
» Proper storage
For use as an antihypertensive
   Importance of diet; possible need for sodium restriction and/or weight
      reduction
» Patient may not experience symptoms of hypertension; importance
      of taking medication even if feeling well
» Does not cure, but helps control hypertension; possible need for
      lifelong therapy; checking with physician before discontinuing
      medication; serious consequences of untreated hypertension

Precautions while using this medication
   Regular visits to physician to check progress
» Possibility of hypokalemia; possible need for additional potassium
      in diet; not changing diet without first checking with physician
   To prevent dehydration, checking with physician if severe nausea,
      vomiting, or diarrhea occurs and continues
   Diabetics: May increase blood sugar levels

Possible photosensitivity; avoiding unprotected exposure to sun; using protective clothing and sun block product; avoiding use of sunlamp, tanning bed, or tanning booth

For use as an antihypertensive

» Not taking other medications, especially nonprescription sympathomimetics, unless discussed with physician

Side/adverse effects

Signs of potential side effects, especially electrolyte imbalance, agranulocytosis, allergic reaction, cholecystitis, pancreatitis, hepatic function impairment, hyperuricemia, gout, and thrombocytopenia

---

▲ For the Patient ▲

912690

ABOUT YOUR MEDICINE

Thiazide diuretics are commonly used to treat high blood pressure (hypertension). They are used also to help reduce the amount of water in the body by increasing the flow of urine. Thiazide diuretics may also be used for other conditions as determined by your doctor.

If any of the information in this leaflet causes you special concern or if you want additional information about your medicine and its use, check with your doctor, nurse, or pharmacist. **Remember, keep this and all other medicines out of the reach of children and never share your medicines with others.**

BEFORE USING THIS MEDICINE

Tell your doctor, nurse, and pharmacist if you . . .

- are allergic to any medicine, either prescription or nonprescription (OTC);
- are pregnant or intend to become pregnant while using this medicine;
- are breast-feeding;
- compete in athletics;
- are taking any other prescription or nonprescription (OTC) medicine, especially cholestyramine, colestipol, digitalis glycosides (heart medicine), or lithium;
- have any other medical problems, especially severe kidney disease.

PROPER USE OF THIS MEDICINE

Thiazide diuretics may cause an unusual feeling of tiredness when you begin to take them. You may also notice an increase in urine or in frequency of urination. To keep this from affecting sleep:

- if you are to take a single dose a day, take it in the morning after breakfast.
- if you are to take more than one dose, take the last one no later than 6 p.m.

For patients taking this medicine for high blood pressure:

- This medicine will not cure your high blood pressure but it does help control it. You must continue to take it—even if you feel well—if you expect to keep your blood pressure down. **You may have to take high blood pressure medicine for the rest of your life.**

If you miss a dose of this medicine, take it as soon as possible. However, if it is almost time for your next dose, skip the missed dose and go back to your regular dosing schedule. Do not double doses.

PRECAUTIONS WHILE USING THIS MEDICINE

This medicine may cause a loss of potassium from your body. To help prevent this, your doctor **may** want you to eat or drink foods that have a high potassium content, take a potassium supplement, or take another medicine to help prevent loss of the potassium in the first place. It is very important to follow these directions. Also, it is important not to change your diet on your own and to check with your doctor if you become sick and have severe or continuing vomiting or diarrhea.

POSSIBLE SIDE EFFECTS OF THIS MEDICINE

Side Effects That Should Be Reported To Your Doctor

> *Rare*—Black, tarry stools; blood in urine or stools; cough or hoarseness; fever or chills; joint pain; lower back or side pain; painful or difficult urination; pinpoint red spots on skin; skin rash or hives; stomach pain (severe) with nausea and vomiting; unusual bleeding or bruising; yellow eyes or skin

> *Signs of too much potassium loss*—Dryness of mouth; increased thirst; mood changes; muscle cramps or pain; nausea or vomiting; unusual tiredness or weakness; weak or irregular heartbeat

> *Signs of too much sodium loss*—Confusion; convulsions; decreased mental activity; irritability; muscle cramps; unusual tiredness or weakness

Side Effects That Usually Do Not Require Medical Attention

These possible side effects may go away during treatment; however, if they continue or are bothersome, check with your doctor, nurse, or pharmacist.

> *Less common*—Decreased sexual ability; diarrhea; dizziness or lightheadedness when standing up; increased sensitivity of skin to sunlight; loss of appetite; upset stomach

Other side effects not listed above may also occur in some patients. If you notice any other effects, check with your doctor, nurse, or pharmacist.

DOXAZOSIN   Systemic

■ For the Pharmacist ■

In providing consultation, consider emphasizing the following selected information (» = major clinical significance):

Before using this medication
» Conditions affecting use, especially:
    Sensitivity to quinazolines
    Use in the elderly—Increased sensitivity to hypotensive effects

Proper use of this medication
    Getting into the habit of taking at same times each day to help increase compliance
» Proper dosing
    Missed dose: Taking as soon as possible; not taking if almost time for next dose; not doubling doses
» Proper storage
For use as an antihypertensive
    Possible need for control of weight and diet, especially sodium intake
» Patient may not experience symptoms of hypertension; importance of taking medication even if feeling well
» Does not cure, but helps control hypertension; possible need for lifelong therapy; serious consequences of untreated hypertension

Precautions while using this medication
    Regular visits to physician to check progress
» Not taking other medications, especially nonprescription sympathomimetics, unless discussed with physician
» Caution if dizziness, lightheadedness, or sudden fainting occurs, especially after initial dose; taking first dose at bedtime
» Caution when getting up suddenly from a lying or sitting position
» Caution in using alcohol, while standing for long periods or exercising, and during hot weather, because of enhanced orthostatic hypotensive effects
» Possibility of drowsiness
» Caution when driving or doing anything else requiring alertness because of possible drowsiness, dizziness, or lightheadedness

Side/adverse effects
    Signs of potential side effects, especially arrhythmias, dizziness, dyspnea, orthostatic hypotension, palpitations, peripheral edema, tachycardia, and vertigo

▲ For the Patient ▲

912587

ALPHA₁-BLOCKERS (Oral): *Including Doxazosin; Prazosin; Terazosin.*

ABOUT YOUR MEDICINE

Alpha₁-blockers are used to treat high blood pressure (hypertension). Terazosin is also used to treat benign enlargement of the prostate (benign prostatic hyperplasia [BPH]). These medicines may also be used for other conditions as determined by your doctor.

If any of the information in this leaflet causes you special concern or if you want additional information about your medicine and its use, check with your doctor, nurse, or pharmacist. **Remember, keep this and all other medicines out of the reach of children and never share your medicines with others.**

BEFORE USING THIS MEDICINE

Tell your doctor, nurse, and pharmacist if you . . .

- are allergic to any medicine, either prescription or non-prescription (OTC);
- are pregnant or intend to become pregnant while using this medicine;
- are breast-feeding;
- are taking any other prescription or nonprescription (OTC) medicine, especially medicines for appetite control, asthma, colds, cough, hay fever, or sinus;
- have any other medical problems, especially heart disease.

PROPER USE OF THIS MEDICINE

For patients taking this medicine for high blood pressure:

- This medicine will not cure your high blood pressure but it does help control it. You must continue to take it—even if you feel well—if you expect to keep your blood pressure down. **You may have to take high blood pressure medicine for the rest of your life.**

For patients taking terazosin for benign enlargement of the prostate:

- Remember that terazosin will not shrink the size of your prostate, but it does help to relieve the symptoms.
- It may take up to 6 weeks before your symptoms get better.

If you miss a dose of this medicine, take it as soon as possible. However, if it is almost time for your next dose, skip the missed dose and go back to your regular dosing schedule. Do not double doses.

PRECAUTIONS WHILE USING THIS MEDICINE

Dizziness, lightheadedness, or sudden fainting may occur after you take this medicine, especially when you get up from a sitting or lying position. These effects are more likely to occur when you take the first dose of this medicine. Taking the first dose at bedtime may prevent problems. However, **be especially careful if you need to get up during the night.** These effects may also occur with any doses you take after the first dose. Getting up slowly may help lessen this problem. **If you feel dizzy, lie down so that you do not faint.** Then sit for a few minutes before standing to prevent the dizziness from returning.

The dizziness, lightheadedness, or fainting is more likely to occur if you drink alcohol, stand for long periods of time, exercise, or if the weather is hot. **While you are taking this medicine, be careful to limit the amount of alcohol you drink.**

Also, use extra care during exercise or hot weather or if you must stand for long periods of time.

This medicine may cause some people to become drowsy or less alert than they are normally. **Make sure you know how you react to this medicine before you drive, use machines, or do other jobs that could be dangerous if you are dizzy, drowsy, or are not alert.** After you have taken several doses of this medicine, these effects should lessen.

POSSIBLE SIDE EFFECTS OF THIS MEDICINE

The following side effects may occur more or less often than listed, depending on which medicine you are taking.

Side Effects That Should Be Reported To Your Doctor

Less common—Dizziness; dizziness or lightheadedness when standing up; fainting (sudden); fast, irregular, or pounding heartbeat; loss of bladder control (prazosin only); shortness of breath; swelling of feet or lower legs

Rare—Chest pain; continuing, painful, inappropriate erection of the penis (prazosin only); shortness of breath (prazosin only)

Side Effects That Usually Do Not Require Medical Attention

These possible side effects may go away during treatment; however, if they continue or are bothersome, check with your doctor, nurse, or pharmacist.

More common—Drowsiness; headache; unusual tiredness or weakness

Less common—Dryness of mouth (prazosin only); nausea; nervousness (doxazosin and prazosin only)

For doxazosin only (in addition to those listed above)— Restlessness; runny nose; unusual irritability

For prazosin only—rare (in addition to those listed above)—Frequent urge to urinate

For terazosin only (in addition to those listed above)— Back or joint pain; blurred vision; stuffy nose

Other side effects not listed above may also occur in some patients. If you notice any other effects, check with your doctor, nurse, or pharmacist.

DRONABINOL   Systemic

■ For the Pharmacist ■

In providing consultation, consider emphasizing the following selected information (» = major clinical significance):

Before using this medication
» Conditions affecting use, especially:
   Sensitivity to marijuana products or sesame oil
   Pregnancy—No studies in humans; increased risk of fetal mortality and resorptions in animal studies with doses many times the usual human dose
   Breast-feeding—Not recommended; distributed into breast milk
   Use in children—Caution recommended because of psychoactive effects and potential for dependence
   Use in the elderly—Caution recommended because of psychoactive effects and potential for dependence
   Other medications, especially CNS depressants

Proper use of this medication
» Importance of not taking more medication than the amount prescribed because of danger of overdose
» Proper dosing
» Missed dose: Taking as soon as possible; not taking if almost time for next dose; not doubling doses
» Proper storage

Precautions while using this medication
» Avoiding use of alcohol or other CNS depressants during therapy
» Caution if dizziness, drowsiness, lightheadedness, or false sense of well-being occurs
» Caution when getting up suddenly from a lying or sitting position
» Suspected overdose: Getting emergency help at once

Side/adverse effects
   Signs of potential side effects, especially psychotomimetic effects and tachycardia

▲ For the Patient ▲

915654

ABOUT YOUR MEDICINE

Dronabinol (droe-NAB-i-nol) is used to prevent the nausea and vomiting that may occur after treatment with cancer medicines. It is used only when other kinds of medicine for nausea and vomiting do not work. Dronabinol is also used to increase appetite in patients with acquired immunodeficiency syndrome (AIDS).

If any of the information in this leaflet causes you special concern or if you want additional information about your medicine and its use, check with your doctor, nurse, or pharmacist. **Remember, keep this and all other medicines out of the reach of children and never share your medicines with others.**

BEFORE USING THIS MEDICINE

Tell your doctor, nurse, and pharmacist if you . . .

- are allergic to any medicine, either prescription or non-prescription (OTC);
- are pregnant or intend to become pregnant while using this medicine;
- are breast-feeding;
- are taking any other prescription or nonprescription (OTC) medicine, especially CNS depressants or tricyclic antidepressants;
- have any other medical problems, especially manic depression or schizophrenia.

PROPER USE OF THIS MEDICINE

Take this medicine only as directed by your physician. Do not take more of it, do not take it more often, and do not take it for a longer time than your doctor ordered. If too much is taken, it may lead to medical problems because of an overdose.

If you miss a dose of this medicine, take it as soon as you remember. However, if it is almost time for your next dose, skip the missed dose and go back to your regular dosing schedule. **Do not double doses.**

PRECAUTIONS WHILE USING THIS MEDICINE

Dronabinol will add to the effects of alcohol and other CNS depressants (medicines that slow down the nervous system). **Check with your doctor before taking any such depressants while you are taking this medicine.**

This medicine may cause some people to become drowsy, dizzy, or lightheaded, or to feel a false sense of well-being. **Make sure you know how you react to this medicine before you drive, use machines, or do other jobs that require you to be alert and clearheaded.**

Dizziness, lightheadedness, or fainting may occur, especially when you get up suddenly from a lying or sitting position. Getting up slowly may help lessen this problem.

If you think you or someone else may have taken an overdose of dronabinol, get emergency help at once. Taking an overdose of this medicine or taking alcohol or CNS depressants with this medicine may lead to severe mental effects. Signs of overdose include changes in mood, confusion, hallucinations, mental depression, nervousness or anxiety, and fast or pounding heartbeat.

POSSIBLE SIDE EFFECTS OF THIS MEDICINE

Side Effects That Should Be Reported To Your Doctor Immediately

> *Less common (may also be signs of overdose)*—Changes in mood; confusion, nervousness, or anxiety; fast or pounding heartbeat; hallucinations; mental depression

Side Effects That Usually Do Not Require Medical Attention

These possible side effects may go away during treatment; however, if they continue or are bothersome, check with your doctor, nurse, or pharmacist.

> *More common*—Clumsiness or unsteadiness; dizziness; drowsiness; trouble thinking

> *Less common or rare*—Blurred vision or any changes in vision; dryness of mouth; feeling faint or lightheaded; restlessness; unusual tiredness or weakness

Other side effects not listed above may also occur in some patients. If you notice any other effects, check with your doctor, nurse, or pharmacist.

EPINEPHRINE   Ophthalmic

■ For the Pharmacist ■

In providing consultation, consider emphasizing the following selected information (» = major clinical significance):

Before using this medication
» Conditions affecting use, especially:
    Sensitivity to epinephrine or sulfites
    Other medical problems, especially cardiovascular disease, angle-closure glaucoma, or predisposition to angle-closure glaucoma

Proper use of this medication
» Importance of not using more medication than the amount prescribed
    Proper administration technique
    Preventing contamination: Not touching applicator tip to any surface; keeping container tightly closed
    Not using if medication becomes discolored or contains a precipitate
» Proper dosing
    Missed dose: Applying as soon as possible; if almost time for next dose, skipping missed dose and returning to regular dosing schedule; not doubling doses
» Proper storage

Precautions while using this medication
    Regular visits to physician to check eye pressure during therapy

Side/adverse effects
    Signs of potential side effects, especially maculopathy in aphakic eyes or signs of systemic absorption

▲ For the Patient ▲

913080

GLAUCOMA EYE MEDICINE—EPINEPHRINE-TYPE: *Including Dipivefrin; Epinephrine; Epinephryl Borate.*

ABOUT YOUR MEDICINE

Epinephrine-type (ep-i-NEF-rin) **glaucoma eye medicines** are used in the eye to treat certain types of glaucoma. Epinephrine and epinephryl borate may also be used in eye surgery.

If any of the information in this leaflet causes you special concern or if you want additional information about your medicine and its use, check with your doctor, nurse, or pharmacist. **Remember, keep this and all other medicines out of the reach of children and never share your medicines with others.**

BEFORE USING THIS MEDICINE
Tell your doctor, nurse, and pharmacist if you . . .
- are allergic to any medicine, either prescription or non-prescription (OTC);
- are pregnant or intend to become pregnant while using this medicine;
- are breast-feeding;
- are taking any other prescription or nonprescription (OTC) medicine;
- have any other medical problems, especially heart or blood vessel disease, or other eye disease.

PROPER USE OF THIS MEDICINE
Use this medicine only as directed. Do not use more of it and do not use it more often than your doctor ordered. To do so may increase the chance of too much medicine being absorbed into the body and the chance of side effects.

To use:
- First, wash your hands. Tilt the head back and, pressing your finger gently on the skin just beneath the lower eyelid, pull the lower eyelid away from the eye to make a space. Drop the medicine into this space. Let go of the eyelid and gently close the eyes. Do not blink. Keep the eyes closed and apply pressure to the inner corner of the eye with your finger for 1 or 2 minutes to allow the medicine to be absorbed by the eye.
- Immediately after using the eye drops, wash your hands to remove any medicine that may be on them.
- To keep the medicine as germ-free as possible, do not touch the applicator tip to any surface (including the eye) and keep the container tightly closed.

For patients using dipivefrin with the compliance cap (C Cap):
- Before using the eye drops for the first time, make sure the number 1 or the correct day of the week appears in the window of the cap.
- Remove the cap and use the eye drops as directed.
- Replace the cap. Holding the cap between your thumb and forefinger, rotate the bottle until the cap clicks to the next position. This will tell you your next dose.
- After every dose, rotate the bottle until the cap clicks to the position that tells you your next dose.

For patients using epinephrine ophthalmic solution:
- Do not use if the solution turns pinkish or brownish in color, or if it becomes cloudy.

For patients using epinephryl borate ophthalmic solution:
- The color of this solution may vary from colorless to amber yellow. Do not use if the solution turns dark brown or becomes cloudy.

If you miss a dose of this medicine, apply the missed dose as soon as possible. However, if it is almost time for your next dose, skip the missed dose and go back to your regular dosing schedule. Do not double doses.

PRECAUTIONS WHILE USING THIS MEDICINE

Your doctor should check your eye pressure at regular visits.

Dipivefrin may cause blurred vision or other vision problems for a short time after each dose is applied. If any of these occur, **do not drive, use machines, or do other jobs that require you to see well.**

POSSIBLE SIDE EFFECTS OF THIS MEDICINE

Side Effects That Should Be Reported To Your Doctor

Less common—Blurred or decreased vision

Possible signs of too much medicine being absorbed into the body—Fast, irregular, or pounding heartbeat; feeling faint; increase in blood pressure; increased sweating; paleness; trembling

Side Effects That Usually Do Not Require Medical Attention

These possible side effects may go away during treatment; however, if they continue or are bothersome, check with your doctor, nurse, or pharmacist.

More common—Headache or browache; stinging, burning, redness, or other eye irritation; watering of eyes

Less common—Eye pain or ache; increased sensitivity of eyes to light

Other side effects not listed above may also occur in some patients. If you notice any other effects, check with your doctor, nurse, or pharmacist.

ERGOLOID MESYLATES Systemic

■For the Pharmacist■

In providing consultation, consider emphasizing the following selected information (» = major clinical significance):

Before using this medication
» Conditions affecting use, especially:
Sensitivity to ergoloid mesylates
Other medical problems, especially bradycardia, hypotension, or acute or chronic psychosis

Proper use of this medication
» Importance of not using more or less medication than the amount prescribed
Proper administration of sublingual tablet: Dissolving tablet under tongue; not eating, drinking or smoking while tablet is dissolving
» Proper dosing
Missed dose: Not taking missed dose; not doubling doses; checking with physician if two or more doses in a row are missed
» Proper storage

Precautions while using this medication
Importance of regular monitoring by physician
» May require several weeks before clinical response is noted; checking with physician before discontinuing medication

Side/adverse effects
Signs of potential side effects, especially bradycardia, orthostatic hypotension, and skin rash

▲ For the Patient ▲

913794

ABOUT YOUR MEDICINE

Ergoloid mesylates (ER-goe-loid MESS-i-lates) belongs to the group of medicines known as ergot alkaloids. It is used to treat some mood, behavior, or other problems that may be due to changes in the brain from Alzheimer's disease or several small strokes. This medicine is different from other ergot alkaloids such as ergotamine and methysergide. It is not useful for treating migraine headache.

If any of the information in this leaflet causes you special concern or if you want additional information about your medicine and its use, check with your doctor, nurse, or pharmacist. **Remember, keep this and all other medicines out of the reach of children and never share your medicines with others.**

BEFORE USING THIS MEDICINE

Tell your doctor, nurse, and pharmacist if you . . .
- are allergic to any medicine, either prescription or non-prescription (OTC);
- are pregnant or intend to become pregnant while using this medicine;

- are breast-feeding;
- are taking any other prescription or nonprescription (OTC) medicine;
- have any other medical problems, especially low blood pressure, other mental problems, or slow heartbeat.

PROPER USE OF THIS MEDICINE
Take this medicine only as directed by your doctor. Do not take more or less of it, and do not take it more often or for a longer period of time than your doctor ordered. To do so may increase the chance of unwanted effects.

For patients taking the sublingual (under-the-tongue) tablets:
- Dissolve the tablet under your tongue. The sublingual tablet should not be chewed or swallowed since it works much faster when absorbed through the lining of the mouth. Do not eat, drink, or smoke while a tablet is dissolving.

If you miss a dose of this medicine, skip the missed dose and go back to your regular dosing schedule. Do not double doses. If you have any questions about this, or if you miss two or more doses in a row, check with your doctor.

PRECAUTIONS WHILE USING THIS MEDICINE
It is important that your doctor check your progress at regular visits to make sure this medicine is working and to check for unwanted effects.

It may take several weeks for this medicine to work. **However, do not stop taking this medicine without first checking with your doctor.**

POSSIBLE SIDE EFFECTS OF THIS MEDICINE
Side Effects That Should Be Reported To Your Doctor

> *Less common or rare*—Dizziness or lightheadedness when getting up from a lying or sitting position; drowsiness; skin rash; slow pulse

Side Effects That Usually Do Not Require Medical Attention

These possible side effects may go away during treatment; however, if they continue or are bothersome, check with your doctor, nurse, or pharmacist.

> *Less common or rare*—Soreness under tongue (with sublingual use)

Other side effects not listed above may also occur in some patients. If you notice any other effects, check with your doctor, nurse, or pharmacist.

ERGONOVINE Systemic

■ For the Pharmacist ■

In providing consultation, consider emphasizing the following selected
information (» = major clinical significance):

Before using this medication
» Conditions affecting use, especially:
   Allergies, hypersensitivity, or intolerance to ergonovine or other
      ergot alkaloids
   Pregnancy—Should not be administered prior to delivery or de-
      livery of the placenta
   Breast-feeding—Ergot alkaloids are excreted in breast milk
   Other medical problems, especially cardiac or vascular disease,
      hepatic function impairment, severe hypertension or history
      of hypertension, renal function impairment, and sepsis

Proper use of this medication
» Importance of not using more medication or for longer than pre-
      scribed; risk of ergotism and gangrene with prolonged use
» Proper dosing
   Missed dose: Not taking at all; not doubling doses
» Proper storage

Precautions while using this medication
   Notifying physician if infection develops, since infection may cause
      increased sensitivity to medication

Side/adverse effects
   Signs of potential side effects, especially allergic reaction, coronary
      vasospasm or other cardiovascular complications, dyspnea, se-
      vere hypertension, or peripheral vasospasm

▲ For the Patient ▲

913808

ERGONOVINE/METHYLERGONOVINE (Oral):
Including Ergonovine; Methylergonovine.

ABOUT YOUR MEDICINE

Ergonovine (er-goe-NOE-veen) and **methylergonovine** (meth-
ill-er-goe-NOE-veen) belong to the group of medicines known
as ergot alkaloids. These medicines are usually given to stop
heavy bleeding that sometimes occurs after the birth of a
baby. Ergonovine and methylergonovine may also be used
for other conditions as determined by your doctor.

If any of the information in this leaflet causes you special
concern or if you want additional information about your
medicine and its use, check with your doctor, nurse, or pharmacist. **Remember, keep this and all other medicines out of
the reach of children and never share your medicines with
others.**

BEFORE USING THIS MEDICINE
Tell your doctor, nurse, and pharmacist if you . . .
- are allergic to any medicine, either prescription or non-prescription (OTC);
- are pregnant or intend to become pregnant while using this medicine;
- are breast-feeding;
- are taking any other prescription or nonprescription (OTC) medicine, especially bromocriptine, nitrates or other medicines for angina, or other ergot alkaloids;
- have any other medical problems, especially angina (chest pain), blood vessel disease, high blood pressure, infection, kidney disease, liver disease, Raynaud's phenomenon, or stroke (history of).

PROPER USE OF THIS MEDICINE
Take this medicine only as directed by your doctor. Do not take more of it, do not take it more often, and do not take it for a longer time than your doctor ordered. If too much is taken or if it is taken for a longer time than your doctor ordered, it may cause serious effects.

If you miss a dose of this medicine, do not take the missed dose at all and do not double the next one. Instead, go back to your regular dosing schedule.

PRECAUTIONS WHILE USING THIS MEDICINE
If you have an infection or illness of any kind, check with your doctor before taking this medicine, since you may be more sensitive to the effects of it.

POSSIBLE SIDE EFFECTS OF THIS MEDICINE
Side Effects That Should Be Reported To Your Doctor Immediately

> *Less common*—Chest pain

> *Rare*—Blurred vision; convulsions (seizures); crushing chest pain; headache (sudden and severe); irregular heartbeat; unexplained shortness of breath

Other Side Effects That Should Be Reported To Your Doctor

> *Less common*—Slow heartbeat

> *Rare*—Itching of skin; pain in arms, legs, or lower back; pale or cold hands or feet; weakness in legs

> *With long-term use*—Dry, shriveled-looking skin on hands, lower legs, or feet; false feeling of insects crawling on the skin; pain and redness in an arm or leg; paralysis of one side of the body

Side Effects That Usually Do Not Require Medical Attention

These possible side effects may go away during treatment; however, if they continue or are bothersome, check with your doctor, nurse, or pharmacist.

> *More common*—Cramping of the uterus; nausea; vomiting

Other side effects not listed above may also occur in some patients. If you notice any other effects, check with your doctor, nurse, or pharmacist.

ERGOTAMINE, BELLADONNA ALKALOIDS, AND PHENOBARBITAL Systemic

■ For the Pharmacist ■

In providing consultation, consider emphasizing the following selected information (» = major clinical significance):

Before using this medication
» Conditions affecting use, especially:
  Allergies to ergotamine, belladonna alkaloids, or barbiturates
  Pregnancy—Use is not recommended because of ergotamine's oxytocic activity; also, belladonna alkaloids and barbiturates cross placenta; phenobarbital may cause fetal abnormalities and neonatal hemorrhage
  Breast-feeding—Ergot alkaloids inhibit lactation; also, they are distributed into breast milk and may cause ergotism in the infant; belladonna alkaloids may also inhibit lactation; phenobarbital is distributed into breast milk and may cause CNS depression in the infant
  Use in children—Increased susceptibility to toxic effects of belladonna alkaloids; increased response to belladonna alkaloids in children with spastic paralysis or brain damage; also, risk of paradoxical phenobarbital-induced excitement in hypersensitive children
  Use in the elderly—Increased risk of hypothermia and other adverse effects associated with peripheral vasoconstriction; also, increased susceptibility to mental and other toxic effects of anticholinergics and barbiturates; danger of precipitating undiagnosed glaucoma; possible memory impairment
  Other medications, especially other anticholinergics, antacids, anticoagulants, antidiarrheals, carbamazepine, CNS depressants, corticosteroids or corticotropin, estrogen- and progestin-containing oral contraceptives, other ergot alkaloids, ketoconazole, monoamine oxidase (MAO) inhibitors, potassium chloride, and other vasoconstrictors (including those present in local anesthetic solutions)
  Other medical problems, especially angina pectoris, coronary artery disease, gastrointestinal obstructive disease, glaucoma, hepatic function impairment, hypertension, severe infection, peripheral vascular disease, pruritus, renal function impairment, urinary retention, and recent or contemplated angioplasty or vascular surgery

Proper use of this medication
» Importance of not using more medication than the amount prescribed; risk of ergotism with overdosage; habit-forming potential
  Proper administration of extended-release tablets: Swallowing whole without crushing, breaking, or chewing
» Proper dosing
  Missed dose: Not taking missed dose at all; not doubling doses
» Proper storage

Precautions while using this medication
» Checking with physician before discontinuing medication after prolonged use; gradual dosage reduction may be necessary to avoid the possibility of withdrawal symptoms

Avoiding antacids and antidiarrheal medication within 1 hour of taking this medication

» Avoiding use of alcohol or other central nervous system (CNS) depressants; alcohol also aggravates headache

» Caution when driving or doing jobs requiring alertness because of possible dizziness, lightheadedness, or drowsiness

Avoiding smoking, since nicotine constricts blood vessels

Avoiding exposure to excessive cold, which may aggravate peripheral vasoconstriction

» Caution during exercise and hot weather; overheating may result in heat stroke

Possible increased sensitivity of eyes to light

Notifying physician if infection develops, since infection may cause increased sensitivity to medication

Possible dryness of mouth, nose, and throat; using sugarless candy or gum, ice or saliva substitute for relief; checking with physician or dentist if dry mouth continues for more than 2 weeks

Side/adverse effects

Signs and symptoms of potential side effects, especially agranulocytosis, allergic reactions, edema, fast or slow heartbeat, gangrene, hepatitis, increased intraocular pressure, cerebral or peripheral ischemia, thrombocytopenia, and coronary or ocular vasospasm

---

▲ For the Patient ▲

913070

ERGOT MEDICINES (Oral): *Including Ergotamine; Ergotamine, Belladonna Alkaloids, and Phenobarbital; Ergotamine and Caffeine; Ergotamine, Caffeine, Belladonna Alkaloids, and Pentobarbital.*

ABOUT YOUR MEDICINE

Ergot medicines are used to treat migraine headaches and some kinds of throbbing headaches. They are not used to prevent headaches but are used to relieve a headache once it has started. Some of these medicines may also be used for other conditions as determined by your doctor.

If any of the information in this leaflet causes you special concern or if you want additional information about your medicine and its use, check with your doctor, nurse, or pharmacist. **Remember, keep this and all other medicines out of the reach of children and never share your medicines with others.**

BEFORE USING THIS MEDICINE

Tell your doctor, nurse, and pharmacist if you . . .

- are allergic to any medicine, either prescription or nonprescription (OTC);
- are pregnant or intend to become pregnant while using this medicine;
- are breast-feeding;
- are taking **any** other prescription or nonprescription (OTC) medicine;

- have **any** other medical problems;
- use cocaine;
- regularly drink large amounts of caffeine-containing beverages such as coffee, tea, soft drinks, or cocoa.

PROPER USE OF THIS MEDICINE

Take this medicine only as directed by your doctor. If the amount you are to take does not relieve your headache, do not take more than your doctor ordered. Instead, check with your doctor. Taking too much of this medicine or taking it too often may cause serious effects such as nausea and vomiting; cold, painful hands or feet; or even gangrene, especially in elderly patients.

This medicine works best if you:
- **Take it at the first sign of headache or migraine attack.**
- **Lie down in a quiet, dark room for at least 2 hours after taking it.**

PRECAUTIONS WHILE USING THIS MEDICINE

Since drinking alcoholic beverages may make headaches worse, it is best to avoid use of alcohol while you are suffering from them.

Since smoking may increase some of the harmful effects of this medicine, it is best to avoid smoking while you are using it.

If you have a serious infection or illness of any kind, check with your doctor before taking this medicine, since you may be more sensitive to its effects.

This medicine may make you more sensitive to cold temperatures, especially if you have blood circulation problems. Dress warmly during cold weather and be careful during prolonged exposure to cold, such as in winter sports. This is especially important for elderly people.

Belladonna alkaloids (may be contained in this medicine) also may cause your eyes to become more sensitive to light than they are normally. Wearing sunglasses may help lessen the discomfort from bright light.

The caffeine in this combination medicine may interfere with the results of a test that uses dipyridamole (e.g., Persantine) to help find out how well your blood is flowing through certain blood vessels. You should not have any caffeine for at least 4 hours before the test.

POSSIBLE SIDE EFFECTS OF THIS MEDICINE

Side Effects That Should Be Reported To Your Doctor Immediately

Changes in vision; confusion; convulsions (seizures); fever; mental depression; muscle twitching; numbness and tingling of fingers, toes, or face; red or violet blisters on skin of hands or feet; ringing or other sounds in ears; seeing flashes of "zig-zag" lights; shortness of breath; stomach pain or bloating; tiredness or weakness; slurred speech; unusually fast, irregular, or slow heartbeat

Other Side Effects That Should Be Reported To Your Doctor

More common—Headaches, more often and/or more severe than before; swelling of feet and lower legs

Less common or rare—Anxiety; chest pain; eye pain; hives or itching of skin; pain in arms, legs, or lower back; pale or cold hands or feet; sore throat and fever; unusual bleeding or bruising; yellow eyes or skin

Side Effects That Usually Do Not Require Medical Attention

These possible side effects may go away during treatment; however, if they continue or are bothersome, check with your doctor, nurse, or pharmacist.

More common—Decreased sweating; diarrhea; dizziness; dryness of mouth, nose, throat, or skin; nausea or vomiting

Other side effects not listed above may also occur in some patients. If you notice any other effects, check with your doctor, nurse, or pharmacist.

After you stop using this medicine, your body may need time to adjust. The length of time this takes depends on the amount of medicine you were using and how long you used it. During this time check with your doctor if your headaches begin again or worsen.

358

ERYTHROMYCINS Systemic

Including Erythromycin; Erythromycin Estolate;
Erythromycin Ethylsuccinate; Erythromycin Gluceptate;
Erythromycin Lactobionate; Erythromycin Stearate.

■ For the Pharmacist ■

In providing consultation, consider emphasizing the following selected
information (» = major clinical significance):

Before using this medication
» Conditions affecting use, especially:
  Hypersensitivity to erythromycins or other macrolides
  Pregnancy—Erythromycins cross the placenta; erythromycin es-
  tolate has been associated with an increased risk of reversible,
  subclinical hepatotoxicity in pregnant women
  Breast-feeding—Erythromycins are distributed into breast milk
  Dental—Oral candidiasis may occur with long-term therapy
  Other medications, especially alfentanil, astemizole, carba-
  mazepine, chloramphenicol, cyclosporine, other hepatotoxic
  medications, lincomycins, terfenadine, warfarin, and xanthines
  Other medical problems, especially a history of cardiac arrhythmias or QT prolongation or hepatic function impairment

Proper use of this medication
  Taking with a full glass of water, on an empty stomach; may be
  taken with food if stomach upset occurs
  Proper administration technique for oral liquids and/or pediatric
  drops, chewable tablets, delayed-release capsules and tablets
  Not using oral liquids and/or pediatric drops after expiration date
» Compliance with full course of therapy, especially in streptococcal
  infections
» Importance of not missing doses and taking at evenly spaced times
» Proper dosing
  Missed dose: Taking as soon as possible; not taking if almost time
  for next dose; not doubling dose
» Proper storage

Precautions while using this medication
  Checking with physician if no improvement within a few days

Side/adverse effects
  Signs of potential side effects, especially, hepatotoxicity, hypersensitivity, inflammation or phlebitis at the injection site, cardiac
  toxicity, loss of hearing, or pancreatitis

▲ For the Patient ▲

912827

ABOUT YOUR MEDICINE

Erythromycins (eh-rith-roe-MYE-sins) are used to treat infections caused by bacteria. They will not work for colds,
flu, or other virus infections. Erythromycins are also used
to prevent "strep" infections in patients with a history of
rheumatic heart disease who may be allergic to penicillin.

These medicines may also be used in Legionnaires' disease and for other problems as determined by your doctor.

If any of the information in this leaflet causes you special concern or if you want additional information about your medicine and its use, check with your doctor, nurse, or pharmacist. **Remember, keep this and all other medicines out of the reach of children and never share your medicines with others.**

BEFORE USING THIS MEDICINE

Tell your doctor, nurse, and pharmacist if you . . .
- are allergic to any medicine, either prescription or non-prescription (OTC);
- are pregnant or intend to become pregnant while using this medicine;
- are breast-feeding;
- are taking **any** other prescription or nonprescription (OTC) medicine;
- are taking astemizole, terfenadine, or terfenadine-containing medicines;
- have any other medical problems, especially liver disease.

PROPER USE OF THIS MEDICINE

Generally, erythromycins are best taken with a full glass (8 ounces) of water on an empty stomach (at least 1 hour before or 2 hours after meals). If stomach upset occurs, erythromycins may be taken with food. If you have any questions about this, check with your doctor or pharmacist.

To help clear up your infection completely, **keep taking this medicine for the full time of treatment** even if you begin to feel better after a few days; **do not miss any doses. This is especially important if you have a "strep" infection since serious heart problems could develop later** if your infection is not cleared up completely.

If you do miss a dose of this medicine, take it as soon as possible. This will help to keep a constant amount of medicine in the blood. However, if it is almost time for your next dose, skip the missed dose and go back to your regular dosing schedule. Do not double doses.

PRECAUTIONS WHILE USING THIS MEDICINE

If your symptoms do not improve within a few days, or if they become worse, check with your doctor.

This medicine must not be given to other people or used for other infections unless you are otherwise directed by your doctor.

POSSIBLE SIDE EFFECTS OF THIS MEDICINE

Side Effects That Should Be Reported To Your Doctor Immediately

Less common—Skin rash, hives, itching

Less common with erythromycin estolate (rare with other erythromycins)—Dark or amber urine; pale stools; stomach pain (severe); unusual tiredness or weakness; yellow eyes or skin

Rare (with liver or kidney disease and high doses)—Fainting; temporary loss of hearing

Side Effects That Usually Do Not Require Medical Attention

These possible side effects may go away during treatment; however, if they continue or are bothersome, check with your doctor, nurse, or pharmacist.

More common—Diarrhea; nausea or vomiting; stomach cramping and discomfort

Less common—Sore mouth or tongue

Other side effects not listed above may also occur in some patients. If you notice any other effects, check with your doctor, nurse, or pharmacist.

ESTROGENS   Systemic

Including Chlorotrianisene; Diethylstilbestrol; Estradiol (Oral); Estradiol (Transdermal); Estrogens, Conjugated; Estrogens, Esterified; Estrone; Estropipate; Ethinyl Estradiol; Quinestrol.

■For the Pharmacist■

In providing consultation, consider emphasizing the following selected information (» = major clinical significance):

Before using this medication
» Conditions affecting use, especially:
    Sensitivity to estrogens
    Carcinogenicity—Increased risk of endometrial cancer for patients with intact uteri placed on unopposed estrogen replacement therapy; decreased risk occurs when used with a progestin; male breast cancer has occurred in association with estrogen use; continuous, long-term estrogen use in animal studies increased frequency of cancers of the breast, cervix, and liver
    Pregnancy—Use of some estrogens suggested to be associated with congenital abnormalities
    Breast-feeding—Use is not recommended because estrogens are distributed into breast milk and may have unpredictable effects
    Use in children—Use in children or growing adolescents may slow or stop growth
    Other medications, especially bromocriptine, cyclosporine, or hepatotoxic medications; smoking tobacco may increase risk of cardiovascular side effects and increase metabolism of estrogen
    Other medical problems, especially some types of breast cancer; abnormal and undiagnosed vaginal bleeding; history of estrogen-induced thrombophlebitis, thrombosis, or thromboembolic disorders; or active thrombophlebitis or thromboembolic disorders
» Reading patient package insert carefully

Proper use of this medication
» Proper storage
For oral or parenteral dosage forms
» Compliance with therapy
    Taking with or immediately after food to reduce nausea
    Missed dose: Taking as soon as possible; not taking if almost time for next dose; not doubling doses
For transdermal estradiol
    Reading patient directions
    Washing and drying hands thoroughly before and after application
    Applying to clean, dry, non-oily, hairless, intact area of skin on the abdomen or buttocks; not applying over cuts or irritation
» Not applying to breasts; not applying to waistline or other areas where tight clothes may rub disk loose
    Pressing the disk firmly in place with palm for about 10 seconds; making sure there is good contact, especially around edges
    Reapplying disk if it comes loose, or discarding and applying a new one

Applying each patch to different area of skin on abdomen or buttocks so at least 1 week elapses before the area is used again to
help prevent skin irritation
» Proper dosing
Missed dose: Using as soon as possible; not using if almost time for
next dose; not doubling doses

Precautions while using this medication
» Regular visits to physician every year, or more often, as determined
by physician
Possibility of dental problems, such as tenderness, swelling, or bleeding of gums; brushing and flossing teeth, massaging gums, and
having dentist clean teeth regularly; checking with dentist if
there are questions about care of teeth or gums or if tenderness,
swelling, or bleeding of gums is noticed
» Stopping medication immediately and checking with physician if
pregnancy is suspected
Importance of not giving medication to anyone else

Side/adverse effects
Withdrawal bleeding will occur in many postmenopausal patients
with an intact uterus who are placed on cyclic estrogen therapy
with a progestin
Signs of potential side effects, especially menstrual irregularities,
chorea, breast pain or tenderness, breast tumors, enlargement of
breasts in females, gynecomastia in males treated for prostatic
cancer, peripheral edema, gallbladder obstruction, hepatitis; for
treatment of prostatic cancer and male breast cancer only—
thromboembolism or thrombus formation

▲ For the Patient ▲

915188

ESTROGENS (Oral): *Including Chlorotrianisene; Diethylstilbestrol; Estradiol (Oral); Estrogens, Conjugated; Estrogens, Esterified; Estropipate; Ethinyl Estradiol; Quinestrol.*

ABOUT YOUR MEDICINE
Estrogens (ESS-troe-jenz) are produced by the body and are
necessary for the normal sexual development of the female
and for the regulation of the menstrual cycle. They are prescribed for several reasons:
- to provide additional hormone when the body does not
produce enough of its own, as during the menopause or
following certain kinds of surgery.
- in the treatment of selected cases of breast cancer in
men and women.
- in the treatment of men with certain kinds of cancer of
the prostate.
- to help prevent osteoporosis in women past menopause.

Estrogens may also be used for other conditions as determined by your doctor.

If any of the information in this leaflet causes you special
concern or if you want additional information about your

medicine and its use, check with your doctor, nurse, or pharmacist. **Remember, keep this and all other medicines out of the reach of children and never share your medicines with others.**

BEFORE USING THIS MEDICINE

Tell your doctor, nurse, and pharmacist if you . . .
- are allergic to any medicine, either prescription or non-prescription (OTC);
- are pregnant or intend to become pregnant while using this medicine;
- are breast-feeding;
- are taking **any** other prescription or nonprescription (OTC) medicine;
- have any other medical problems, especially blood clots (or history of during estrogen therapy), breast cancer (active or suspected), changes in vaginal bleeding, heart or circulation disease, or stroke (for men); or if you smoke.

PROPER USE OF THIS MEDICINE

Most patients will receive an information sheet regarding the benefits and risks of this medicine. **Be sure you have read and understand that information.** This leaflet is not intended to replace that information sheet.

Take this medicine only as directed. Do not take more of it and do not take it for a longer time than your doctor ordered. Try to take the medicine at the same time each day to reduce the possibility of side effects.

If you miss a dose of this medicine, take it as soon as possible. However, if it is almost time for your next dose, skip the missed dose. Do not double doses.

PRECAUTIONS WHILE USING THIS MEDICINE

It is very important that your doctor check your progress at regular visits. These visits will usually be every year.

It is not yet known whether the use of estrogens increases the risk of breast cancer in women. Breast cancer has occurred rarely in men taking estrogens.

Cigarette smoking when using birth control pills containing estrogen has been found to increase the risk of serious side effects affecting the heart or circulation. **To reduce the risk, do not smoke cigarettes while using estrogens.**

If you think that you may be pregnant, stop using the medicine immediately and check with your doctor. Continued use of some estrogens during pregnancy may cause birth defects in the child. Diethylstilbestrol may also increase the risk of vaginal cancer developing in daughters when they reach childbearing age.

POSSIBLE SIDE EFFECTS OF THIS MEDICINE

Along with their wanted effects, **estrogens sometimes cause some serious unwanted effects.** Rarely, they have caused blood clots, stroke, and heart attack in men being treated with high doses for cancer. The prolonged use of estrogens has been reported to increase the risk of endometrial cancer (cancer of the lining of the uterus) in women after menopause. When estrogens are used in low doses for less than 1 year, there is less risk. The risk is also reduced if a progestin (another female hormone) is added to, or replaces part of, the estrogen dose. If the uterus has been removed, there is no risk of endometrial cancer.

Side Effects That Should Be Reported To Your Doctor Immediately

Stop taking this medicine and get emergency help immediately if any of the following side effects occur:

> *Rare (for males being treated for breast or prostate cancer only)*—Headache (sudden or severe); loss of coordination; change in vision (sudden); pains in chest, groin, or leg, especially in calf of leg; shortness of breath; slurring of speech; weakness or numbness in arm or leg

Other Side Effects That Should Be Reported To Your Doctor

> *More common*—Breast pain (in females and males); increased breast size (in females and males); swelling of feet and lower legs

> *Less common or rare*—Changes in vaginal bleeding; lumps in, or discharge from, breast (in females and males); pains in stomach, side, or abdomen; uncontrolled, jerky muscle movements; yellow eyes or skin

Also, many women who are taking estrogens with a progestin (another female hormone) and have not had their uterus removed will start having monthly vaginal bleeding, similar to menstrual periods, again.

Other side effects not listed above may also occur in some patients. If you notice any other effects, check with your doctor, nurse, or pharmacist.

▲ For the Patient ▲

917161

ESTRADIOL (Transdermal)

ABOUT YOUR MEDICINE

Estradiol (es-tra-DYE-ol) is an estrogen (a type of female hormone). It is necessary for sexual development of the female and regulation of the menstrual cycle during childbearing years.

Transdermal estradiol is used as a skin patch and is prescribed to provide additional hormone when the body does not produce enough of its own, as after menopause or certain kinds of surgery in females. Estradiol may also be used for other conditions as determined by your doctor.

If any of the information in this leaflet causes you special concern or if you want additional information about your medicine and its use, check with your doctor, nurse, or pharmacist. **Remember, keep this and all other medicines out of the reach of children and never share your medicines with others.**

BEFORE USING THIS MEDICINE

Tell your doctor, nurse, and pharmacist if you . . .

- are allergic to any medicine, either prescription or non-prescription (OTC);
- are pregnant or intend to become pregnant while using this medicine;
- are breast-feeding;
- are taking **any** other prescription or nonprescription (OTC) medicine;
- have any other medical problems, especially blood clots (or history of), breast cancer (active or suspected), or changes in vaginal bleeding;
- are a smoker.

PROPER USE OF THIS MEDICINE

This medicine usually comes with patient instructions. Read them carefully before using this medicine.

Wash and dry your hands thoroughly before and after handling the patch.

Do not trim or cut the patch to change the dose.

Put the patch on a clean, dry area of your abdomen (stomach) or buttocks that has little hair. Do not put it on scars, cuts, or irritations. **Do not apply the patch to the breasts** or to areas where clothes may rub it loose. Press the patch firmly in place to make sure it sticks. Put each patch on a different area of skin to prevent skin problems. Wait at least 1 week before you use the same area again.

With normal activity, the patch will stay in place, even during swimming, showering, or bathing. If a patch becomes loose or falls off, reapply it or discard it and apply a new one.

After taking off a used patch, fold it in half with sticky sides together. Discard carefully out of the reach of children.

If you forget to apply a new patch when you are supposed to, apply it as soon as possible. However, if it is almost time for the next patch, skip the missed one and go back to your regular schedule. Do not apply more than one patch at a time.

PRECAUTIONS WHILE USING THIS MEDICINE
It is very important that your doctor check your progress at regular visits to make sure this medicine does not cause unwanted effects.

It is not yet known whether the use of estrogens increases the risk of breast cancer in women. Check your breasts regularly for any unusual lumps or discharge and have a mammogram done if your doctor recommends it.

If you think that you may be pregnant, stop using the medicine immediately and check with your doctor. Continued use of some estrogens during pregnancy may cause birth defects in the child.

POSSIBLE SIDE EFFECTS OF THIS MEDICINE
Side Effects That Should Be Reported To Your Doctor

> *More common*—Breast pain; increased breast size; swelling of feet and lower legs; weight gain (rapid)

> *Less common or rare*—Changes in vaginal bleeding; lumps in, or discharge from, breast; pains in stomach, side, or abdomen; uncontrolled jerky muscle movements; yellow eyes or skin

Side Effects That Usually Do Not Require Medical Attention

These possible side effects may go away during treatment; however, if they continue or are bothersome, check with your doctor, nurse, or pharmacist.

> *More common*—Bloating of stomach; cramps of lower stomach; loss of appetite; nausea; skin irritation or redness where skin patch was worn

> *Less common*—Diarrhea (mild); dizziness (mild); headaches (mild); migraine headaches; problems in wearing contact lenses; unusual increase in sexual desire; vomiting (usually with high doses)

Many women who take estrogens with a progestin (another female hormone) start having monthly vaginal bleeding, similar to menstrual periods again. This effect continues for as long as the medicine is taken. However, monthly bleeding will not occur if the uterus has been removed by surgery (total hysterectomy).

Other side effects not listed above may also occur in some patients. If you notice any other effects, check with your doctor, nurse, or pharmacist.

ESTROGENS Vaginal

Including Dienestrol; Estradiol; Estrogens, Conjugated; Estrone; Estropipate.

■For the Pharmacist■

In providing consultation, consider emphasizing the following selected information (» = major clinical significance):

Before using this medication
» Conditions affecting use, especially:
  Sensitivity to estrogens
  Carcinogenicity—Increased risk of endometrial cancer for patients with an intact uterus placed on unopposed estrogen replacement therapy; decreased risk occurs when used with a progestin; continuous, long-term estrogen use in animal studies increased frequency of cancers of the breast, cervix, and liver
  Pregnancy—Use of some estrogens suggested to be associated with congenital abnormalities
  Breast-feeding—Use is not recommended because estrogens are excreted in breast milk and may have unpredictable effects
  Other medications, especially bromocriptine, cyclosporine, hepatotoxic medications; smoking tobacco may increase risk of cardiovascular side effects and increase metabolism of estrogen
  Other medical problems, especially some types of breast cancer; abnormal and undiagnosed vaginal bleeding; history of estrogen-induced thrombophlebitis, thrombosis, or thromboembolic disorders; or active thrombophlebitis or thromboembolic disorders

Proper use of this medication
» Reading patient package insert carefully
» Compliance with therapy
  Using medication at bedtime to increase effectiveness; wearing sanitary napkin to protect clothing
  Proper administration technique
» Proper dosing
  Missed dose: Not using missed dose at all but returning to regular dosing schedule
» Proper storage

Precautions while using this medication
» Regular visits to physician at least every year, or more often, as determined by physician
  Possibility of dental problems, such as tenderness, swelling, or bleeding of gums; brushing and flossing teeth, massaging gums, and having dentist clean teeth regularly; checking with dentist if there are questions about care of teeth or gums or if tenderness, swelling, or bleeding of gums is noticed
» Stopping medication immediately and checking with physician if pregnancy is suspected
  Importance of not giving medication to anyone else

Side/adverse effects
  Withdrawal bleeding will occur in many postmenopausal patients with an intact uterus who are placed on cyclic estrogen therapy with a progestin

Signs of potential side effects, especially menstrual irregularities, chorea, breast tumors, peripheral edema, gallbladder obstruction, or hepatitis

---

▲ For the Patient ▲

913885

ABOUT YOUR MEDICINE

Estrogens (ESS-troe-jenz) are female hormones. They are produced by the body and are necessary for the normal sexual development of the female and for the regulation of the menstrual cycle during the childbearing years.

Uncomfortable changes may occur in vaginal tissues when the body does not produce enough estrogens, as during the menopause. In order to relieve such uncomfortable conditions, estrogens are prescribed for vaginal use.

If any of the information in this leaflet causes you special concern or if you want additional information about your medicine and its use, check with your doctor, nurse, or pharmacist. **Remember, keep this and all other medicines out of the reach of children and never share your medicines with others.**

BEFORE USING THIS MEDICINE

Since vaginal estrogens may be absorbed into the body, the following should be kept in mind:
- Most patients will receive an information sheet regarding the benefits and risks of this medicine. **Be sure you have read and understand that information.** This leaflet is not intended to replace that information sheet.
- The prolonged use of estrogens has been reported to increase the risk of endometrial cancer (cancer of the lining of the uterus) in women after the menopause. When estrogens are used in low doses for less than 1 year, there is less risk. The risk is also reduced if a progestin (another female hormone) is added to, or replaces part of, the estrogen dose. If the uterus has been removed by surgery (hysterectomy), there is no risk of endometrial cancer.
- Cigarette smoking when using birth control pills containing estrogen has been found to increase the risk of serious side effects affecting the heart or circulation. **To reduce the risk, do not smoke cigarettes while using estrogens.**

Tell your doctor, nurse, and pharmacist if you . . .
- are allergic to any medicine, either prescription or nonprescription (OTC);
- are pregnant or intend to become pregnant while using this medicine;
- are breast-feeding;
- are taking **any** other prescription or nonprescription (OTC) medicine;

- have any other medical problems, especially blood clots (or history of during estrogen therapy), breast cancer (active or suspected), or changes in vaginal bleeding.

PROPER USE OF THIS MEDICINE

Use this medicine only as directed. Do not use more of it and do not use it for a longer time than your doctor ordered.

If you miss a dose of this medicine and do not remember it until the next day, do not use the missed dose at all. Instead, go back to your regular schedule.

PRECAUTIONS WHILE USING THIS MEDICINE

It is very important that your doctor check your progress at regular visits. These visits will usually be every year.

Certain brands of vaginal estrogens contain oils that can weaken latex (rubber) condoms, diaphragms, or cervical caps. This increases the chance of a condom breaking during sexual intercourse. The rubber in cervical caps or diaphragms may break down faster and wear out sooner. Check with your doctor, nurse, or pharmacist to make sure the vaginal estrogen product you are using can be used with latex (rubber) birth control devices.

It is not yet known whether the use of estrogens increases the risk of breast cancer in women.

If you think that you may be pregnant, stop using the medicine immediately and check with your doctor. Continued use of some estrogens during pregnancy may cause birth defects in the child.

POSSIBLE SIDE EFFECTS OF THIS MEDICINE
Side Effects That Should Be Reported To Your Doctor

More common—Pain, tenderness, or enlargement of breasts; swelling of feet and lower legs; weight gain (rapid)

Less common or rare—Changes in vaginal bleeding; lumps in, or discharge from, breast; pains in stomach, side, or abdomen; swelling, redness, or itching around vaginal area; uncontrolled, jerky muscle movements; yellow eyes or skin

Side Effects That Usually Do Not Require Medical Attention

These possible side effects may go away during treatment; however, if they continue or are bothersome, check with your doctor, nurse, or pharmacist.

More common—Bloating of stomach; cramps of lower stomach; loss of appetite

Also, many women who are using estrogens with a progestin (another female hormone) and have not had their uterus removed will start having monthly vaginal bleeding, similar to menstrual periods, again.

Other side effects not listed above may also occur in some patients. If you notice any other effects, check with your doctor, nurse, or pharmacist.

ESTROGENS AND PROGESTINS   Oral Contraceptives   Systemic

■ For the Pharmacist ■

In providing consultation, consider emphasizing the following selected information (» = major clinical significance):

Before using this medication
» Conditions affecting use, especially:
   Sensitivity to estrogens or progestins
   Pregnancy—Not recommended for use during pregnancy
   Breast-feeding—Oral contraceptives are distributed into breast milk
   Use in adolescents—Careful counseling may be required to increase possibility of compliance
   Dental—May increase possibility of bleeding of gingival tissues, gingival hyperplasia, or local alveolar osteitis (dry socket)
   Other medications, especially hepatic enzyme inducers, coumarin- or indandione-derivative anticoagulants, tricyclic antidepressants, bromocriptine, hepatotoxic medications (especially dantrolene), or tobacco smoking
   Other medical problems, especially known or suspected breast cancer; carcinoma of the uterus, cervix, or vagina; history of cerebrovascular accidents (especially if patient smokes cigarettes); cerebrovascular disease; history of cholestatic jaundice; coronary artery disease; benign or malignant hepatic tumors (active or history of); known or suspected estrogen-dependent neoplasms; known or suspected pregnancy; thrombophlebitis, thrombosis, or thromboembolic disorders (active, history of, or history of associated with previous estrogen use); endometriosis; gallbladder disease (or history of); hypercalcemia associated with tumors or metabolic bone disease; scanty or irregular menstrual periods; hepatic porphyria (acute, intermittent, or variegate); or uterine fibroids
» Reading patient package insert carefully

Proper use of this medication
» Compliance with therapy; taking medication at the same time each day, at 24-hour intervals
   Taking with or immediately after food to reduce nausea
   Keeping an extra 1-month supply available
   Keeping tablets in original container
   Taking tablets in proper (color-coded) sequence
» Proper dosing
   Missed doses for the monophasic, biphasic, or triphasic cycles:
   Missing the first tablet of a new cycle—Taking as soon as possible; if not remembered until next day, taking 2 tablets; continuing on regular dosing schedule and using another birth control method for seven days after the last missed dose
   Missing one day—Taking as soon as possible; if not remembered until next day, taking 2 tablets; continuing on regular dosing schedule
   Missing two days in a row in the first or second week—Taking 2 tablets a day for next 2 days, then continuing on regular dosing schedule; using second method of birth control for remainder of cycle
   Missing two days in a row in the third week; or

Missing three days in a row—
>   Using day-1 start: Discarding remaining doses for current cycle; beginning a new cycle following its dosing schedule and using a second method of birth control for seven days after the last missed dose; may miss one menstrual period but contacting health care professional if second menstrual period is missed
>   Using day-5 start: Continuing on regular dosing schedule for current cycle and using a second method of birth control until menstrual period begins; contacting health care professional if menstrual period is missed
>   Using Sunday start: Continuing on regular dosing schedule for current cycle until Sunday; on Sunday, throwing out remaining doses for current cycle and beginning a new cycle; using a second method of birth control for seven days after the last missed dose; may miss one menstrual period but contacting health care professional if second menstrual period is missed
> Missing any of the last seven tablets of a 28-day cycle is not important but beginning new cycle on time is essential

» Proper storage

Precautions while using this medication
» Regular visits to physician at least every 6 to 12 months to check progress
» Using a second method of contraception during the first 3 weeks when beginning use of oral contraceptives
» Caution if medical or dental surgery or emergency treatment is required—increased risk of thrombotic complications
» Using second method of birth control during each cycle in which the following medications are used: ampicillin, bacampicillin, chloramphenicol, dihydroergotamine, hepatic enzyme inducers, mineral oil, oral neomycin, penicillin V, sulfonamides, tetracyclines, or certain tranquilizers

What to expect and do if vaginal bleeding occurs

What to expect and do if menstrual period is missed

Possibility of dental problems, such as tenderness, swelling, or bleeding of gums; brushing and flossing teeth, massaging gums, and having dentist clean teeth regularly; checking with dentist if there are questions about care of teeth or gums or if tenderness, swelling, or bleeding of gums is noticed

Possibility of photosensitivity

Potential intolerance of contact lenses; contacting physician if wearing contact lenses and notice a change in vision or an inability to wear lenses

» Stopping medication immediately and checking with physician if pregnancy is suspected

If scheduled for laboratory tests, telling physician if taking birth control pills; certain blood tests may be affected by oral contraceptives

Caution about improper use of this type of medication

Not taking leftover oral contraceptives from an old prescription, especially after a pregnancy

Side/adverse effects
Signs of potential side effects, especially blood clots; possible breast tumors; changes in vaginal bleeding pattern; cystitis-like syndrome; fainting; hepatitis or gallbladder obstruction, or liver tumor; hepatoma; gradual increase in blood pressure; malignant melanoma; mental depression; retinal thrombosis or cataracts;

skin rash, redness, or other irritation; or vaginal candidiasis or vaginitis

Cigarette smoking combined with oral contraceptive use causes increased risk of serious side effects, especially for heavy smokers or women over age 35

▲ For the Patient ▲

913896

ABOUT YOUR MEDICINE

Most **oral contraceptives** (birth control pills) contain two types of female hormones, **estrogens** (ESS-troe-jenz) and **progestins** (proe-JESS-tins). They are taken by mouth on a regular schedule to prevent pregnancy. Some brands may also be used for other conditions as determined by your doctor. Oral contraceptives do not prevent venereal or sexually transmitted diseases (VD or STDs).

If any of the information in this leaflet causes you special concern or if you want additional information about your medicine and its use, check with your doctor, nurse, or pharmacist. **Remember, keep this and all other medicines out of the reach of children and never share your medicines with others.**

BEFORE USING THIS MEDICINE

Tell your doctor, nurse, and pharmacist if you . . .
- are allergic to any medicine, either prescription or non-prescription (OTC);
- suspect that you are pregnant;
- are breast-feeding;
- are taking **any** other prescription or nonprescription (OTC) medicine;
- smoke cigarettes;
- have **any** other medical problems.

PROPER USE OF THIS MEDICINE

You should get a paper (package insert) about the use of this medicine as well as risks of using it. **Be sure you have read and understand that information.** This leaflet does not replace that information.

Oral contraceptives must be taken exactly on schedule to prevent pregnancy. Take them at the same time each day, not more than 24 hours apart.

If you miss a dose of this medicine:
- **For one day**—Take the missed tablet as soon as you remember. If it is not remembered until the next day, take the missed tablet plus the tablet that is regularly scheduled for that day. With some products, you will need to use a second method of birth control to make sure that you are protected for the rest of the cycle (pill

packet). The package insert you got with your prescription should tell you if you need to take this extra precaution. If you have any questions about this, check with your doctor, nurse, or pharmacist.

- **For more than one day—Check with your doctor or the package insert for your product.** With certain brands, your doctor may need to tell you how to get back on a regular dosing schedule and how to avoid pregnancy.

PRECAUTIONS WHILE USING THIS MEDICINE

It is very important that your doctor check your progress at regular visits to make sure this medicine does not cause unwanted effects.

Tell the physician or dentist in charge that you are taking this medicine before having any kind of surgery or dental or emergency treatment.

Certain medicines may reduce the effectiveness of oral contraceptives. **Use a second method of birth control during each cycle (pill packet) in which any of the following medicines are used:** ampicillin, adrenocorticoids (cortisone-like medicine), bacampicillin, barbiturates, carbamazepine, chloramphenicol, dihydroergotamine, griseofulvin, mineral oil, neomycin (oral), penicillin V, phenylbutazone, phenytoin, primidone, rifampin, sulfonamides (sulfa medicine), tetracyclines, tranquilizers, valproic acid.

When you begin to use oral contraceptives, your body needs at least 7 days to adjust before pregnancy will be prevented. **Use a second method of birth control for the first cycle (pill packet) to be sure you are protected.**

Cigarette smoking when using oral contraceptives has been found to increase the risk of serious side effects affecting the heart and circulation. **To reduce the risk, do not smoke cigarettes while using oral contraceptives.**

If you think that you are pregnant, stop taking this medicine immediately and check with your doctor.

POSSIBLE SIDE EFFECTS OF THIS MEDICINE

Rarely, birth control pills cause serious effects such as benign (not cancerous) liver tumors, liver cancer, blood clots, heart attack and stroke, and problems of the gallbladder, liver, and uterus. These effects can be very serious and may cause death. **Carefully read the package insert you received with this medicine and discuss these effects with your doctor.**

Side Effects That Should Be Reported To Your Doctor Immediately

The following side effects may be caused by blood clots but rarely occur. However, **if they do occur, they require immediate medical attention. Get emergency help immediately if you have** abdominal or stomach pain (sudden, severe, or continuing); coughing up blood; headache (severe); loss of coordination; loss of or change in vision (sudden); shortness of breath (sudden or unexplained); slurring of speech; pains in chest, groin, or leg (especially in calf); unexplained weakness, numbness, or pain in arm or leg.

Other Side Effects That Should Be Reported To Your Doctor

> *Less common or rare*—Bulging eyes; changes in vaginal bleeding; double vision; fainting; frequent urge to urinate or painful urination; increased blood pressure; loss of vision; lumps in or discharge from breast; mental depression; skin rash, redness, or other skin irritation; swelling, pain, or tenderness in stomach, side, or abdomen; unusual or dark-colored mole; vaginal discharge (thick, white, or curd-like); vaginal itching or irritation; yellow eyes or skin

Side Effects That Usually Do Not Require Medical Attention

These possible side effects may go away during treatment; however, if they continue or are bothersome, check with your doctor, nurse, or pharmacist.

> *More common*—Acne; bloating of stomach; changes in appetite; cramps of lower stomach; nausea; swelling of ankles and feet; swelling and increased tenderness of breasts; unusual tiredness or weakness; unusual weight gain

Other side effects not listed above may also occur in some patients. If you notice any other effects, check with your doctor, nurse, or pharmacist.

ETHAMBUTOL   Systemic

■ For the Pharmacist ■

In providing consultation, consider emphasizing the following selected information (» = major clinical significance):

Before using this medication
» Conditions affecting use, especially:
    Pregnancy—Ethambutol crosses the placenta. However, problems in humans have not been documented
    Breast-feeding—Ethambutol is distributed into breast milk
    Use in children—Appropriate studies have not been done in children up to 13 years of age. Ethambutol is generally not recommended in children whose visual acuity cannot be monitored (younger than 6 years of age)
    Other medical problems, especially optic neuritis and renal function impairment

Proper use of this medication
    Taking with food if gastrointestinal irritation occurs
» Compliance with full course of therapy, which may take months or years
» Proper dosing
    Missed dose: Taking as soon as possible; not taking if almost time for next dose; not doubling doses
» Proper storage

Precautions while using this medication
    Checking with physician if no improvement within 2 or 3 weeks
» Regular visits to physician to check progress; need to report promptly to physician signs of optic neuritis and prodromal signs of peripheral neuritis; need for ophthalmologic examinations if signs of optic neuritis occur
» Caution if blurred vision or loss of vision occurs

Side/adverse effects
    Signs of potential side effects, especially acute gouty arthritis, hypersensitivity, peripheral neuritis, or retrobulbar optic neuritis

▲ For the Patient ▲

913900

ABOUT YOUR MEDICINE

Ethambutol (e-THAM-byoo-tole) is used to treat tuberculosis (TB). It is used with other medicines for TB. This medicine may also be used for other medical problems as determined by your doctor.

To help clear up your tuberculosis (TB) completely, you must keep taking this medicine for the full time of treatment, even if you begin to feel better. This is very important. It is also important that you do not miss any doses.

If any of the information in this leaflet causes you special concern or if you want additional information about your medicine and its use, check with your doctor, nurse, or pharmacist. **Remember, keep this and all other medicines out of**

the reach of children and never share your medicines with others.

BEFORE USING THIS MEDICINE

Tell your doctor, nurse, and pharmacist if you . . .

- are allergic to any medicine, either prescription or non-prescription (OTC);
- are pregnant or intend to become pregnant while using this medicine;
- are breast-feeding;
- are taking any other prescription or nonprescription (OTC) medicine;
- have any other medical problems, especially kidney disease or optic neuritis (eye nerve damage).

PROPER USE OF THIS MEDICINE

Ethambutol may be taken with food if this medicine upsets your stomach.

To help clear up your tuberculosis (TB) completely, **it is very important that you keep taking ethambutol for the full time of treatment** even if you begin to feel better after a few weeks. You may have to take it every day for as long as 1 to 2 years or more. **It is important that you do not miss any doses.**

If you do miss a dose of this medicine, take it as soon as possible. However, if it is almost time for your next dose, skip the missed dose and go back to your regular dosing schedule. Do not double doses.

PRECAUTIONS WHILE USING THIS MEDICINE

If your symptoms do not improve within 2 to 3 weeks, or if they become worse, check with your doctor.

It is very important that your doctor check your progress at regular visits.

Check with your doctor immediately if blurred vision, eye pain, red-green color blindness, or any loss of vision occurs during treatment. Your doctor may want you to have your eyes checked by an ophthalmologist (eye doctor).

Make sure you know how you react to this medicine before you drive, use machines, or do other jobs that require you to be alert or able to see well. If these reactions are especially bothersome, check with your doctor.

POSSIBLE SIDE EFFECTS OF THIS MEDICINE

Side Effects That Should Be Reported To Your Doctor Immediately

> *Less common*—Chills; pain and swelling of joints, especially big toe, ankle, knee; tense, hot skin over affected joints

Rare—Any loss of vision; blurred vision; eye pain; fever; joint pain; numbness, tingling, burning pain, or weakness in the hands or feet; red-green color blindness; skin rash

Other side effects not listed above may also occur in some patients. If you notice any other effects, check with your doctor, nurse, or pharmacist.

ETHCHLORVYNOL Systemic

■ For the Pharmacist ■

In providing consultation, consider emphasizing the following selected information (» = major clinical significance):

Before using this medication
» Conditions affecting use, especially:
Sensitivity to ethchlorvynol
Carcinogenicity/tumorigenicity—A study in mice showed eth-chlorvynol, at doses up to 7 times the maximum human daily dose for 22 to 24 months, to significantly increase total lung tumors in female mice
Pregnancy—Ethchlorvynol crosses placenta; use not recommended during first and second trimesters, because studies in animals have shown a higher percentage of stillbirths and a lower survival rate of offspring when ethchlorvynol was given in doses of 40 mg per kg of body weight (mg/kg) per day; also, use during third trimester may produce CNS depression and withdrawal symptoms in neonate
Use in the elderly—Elderly patients may be more sensitive to effects of ethchlorvynol
Other medications, especially alcohol or other CNS depression–producing medications or coumarin- or indandione-derivative anticoagulants
Other medical problems, especially alcohol or drug abuse or dependence, mental depression, or porphyria

Proper use of this medication
» Taking medication with food or milk to minimize dizziness or ataxia
» Importance of not taking more medication than the amount prescribed because of habit-forming potential
» Proper dosing
» Proper storage

Precautions while using this medication
Regular visits to physician to check progress during prolonged therapy
Checking with physician before discontinuing medication after prolonged use; gradual dosage reduction may be necessary to avoid possibility of withdrawal symptoms
» Avoiding use of alcohol or other CNS depressants
» Suspected overdose: Getting emergency help at once
» Caution if dizziness, lightheadedness, or daytime drowsiness occurs

Side/adverse effects
Signs of potential side effects, especially allergic reaction, cholestatic jaundice, paradoxical reaction, and thrombocytopenia
Side/adverse effects more likely to occur in elderly patients, who may be more sensitive to effects of ethchlorvynol

▲ For the Patient ▲

913910

ABOUT YOUR MEDICINE

Ethchlorvynol (eth-klor-VI-nole) is used to treat insomnia (trouble in sleeping). However, it has generally been replaced by other medicines for the treatment of insomnia. If ethchlorvynol is used regularly (for example, every day) to help produce sleep, it is usually not effective for more than 1 week.

If any of the information in this leaflet causes you special concern or if you want additional information about your medicine and its use, check with your doctor, nurse, or pharmacist. **Remember, keep this and all other medicines out of the reach of children and never share your medicines with others.**

BEFORE USING THIS MEDICINE

Tell your doctor, nurse, and pharmacist if you . . .
- are allergic to any medicine, either prescription or non-prescription (OTC);
- are pregnant or intend to become pregnant while using this medicine;
- are breast-feeding;
- are taking any other prescription or nonprescription (OTC) medicine, especially other CNS depressants, or anticoagulants (blood thinners);
- have any other medical problems, especially mental depression, history of drug abuse or dependence, or porphyria.

PROPER USE OF THIS MEDICINE

Ethchlorvynol is best taken with food or a glass of milk to lessen the possibility of dizziness, clumsiness, or unsteadiness, which may occur shortly after you take this medicine.

Take this medicine only as directed by your doctor. Do not take more of it, do not take it more often, and do not take it for a longer time than your doctor ordered. If too much is taken, it may become habit-forming.

Keep this medicine out of the reach of children since overdose is especially dangerous in children.

PRECAUTIONS WHILE USING THIS MEDICINE

If you will be taking this medicine regularly for a long time:
- Your doctor should check your progress at regular visits.
- Do not stop taking it without first checking with your doctor. Your doctor may want you to reduce gradually the amount you are taking before stopping completely.

This medicine will add to the effects of alcohol and other CNS depressants (medicines that slow down the nervous system). **Check with your doctor before taking any such depressants while you are taking this medicine.**

If you think you or someone else may have taken an overdose, get emergency help at once. Taking an overdose of ethchlorvynol or taking alcohol or other CNS depressants with ethchlorvynol may lead to unconsciousness and possibly death. Some signs of an overdose are continuing confusion, severe weakness, shortness of breath or slow or troubled breathing, slow heartbeat, slurred speech, and staggering.

This medicine may cause some people to become dizzy, light-headed, drowsy, or less alert than they are normally. Even if taken at bedtime, it may cause some people to feel drowsy or less alert on arising. **Make sure you know how you react to this medicine before you drive, use machines, or do other jobs that require you to be alert.**

POSSIBLE SIDE EFFECTS OF THIS MEDICINE
Side Effects That Should Be Reported To Your Doctor

> *Less common*—Skin rash or hives; unusual bleeding or bruising; unusual excitement, nervousness, or restless-ness
>
> *Rare*—Darkening of urine; itching; pale stools; yellow eyes or skin

Side Effects That Usually Do Not Require Medical Attention

> *More common*—Blurred vision; dizziness or lighthead-edness; indigestion; nausea or vomiting; numbness of face; stomach pain; unpleasant aftertaste; unusual tiredness or weakness

Other side effects not listed above may also occur in some patients. If you notice any other effects, check with your doctor, nurse, or pharmacist.

After you stop using this medicine, your body may need time to adjust. If you took this medicine in high doses or for a long time, this may take up to 2 weeks. During this period of time check with your doctor if you notice any unusual effects, especially convulsions (seizures); halluci-nations; muscle twitching; nausea or vomiting; restlessness, nervousness, or irritability; sweating; trembling; trouble in sleeping; or weakness.

ETHINAMATE   Systemic

■For the Pharmacist■

In providing consultation, consider emphasizing the following selected
   information (» = major clinical significance):

Before using this medication
» Conditions affecting use, especially:
      Sensitivity to ethinamate
      Use in the elderly—Elderly patients may be more sensitive to
         effects of ethinamate
      Other medications, especially alcohol or other CNS depression–
         producing medications

Proper use of this medication
» Importance of not using more medication than the amount pre-
      scribed because of habit-forming potential
» Proper storage

Precautions while using this medication
   Regular visits to physician to check progress during prolonged ther-
      apy
   Checking with physician before discontinuing medication after pro-
      longed use; gradual dosage reduction may be necessary to avoid
      possibility of withdrawal symptoms
» Avoiding use of alcohol or other CNS depressants
» Suspected overdose: Getting emergency help at once
» Caution if daytime drowsiness occurs

Side/adverse effects
   Signs of potential side effects, especially allergic reaction, paradox-
      ical reaction, and thrombocytopenia
   Side/adverse effects more likely to occur in elderly patients, who
      may be more sensitive to effects of ethinamate

▲ For the Patient ▲

913921

ABOUT YOUR MEDICINE

Ethinamate (e-THIN-a-mate) is used to treat insomnia (trouble in sleeping). However, it has generally been replaced by
other medicines for the treatment of insomnia. If ethinamate
is used regularly (for example, every day) to help produce
sleep, it is usually not effective for more than 1 week.

If any of the information in this leaflet causes you special
concern or if you want additional information about your
medicine and its use, check with your doctor, nurse, or pharmacist. **Remember, keep this and all other medicines out of
the reach of children and never share your medicines with
others.**

BEFORE USING THIS MEDICINE

Tell your doctor, nurse, and pharmacist if you . . .
   • are allergic to any medicine, either prescription or non-
      prescription (OTC);

- are pregnant or intend to become pregnant while using this medicine;
- are breast-feeding;
- are taking any other prescription or nonprescription (OTC) medicine, especially other CNS depressants;
- have any other medical problems.

PROPER USE OF THIS MEDICINE

Take this medicine only as directed by your doctor. Do not take more of it, do not take it more often, and do not take it for a longer time than your doctor ordered. If too much is taken, it may become habit-forming.

Keep this medicine out of the reach of children. Overdose of ethinamate is especially dangerous in children.

PRECAUTIONS WHILE USING THIS MEDICINE

If you will be taking this medicine regularly for a long time:
- Your doctor should check your progress at regular visits.
- Do not stop taking it without first checking with your doctor. Your doctor may want you to reduce gradually the amount you are taking before stopping completely.

This medicine will add to the effects of alcohol and other CNS depressants (medicines that slow down the nervous system). **Check with your doctor before taking any such depressants while you are taking this medicine.**

If you think you or someone else may have taken an overdose, get emergency help at once. Taking an overdose of ethinamate or taking alcohol or other CNS depressants with ethinamate may lead to unconsciousness and possibly death. Some signs of an overdose are confusion, severe weakness, shortness of breath or slow or troubled breathing, slow heartbeat, slurred speech, and staggering.

This medicine may cause some people to become drowsy or less alert than they are normally. Even if taken at bedtime, it may cause some people to feel drowsy or less alert on arising. **Make sure you know how you react to this medicine before you drive, use machines, or do other jobs that require you to be alert.**

POSSIBLE SIDE EFFECTS OF THIS MEDICINE
Side Effects That Should Be Reported To Your Doctor

> *Less common*—Skin rash; unusual excitement (especially in children)

> *Rare*—Unusual bleeding or bruising

Other side effects not listed above may also occur in some patients. If you notice any other effects, check with your doctor, nurse, or pharmacist.

After you stop using this medicine, your body may need time to adjust. The length of time this takes depends on the amount of medicine you were using and how long you used it. During this period of time check with your doctor if you notice any unusual effects, especially confusion; convulsions (seizures); hallucinations; restlessness, nervousness, or irritability; trembling; trouble in sleeping.

ETHIONAMIDE Systemic

■ For the Pharmacist ■

In providing consultation, consider emphasizing the following selected information (» = major clinical significance):

Before using this medication
» Conditions affecting use, especially:
  Hypersensitivity to ethionamide
  Pregnancy—Ethionamide crosses the placenta
  Dental—Ethionamide may cause a metallic taste and stomatitis
  Other medications, especially cycloserine
  Other medical problems, especially diabetes mellitus or hepatic
    function impairment

Proper use of this medication
  Taking with or after meals if gastrointestinal irritation occurs
» Compliance with full course of therapy, which may take months or
    years
» Taking pyridoxine concurrently to prevent or minimize signs of pe-
    ripheral neuritis
» Proper dosing
  Missed dose: Taking as soon as possible; not taking if almost time
    for next dose; not doubling doses
» Proper storage

Precautions while using this medication
  Checking with physician if no improvement within 2 or 3 weeks
» Regular visits to physician to check progress, as well as ophthal-
    mologic examinations if signs of optic neuritis occur
» Caution if blurred vision or loss of vision occurs
» Need to report promptly to physician signs of optic neuritis and
    prodromal signs of peripheral neuritis

Side/adverse effects
  Signs of potential side effects, especially hepatitis or jaundice, pe-
    ripheral neuritis, psychiatric disturbances, goiter or hypothy-
    roidism, hypoglycemia, optic neuritis, and skin rash

▲ For the Patient ▲

913932

ABOUT YOUR MEDICINE

Ethionamide (e-thye-ON-am-ide) is used with other medicines to treat tuberculosis (TB). Ethionamide may also be
used for other problems as determined by your doctor.
**To help clear up your tuberculosis (TB) completely, you must
keep taking this medicine for the full time of treatment, even
if you begin to feel better. This is very important. It is also
very important that you do not miss any doses.**

If any of the information in this leaflet causes you special
concern or if you want additional information about your
medicine and its use, check with your doctor, nurse, or pharmacist. **Remember, keep this and all other medicines out of
the reach of children and never share your medicines with
others.**

BEFORE USING THIS MEDICINE
Tell your doctor, nurse, and pharmacist if you . . .
- are allergic to any medicine, either prescription or non-prescription (OTC);
- are pregnant or intend to become pregnant while using this medicine;
- are breast-feeding;
- are taking any other prescription or nonprescription (OTC) medicine, especially cycloserine;
- have any other medical problems, especially sugar diabetes or liver disease.

PROPER USE OF THIS MEDICINE
Ethionamide may be taken with or after meals if it upsets your stomach.

To help clear up your TB completely, **it is very important that you keep taking this medicine for the full time of treatment** even if you begin to feel better after a few weeks. You may have to take it every day for as long as 1 to 2 years or more. **It is important that you do not miss any doses.**

Your doctor may also want you to take pyridoxine (vitamin B₆) every day to help prevent or lessen some of the side effects of ethionamide. If so, **it is very important to take pyridoxine every day along with this medicine.**

If you miss a dose of either of these medicines, take it as soon as possible. However, if it is almost time for your next dose, skip the missed dose and go back to your regular dosing schedule. Do not double doses.

PRECAUTIONS WHILE USING THIS MEDICINE
If your symptoms do not improve within 2 to 3 weeks, or if they become worse, check with your doctor.

It is very important that your doctor check your progress at regular visits. Also, **check with your doctor immediately if blurred vision or any loss of vision, with or without eye pain, occurs during treatment.** Your doctor may want you to have your eyes checked by an ophthalmologist (eye doctor).

This medicine may cause blurred vision or loss of vision. **Make sure you know how you react to this medicine before you drive, use machines, or do other jobs that require you to be alert or able to see well.**

If this medicine causes clumsiness; unsteadiness; or numbness, tingling, burning, or pain in the hands and feet, check with your doctor immediately. These may be early warning signs of more serious nerve problems that could develop later.

This medicine must not be given to other people or used for other infections unless you are otherwise directed by your doctor.

POSSIBLE SIDE EFFECTS OF THIS MEDICINE
Side Effects That Should Be Reported To Your Doctor Immediately

Less common—Clumsiness or unsteadiness; confusion; mental depression; mood or other mental changes; numbness, tingling, burning, or pain in hands and feet; yellow eyes or skin

Rare—Blurred vision or loss of vision, with or without eye pain; changes in menstrual periods; coldness; decreased sexual ability (males); difficulty in concentrating; dry, puffy skin; fast heartbeat; increased hunger; nervousness; shakiness; skin rash; swelling of front part of neck; weight gain

Side Effects That Usually Do Not Require Medical Attention

These possible side effects may go away during treatment; however, if they continue or are bothersome, check with your doctor, nurse, or pharmacist.

More common—Dizziness (especially when getting up from a lying or sitting position); loss of appetite; metallic taste; nausea or vomiting; sore mouth

Other side effects not listed above may also occur in some patients. If you notice any other effects, check with your doctor, nurse, or pharmacist.

388

ETIDRONATE Systemic

■ For the Pharmacist ■

In providing consultation, consider emphasizing the following selected
information (» = major clinical significance):

Before using this medication
» Conditions affecting use, especially:
  Sensitivity to etidronate
  Use in children—Children given adult dosages for nearly a year
    or more were reported to have signs of a rachitic syndrome
    that were reversible upon discontinuation of etidronate
  Use in the elderly—Elderly patients may be more prone to over-
    hydration when treated with parenteral etidronate in con-
    junction with hydration therapy
  Other medications, especially antacids or mineral supplements
  Other medical problems, especially renal function impairment,
    bone fractures, cardiac failure, or enterocolitis

Proper use of this medication
» Taking with water on an empty stomach, at least 2 hours before or
  after food (upon arising, midmorning, or at bedtime)
» Compliance with therapy; not taking more or less medication or for
  longer period of time than prescribed
  Checking with physician before discontinuing medication; may re-
    quire 1 to 3 months for symptomatic improvement
» Maintaining a well-balanced diet with adequate intake of calcium
  and vitamin D; not taking within 2 hours of milk or milk prod-
  ucts, antacids, mineral supplements, or other medicines high in
  calcium, magnesium, iron, or aluminum
» Proper dosing
  Missed dose: Taking as soon as possible; not taking if almost time
    for next dose; not doubling doses
» Proper storage

Precautions while using this medication
» Regular visits to physician to check progress even if between treat-
  ments
  Checking with physician if nausea or diarrhea occurs and continues;
    dosage adjustment may be necessary
» Checking with physician if bone pain appears or worsens during
  treatment

Side/adverse effects
  Signs of potential side effects, especially increased or continuing
    bone pain, fractures, or allergic reaction

▲ For the Patient ▲

918299

ABOUT YOUR MEDICINE

Etidronate (eh-tih-DROE-nate) is used to treat Paget's disease of bone. It may also be used to treat or prevent a certain
type of bone problem that may occur after hip replacement
surgery or spinal injury.

Etidronate is also used to treat hypercalcemia (too much calcium in the blood) that may occur with some types of cancer.

If any of the information in this leaflet causes you special concern or if you want additional information about your medicine and its use, check with your doctor, nurse, or pharmacist. **Remember, keep this and all other medicines out of the reach of children and never share your medicines with others.**

BEFORE USING THIS MEDICINE

Tell your doctor, nurse, and pharmacist if you . . .
- are allergic to any medicine, either prescription or non-prescription (OTC);
- are pregnant or intend to become pregnant while using this medicine;
- are breast-feeding;
- are taking any other prescription or nonprescription (OTC) medicine, especially antacids containing calcium, magnesium, or aluminum; or mineral supplements or other medicines containing calcium, iron, magnesium, or aluminum;
- have any other medical problems, especially bone fracture, intestinal or bowel disease, or kidney disease.

PROPER USE OF THIS MEDICINE

Take etidronate with water on an empty stomach at least 2 hours before or after food (midmorning is best) or at bedtime. Food may decrease the amount of etidronate absorbed by your body.

Take etidronate only as directed. Do not take more of it, do not take it more often, and do not take it for a longer time than your doctor ordered. To do so may increase the chance of side effects.

In some patients, etidronate takes up to 3 months to work. If you feel that the medicine is not working, do not stop taking it on your own. Instead, check with your doctor.

It is important that you eat a well-balanced diet with an adequate amount of calcium and vitamin D (found in milk or other dairy products). Too much or too little of either may increase the chance of side effects while you are taking etidronate. Your doctor can help you choose the meal plan that is best for you. **However, do not take any food, especially milk, milk formulas, or other dairy products, or antacids, mineral supplements, or other medicines that are high in calcium or iron (high amounts of these minerals may also be in some vitamin preparations), magnesium, or aluminum** within 2 hours of taking etidronate. To do so may keep this medicine from working properly.

If you miss a dose of this medicine, take it as soon as possible. However, if it is almost time for your next dose, skip the

missed dose and go back to your regular dosing schedule.
Do not double doses.

PRECAUTIONS WHILE USING THIS MEDICINE

It is important that your doctor check your progress at regular visits even if you are between treatments and are not taking this medicine. If your condition has improved and your doctor has told you to stop taking etidronate, your progress must still be checked. The results of laboratory tests or the occurrence of certain symptoms will tell your doctor if more medicine must be taken. Your doctor may want you to begin another course of treatment after you have been off the medicine for at least 3 months.

If this medicine causes you to have nausea or diarrhea and it continues, check with your doctor. The dose may need to be changed.

If bone pain occurs or worsens during treatment, check with your doctor.

POSSIBLE SIDE EFFECTS OF THIS MEDICINE
Side Effects That Should Be Reported To Your Doctor

> *More common*—Bone pain or tenderness (increased, continuing, or returning—in patients with Paget's disease)

> *Less common*—Bone fractures, especially of the thigh bone

> *Rare*—Hives; skin rash or itching; swelling of the arms, legs, face, lips, tongue, or throat

Side Effects That Usually Do Not Require Medical Attention

These possible side effects may go away during treatment; however, if they continue or are bothersome, check with your doctor, nurse, or pharmacist.

> *More common—at higher doses*—Diarrhea; nausea

Other side effects not listed above may also occur in some patients. If you notice any other effects, check with your doctor, nurse, or pharmacist.

ETRETINATE   Systemic

■For the Pharmacist■

In providing consultation, consider emphasizing the following selected information (» = major clinical significance):

Before using this medication
» Conditions affecting use, especially:

Sensitivity to etretinate, isotretinoin, tretinoin, or vitamin A–like preparations

Pregnancy—Not taking etretinate during pregnancy, because it causes birth defects in humans. In addition, since it is not known how long pregnancy should be avoided after treatment stops, planning on never having children after treatment with etretinate. Not taking etretinate unless an effective form of contraception is used for at least 1 month before beginning treatment. Continuing contraception during treatment and for as long as pregnancy is possible after etretinate is stopped. Discussing this information with doctor

Breast-feeding—Although it is not known whether etretinate passes into the breast milk, etretinate is not recommended during breast-feeding, or if breast-feeding is planned in the future, because it may cause unwanted effects in nursing babies

Use in children—Because of the shortage of data on etretinate treatment in children and the possibility that children may be more sensitive to the effects of the medication, etretinate should not be used in children unless all alternative therapies have been exhausted

Other medications, especially alcohol, methotrexate or other hepatotoxic medications, isotretinoin, tretinoin, vitamin A, and tetracyclines

Other medical problems, especially personal or family history of cardiovascular risk or disease or hypertriglyceridemia or conditions predisposing to hypertriglyceridemia, such as high alcohol intake or history of high alcohol intake, family history of hypertriglyceridemia, or obesity

Proper use of this medication
» Taking each dose with milk or fatty food because fats help medication to be absorbed better; rest of time following low-fat diet because of possible hypertriglyceridemia and consequent cardiovascular risks
» Importance of not taking more medication than the amount prescribed
» Proper dosing

Missed dose: Taking as soon as possible with milk or fatty food; not taking if almost time for next dose; not doubling doses
» Proper storage

Precautions while using this medication
» Regular visits to physician to check progress during therapy
» Using a reliable form of contraception and not changing contraception method during therapy and for as long as able to become pregnant after therapy ends, since etretinate causes birth defects in humans during its use and for at least several years afterwards (it is not known how long after therapy is discontinued that birth

defects may occur); stopping medication immediately and checking with physician if pregnancy is suspected during therapy;
checking with physician as soon as possible if pregnancy occurs
anytime in the future after therapy is discontinued; talking to
physician in either case about the risks of continuing the pregnancy

» To prevent the possibility of a pregnant patient receiving blood
containing etretinate, never donating blood to a blood bank during or after treatment with etretinate, since it is not known how
long etretinate stays in the body

» Avoiding concurrent use of vitamin A and vitamin supplements
containing vitamin A

» Not drinking, or at least reducing consumption of, alcoholic beverages, because of possible hypertriglyceridemia and consequent
cardiovascular risks

Diabetics: May alter blood sugar concentrations

» Caution if decrease in night vision, which may be sudden, occurs;
not driving, using machines, or doing other things that could be
dangerous if unable to see well; checking with physician if this
occurs

Possibility of dryness of eyes; may decrease tolerance to contact
lenses during therapy and for several weeks or longer after discontinuation of therapy; checking with physician if inflammation
occurs and about using ocular lubricant to relieve dryness of eyes

Possibility of photosensitivity; avoiding unprotected exposure to sunlight and not using sunlamp; checking with physician if severe
reaction occurs

Possible dryness of mouth and nose; for relief of mouth dryness,
using sugarless gum or candy, ice, or saliva substitute for relief;
checking with dentist if dry mouth continues for more than 2
weeks

Possibility that psoriasis may appear to worsen, with increased redness or itching, during initial therapy; checking with physician
if irritation or other symptoms of condition become severe; possibly having to take medication for 2 or 3 months before full
effects are seen

Side/adverse effects

Signs of potential side effects, especially abnormalities of conjunc-
tiva, cornea, lens, retina, extraocular musculature, ocular tension, pupil, or vitreous humor; amnesia; anxiety; bleeding or inflammation of gums; blot retinal hemorrhage; bone or joint pain,
tenderness, or stiffness; conjunctivitis; cramps or pain in upper
abdomen or stomach area; depression; ear infection; eyelid abnormalities; hepatitis; iritis; mucous membrane abnormalities;
muscle cramps; otitis externa; photophobia; posterior subcap-
sular cataract; pseudotumor cerebri; scotoma; or unusual bruising

▲ For the Patient ▲

915665

ABOUT YOUR MEDICINE

Etretinate (e-TRET-i-nate) is used to treat severe psoriasis.
It is usually used only after other medicines have been tried
and have failed to help.

**Etretinate must not be used in women who are able to bear
children unless other forms of treatment have been tried first**

and have failed. Etretinate must not be taken during pregnancy, because it causes birth defects. In addition, if you take etretinate, you must plan on never having children in the future. It is very important that you read, understand, and follow the pregnancy warnings for etretinate.

If any of the information in this leaflet causes you special concern or if you want additional information about your medicine and its use, check with your doctor, nurse, or pharmacist. **Remember, keep this and all other medicines out of the reach of children and never share your medicines with others.**

BEFORE USING THIS MEDICINE

Etretinate must not be taken during pregnancy, because it causes birth defects. In addition, since it is not known how long pregnancy should be avoided after treatment stops, you must plan on never having children if you take etretinate. Etretinate must not be taken unless an effective form of contraception (birth control) is used for at least 1 month before beginning treatment. Contraception must be continued during treatment and for as long as you are able to become pregnant after etretinate is stopped.

Tell your doctor, nurse, and pharmacist if you . . .
- are allergic to any medicine, either prescription or non-prescription (OTC);
- **are pregnant or may become pregnant while using this medicine;**
- are breast-feeding;
- are using any other prescription or nonprescription (OTC) medicine, especially isotretinoin, methotrexate, tetracyclines, tretinoin, or vitamin A;
- have **any** other medical problems.

PROPER USE OF THIS MEDICINE

It is very important that you take etretinate only as directed. Take each dose of etretinate with milk or a fatty food to help your body absorb the medicine better. **However, follow a low-fat diet during the rest of the day.**

PRECAUTIONS WHILE USING THIS MEDICINE

Your doctor should check your progress at regular visits.

Since etretinate causes birth defects and it is not known how long pregnancy should be avoided after treatment stops, you must plan on never having children if you take etretinate. For as long as you are able to become pregnant, you must use a reliable form of birth control. In addition, you must not change your birth control method unless you have checked with your doctor first. If you think you have become pregnant while taking etretinate, or at any time after you have stopped taking it, check with your doctor as soon as possible. Stop taking the medicine at once if you are still taking it.

To prevent the possibility of a pregnant patient receiving your blood, you must plan on never donating blood during or after treatment with etretinate.

Do not take vitamin A–containing supplements while taking this medicine.

Drinking too much alcohol while taking etretinate may increase the chance of heart and blood vessel disease. It is best that you **do not drink alcoholic beverages or that you at least reduce the amount you usually drink.**

In some patients, etretinate may cause a decrease in night vision. This decrease may occur suddenly. If it does occur, **do not drive, use machines, or do other jobs that require you to see well.** Also, check with your doctor.

When you first begin taking this medicine, avoid too much sun and do not use a sunlamp until you see how you react to the sun, especially if you tend to burn easily. **If you have a severe reaction, check with your doctor.**

POSSIBLE SIDE EFFECTS OF THIS MEDICINE
Side Effects That Should Be Reported To Your Doctor Immediately

> *Less common*—Blurred, double, or other vision changes; dark-colored urine; flu-like symptoms; yellow eyes or skin
>
> *Rare*—Headache (severe or continuing), nausea and vomiting

Other Side Effects That Should Be Reported To Your Doctor

> *More common*—Bone or joint pain, tenderness, or stiffness; bruising (unusual); burning, redness, itching, or other sign of inflammation or irritation of eyes; cramps or pain in upper abdomen or stomach area; muscle cramps
>
> *Less common or rare*—Bleeding or redness of gums; change in hearing or other ear problems; confusion; mood or mental changes

Side Effects That Usually Do Not Require Medical Attention

These possible side effects may go away during treatment; however, if they continue or are bothersome, check with your doctor, nurse, or pharmacist.

> *More common*—Changes in appetite; dryness or irritation of lips, nose, or skin; headache (mild); thinning of hair; unusual thirst; unusual tiredness

Other side effects not listed above may also occur in some patients. If you notice any other effects, check with your doctor, nurse, or pharmacist.

FINASTERIDE   Systemic

■ For the Pharmacist ■

In providing consultation, consider emphasizing the following selected information (» = major clinical significance):

Before using this medication
» Conditions affecting use, especially:
>> Sensitivity to finasteride
>> Carcinogenicity—Increased incidence of testicular tumors in mice and rats receiving very high doses
>> Pregnancy—When sexual partner is or may become pregnant, patient should either avoid exposure of sexual partner to semen or discontinue finasteride
>> Other medications, especially anticholinergics or medications with anticholinergic effects, adrenergic bronchodilators, xanthine bronchodilators, or sympathomimetic decongestants

Proper use of this medication
>> Getting into the habit of taking at same time each day to help increase compliance
» Does not cure, but helps control BPH; possible need for lifelong therapy; checking with physician before discontinuing medication
>> Tablets may be crushed
>> All patients with BPH should avoid drinking fluids, especially coffee or alcohol, in the evening, to reduce nocturia
» Proper dosing
>> Missed dose: Taking as soon as possible; not taking if almost time for next dose; not doubling doses
» Proper storage

Precautions while using this medication
» Not taking other medications, especially nonprescription sympathomimetics, unless discussed with physician
>> Women who are or who may become pregnant should not handle crushed tablets

Side/adverse effects
>> Signs of potential side effects, especially decreased libido, decreased volume of ejaculate, or impotence (these side effects occur less frequently or rarely, and usually do not need medical attention)

▲ For the Patient ▲

918630

ABOUT YOUR MEDICINE

Finasteride (fi-NAS-teer-ide) belongs to the group of medicines called enzyme inhibitors. It is used to treat enlargement of the prostate (benign prostatic hyperplasia or BPH), a condition that causes urinary problems in men.

If any of the information in this leaflet causes you special concern or if you want additional information about your medicine and its use, check with your doctor, nurse, or pharmacist. **Remember, keep this and all other medicines out of**

the reach of children and never share your medicines with others.

BEFORE USING THIS MEDICINE

Tell your doctor, nurse, and pharmacist if you . . .
- are allergic to any medicine, either prescription or non-prescription (OTC);
- intend to have children;
- are taking **any** other prescription or nonprescription (OTC) medicine;
- have any other medical problems, especially liver disease.

PROPER USE OF THIS MEDICINE

To help you remember to take your medicine, try to get into the habit of taking it at the same time each day.

Remember that this medicine does not cure BPH but it does help reduce the size of the prostate. **You may have to take medicine for the rest of your life.** Do not stop taking this medicine without first checking with your doctor.

Finasteride tablets may be crushed to make them easier to swallow.

This medicine helps to reduce urinary problems in men with BPH. In general, it is best to avoid drinking fluids, especially coffee or alcohol, in the evening. This will help keep your sleep from being disturbed by the need to urinate.

If you miss a dose of this medicine, take the missed dose as soon as you remember it. However, if it is almost time for your next dose, skip the missed dose and go back to your regular dosing schedule. Do not double doses.

PRECAUTIONS WHILE USING THIS MEDICINE

Do not take other medicines unless they have been discussed with your doctor. This especially includes over-the-counter (nonprescription) medicines for appetite control, asthma, colds, cough, hay fever, or sinus problems, since they may cause problems with urination and could reduce the effects of finasteride.

Women who are or may become pregnant should not handle crushed finasteride tablets. There is a risk that the medicine could be absorbed into the body and harm the fetus.

POSSIBLE SIDE EFFECTS OF THIS MEDICINE

Side Effects That Usually Do Not Require Medical Attention

These possible side effects may go away during treatment; however, if they continue or are bothersome, check with your doctor, nurse, or pharmacist.

> *Less common or rare*—Decreased libido (decreased interest in sex); decreased volume of ejaculate (amount

of semen); impotence (inability to have or keep an erection)

Other side effects not listed above may also occur in some patients. If you notice any other effects, check with your doctor, nurse, or pharmacist.

FLECAINIDE   Systemic

■ For the Pharmacist ■

In providing consultation, consider emphasizing the following selected
   information (» = major clinical significance):

Before using this medication
» Conditions affecting use, especially:
   Sensitivity to flecainide or amide-type anesthetics
   Pregnancy—Teratogenic in rabbits
   Use in the elderly—Increased duration of action; increased risk
      of proarrhythmic effects
   Other medications, especially other antiarrhythmics
   Other medical problems, especially hepatic function impairment

Proper use of this medication
» Compliance with therapy; taking as directed even if feeling well
» Importance of not missing doses and taking at evenly spaced inter-
   vals
» Proper dosing
   Missed dose: Taking as soon as possible if remembered within 6
      hours; not taking if remembered later; not doubling doses
» Proper storage

Precautions while using this medication
   Regular visits to physician to check progress
   Carrying medical identification card or bracelet
» Caution if any kind of surgery (including dental surgery) or emer-
   gency treatment is required
» Caution when driving or doing things requiring alertness because
   of possible dizziness
   Checking with physician before discontinuing medication; gradual
      dosage reduction may be necessary

Side/adverse effects
   Signs of potential side effects, especially arrhythmias, chest pain,
      congestive heart failure, trembling or shaking, and hepatic func-
      tion impairment

▲ For the Patient ▲

913036

ANTIARRHYTHMICS, TYPE I (Oral): *Including
Disopyramide; Encainide; Flecainide; Mexiletine;
Moricizine; Procainamide; Propafenone; Quinidine;
Tocainide.*

ABOUT YOUR MEDICINE

Type I antiarrhythmics are used to correct irregular heartbeats to a normal rhythm and to slow an overactive heart.

There is a chance that these medicines may cause new heart
rhythm problems when they are used. Usually this effect is
rare and mild. However, some of these medicines are more
likely than others to cause this effect. For example, encainide
and flecainide have been shown to cause severe problems in

some patients, and so they are only used to treat serious heart rhythm problems. Discuss this possible effect with your doctor.

If any of the information in this leaflet causes you special concern or if you want additional information about your medicine and its use, check with your doctor, nurse, or pharmacist. **Remember, keep this and all other medicines out of the reach of children and never share your medicines with others.**

BEFORE USING THIS MEDICINE

Tell your doctor, nurse, and pharmacist if you . . .
- are allergic to any medicine, either prescription or nonprescription (OTC);
- are pregnant or intend to become pregnant while using this medicine;
- are breast-feeding;
- are taking **any** other prescription or nonprescription (OTC) medicine;
- have **any** other medical problems.

PROPER USE OF THIS MEDICINE

Take this medicine exactly as directed by your doctor, even though you may feel well. Do not take more medicine than ordered.

For patients taking the extended-release capsules or tablets:
- Swallow whole without breaking, crushing, or chewing.

It is best to take each dose at evenly spaced times day and night.

For patients taking mexiletine:
- To lessen the possibility of stomach upset, this medicine should be taken with food or immediately after meals or with milk or an antacid.

If you miss a dose of this medicine, take it as soon as possible. However, if you do not remember until it is almost time for the next dose, skip the missed dose and go back to your regular dosing schedule. Do not double doses.

PRECAUTIONS WHILE USING THIS MEDICINE

It is important that your doctor check your progress at regular visits to make sure the medicine is working properly to help your heart.

Do not suddenly stop taking this medicine without first checking with your doctor. Stopping it suddenly may cause a serious change in heart activity.

Dizziness or lightheadedness or blurred vision may occur. **Make sure you know how you react to this medicine before you drive, use machines, or do other jobs that require you to be alert and able to see well.**

For patients taking disopyramide:
- **If signs of hypoglycemia (low blood sugar) such as chills, hunger, nausea, nervousness, or sweating appear, eat or drink a food containing sugar and call your doctor right away.**
- **Use extra care not to become overheated during exercise or hot weather,** since this medicine will often make you sweat less and could possibly result in heatstroke.

POSSIBLE SIDE EFFECTS OF THIS MEDICINE

Side Effects That Should Be Reported To Your Doctor Immediately

> *For quinidine only, especially after the first dose or first few doses*—Breathing difficulty; changes in vision; dizziness, lightheadedness, or fainting; fever; severe headache; ringing in ears; skin rash

Other Side Effects That Should Be Reported To Your Doctor

> *For all antiarrhythmics*—Chest pain; fast or irregular heartbeat; fever or chills; shortness of breath or painful breathing; skin rash or itching; unusual bleeding or bruising

> *For disopyramide (in addition to above)*—Difficult urination; swelling of feet or lower legs

> *For encainide, flecainide, moricizine, and propafenone (in addition to above)*—Swelling of feet or lower legs; trembling or shaking

Side Effects That Usually Do Not Require Medical Attention

These possible side effects may go away during treatment; however, if they continue or are bothersome, check with your doctor, nurse, or pharmacist.

> *For all antiarrhythmics*—Blurred or double vision; dizziness or lightheadedness

> *For disopyramide (in addition to above)*—Dry mouth and throat

> *For flecainide (in addition to above)*—Seeing spots

> *For mexiletine (in addition to above)*—Heartburn; nausea and vomiting; nervousness; trembling or shaking of hands; unsteadiness or trouble walking

> *For procainamide (in addition to above)*—Diarrhea; loss of appetite

> *For propafenone (in addition to above)*—Change in taste

> *For quinidine (in addition to above)*—Bitter taste; diarrhea; flushing of skin with itching; loss of appetite; nausea or vomiting; stomach pain or cramps

> *For tocainide (in addition to above)*—Loss of appetite; nausea

Other side effects not listed above may also occur in some patients. If you notice any other effects, check with your doctor, nurse, or pharmacist.

FLUDROCORTISONE   Systemic

■For the Pharmacist■

In providing consultation, consider emphasizing the following selected
   information (» = major clinical significance):

Before using this medication
» Conditions affecting use, especially:
      Sensitivity to fludrocortisone
      Pregnancy—Infants born to mothers who received substantial
         doses of corticosteroids during pregnancy require close ob-
         servation for signs of hypoadrenalism
      Use in children and growing adolescents—May cause growth
         suppression and inhibition of endogenous steroid production
      Other medications, especially hypokalemia-causing medications,
         digitalis glycosides, hepatic enzyme inducers, or sodium-con-
         taining medications or food
      Other medical problems, especially cardiac disease, congestive
         heart failure, hypertension, or renal function impairment

Proper use of this medication
» Importance of not taking more medication than the amount pre-
      scribed
   Missed dose: Taking as soon as possible; not taking if almost time
      for next dose; not doubling doses
» Proper dosing
» Proper storage

Precautions while using this medication
» Regular visits to physician to check progress during therapy
   Carrying medical identification card during long-term therapy

Side/adverse effects
   Signs of potential side effects, especially anaphylaxis, congestive
      heart failure, dizziness, severe headache, hypokalemic syndrome,
      or peripheral edema

▲ For the Patient ▲

917285

ABOUT YOUR MEDICINE

Fludrocortisone (floo-droe-KOR-ti-sone) is a corticosteroid
(kor-ti-koh-STER-oid) (cortisone-like medicine). It belongs
to the family of medicines called steroids. If your body does
not produce enough corticosteroids, your doctor may have
prescribed this medicine to help make up the difference.
Fludrocortisone may also be used to treat other medical
conditions as determined by your doctor.

If any of the information in this leaflet causes you special
concern or if you want additional information about your
medicine and its use, check with your doctor, nurse, or pharmacist. **Remember, keep this and all other medicines out of
the reach of children and never share your medicines with
others.**

BEFORE USING THIS MEDICINE
Tell your doctor, nurse, and pharmacist if you . . .

- are allergic to any medicine, either prescription or non-prescription (OTC);
- are pregnant or intend to become pregnant while using this medicine;
- are breast-feeding;
- are taking **any** other prescription or nonprescription (OTC) medicine;
- have any other medical problems, especially heart disease, high blood pressure, or kidney disease.

PROPER USE OF THIS MEDICINE
Take this medicine only as directed by your doctor. Do not take more or less of it, do not take it more often, and do not take it for a longer time than your doctor ordered. To do so may increase the chance of side effects.

If you miss a dose of this medicine, take it as soon as you remember. However, if it is almost time for your next dose, skip the missed dose and go back to your regular dosing schedule. Do not double doses.

PRECAUTIONS WHILE USING THIS MEDICINE
Your doctor should check your progress at regular visits to make sure this medicine does not cause unwanted effects.

If you will be using this medicine for a long time, your doctor may want you to carry a medical identification card stating that you are using this medicine.

While you are taking fludrocortisone, be careful to limit the amount of alcohol you drink.

POSSIBLE SIDE EFFECTS OF THIS MEDICINE
Side Effects That Should Be Reported To Your Doctor Immediately

Less common or rare—Cough; difficulty swallowing; hives; irregular breathing or shortness of breath; irregular heartbeat; redness and itching of skin; redness of eyes; swelling of nasal passages, face, or eyelids; swollen neck veins; unusual tiredness or weakness

Other Side Effects That Should Be Reported To Your Doctor

Less common or rare—Dizziness; headache (severe or continuing); loss of appetite; muscle cramps or pain; nausea; swelling of feet or lower legs; weakness in arms, legs, or trunk (severe); weight gain (rapid); vomiting

Other side effects not listed above may also occur in some patients. If you notice any other effects, check with your doctor, nurse, or pharmacist.

FLUOROQUINOLONES   Systemic

Including Fluoroquinolones (Injection); Fluroquinolones (Oral).

■ For the Pharmacist ■

In providing consultation, consider emphasizing the following selected information (» = major clinical significance):

Before using this medication
» Conditions affecting use, especially:
   Allergies to fluoroquinolones or other quinolone derivatives
   Pregnancy—Fluoroquinolones are not recommended for use during pregnancy because they have been shown to cause arthropathy in immature animals
   Breast-feeding—Not recommended since fluoroquinolones have been shown to cause arthropathy in immature animals
   Use in children—Use of fluoroquinolones is not recommended in infants and children since these medications have been shown to cause arthropathy in immature animals
   Use in adolescents—Use of fluoroquinolones is not recommended in adolescents since these medications have been shown to cause arthropathy in immature animals
   Other medications, especially aluminum-, calcium-, and/or magnesium-containing antacids, caffeine-containing products, didanosine, ferrous sulfate, sucralfate, aminophylline, oxtriphylline, theophylline, or warfarin
   Other medical problems, especially allergy to quinolones and renal function impairment

Proper use of this medication
» Not giving to infants, children, adolescents, or pregnant women; fluoroquinolones have been shown to cause arthropathy in immature animals
» Taking with full glass (240 mL) of water; maintaining adequate fluid intake
» For enoxacin, norfloxacin, and ofloxacin—taking on an empty stomach
» For ciprofloxacin and lomefloxacin—taking with meals or on an empty stomach
» Compliance with full course of therapy
» Importance of not missing doses and taking at evenly spaced times
» Proper dosing
   Missed dose: Taking as soon as possible; not taking if almost time for next dose; not doubling doses
» Proper storage

Precautions while using this medication
   Checking with physician if no improvement within a few days
» Avoiding concurrent use of antacids or sucralfate and fluoroquinolones; taking antacids or sucralfate at least 6 hours before or 2 hours after administration of ciprofloxacin or lomefloxacin, 2 hours before or after administration of norfloxacin or ofloxacin, and 8 hours before or 2 hours after administration of enoxacin
» Possible photosensitivity reactions
» Caution if blurred vision or other vision problems, dizziness, lightheadedness, or drowsiness occurs

Side/adverse effects
> Signs of potential side effects, especially central nervous system stimulation, hypersensitivity reactions, interstitial nephritis, and phlebitis

---

▲ For the Patient ▲

918890

FLUOROQUINOLONES (Injection): *Including Ciprofloxacin; Ofloxacin.*

ABOUT YOUR MEDICINE

Fluoroquinolones (flu-roe-KWIN-a-lones) are used to treat bacterial infections in many different parts of the body. These medicines will not work for colds, flu, or other virus infections. Fluoroquinolones may also be used for other conditions as determined by your doctor.

If any of the information in this leaflet causes you special concern or if you want additional information about your medicine and its use, check with your doctor, nurse, or pharmacist. **Remember, keep this and all other medicines out of the reach of children and never share your medicines with others.**

BEFORE USING THIS MEDICINE

Tell your doctor, nurse, and pharmacist if you . . .
- are allergic to any medicine, either prescription or non-prescription (OTC);
- are pregnant or intend to become pregnant while using this medicine;
- are breast-feeding;
- are taking any other prescription or nonprescription (OTC) medicine, especially aminophylline, antacids, anticoagulants (blood thinners), iron supplements, oxtriphylline, sucralfate, or theophylline;
- have any other medical problems, especially kidney disease.

PROPER USE OF THIS MEDICINE

This medicine should not be used in infants, children, adolescents, or pregnant or breast-feeding women unless otherwise directed by your doctor.

Some medicines given by injection may sometimes be given at home to patients who do not need to be in the hospital for the full time of treatment. If you are using this medicine at home, **make sure you clearly understand and carefully follow your doctor's instructions.**

You should drink several glasses of water every day while using this medicine, unless otherwise directed.

To help clear up your infection completely, **keep using this medicine for the full time of treatment,** even if you begin to feel better after a few days.

This medicine works best when there is a constant amount in the blood or urine. **To help keep the amount constant, do not miss any doses. Also, it is best to use the medicine at evenly spaced times, day and night.**

If you do miss a dose of this medicine, use it as soon as possible. However, if it is almost time for your next dose, skip the missed dose and go back to your regular dosing schedule. Do not double doses.

PRECAUTIONS WHILE USING THIS MEDICINE

If your symptoms do not improve within a few days, check with your doctor.

Some people who use fluoroquinolones may become more sensitive to sunlight than they are normally. When you first begin using this medicine, avoid too much sun and do not use a sunlamp until you see how you react to the sun, especially if you tend to burn easily. **If you have a severe reaction, check with your doctor.**

This medicine may cause some people to become dizzy, light-headed, drowsy, or less alert than they are normally. **Make sure you know how you react before you drive, use machines, or do other jobs that require you to be alert.**

This medicine must not be given to other people or used for other infections unless you are otherwise directed by your doctor.

POSSIBLE SIDE EFFECTS OF THIS MEDICINE

Side Effects That Should Be Reported To Your Doctor Immediately

Rare—Agitation; confusion; fever; hallucinations; pain at place of injection; peeling of the skin; shakiness or tremors; shortness of breath; skin rash, itching, or redness; swelling of face or neck

Side Effects That Usually Do Not Require Medical Attention

These possible side effects may go away during treatment; however, if they continue or are bothersome, check with your doctor, nurse, or pharmacist.

More common—Abdominal or stomach pain or discomfort; diarrhea; dizziness; drowsiness; headache; lightheadedness; nausea or vomiting; nervousness; trouble in sleeping

Less common or rare—Increased sensitivity of skin to sunlight

Other side effects not listed above may also occur in some patients. If you notice any other effects, check with your doctor, nurse, or pharmacist.

▲ For the Patient ▲

916136

FLUOROQUINOLONES (Oral): *Including*
Ciprofloxacin; Enoxacin; Lomefloxacin; Norfloxacin;
Ofloxacin.

ABOUT YOUR MEDICINE

Fluoroquinolones (flu-roe-KWIN-a-lones) are used to treat
bacterial infections in many different parts of the body. These
medicines will not work for colds, flu, or other virus infections. Fluoroquinolones may also be used for other problems
as determined by your doctor.

If any of the information in this leaflet causes you special
concern or if you want additional information about your
medicine and its use, check with your doctor, nurse, or pharmacist. **Remember, keep this and all other medicines out of
the reach of children and never share your medicines with
others.**

BEFORE USING THIS MEDICINE

Tell your doctor, nurse, and pharmacist if you . . .
- are allergic to any medicine, either prescription or nonprescription (OTC);
- are pregnant or intend to become pregnant while using
  this medicine;
- are breast-feeding;
- are taking any other prescription or nonprescription
  (OTC) medicine, especially aminophylline, antacids,
  anticoagulants (blood thinners), oxtriphylline, sucralfate, or theophylline;
- have any other medical problems, especially brain or
  spinal cord damage, history of convulsive disorders (seizures, epilepsy), or kidney disease.

PROPER USE OF THIS MEDICINE

**This medicine should not be used in infants, children, ado-
lescents, or pregnant or breast-feeding women** unless otherwise directed by your doctor.

**This medicine is best taken with a full glass (8 ounces) of
water** on an empty stomach (either 1 hour before or 2 hours
after meals). However, if this medicine upsets your stomach,
your doctor may want you to take it with food; **but do not
take milk or other dairy products within 1 or 2 hours of the
time you take this medicine. Several additional glasses of
water should be taken every day,** unless otherwise directed.

To help clear up your infection completely, **keep taking this
medicine for the full time of treatment,** even if you begin to
feel better after a few days.

This medicine works best when there is a constant amount
in the blood or urine. **To help keep the amount constant, do**

not miss any doses. Also, it is best to take the doses at evenly spaced times, day and night.

If you do miss a dose of this medicine, take it as soon as possible. However, if it is almost time for your next dose, skip the missed dose and go back to your regular dosing schedule. Do not double doses.

PRECAUTIONS WHILE USING THIS MEDICINE

If your symptoms do not improve within a few days, check with your doctor.

If you are taking antacids or sucralfate, do not take them at the same time that you take this medicine. It is best to take antacids or sucralfate 2 to 3 hours before or after taking this medicine.

Some people who take fluoroquinolones may become more sensitive to sunlight than they are normally. When you first begin taking this medicine, avoid too much sun and do not use a sunlamp until you see how you react to the sun, especially if you tend to burn easily. **If you have a severe reaction, check with your doctor.**

This medicine may cause vision problems. It may also cause some people to become dizzy, lightheaded, drowsy, or less alert than they are normally. **Make sure you know how you react before you drive, use machines, or do other jobs that could be dangerous if you are not alert or able to see well.**

This medicine must not be given to other people or used for other infections unless you are otherwise directed by your doctor.

POSSIBLE SIDE EFFECTS OF THIS MEDICINE
Side Effects That Should Be Reported To Your Doctor Immediately

> *Rare*—Agitation; confusion; fever; hallucinations; peeling of the skin; shakiness or tremors; shortness of breath; skin rash, itching, or redness; swelling of face or neck

Side Effects That Usually Do Not Require Medical Attention

These possible side effects may go away during treatment; however, if they continue or are bothersome, check with your doctor, nurse, or pharmacist.

> *More common*—Abdominal or stomach pain or discomfort; diarrhea; dizziness; drowsiness; headache; lightheadedness; nausea or vomiting; nervousness; trouble in sleeping

> *Less common or rare*—Increased sensitivity of skin to sunlight

Other side effects not listed above may also occur in some patients. If you notice any other effects, check with your doctor, nurse, or pharmacist.

FLUOXETINE   Systemic

■ For the Pharmacist ■

In providing consultation, consider emphasizing the following selected
information (» = major clinical significance):

Before using this medication
» Conditions affecting use, especially:
>Recent anecdotal reports of fluoxetine use possibly related to
suicidal ideation in a few patients
>Sensitivity to fluoxetine
>Breast-feeding—Not recommended
>Other medications, especially CNS depression–causing medi-
cations; highly protein-bound medications such as anticoagulants, digitalis, or digitoxin; monoamine oxidase (MAO) inhibitors; phenytoin; or tryptophan
>Other medical problems, especially hepatic or renal function
impairment

Proper use of this medication
» Compliance with therapy; not taking more or less medicine than
prescribed
>May be taken with food to lessen possible stomach upset
» May require up to 4 weeks or longer of therapy to obtain antide-
pressant effects
» Proper dosing
>Missed dose: Skipping the missed dose and continuing on regular
schedule with next dose; not doubling doses
» Proper storage

Precautions while using this medication
>Regular visits to physician to check progress of therapy
» Avoiding use of alcoholic beverages; not taking other CNS depressants unless prescribed by physician
» Stopping fluoxetine and checking with physician as soon as possible
if skin rash or hives occurs
» Possible drowsiness, impairment of judgment, thinking, or motor
skills; caution when driving or doing jobs requiring alertness
» Possible dizziness or lightheadedness; caution when getting up suddenly from a lying or sitting position
» Possible dryness of mouth; using sugarless gum or candy, ice, or
saliva substitute for relief; checking with physician or dentist if
dry mouth continues for more than 2 weeks

Side/adverse effects
>Signs of potential side effects, especially chills or fever, swollen
glands, joint or muscle pain, skin rash, hives, or itching, trouble
in breathing, allergic reaction, serum sickness–like syndrome,
convulsions, mania, or hypomania

▲ For the Patient ▲

916147

ABOUT YOUR MEDICINE

Fluoxetine (floo-OX-uh-teen) is used to treat mental depression. It is also used to treat obsessive-compulsive disorder.

If any of the information in this leaflet causes you special concern or if you want additional information about your medicine and its use, check with your doctor, nurse, or pharmacist. **Remember, keep this and all other medicines out of the reach of children and never share your medicines with others.**

BEFORE USING THIS MEDICINE

Tell your doctor, nurse, and pharmacist if you . . .
- are allergic to any medicine, either prescription or non-prescription (OTC);
- are pregnant or intend to become pregnant while using this medicine;
- are breast-feeding;
- are taking any other prescription or nonprescription (OTC) medicine, especially anticoagulants (blood thinners), CNS depressants, digitalis glycosides (heart medicine), MAO inhibitors, phenytoin, or tryptophan;
- have any other medical problems, especially kidney disease or liver disease, or a history of seizure disorders.

PROPER USE OF THIS MEDICINE

Take this medicine only as directed by your doctor, to benefit your condition as much as possible. Do not take more of it, do not take it more often, and do not take it for a longer time than your doctor ordered.

If this medicine upsets your stomach, it may be taken with food.

Sometimes fluoxetine must be taken for up to 4 weeks or longer before you begin to feel better. Your doctor should check your progress at regular visits during this time.

If you miss a dose of this medicine, it is not necessary to make up the missed dose. Skip the missed dose and continue with your next scheduled dose. Do not double doses.

PRECAUTIONS WHILE USING THIS MEDICINE

It is important that your doctor check your progress at regular visits, to allow dosage adjustments and help reduce any side effects.

This medicine will add to the effects of alcohol and other CNS depressants (medicines that slow down the nervous system). **Check with your doctor before taking any such depressants while you are using this medicine.**

If you develop a skin rash or hives, stop taking fluoxetine and check with your doctor as soon as possible.

This medicine may cause some people to become drowsy. **Make sure you know how you react to fluoxetine before you drive, use machines, or do other jobs that could be dangerous if you are not alert.**

Dizziness, lightheadedness, or fainting may occur, especially when you get up from a lying or sitting position. Getting up

slowly may help. If this problem continues or gets worse, check with your doctor.

This medicine may cause dryness of the mouth. For temporary relief, use sugarless gum or candy, melt bits of ice in your mouth, or use a saliva substitute. However, if your mouth continues to feel dry for more than 2 weeks, check with your physician or dentist. Continuing dryness of the mouth may increase the chance of dental disease, including tooth decay, gum disease, and fungus infections.

POSSIBLE SIDE EFFECTS OF THIS MEDICINE
Side Effects That Should Be Reported To Your Doctor

Less common—Chills or fever; joint or muscle pain; skin rash, hives, or itching; trouble in breathing

Rare—Anxiety or nervousness; burning or tingling in fingers, hands, or arms; cold sweats; confusion; convulsions (seizures); cool, pale skin; difficulty in concentration; drowsiness; excessive hunger; fast heartbeat; headache; shakiness or unsteady walk; swelling of feet or lower legs; swollen glands; unusual tiredness or weakness

Side Effects That Usually Do Not Require Medical Attention

These possible side effects may go away during treatment; however, if they continue or are bothersome, check with your doctor, nurse, or pharmacist.

More common—Anxiety and nervousness; diarrhea; drowsiness; headache; increased sweating; nausea; trouble in sleeping

Less common—Abnormal dreams; change in taste; changes in vision; chest pain; constipation; cough; decreased appetite or weight loss; decreased sexual drive or ability; decrease in concentration; dizziness or lightheadedness; dryness of mouth; fast or irregular heartbeat; feeling of warmth or heat; flushing or redness of skin, especially on face and neck; frequent urination; increased appetite; menstrual pain; stomach cramps, gas, or pain; stuffy nose; tiredness or weakness; tremor; vomiting

Other side effects not listed above may also occur in some patients. If you notice any other effects, check with your doctor, nurse, or pharmacist.

GEMFIBROZIL   Systemic

■ For the Pharmacist ■

In providing consultation, consider emphasizing the following selected information (» = major clinical significance):

Before using this medication
Potential serious toxicity because of similarity to clofibrate
» Diet as preferred therapy
» Conditions affecting use especially:
    Sensitivity to gemfibrozil
    Pregnancy—High doses in animals cause birth defects and an increase in fetal deaths
    Breast-feeding—High doses associated with increased incidence of tumors in rats; consider when deciding whether to breast-feed
    Use in children—Not recommended in children under 2 years of age since cholesterol is required for normal development
    Other medications, especially lovastatin or oral anticoagulants
    Other medical problems, especially primary biliary cirrhosis, hepatic function impairment, or severe renal function impairment

Proper use of this medication
» Importance of not taking more or less medication than the amount prescribed
Taking 30 minutes before morning and evening meal
» Compliance with prescribed diet
» Proper dosing
Missed dose: Taking as soon as possible; not taking if almost time for next dose; not doubling doses
» Proper storage

Precautions while using this medication
» Importance of close monitoring by physician
» Checking with physician before discontinuing medication; blood lipid concentrations may increase significantly

Side/adverse effects
Signs of potential side effects, especially gallstones, leukopenia, anemia, and myositis

▲ For the Patient ▲

913954

ABOUT YOUR MEDICINE

Gemfibrozil (gem-FI-broe-zil) is used to lower levels of cholesterol and triglyceride (fat-like substances) in the blood. This may help prevent medical problems caused by such substances clogging the blood vessels.

If any of the information in this leaflet causes you special concern or if you want additional information about your medicine and its use, check with your doctor, nurse, or pharmacist. **Remember, keep this and all other medicines out of the reach of children and never share your medicines with others.**

BEFORE USING THIS MEDICINE

In addition to its helpful effects in treating your medical problem, this type of medicine may have some harmful effects.

Results of a large study using gemfibrozil seem to show that it may cause a higher rate of some cancers in humans. In addition, the action of gemfibrozil is similar to that of another medicine called clofibrate. Studies with clofibrate have suggested that it may increase the patient's risk of cancer, liver disease, and pancreatitis (inflammation of the pancreas), gallstones, and problems from gallbladder surgery. However, it may also decrease the risk of heart attacks. Other studies have not found all of these effects. Be sure you have discussed this with your doctor before taking this medicine.

Importance of diet—Your doctor will probably try to control your condition by prescribing a personal diet for you. Such a diet may be low in fats, sugars, and/or cholesterol. Also, it may be very important for you to go on a reducing diet. **Medicine is prescribed only when additional help is needed** and is effective only when a schedule of diet and exercise is properly followed. However, check with your doctor before going on any diet.

Tell your doctor, nurse, and pharmacist if you . . .
- are allergic to any medicine, either prescription or non-prescription (OTC);
- are pregnant or intend to become pregnant while using this medicine;
- are breast-feeding;
- are taking any other prescription or nonprescription (OTC) medicine, especially anticoagulants (blood thinners) or lovastatin;
- have any other medical problems, especially kidney disease or liver disease.

PROPER USE OF THIS MEDICINE

Use this medicine only as directed by your doctor. Do not use more or less of it, and do not use it more often or for a longer time than your doctor ordered.

This medicine is usually taken twice a day. If you are taking 2 doses a day, it is best to take the medicine 30 minutes before your breakfast and evening meals.

If you miss a dose of this medicine, take it as soon as possible. However, if it is almost time for your next dose, skip the missed dose and go back to your regular dosing schedule. Do not double doses.

PRECAUTIONS WHILE USING THIS MEDICINE

It is very important that your doctor check your progress at regular visits. This will allow your doctor to see if the medicine is working properly to lower your cholesterol and triglyceride levels and if you should continue to take it.

Do not stop taking this medication without first checking with your doctor. When you stop taking this medicine, your blood cholesterol levels may increase again. Your doctor may want you to follow a special diet to help prevent this from happening.

POSSIBLE SIDE EFFECTS OF THIS MEDICINE
Side Effects That Should Be Reported To Your Doctor Immediately

  Rare—Cough or hoarseness; fever or chills; lower back or side pain; painful or difficult urination; stomach pain (severe) with nausea and vomiting

Other Side Effects That Should Be Reported To Your Doctor

  Rare—Muscle pain; unusual tiredness or weakness

Side Effects That Usually Do Not Require Medical Attention

These possible side effects may go away during treatment; however, if they continue or are bothersome, check with your doctor, nurse, or pharmacist.

  More common—Stomach pain, gas, or heartburn

  Less common—Diarrhea; nausea or vomiting; skin rash

Other side effects not listed above may also occur in some patients. If you notice any other effects, check with your doctor, nurse, or pharmacist.

GOLD COMPOUNDS   Systemic

Including Auranofin; Aurothioglucose; Gold Sodium Thiomalate.

■For the Pharmacist■

In providing consultation, consider emphasizing the following selected information (**»** = major clinical significance):

Before using this medication
» Conditions affecting use, especially:

    Sensitivity to gold, other heavy metals, or sesame products

    Pregnancy—Studies in humans have not been done, but gold compounds have caused teratogenic and fetotoxic effects in animal studies

    Breast-feeding—Use is not recommended because of potential adverse effects in the nursing infant; aurothioglucose and gold sodium thiomalate are excreted in human breast milk; it is not known whether auranofin is excreted in human breast milk

    Dental—Risk of adverse effects such as infection, delayed healing, and gingival bleeding associated with blood dyscrasias, as well as gold compound–induced gingivitis, glossitis, and/or stomatitis

    Other medications, especially penicillamine

    Other medical problems, especially serious adverse effects to prior gold therapy, blood dyscrasias (especially hemorrhagic or caused by sensitivity to a medication), severe debilitation, Sjögren's syndrome, systemic lupus erythematosus, eczema, or urticaria

Proper use of this medication

    Compliance with therapy; symptomatic relief may not occur until after three to six months of continuous use

» Proper dosing

For auranofin (oral dosage form) only

» Not taking more medication than amount prescribed

    Missed dose: If dosing schedule is—

    Once a day: Taking as soon as possible; not taking if not remembered until next day; not doubling doses

    More than once a day: Taking as soon as possible; not taking if almost time for next dose; not doubling doses

» Proper storage

Precautions while using this medication

    Possibility of phototoxicity

For oral dosage form only

    Regular visits to physician to check progress during therapy; blood and urine tests may be required to detect possible adverse effects

For parenteral dosage forms only

    Possibility of nitritoid reactions immediately following injection

    Possibility of joint pain occurring for 1 or 2 days after injection

Side/adverse effects

    Signs and symptoms of potential side effects, especially allergic reactions, blood dyscrasias, central nervous system or neurologic effects, cutaneous or dermatologic effects, difficulty in swallowing, fever, ulcerative enterocolitis, gastrointestinal bleeding, hepatotoxicity, mucous membrane reactions, ocular effects, pulmonary effects, and renal effects

Possibility of side effects occurring up to many months after discontinuation of medication

---

▲ For the Patient ▲

914006

ABOUT YOUR MEDICINE

Gold compounds are used in the treatment of rheumatoid arthritis. They may also be used for other conditions as determined by your doctor. Auranofin is taken by mouth; the other gold compounds are given by injection.

If any of the information in this leaflet causes you special concern or if you want additional information about your medicine and its use, check with your doctor, nurse, or pharmacist. **Remember, keep this and all other medicines out of the reach of children and never share your medicines with others.**

BEFORE USING THIS MEDICINE

Tell your doctor, nurse, and pharmacist if you . . .
- are allergic to any medicine, either prescription or non-prescription (OTC);
- are pregnant or intend to become pregnant while using this medicine;
- are breast-feeding;
- are taking **any** other prescription or nonprescription (OTC) medicine;
- have **any** other medical problems.

PROPER USE OF THIS MEDICINE

In order for this medicine to work, it must be taken regularly as ordered by your doctor. Continue receiving the injections or taking auranofin even if you think the medicine is not working. You may not notice the effects of this medicine until after 3 to 6 months of regular use.

For patients taking auranofin:
- **Do not take more of this medicine than ordered by your doctor.** Taking too much auranofin may increase the chance of serious unwanted effects.
- **If you miss a dose of this medicine,** take it as soon as possible. However, if you do not remember until the next day, or if it is almost time for your next dose, skip the missed dose and go back to your regular dosing schedule. Do not double doses.

PRECAUTIONS WHILE USING THIS MEDICINE

Gold compounds may cause some people to become more sensitive to sunlight than they are normally. It is best to avoid too much sun or use of a sunlamp while being treated with a gold compound. You may protect yourself against sunlight with clothing, or ask your doctor if you may use a factor-15 sunscreen.

For patients taking auranofin:
- Your doctor should check your progress at regular visits. Blood and urine tests may be needed to check for unwanted effects.

For patients receiving gold injections:
- Dizziness, feeling faint, flushing or redness of the face, nausea or vomiting, increased sweating, or unusual weakness may occur after an injection. These will usually go away after you lie down for a few minutes.
- Joint pain may occur for 1 or 2 days after you receive an injection of this medicine. This effect usually disappears after the first few injections.

POSSIBLE SIDE EFFECTS OF THIS MEDICINE

Although not all of these side effects appear very often, they may occur at any time during treatment with this medicine **and up to many months after treatment has ended,** and they may require medical attention.

Side Effects That Should Be Reported To Your Doctor

More common—Irritation or soreness of tongue; metallic taste; redness, soreness, swelling, or bleeding of gums; skin rash or itching; ulcers, sores, or white spots on lips or in mouth or throat

Less common—Bloody or cloudy urine; hives; sore throat and fever with or without chills; spitting blood; unusual bleeding or bruising

Rare—Bloody or black tarry stools; confusion; convulsions (seizures); coughing; decreased urination; decreased vision; difficulty in swallowing; fever; hallucinations; irritation of nose, throat, or upper chest area; irritation of vagina; numbness, tingling, pain, or weakness, especially in the face, hands, arms, or feet; pain, redness, itching, or tearing of eyes; problems with muscle coordination; red, thickened, or scaly skin; swelling of face, fingers, ankles, lower legs, or feet; swellings (large) on face, eyelids, mouth, lips, and/or tongue; swollen and/or painful glands; vomiting of blood or material that looks like coffee grounds; wheezing or difficulty breathing; yellow eyes or skin

Side Effects That Usually Do Not Require Medical Attention

These possible side effects may go away during treatment; however, if they continue or are bothersome, check with your doctor, nurse, or pharmacist.

More common with auranofin; rare with injections—Abdominal or stomach cramps or pain; bloated feeling, gas, or indigestion; diarrhea or loose stools; nausea or vomiting

Other side effects not listed above may also occur in some patients. If you notice any other effects, check with your doctor, nurse, or pharmacist.

GRISEOFULVIN   Systemic

■ For the Pharmacist ■

In providing consultation, consider emphasizing the following selected information (**»** = major clinical significance):

Before using this medication
» Conditions affecting use, especially:
  Hypersensitivity to griseofulvin; theoretic cross-sensitivity with penicillin, however, penicillin-sensitive patients have received griseofulvin without difficulty
  Pregnancy—Griseofulvin crosses the placenta; use is not recommended during pregnancy since griseofulvin has been shown to be embryotoxic and teratogenic in rats
  Dental—Griseofulvin may cause oral thrush
  Other medications, especially coumarin- or indandione-derivative anticoagulants or estrogen-containing oral contraceptives
  Other medical problems, especially hepatic dysfunction or porphyria

Proper use of this medication
» Taking with or after meals, especially fatty ones, to minimize gastrointestinal irritation and to increase absorption; checking with physician if on low-fat diet
  Proper administration technique for oral suspension
» Compliance with full course of therapy
» Proper dosing
  Missed dose: Taking as soon as possible; not taking if almost time for next dose; not doubling doses
» Proper storage

Precautions while using this medication
  Regular visits to physician to check progress during therapy
» Use of an alternate or additional means of contraception if taking estrogen-containing oral contraceptives concurrently and for 1 month after stopping griseofulvin
  Caution in drinking alcoholic beverages during griseofulvin therapy
» Caution if dizziness occurs
» Possible photosensitivity reactions

Side/adverse effects
  Signs of potential side effects, especially confusion, hypersensitivity, photosensitivity, oral thrush, granulocytopenia, leukopenia, and peripheral neuritis

▲ For the Patient ▲

914017

ABOUT YOUR MEDICINE

Griseofulvin (gri-see-oh-FUL-vin) belongs to the group of medicines called antifungals. It is used to treat fungus infections of the skin, hair, fingernails, and toenails. This medicine may be taken alone or used along with medicines that are applied to the skin for fungus infections.

If any of the information in this leaflet causes you special concern or if you want additional information about your

medicine and its use, check with your doctor, nurse, or pharmacist. **Remember, keep this and all other medicines out of the reach of children and never share your medicines with others.**

BEFORE USING THIS MEDICINE

Discuss with your doctor the possible side effects that may be caused by this medicine. Some of them may be serious and/or long-term.

Tell your doctor, nurse, and pharmacist if you . . .
- are allergic to any medicine, either prescription or nonprescription (OTC);
- are pregnant or intend to become pregnant while using this medicine;
- are breast-feeding;
- are taking any other prescription or nonprescription (OTC) medicine, especially anticoagulants (blood thinners) or oral contraceptives (birth control pills) containing estrogen;
- have any other medical problems, especially liver disease or porphyria.

PROPER USE OF THIS MEDICINE

Griseofulvin is best taken with or after meals, especially fatty ones (for example, whole milk or ice cream). This lessens possible stomach upset and helps to clear up the infection by helping your body absorb the medicine better. **However, if you are on a low-fat diet, check with your doctor.**

To help clear up your infection completely, **keep taking this medicine for the full time of treatment** even if you begin to feel better after a few days; do not miss any doses.

If you do miss a dose of this medicine, take it as soon as possible. However, if it is almost time for your next dose, skip the missed dose and go back to your regular dosing schedule. Do not double doses.

PRECAUTIONS WHILE USING THIS MEDICINE

Your doctor should check your progress at regular visits to make sure that griseofulvin does not cause unwanted effects.

Oral contraceptives (birth control pills) containing estrogen may not work properly if you take them while you are taking griseofulvin. Unplanned pregnancies may occur. You should use a different or additional means of birth control while you are taking griseofulvin and for one month after stopping griseofulvin. If you have any questions about this, check with your doctor or pharmacist.

Griseofulvin may increase the effects of alcohol. If taken with alcohol it may also cause fast heartbeat, flushing, increased sweating, or redness of the face. Therefore, if you have this reaction, do not drink alcoholic beverages while you are taking this medicine, unless you have first checked with your doctor.

This medicine may cause some people to become dizzy or less alert than they are normally. **Make sure you know how you react to this medicine before you drive, use machines, or do other jobs that require you to be alert.** If these reactions are especially bothersome, check with your doctor.

Griseofulvin may cause your skin to be more sensitive to sunlight than it is normally. When you first begin taking this medicine, avoid too much sun and do not use a sunlamp until you see how you react to the sun, especially if you tend to burn easily. **If you have a severe reaction, check with your doctor.**

This medicine must not be given to other people or used for other infections unless otherwise directed by your doctor.

POSSIBLE SIDE EFFECTS OF THIS MEDICINE
Side Effects That Should Be Reported To Your Doctor

> *Less common*—Confusion; increased sensitivity of skin to sunlight; skin rash, hives, or itching; soreness or irritation of mouth or tongue
>
> *Rare*—Numbness, tingling, pain, or weakness in hands or feet; sore throat and fever; yellow eyes or skin

Side Effects That Usually Do Not Require Medical Attention

These possible side effects may go away during treatment; however, if they continue or are bothersome, check with your doctor, nurse, or pharmacist.

> *More common*—Headache

Other side effects not listed above may also occur in some patients. If you notice any other effects, check with your doctor, nurse, or pharmacist.

GUANABENZ   Systemic

■ For the Pharmacist ■

In providing consultation, consider emphasizing the following selected
   information (» = major clinical significance):

Before using this medication
» Conditions affecting use, especially:
      Sensitivity to guanabenz
      Pregnancy—High doses in animals cause decreased fertility, birth
         defects, and fetal death
      Use in the elderly—Increased sensitivity to hypotensive and sed-
         ative effects
      Dental—May decrease or inhibit salivary flow
      Other medications, especially systemic beta-adrenergic blocking
         agents

Proper use of this medication
   Possible need for control of weight and diet, especially sodium intake
» Patient may not experience symptoms of hypertension; importance
      of taking medication even if feeling well
» Does not cure but helps control hypertension; possible need for life-
      long therapy; serious consequences of untreated hypertension
   Getting into the habit of taking at same time each day to help
      increase compliance
» Proper dosing
   Missed dose: Taking as soon as possible; not taking if almost time
      for next dose; checking with physician if two or more doses in
      a row are missed; possible unpleasant effects if stopped abruptly
» Proper storage

Precautions while using this medication
   Regular visits to physician to check progress
   Checking with physician before discontinuing medication; possible
      need for gradual dosage reduction
   Caution if any kind of surgery (including dental surgery) or emer-
      gency treatment is required
» Not taking other medications, especially nonprescription sympatho-
      mimetics, unless discussed with physician
» Caution in taking alcohol or other CNS depressants
» Caution when driving or doing things requiring alertness because of
      possible dizziness or drowsiness
   Possible dryness of mouth; using sugarless candy or gum, ice, or
      saliva substitute for relief; checking with physician or dentist if
      dry mouth continues for more than 2 weeks

Side/adverse effects
   Signs of potential side effects, especially signs and symptoms of
      overdose or withdrawal reaction

▲ For the Patient ▲

ABOUT YOUR MEDICINE

Guanabenz (GWAHN-a-benz) belongs to the general class
of medicines called antihypertensives. It is used to treat high
blood pressure (hypertension).

If any of the information in this leaflet causes you special concern or if you want additional information about your medicine and its use, check with your doctor, nurse, or pharmacist. **Remember, keep this and all other medicines out of the reach of children and never share your medicines with others.**

BEFORE USING THIS MEDICINE
Tell your doctor, nurse, and pharmacist if you . . .
- are allergic to any medicine, either prescription or nonprescription (OTC);
- are pregnant or intend to become pregnant while using this medicine;
- are breast-feeding;
- are taking any other prescription or nonprescription (OTC) medicine, especially one that contains beta-blockers;
- have any other medical problems.

PROPER USE OF THIS MEDICINE
Importance of diet—When prescribing medicine for your condition, your doctor will probably try to control your condition by prescribing a personal diet for you. Such a diet may be low in sodium (salt). Medicine is usually more effective when such a diet is properly followed.

Many patients who have high blood pressure will not notice any signs of the problem. In fact, many may feel normal. It is very important that you **take your medicine exactly as directed** and that you keep your doctor's appointments even if you feel well.

This medicine will not cure your high blood pressure but it does help control it. You must continue to take it—even if you feel well—if you expect to keep your blood pressure down. **You may have to take high blood pressure medicine for the rest of your life.**

If you miss a dose of this medicine, take it as soon as possible. However, if it is almost time for your next dose, skip the missed dose and go back to your regular dosing schedule. Do not double doses. If you miss two or more doses in a row, check with your doctor. If your body suddenly goes without this medicine, some unpleasant effects may occur.

PRECAUTIONS WHILE USING THIS MEDICINE
Do not take other medicines unless they have been discussed with your doctor. This especially includes over-the-counter (nonprescription) medicines for appetite control, asthma, colds, cough, hay fever, or sinus problems, since they may tend to increase your blood pressure.

Check with your doctor before you stop taking this medicine. Your doctor may want you to reduce gradually the amount you are taking before stopping completely.

This medicine will add to the effects of alcohol and other CNS depressants (medicines that slow down the nervous system). **Check with your doctor before taking any such depressants while you are using this medicine.**

Guanabenz may cause some people to become dizzy, drowsy, or less alert than they are normally. **Make sure you know how you react to this medicine before you drive, use machines, or do other jobs that require you to be alert.**

POSSIBLE SIDE EFFECTS OF THIS MEDICINE
Side Effects That Usually Do Not Require Medical Attention

These possible side effects may go away during treatment; however, if they continue or are bothersome, check with your doctor, nurse, or pharmacist.

> *More common*—Dizziness; drowsiness; dry mouth; weakness

Other side effects not listed above may also occur in some patients. If you notice any other effects, check with your doctor, nurse, or pharmacist.

After you have been using this medicine for a while, unpleasant effects may occur if you stop taking it too suddenly. After you stop taking this medicine, check with your doctor if any unusual effects occur, especially anxiety or tenseness, chest pain, fast or irregular heartbeat, headache, increased salivation, increased sweating, nausea or vomiting, nervousness or restlessness, shaking or trembling of hands or fingers, stomach cramps, or trouble in sleeping.

GUANADREL Systemic

■ For the Pharmacist ■

In providing consultation, consider emphasizing the following selected information (» = major clinical significance):

Before using this medication
» Conditions affecting use, especially:
 Sensitivity to guanadrel
 Use in the elderly—Increased sensitivity to hypotensive effects
 Other medications, especially tricyclic antidepressants, loxapine, thioxanthenes, trimeprazine, or MAO inhibitors
 Other medical problems, especially congestive heart failure or pheochromocytoma

Proper use of this medication
 Importance of diet; possible need for sodium restriction and/or weight reduction
» Patients may not experience symptoms of hypertension; importance of taking medication even if feeling well
» Does not cure, but helps control hypertension; possible need for lifelong therapy; checking with physician before discontinuing medication; serious consequences of untreated hypertension
 Getting into the habit of taking at same time each day to help increase compliance
» Proper dosing
 Missed dose: Taking as soon as possible; not taking if almost time for next dose; not doubling doses
» Proper storage

Precautions while using this medication
 Regular visits to physician to check progress
» Caution when getting up suddenly from a lying or sitting position, especially in the morning
» Caution in using alcohol, while standing for long periods or exercising, and during hot weather because of enhanced orthostatic hypotensive effects
» Not taking other medications, especially nonprescription sympathomimetics, unless discussed with physician
 Caution if any kind of surgery (including dental surgery) or emergency treatment is required
 Reporting fever to physician; dosage adjustment may be required

Side/adverse effects
 Signs of potential side effects, especially peripheral edema, dyspnea, and angina

▲ For the Patient ▲

914039

ABOUT YOUR MEDICINE

Guanadrel (GWAHN-a-drel) belongs to the general class of medicines called antihypertensives. It is used to treat high blood pressure (hypertension).

If any of the information in this leaflet causes you special concern or if you want additional information about your

medicine and its use, check with your doctor, nurse, or pharmacist. **Remember, keep this and all other medicines out of the reach of children and never share your medicines with others.**

BEFORE USING THIS MEDICINE

Tell your doctor, nurse, and pharmacist if you . . .
- are allergic to any medicine, either prescription or non-prescription (OTC);
- are pregnant or intend to become pregnant while using this medicine;
- are breast-feeding;
- are taking **any** other prescription or nonprescription (OTC) medicine;
- have any other medical problems, especially heart disease or pheochromocytoma.

PROPER USE OF THIS MEDICINE

Importance of diet—When prescribing medicine for your condition, your doctor may also prescribe a personal diet for you. Such a diet may be low in sodium (salt). Medicine is usually more effective when such a diet is properly followed.

Many patients who have high blood pressure will not notice any signs of the problem. In fact, many may feel normal. It is very important that you **take your medicine exactly as directed** and that you keep your doctor's appointments even if you feel well.

This medicine will not cure your high blood pressure but it does help control it. You must continue to take it—even if you feel well—if you expect to keep your blood pressure down. **You may have to take high blood pressure medicine for the rest of your life.**

If you miss a dose of guanadrel, take it as soon as possible. However, if it is almost time for your next dose, skip the missed dose and go back to your regular dosing schedule. Do not double doses.

PRECAUTIONS WHILE USING THIS MEDICINE

Dizziness, lightheadedness, or fainting may occur, especially when you get up from a lying or sitting position. This may be more likely to occur in the morning. **Getting up slowly may help.** If you feel dizzy, sit or lie down. When you get up from lying down, sit on the edge of the bed with your feet dangling for 1 or 2 minutes. Then stand up slowly. If the problem continues or gets worse, check with your doctor.

The dizziness, lightheadedness, or fainting is also more likely to occur if you drink alcohol, stand for long periods of time, or exercise, or if the weather is hot. **While you are taking guanadrel, be careful in the amount of alcohol you drink. Also, use extra care during exercise or hot weather or if you must stand for long periods of time.**

Do not take other medicines unless they have been discussed with your doctor. This especially includes over-the-counter (nonprescription) medicines for appetite control, asthma, colds, cough, hay fever, or sinus problems, since they may tend to increase your blood pressure.

Tell your doctor if you get a fever since that may change the amount of medicine you have to take.

POSSIBLE SIDE EFFECTS OF THIS MEDICINE
Side Effects That Should Be Reported To Your Doctor Immediately

   Rare—Blurred vision; dizziness or faintness (severe)

Other Side Effects That Should Be Reported To Your Doctor

   More common—Swelling of feet or lower legs

   Less common or rare—Chest pain; shortness of breath

Side Effects That Usually Do Not Require Medical Attention

These possible side effects may go away during treatment; however, if they continue or are bothersome, check with your doctor, nurse, or pharmacist.

   More common—Difficulty in ejaculating; dizziness, lightheadedness, or fainting, especially when standing up; drowsiness or tiredness

Other side effects not listed above may also occur in some patients. If you notice any other effects, check with your doctor, nurse, or pharmacist.

GUANETHIDINE   Systemic

■ For the Pharmacist ■

In providing consultation, consider emphasizing the following selected information (» = major clinical significance):

Before using this medication
» Conditions affecting use, especially:
   Sensitivity to guanethidine
   Fertility—Reversible inhibition of ejaculation
   Breast-feeding—Small quantities distributed into breast milk
   Use in the elderly—Increased sensitivity to hypotensive effects
   Other medications, especially tricyclic antidepressants, loxapine, thioxanthenes, trimeprazine, minoxidil, MAO inhibitors, oral antidiabetic agents, or metaraminol
   Other medical problems, especially congestive heart failure or pheochromocytoma

Proper use of this medication
   Possible need for control of weight and diet, especially sodium intake
» Patient may not experience symptoms of hypertension; importance of taking medication even if feeling well
» Does not cure, but helps control hypertension; possible need for lifelong therapy; checking with physician before discontinuing medication; serious consequences of untreated hypertension
   Getting into the habit of taking at same time each day to help increase compliance
» Proper dosing
   Missed dose: Taking as soon as possible; not taking if almost time for next dose; not doubling doses
» Proper storage

Precautions while using this medication
   Regular visits to physician to check progress
» Caution when getting up suddenly from a lying or sitting position, especially in the morning
» Caution in using alcohol, while standing for long periods or exercising, and during hot weather because of enhanced orthostatic hypotensive effects
» Not taking other medications, especially nonprescription sympathomimetics, unless discussed with physician
   Caution if any kind of surgery (including dental surgery) or emergency treatment is required
   Reporting fever to physician; dosage adjustment may be required

Side/adverse effects
   Signs of potential side effects, especially peripheral and pulmonary edema and angina

▲ For the Patient ▲

914040

ABOUT YOUR MEDICINE

Guanethidine (gwahn-ETH-i-deen) belongs to the general class of medicines called antihypertensives. It is used to treat high blood pressure (hypertension).

If any of the information in this leaflet causes you special concern or if you want additional information about your medicine and its use, check with your doctor, nurse, or pharmacist. **Remember, keep this and all other medicines out of the reach of children and never share your medicines with others.**

BEFORE USING THIS MEDICINE

Tell your doctor, nurse, and pharmacist if you . . .
- are allergic to any medicine, either prescription or non-prescription (OTC);
- are pregnant or intend to become pregnant while using this medicine;
- are breast-feeding;
- are taking **any** other prescription or nonprescription (OTC) medicine;
- have any other medical problems, especially heart disease or pheochromocytoma.

PROPER USE OF THIS MEDICINE

Many patients who have high blood pressure will not notice any signs of the problem. In fact, many may feel normal. It is very important that you **take your medicine exactly as directed** and that you keep your doctor's appointments even if you feel well.

This medicine will not cure your high blood pressure but it does help control it. You must continue to take it—even if you feel well—if you expect to keep your blood pressure down. **You may have to take high blood pressure medicine for the rest of your life.**

If you miss a dose of guanethidine, take it as soon as possible. However, if it is almost time for your next dose, skip the missed dose and go back to your regular dosing schedule. Do not double doses.

PRECAUTIONS WHILE USING THIS MEDICINE

Dizziness, lightheadedness, or fainting may occur, especially when you get up from a lying or sitting position. This is more likely to occur in the morning. **Getting up slowly may help.** When you get up from lying down, sit on the edge of the bed with your feet dangling for 1 or 2 minutes. Then stand up slowly. If the problem continues or gets worse, check with your doctor.

The dizziness, lightheadedness, or fainting is also more likely to occur if you drink alcohol, stand for long periods of time, exercise, or if the weather is hot. **While you are taking this medicine, be careful in the amount of alcohol you drink. Also, use extra care during exercise or hot weather or if you must stand for long periods of time.**

Do not take other medicines unless they have been discussed with your doctor. This especially includes over-the-counter (nonprescription) medicines for appetite control, asthma, colds, cough, hay fever, or sinus problems, since they may tend to increase your blood pressure.

Tell your doctor if you get a fever since that may change the amount of medicine you have to take.

POSSIBLE SIDE EFFECTS OF THIS MEDICINE
Side Effects That Should Be Reported To Your Doctor

> *More common*—Swelling of feet or lower legs

> *Less common or rare*—Chest pain; shortness of breath

Side Effects That Usually Do Not Require Medical Attention

These possible side effects may go away during treatment; however, if they continue or are bothersome, check with your doctor, nurse, or pharmacist.

> *More common*—Diarrhea or increase in bowel movements; dizziness, lightheadedness, or fainting when standing up; sexual problems in males; slow heartbeat; stuffy nose; unusual tiredness or weakness

> *Less common*—Blurred vision, drooping eyelids; dryness of mouth; headache; loss of hair on scalp; muscle pain or tremors; nausea or vomiting; nighttime urination; skin rash

Other side effects not listed above may also occur in some patients. If you notice any other effects, check with your doctor, nurse, or pharmacist.

GUANFACINE   Systemic

■ For the Pharmacist ■

In providing consultation, consider emphasizing the following selected
information (» = major clinical significance):

Before using this medication
» Conditions affecting use, especially:
    Sensitivity to guanfacine
    Pregnancy—Use of extremely high doses in animals caused in-
    creased fetal deaths
    Use in the elderly—Increased sensitivity to hypotensive effects

Proper use of this medication
    Possible need for control of weight and diet, especially sodium intake
» Patient may not experience symptoms of hypertension; importance
    of taking medication even if feeling well
» Does not cure, but helps control hypertension; possible need for
    lifelong therapy; serious consequences of untreated hypertension
    Taking at bedtime to reduce daytime drowsiness
» Proper dosing
» Missed dose: Taking as soon as possible; checking with physician if
    two or more doses in a row are missed; possible reaction if stopped
    abruptly
» Proper storage

Precautions while using this medication
    Regular visits to physician to check progress
    Checking with physician before discontinuing medication; gradual
    dosage reduction may be necessary to avoid rebound hyperten-
    sion
    Having enough medication on hand to get through weekends, hol-
    idays, and vacations; possibly carrying second prescription for
    emergency use
    Caution if any kind of surgery (including dental surgery) or emer-
    gency treatment is required
» Not taking other medications, especially nonprescription sympatho-
    mimetics, unless discussed with physician
» Avoiding use of alcohol or other CNS depressants
» Caution when driving or doing things requiring alertness because of
    possible drowsiness
    Possible dryness of mouth; using sugarless gum or candy, ice, or
    saliva substitute for relief; checking with dentist if dry mouth
    continues for more than 2 weeks

Side/adverse effects
    Signs of potential side effects, especially confusion, mental depres-
    sion, and withdrawal reaction

▲ For the Patient ▲

915235

ABOUT YOUR MEDICINE

Guanfacine (GWAHN-fa-seen) belongs to the general class
of medicines called antihypertensives. It is used to treat high
blood pressure (hypertension).

If any of the information in this leaflet causes you special concern or if you want additional information about your medicine and its use, check with your doctor, nurse, or pharmacist. **Remember, keep this and all other medicines out of the reach of children and never share your medicines with others.**

BEFORE USING THIS MEDICINE

Tell your doctor, nurse, and pharmacist if you . . .
- are allergic to any medicine, either prescription or non-prescription (OTC);
- are pregnant or intend to become pregnant while using this medicine;
- are breast-feeding;
- are taking **any** other prescription or nonprescription (OTC) medicine;
- have any other medical problems.

PROPER USE OF THIS MEDICINE

This medicine will not cure your high blood pressure but it does help control it. You must continue to take it—even if you feel well—if you expect to keep your blood pressure down. **You may have to take high blood pressure medicine for the rest of your life.**

Take your daily dose of guanfacine at bedtime. (If you are taking more than one dose a day, take your last dose at bedtime.) Taking it this way will help lessen daytime drowsiness.

If you miss a dose of this medicine, take it as soon as possible. However, if it is almost time for your next dose, skip the missed dose and go back to your regular dosing schedule. Do not double doses. **If you miss taking guanfacine for two or more days in a row, check with your doctor.** If your body suddenly goes without this medicine, some unwanted effects may occur.

PRECAUTIONS WHILE USING THIS MEDICINE

It is important that your doctor check your progress at regular visits to make sure this medicine is working properly.

Check with your doctor before you stop taking guanfacine. Your doctor may want you to reduce gradually the amount you are taking before stopping completely.

Make sure that you have enough guanfacine on hand to last through weekends, holidays, and vacations. You should not miss any doses.

Before having any kind of surgery or dental or emergency treatment, tell the physician or dentist in charge that you are using this medicine.

Do not take other medicines unless they have been discussed with your doctor. This especially includes over-the-counter (nonprescription) medicines for appetite control, asthma, colds, cough, hay fever, or sinus problems, since they may tend to increase your blood pressure.

Guanfacine will add to the effects of alcohol and other CNS depressants (medicines that slow down the nervous system). **Check with your doctor before taking any such depressants while you are taking this medicine.**

Guanfacine may cause some people to become dizzy, drowsy, or less alert than they are normally. **Make sure you know how you react to this medicine before you drive, use machines, or do other jobs that require you to be alert.**

POSSIBLE SIDE EFFECTS OF THIS MEDICINE
Side Effects That Should Be Reported To Your Doctor

    Less common—Confusion; mental depression

Side Effects That Usually Do Not Require Medical Attention

These possible side effects may go away during treatment; however, if they continue or are bothersome, check with your doctor, nurse, or pharmacist.

    More common—Constipation; dizziness; drowsiness; dry mouth

    Less common—Decreased sexual ability; dry, itching, or burning eyes; headache; nausea or vomiting; trouble in sleeping; unusual tiredness or weakness

Other side effects not listed above may also occur in some patients. If you notice any other effects, check with your doctor, nurse, or pharmacist.

After you have been using this medicine for a while, unwanted effects may occur if you stop taking it too suddenly. After you stop taking this medicine, check with your doctor if you notice anxiety or tenseness, chest pain, fast or irregular heartbeat, headache, increased salivation, nausea or vomiting, nervousness or restlessness, shaking or trembling of hands and fingers, stomach cramps, sweating, or trouble in sleeping.

HISTAMINE H$_2$-RECEPTOR ANTAGONISTS Systemic

Including Cimetidine; Famotidine; Nizatidine; Ranitidine.

■ For the Pharmacist ■

In providing consultation, consider emphasizing the following selected information (» = major clinical significance):

Before using this medication
» Conditions affecting use, especially:
  Sensitivity to any of the H$_2$-receptor antagonists
  Pregnancy—All cross placenta
  Breast-feeding—Cimetidine, famotidine, nizatidine, and ranitidine distributed into breast milk; nursing not recommended during cimetidine therapy, because of high concentration in breast milk
  Use in the elderly—Confusion more likely with cimetidine, famotidine, and ranitidine in elderly patients with impaired hepatic or renal function
  Other medications, especially ketoconazole (with all H$_2$-receptor antagonists); anticoagulants, metoprolol, phenytoin, xanthines (with cimetidine and possibly ranitidine only); propranolol or tricyclic antidepressants (with cimetidine only)
  Other medical problems, especially renal function impairment

Proper use of this medication
  Dosing schedule:
    1 dose a day—Taking at bedtime
    2 doses a day—Taking in the morning and at bedtime
    Several doses a day—Taking with meals and at bedtime
  Taking antacids for relief of ulcer pain; not taking within ½ to 1 hour of histamine H$_2$-receptor antagonists
» Compliance with full course of therapy
» Proper dosing
  Missed dose: Taking as soon as possible; not taking if almost time for next dose; not doubling doses
» Proper storage

Precautions while using this medication
  Possible interference with gastric acid secretion tests or skin tests using allergens; need to inform physician of use of medication
  Avoiding use of foods, drinks, or other medication that may cause gastrointestinal irritation
  Discontinuing smoking or at least avoiding smoking after last dose of day
  Avoiding alcoholic beverages
  Checking with physician if condition does not improve or worsens

Side/adverse effects
  Signs of possible side effects, especially allergic reaction, bradycardia or tachycardia, bronchospasm, confusion, fever, and neutropenia or other blood dyscrasias

▲ For the Patient ▲

913091

ABOUT YOUR MEDICINE

H$_2$-blockers are used in the treatment and prevention of duodenal ulcers. Some of the H$_2$-blockers are used also to treat gastric ulcers. In addition, H$_2$-blockers are used in some conditions in which the stomach produces too much acid. These medicines may also be used for other conditions as determined by your doctor.

If any of the information in this leaflet causes you special concern or if you want additional information about your medicine and its use, check with your doctor, nurse, or pharmacist. **Remember, keep this and all other medicines out of the reach of children and never share your medicines with others.**

BEFORE USING THIS MEDICINE

Tell your doctor, nurse, and pharmacist if you . . .
  • are allergic to any medicine, either prescription or non-prescription (OTC);
  • are pregnant or intend to become pregnant while using this medicine;
  • are breast-feeding;
  • are taking any other prescription or nonprescription (OTC) medicine, especially ketoconazole;
  • are taking cimetidine and are also taking aminophylline, amitriptyline, amoxapine, anticoagulants (blood thinners), caffeine, clomipramine, desipramine, doxepin, imipramine, metoprolol, nortriptyline, oxtriphylline, phenytoin, propranolol, protriptyline, theophylline, or trimipramine;
  • are taking ranitidine and are also taking anticoagulants (blood thinners), caffeine, metoprolol, phenytoin, or theophylline;
  • have any other medical problems, especially severe kidney disease.

PROPER USE OF THIS MEDICINE

It may take several days for this medicine to begin to relieve stomach pain. To help relieve pain, antacids may be taken with this medicine, unless your doctor has told you not to use them. However, you should wait one-half to one hour between taking the antacid and this medicine.

Take this medicine for the full time of treatment, even if you begin to feel better. Also, it is important that you keep your doctor's appointments for check-ups so that your doctor will be better able to tell you when to stop taking this medicine.

For patients taking:
  • One dose a day—Take it at bedtime, unless otherwise directed.

- Two doses a day—Take one in the morning and one at bedtime.
- Several doses a day—Take them with meals and at bedtime for best results.

If you miss a dose of this medicine, take it as soon as possible. However, if it is almost time for your next dose, skip the missed dose and go back to your regular dosing schedule. Do not double doses.

PRECAUTIONS WHILE USING THIS MEDICINE
Some tests may be affected by this medicine. Tell the doctor in charge that you are taking this medicine before:
- You have any skin tests for allergies.
- You have any tests to determine how much acid your stomach produces.

Remember that certain medicines, such as aspirin, as well as certain foods and drinks (e.g., citrus products, carbonated drinks, etc.) irritate the stomach and may make your problem worse.

Cigarette smoking tends to decrease the effect of H₂-blockers by increasing the amount of acid produced by the stomach. This is more likely to affect the stomach's nighttime production of acid. While taking this medicine, stop smoking completely, or at least do not smoke after the last dose of the day.

Check with your doctor if your ulcer pain continues or gets worse.

POSSIBLE SIDE EFFECTS OF THIS MEDICINE
Side Effects That Should Be Reported To Your Doctor

Rare—Confusion; fast, pounding, or irregular heartbeat; slow heartbeat; sore throat and/or fever; swelling of eyelids; tightness in chest; unusual bleeding or bruising; unusual tiredness or weakness

Other side effects not listed above may also occur in some patients. If you notice any other effects, check with your doctor, nurse, or pharmacist.

HMG-CoA REDUCTASE INHIBITORS   Systemic

Including Lovastatin; Pravastatin; Simvastatin.

■ For the Pharmacist ■

In providing consultation, consider emphasizing the following selected information (» = major clinical significance):

Before using this medication
Diet as preferred therapy; importance of following prescribed diet
» Conditions affecting use, especially:
   Sensitivity to any HMG-CoA reductase inhibitor
   Pregnancy—Use not recommended in pregnancy or in women who plan to become pregnant, because inhibited formation of cholesterol may impair fetal development
   Breast-feeding—Use not recommended, because of potentially serious adverse effects in nursing infants
   Use in children—Safety and efficacy have not been established
   Other medications, especially cyclosporine, gemfibrozil, or niacin
   Other medical problems, especially uncontrolled seizures; recent major surgery; organ transplant with immunosuppressant therapy; hypotension; severe infection; severe metabolic, endocrine, or electrolyte disorders; major surgery; trauma; active hepatic disease

Proper use of this medication
For all HMG-CoA reductase inhibitors
» Importance of not taking more or less medication than the amount prescribed
   This medication does not cure the condition but instead helps control it
» Compliance with prescribed diet
» Proper dosing
   Missed dose: Taking as soon as possible; not taking if almost time for next dose; not doubling doses
» Proper storage
For lovastatin
   Taking with meals, since medication is more effective with food

Precautions while using this medication
» Importance of close monitoring by physician
» Checking with physician before discontinuing medications; blood lipid levels may increase significantly
» Caution if any kind of surgery (including dental surgery) or emergency treatment is required

Side/adverse effects
   Signs of potential side effects, especially myalgia, myositis, or rhabdomyolysis (for all HMG-CoA reductase inhibitors); blurred vision (for lovastatin)

▲ For the Patient ▲

915687

ABOUT YOUR MEDICINE

Lovastatin (LOE-va-sta-tin), **pravastatin** (PRA-va-stat-in), and **simvastatin** (SIM-va-stat-in) are used to lower levels of cholesterol and other fats in the blood. This may help prevent medical problems caused by cholesterol clogging the blood vessels.

These medicines belong to the group of medicines called HMG-CoA reductase inhibitors.

If any of the information in this leaflet causes you special concern or if you want additional information about your medicine and its use, check with your doctor, nurse, or pharmacist. **Remember, keep this and all other medicines out of the reach of children and never share your medicines with others.**

BEFORE USING THIS MEDICINE

Importance of diet—Before prescribing medicine to lower your cholesterol, your doctor will probably try to control your condition by prescribing a personal diet for you. Such a diet may be low in fats, sugars, and/or cholesterol. Many people are able to control their condition by carefully following their doctor's orders for proper diet and exercise. **Medicine is prescribed only when additional help is needed** and is effective only when a schedule of diet and exercise is properly followed.

Also, this medicine is less effective if you are greatly overweight. It may be very important for you to go on a reducing diet. However, check with your doctor before going on any diet.

Tell your doctor, nurse, and pharmacist if you . . .
- are allergic to any medicine, either prescription or nonprescription (OTC);
- **are pregnant or intend to become pregnant while using this medicine;**
- are breast-feeding;
- are taking any other prescription or nonprescription (OTC) medicine, especially cyclosporine, gemfibrozil, or niacin;
- have had major surgery, especially a heart transplant;
- have any other medical problems, especially convulsions (seizures) or liver disease.

PROPER USE OF THIS MEDICINE

Use this medicine only as directed by your doctor. Do not use more or less of it, and do not use it more often or for a longer time than ordered.

Remember that this medicine will not cure your condition but it does help control it. Therefore, you must continue to take it as directed if you expect to keep your cholesterol levels down.

For patients taking lovastatin:
• This medicine works better when it is taken with food. If you are taking this medicine once a day, take it with the evening meal. If you are taking more than one dose a day, take with meals or snacks.

If you miss a dose of this medicine, take it as soon as possible. However, if it is almost time for your next dose, skip the missed dose and go back to your regular dosing schedule. Do not double doses.

PRECAUTIONS WHILE USING THIS MEDICINE
It is very important that your doctor check your progress at regular visits. This will allow your doctor to see if the medicine is working properly to lower your cholesterol levels and that it does not cause unwanted effects.

Do not stop taking this medicine without first checking with your doctor. When you stop taking this medicine, your blood cholesterol levels may increase again. Your doctor may want you to follow a special diet to help prevent this from happening.

Before having any kind of surgery or dental or emergency treatment, tell the physician or dentist in charge that you are taking this medicine.

POSSIBLE SIDE EFFECTS OF THIS MEDICINE
Side Effects That Should Be Reported To Your Doctor

Less common—Blurred vision (lovastatin and pravastatin only); fever; muscle aches or cramps; unusual tiredness or weakness

Side Effects That Usually Do Not Require Medical Attention

These possible side effects may go away during treatment; however, if they continue or are bothersome, check with your doctor, nurse, or pharmacist.

Less common—Constipation, diarrhea, gas, heartburn, or stomach pain; decreased sexual ability (lovastatin only); dizziness; headache; nausea; skin rash; trouble in sleeping (lovastatin only)

Other side effects not listed above may also occur in some patients. If you notice any other effects, check with your doctor, nurse, or pharmacist.

HYDRALAZINE   Systemic

■ For the Pharmacist ■

In providing consultation, consider emphasizing the following selected
  information (» = major clinical significance):

Before using this medication
» Conditions affecting use, especially:
  Sensitivity to hydralazine
  Pregnancy—Blood problems reported in infants of mothers who
    took hydralazine; causes birth defects in animals
  Use in the elderly—Increased sensitivity to hypotensive effects
  Other medications, especially diazoxide
  Other medical problems, especially coronary artery disease or
    rheumatic heart disease

Proper use of this medication
  Getting into the habit of taking at same times each day to help
    increase compliance
» Proper dosing
  Missed dose: Taking as soon as possible; not taking if almost time
    for next dose; not doubling doses
» Proper storage
For use as an antihypertensive
  Possible need for control of weight and diet, especially sodium intake
» Patient may not experience symptoms of hypertension; importance
    of taking medication even if feeling well
» Does not cure, but helps control hypertension; possible need for
    lifelong therapy; checking with physician before discontinuing
    medication; serious consequences of untreated hypertension

Precautions while using this medication
  Regular visits to physician to check progress
» Caution when driving or doing things requiring alertness because of
    possible headache or dizziness
For use as an antihypertensive
» Not taking other medications, especially nonprescription sympatho-
    mimetics, unless discussed with physician

Side/adverse effects
  Signs of potential side effects, especially allergic reaction, angina
    pectoris, cutaneous vasculitis, lymphadenopathy, peripheral neu-
    ritis, sodium and water retention, edema, and SLE-like syndrome

▲ For the Patient ▲

912339

ABOUT YOUR MEDICINE

Hydralazine (hye-DRAL-a-zeen) belongs to the general class
of medicines called antihypertensives. It is used to treat high
blood pressure (hypertension). Hydralazine may also be used
for other conditions as determined by your doctor.

If any of the information in this leaflet causes you special
concern or if you want additional information about your
medicine and its use, check with your doctor, nurse, or pharmacist. **Remember, keep this and all other medicines out of**

the reach of children and never share your medicines with others.

BEFORE USING THIS MEDICINE

Tell your doctor, nurse, and pharmacist if you . . .
- are allergic to any medicine, either prescription or nonprescription (OTC);
- are pregnant or intend to become pregnant while using this medicine;
- are breast-feeding;
- are taking any other prescription or nonprescription (OTC) medicine, especially diazoxide or medicines for appetite control, asthma, colds, cough, hay fever, or sinus;
- have any other medical problems, especially heart or blood vessel disease.

PROPER USE OF THIS MEDICINE

Hydralazine will not cure your high blood pressure but it does help control it. You must continue to take it—even if you feel well—if you expect to keep your blood pressure down. **You may have to take high blood pressure medicine for the rest of your life.**

If you miss a dose of this medicine, take it as soon as possible. However, if it is almost time for your next dose, skip the missed dose and go back to your regular dosing schedule. Do not double doses.

PRECAUTIONS WHILE USING THIS MEDICINE

It is important that your doctor check your progress at regular visits while you are taking this medicine.

Hydralazine may cause some people to have headaches or to feel dizzy. **Make sure you know how you react to this medicine before you drive, use machines, or do other jobs that require you to be alert.**

POSSIBLE SIDE EFFECTS OF THIS MEDICINE
Side Effects That Should Be Reported To Your Doctor

   Less common—Blisters on skin; chest pain; general feeling of discomfort, illness, or weakness; joint pain; numbness, tingling, pain, or weakness in hands or feet; skin rash or itching; sore throat and fever; swelling of feet or lower legs; swelling of the lymph glands

Side Effects That Usually Do Not Require Medical Attention

These possible side effects may go away during treatment; however, if they continue or are bothersome, check with your doctor, nurse, or pharmacist.

   More common—Diarrhea; fast or irregular heartbeat; headache; loss of appetite; nausea or vomiting; pounding heartbeat

Other side effects not listed above may also occur in some patients. If you notice any other effects, check with your doctor, nurse, or pharmacist.

INDAPAMIDE   Systemic

■ For the Pharmacist ■

In providing consultation, consider emphasizing the following selected information (» = major clinical significance):

Before using this medication
» Conditions affecting use, especially:
    Sensitivity to indapamide or other sulfonamide-type medications
    Pregnancy—Routine use not recommended
    Use in the elderly—Increased sensitivity to hypotensive and electrolyte effects
    Other medications, especially digitalis glycosides or lithium
    Other medical problems, especially anuria or severe renal function impairment

Proper use of this medication
    Diuretic effects of the medication and timing of doses to minimize inconvenience of diuresis
    Getting into habit of taking at same time each day to help increase compliance
» Proper dosing
    Missed dose: Taking as soon as possible; not taking if almost time for next dose; not doubling doses
» Proper storage
For use as an antihypertensive
    Possible need for control of weight and diet, especially sodium intake
» Patients may not experience symptoms of hypertension; importance of taking medication even if feeling well
» Does not cure but helps control hypertension; possible need for lifelong therapy; checking with physician before discontinuing therapy; serious consequences of untreated hypertension

Precautions while using this medication
    Regular visits to physician to check progress
» Possibility of hypokalemia; possible need for additional potassium in diet; not changing diet without first checking with physician
    To prevent dehydration, checking with physician if severe nausea, vomiting, or diarrhea occurs and continues
For use as an antihypertensive
» Not taking other medications, especially nonprescription sympathomimetics, unless discussed with physician

Side/adverse effects
    Signs of potential side effects, especially allergic reaction and electrolyte imbalance

▲ For the Patient ▲

914120

ABOUT YOUR MEDICINE

Indapamide (in-DAP-a-mide) belongs to the group of medicines known as diuretics. It is commonly used to treat high blood pressure (hypertension). Indapamide is also used to help reduce the amount of water in the body by increasing the flow of urine.

If any of the information in this leaflet causes you special concern or if you want additional information about your medicine and its use, check with your doctor, nurse, or pharmacist. **Remember, keep this and all other medicines out of the reach of children and never share your medicines with others.**

BEFORE USING THIS MEDICINE

Tell your doctor, nurse, and pharmacist if you . . .
- are allergic to any medicine, either prescription or non-prescription (OTC);
- are pregnant or intend to become pregnant while using this medicine;
- are breast-feeding;
- are taking any other prescription or nonprescription (OTC) medicine, especially digitalis glycosides (heart medicine), or lithium;
- have any other medical problems, especially kidney disease.

PROPER USE OF THIS MEDICINE

Indapamide may cause you to have an unusual feeling of tiredness when you begin to take it. You may also notice an increase in urine or in your frequency of urination. To keep this from affecting sleep:
- if you are to take a single dose a day, take it in the morning after breakfast.
- if you are to take more than one dose, take the last one no later than 6 p.m.

For patients taking indapamide for high blood pressure:
- Many patients who have high blood pressure will not notice any signs of the problem. In fact, many may feel normal. It is very important that you **take your medicine exactly as directed** and that you keep your appointments with your doctor even if you feel well.
- This medicine will not cure your high blood pressure but it does help control it. You must continue to take it—even if you feel well—if you expect to keep your blood pressure down. **You may have to take high blood pressure medicine for the rest of your life.**

If you miss a dose of this medicine, take it as soon as possible. However, if it is almost time for your next dose, skip the missed dose and go back to your regular dosing schedule. Do not double doses.

PRECAUTIONS WHILE USING THIS MEDICINE

It is important that your doctor check your progress at regular visits in order to make sure that indapamide is working properly.

This medicine may cause a loss of potassium from your body. To help prevent this, your doctor may want you to eat or drink foods that have a high potassium content (for example, orange or other citrus fruit juices), or take a potassium supplement, or take another medication to help prevent the loss of the potassium in the first place. It is very important to follow these directions, but do not change your diet on your own, since too much potassium could be harmful.

Check with your doctor if you become sick and have severe or continuing vomiting or diarrhea. These problems may cause you to lose additional water and potassium.

For patients taking this medicine for high blood pressure:

* **Do not take other medicines unless they have been discussed with your doctor.** This especially includes over-the-counter (nonprescription) medicines for appetite control, asthma, colds, hay fever, or sinus problems, since they may tend to increase your blood pressure.

POSSIBLE SIDE EFFECTS OF THIS MEDICINE

Side Effects That Should Be Reported To Your Doctor

> *Rare*—Skin rash, itching, or hives

> *Signs of too much potassium loss*—Dryness of mouth; increased thirst; irregular heartbeat; mood or mental changes; muscle cramps or pain; nausea or vomiting; unusual tiredness; weak pulse

Side Effects That Usually Do Not Require Medical Attention

These possible side effects may go away during treatment; however, if they continue or are bothersome, check with your doctor, nurse, or pharmacist.

> *Less common or rare*—Diarrhea; dizziness or lightheadedness, especially when standing up; headache; loss of appetite; trouble in sleeping; upset stomach

Other side effects not listed above may also occur in some patients. If you notice any other effects, check with your doctor, nurse, or pharmacist.

INSULIN   Systemic

∎For the Pharmacist∎

In providing consultation, consider emphasizing the following selected information (» = major clinical significance):

Before using this medication
» Conditions affecting use, especially:
　　Sensitivity to insulins
　　Other medications, especially alcohol; beta-adrenergic blocking
　　　agents; or corticosteroids
　　Other medical problems, especially high fever, hyperthyroidism,
　　　severe infections, diabetic ketoacidosis, trauma, surgery,
　　　diarrhea, hypothyroidism, nausea, vomiting, or renal function
　　　impairment
» Emphasis on diabetic meal plan

Proper use of this medication
» Using correct insulin and syringe
　　How insulin syringes are marked
» Proper preparation of medication; gently shaking, inverting, or roll-
　　ing contents of insulin vial immediately before use; not shaking
　　hard; not using if contents are lumpy or grainy or if they stick
　　to bottle; not using regular insulin that is cloudy or discolored;
　　drawing insulin into syringe
　　Mixing types of insulin (only when directed by physician); always
　　　drawing in same order; if using regular insulin, drawing it first;
　　　knowing whether injection must be given right after mixing; if
　　　not using mixed insulins right after mixing, gently shaking or
　　　rolling syringe prior to use in order to remix
» Proper administration technique
» Carefully reading patient instruction sheet contained in insulin pack-
　　age
　　Use of disposable syringes
　　Use of glass syringe and metal needle
　　Use of insulin infusion pump; always using clear and colorless in-
　　　sulin; not mixing buffered regular insulin with any other insulin;
　　　following pump manufacturer's directions on filling syringe or
　　　reservoir; checking tubing and infusion-site dressing frequently
　　　for improper infusion
» Compliance with therapy
» Proper dosing
　　Storage and expiration date of insulin

Precautions while using this medication
» Regular visits to physician to check progress, especially during the
　　first few weeks of treatment
» Carefully following special instructions of physician:
　　Discussing use of alcohol with physician
　　Carefully following diabetic meal plan
　　Exercising as directed by physician
　　Testing for acetone in urine
　　Testing for blood glucose levels
　　Carefully selecting and rotating injection sites, following phy-
　　　sician's recommendations
» Not taking other medications unless discussed with physician
» Preparing for emergency

» Recognizing symptoms of hypoglycemia and knowing what to do if
   they occur:
   Anxious feeling
   Cold sweats
   Confusion
   Cool, pale skin
   Difficulty in concentration
   Drowsiness
   Excessive hunger
   Headache
   Nausea
   Nervousness
   Rapid pulse
   Shakiness
   Unusual tiredness or weakness
   Vision changes
   Knowing what to do if nausea, vomiting, or fever develops; contin-
   uing use of insulin even if patient cannot eat regular diet; check-
   ing with physician if vomiting is severe or if blood sugar levels
   are not controlled
» Recognizing symptoms of hyperglycemia and ketoacidosis:
   Drowsiness
   Dry mouth
   Flushed, dry skin
   Fruit-like breath odor
   Increased blood sugar concentration
   Increased urination
   Loss of appetite
   Stomachache, nausea, or vomiting
   Tiredness
   Trouble in breathing (rapid and deep)
   Unusual thirst
» Suggestions when traveling

▲ For the Patient ▲

912361

ABOUT YOUR MEDICINE

Insulin (IN-su-lin) is a hormone that helps the body turn the
food we eat into energy. This occurs whether we make our
own insulin in the pancreas gland or take it by injection.
Diabetes mellitus (sugar diabetes) is a condition in which
the body does not make enough insulin to meet its needs or
does not properly use the insulin it makes. One or more
injections of insulin a day may be needed to control your
diabetes. Insulin is usually injected before meals or at bedtime. Your doctor will discuss the number of injections you
will need, the kind of insulin to use, the correct dose, and
the right time to take it.

If any of the information in this leaflet causes you special
concern or if you want additional information about your
medicine and its use, check with your doctor, nurse, or pharmacist. **Remember, keep this and all other medicines out of
the reach of children and never share your medicines with
others.**

BEFORE USING THIS MEDICINE

Tell your doctor, nurse, and pharmacist if you . . .

- are allergic to insulins made from beef or pork;
- are pregnant or intend to become pregnant while using this medicine;
- are taking any other prescription or nonprescription (OTC) medicine, especially adrenocorticoids (cortisone-like medicine); aspirin, medicines for appetite control, asthma, colds, cough, hay fever, or sinus problems; or beta-blockers;
- have any other medical problems, especially infections, kidney disease, liver disease, or thyroid disease.

PROPER USE OF THIS MEDICINE

Do not change the strength, brand, or type of insulin you are using unless told to do so by your doctor.

Each package of insulin contains a patient information sheet. Read this sheet carefully.

Follow carefully the special meal plan your doctor gave you. This is the most important part of controlling your condition. Also, **test for sugar in your blood or urine as directed and follow directions for exercise and care of your feet.**

An unopened bottle of insulin should be refrigerated without freezing until needed. However, insulin you are now using regularly may be kept at room temperature if it will be used up within a month. Insulin that has been kept at room temperature for longer than a month should be thrown away. Do not expose insulin to very hot temperatures or sunlight.

PRECAUTIONS WHILE USING THIS MEDICINE

Drinking alcohol while you are using insulin may cause you to have dangerously low blood sugar. **Avoid alcoholic beverages until you have discussed this with your doctor.**

Eat or drink something containing sugar and check with your doctor right away if mild symptoms of low blood sugar (hypoglycemia) appear. Good sources of sugar are glucose tablets or gel, fruit juice, corn syrup, honey, regular (non-diet) soft drinks, or sugar dissolved in water. It is a good idea to check your blood sugar to confirm that it is low.

If severe symptoms such as convulsions (seizures) or unconsciousness occur, diabetics should not eat or drink anything. There is a chance that they could choke from not swallowing correctly. Emergency medical help should be obtained immediately.

Hypoglycemia (low blood sugar) may occur if you use too much insulin, skip or delay meals, exercise more than usual, have any sickness, especially with vomiting or diarrhea, or drink a significant amount of alcohol.

Signs of low blood sugar include abdominal or stomach pain; anxious feeling; chills; cold sweats; confusion; convulsions (seizures); cool pale skin; difficulty in thinking; drowsiness; excessive hunger; headache; nausea or vomiting (continuing); nervousness; rapid heartbeat; shakiness; unconsciousness; unsteady walk; unusual tiredness or weakness; or vision changes.

Low blood sugar must be treated before it leads to unconsciousness (passing out). Glucagon is also used in emergency situations such as unconsciousness. Have a glucagon kit available, along with a syringe and needle. Make sure you and people in your household know how and when to prepare and use it.

Hyperglycemia (high blood sugar) symptoms may occur if you do not take enough insulin; if you skip a dose of insulin; if you overeat or do not follow your meal plan; if you have a fever, diarrhea, or infection; or do not exercise as much as usual.

Signs of high blood sugar appear more slowly than those for low blood sugar, and usually include dry mouth; drowsiness; flushed, dry skin; fruit-like breath odor; increased urination; loss of appetite; stomachache, nausea, or vomiting; tiredness; troubled breathing (rapid and deep); unusual thirst

Symptoms of both low blood sugar and high blood sugar must be corrected before they progress to a more serious condition. In either situation, you should check with your doctor immediately. Also, **if you become sick,** especially with nausea, vomiting, or fever, call your doctor for instructions.

INTERFERONS, ALPHA   Systemic

■For the Pharmacist■

In providing consultation, consider emphasizing the following selected information (» = major clinical significance):

Before using this medication
» Conditions affecting use, especially:
  Sensitivity to alpha interferons
  Pregnancy—Abortifacient effects found in rhesus monkeys
  Breast-feeding—Possible need to avoid during alpha interferon therapy because of risk of serious adverse effects
  Use in teenagers—Possible effects on menstrual cycle
  Use in the elderly—Risk of cardiotoxic and neurotoxic effects may be increased
  Other medical problems, especially history of autoimmune disease, severe cardiac disease, chicken pox, compromised CNS function, diabetes mellitus, herpes zoster, history of psychiatric disease, pulmonary disease, seizure disorders, and thyroid function impairment

Proper use of this medication
» Compliance with therapy
» Reading patient directions carefully with regard to:
  —Preparation of the injection
  —Use of disposable syringes
  —Proper administration technique
  —Stability of the injection
  Importance of ample fluid intake to reduce risk of hypotension
  Administration at bedtime to minimize inconvenience of fatigue
» Proper dosing
  Missed dose: Skipping missed dose and going back to regular schedule; not doubling doses; checking with physician
» Proper storage

Precautions while using this medication
» Importance of close monitoring by physician
» Not changing brands of interferon without consulting physician, because of differences in dosage
» Caution in taking alcohol or other CNS depressants during therapy
» Caution when driving or doing anything else requiring alertness because of possible fatigue and dizziness
» Frequency of fever and flu-like symptoms; possible need for acetaminophen before and after a dose is given
  Caution if bone marrow depression occurs:
» Avoiding exposure to persons with bacterial infections, especially during periods of low blood counts; checking with physician immediately if fever or chills, cough or hoarseness, lower back or side pain, or painful or difficult urination occur
» Checking with physician immediately if unusual bleeding or bruising; black, tarry stools; blood in urine or stools; or pinpoint red spots on skin occur
  Caution in use of regular toothbrush, dental floss, or toothpick; physician, dentist, or nurse may suggest alternatives; checking with physician before having dental work done
  Not touching eyes or inside of nose unless hands washed immediately before

Using caution to avoid accidental cuts with use of sharp objects such as safety razor or fingernail or toenail cutters

Avoiding contact sports or other situations where bruising or injury could occur

Side/adverse effects

Signs of potential side effects, especially cardiotoxicity, neurotoxicity, peripheral neuropathy, leukopenia, and thrombocytopenia

Possibility of minor hair loss; hair should return after treatment has ended

---

▲ For the Patient ▲

916169

ABOUT YOUR MEDICINE

Alpha interferons (in-ter-FEER-ons) are used to treat hairy cell leukemia and AIDS–related Kaposi's sarcoma. They are also used to treat laryngeal papillomatosis (growths in the respiratory tract) in children, genital warts, and some kinds of hepatitis. Alpha interferons may also be used for other conditions as determined by your doctor.

If any of the information in this leaflet causes you special concern or if you want additional information about your medicine and its use, check with your doctor, nurse, or pharmacist. **Remember, keep this and all other medicines out of the reach of children and never share your medicines with others.**

BEFORE USING THIS MEDICINE

Tell your doctor, nurse, and pharmacist if you . . .

- are allergic to any medicine, either prescription or nonprescription (OTC);
- are pregnant or intend to become pregnant while using this medicine;
- are breast-feeding;
- are taking any other prescription or nonprescription (OTC) medicine;
- have any other medical problems, especially chickenpox (including recent exposure), convulsions (seizures), diabetes mellitus (sugar diabetes), heart disease, herpes zoster (shingles), lung disease, mental problems (or history of), problems with overactive immune system, or thyroid disease;
- have recently had a heart attack.

PROPER USE OF THIS MEDICINE

If you are injecting this medicine yourself, **use it exactly as directed.**

Each package of alpha interferon contains a patient instruction sheet. Read this sheet carefully and make sure you understand:

- How to prepare and give the injection.
- Proper use of disposable syringes.
- How long the injection is stable.

If you have any questions about any of this, check with your doctor, nurse, or pharmacist.

If you miss a dose of this medicine, do not give the missed dose at all and do not double the next one. Check with your doctor for further instructions.

PRECAUTIONS WHILE USING THIS MEDICINE
It is very important that your doctor check your progress at regular visits.

Do not change to another brand of alpha interferon without checking with your doctor.

This medicine will add to the effects of alcohol and other CNS depressants (medicines that slow down the nervous system). **Check with your doctor before taking any such depressants while you are using this medicine.**

Alpha interferon may cause some people to become unusually tired or dizzy, or less alert than they are normally. **Make sure you know how you react before you drive, use machines, or do other jobs that require you to be alert.**

This medicine commonly causes a flu-like reaction, with aching muscles, fever and chills, and headache. **Follow your doctor's instructions carefully about taking your temperature, and how much and when to take acetaminophen.**

Alpha interferon can lower the number of white blood cells in your blood, increasing the chance of getting an infection. It can also lower the number of platelets, which are necessary for proper blood clotting. If this occurs:
- Avoid people with infections.
- Be careful when using a regular toothbrush, dental floss, or toothpick.
- Do not touch your eyes or the inside of your nose unless you have just washed your hands and have not touched anything else in the meantime.
- Be careful not to cut, bruise, or injure yourself.

POSSIBLE SIDE EFFECTS OF THIS MEDICINE
Side Effects That Should Be Reported To Your Doctor

Less common—Confusion; mental depression; nervousness; numbness or tingling of fingers, toes, and face; trouble in sleeping; trouble in thinking or concentrating

Rare—Black, tarry stools; blood in urine or stools; chest pain; cough or hoarseness; fever or chills (beginning after 3 weeks of treatment); irregular heartbeat; lower back or side pain; painful or difficult urination; pinpoint red spots on skin; unusual bleeding or bruising

Side Effects That Usually Do Not Require Medical Attention

These possible side effects may go away during treatment; however, if they continue or are bothersome, check with your doctor, nurse, or pharmacist.

More common—Aching muscles; change in taste or metallic taste; fever and chills (should lessen after the first 1 or 2 weeks of treatment); general feeling of discomfort or illness; headache; loss of appetite; nausea and vomiting; skin rash; unusual tiredness

Alpha interferon may cause a temporary loss of some hair. After treatment has ended, normal hair growth should return.

Other side effects not listed above may also occur in some patients. If you notice any other effects, check with your doctor, nurse, or pharmacist.

IPRATROPIUM   Inhalation-Local

▮ For the Pharmacist ▮

In providing consultation, consider emphasizing the following selected information (» = major clinical significance):

Before using this medication
» Conditions affecting use, especially:
   Sensitivity to ipratropium or belladonna alkaloids

Proper use of this medication
» Helps control symptoms of lung disease; inhalation solution used only with other bronchodilators when treating acute asthma attacks
» Importance of not using more medication than the amount prescribed
» Avoiding contact with the eyes; closing eyes if necessary when inhaling; if accidentally sprayed into the eyes or if nebulized solution escapes into the eyes, irritation or blurring of vision may occur; rinsing eyes with cool water if necessary
   Reading patient instructions carefully before using
» If using regularly, importance of using every day at regularly spaced times.
» Proper dosing
   Missed dose: If used regularly, using as soon as possible; using any remaining doses for that day at regularly spaced intervals
» Proper storage
For inhalation aerosol dosage form
   Checking periodically with health care professional for proper use of inhaler to prevent improper technique and incorrect dosage
   Testing inhaler before using first time or first time in a while
   Proper administration technique without spacer device
   Proper administration technique with spacer device
   Proper cleaning procedure for inhaler
   Checking fullness of canister by placing it in water
For inhalation solution dosage form
   Using only in nebulizer as instructed by physician
   Preparing solution for nebulizer
   Proper administration technique: Using in a power-operated nebulizer with an adequate flow rate and equipped with a face mask or mouthpiece

Precautions while using this medication
» Checking with physician immediately if symptoms do not improve within 30 minutes after using this medication or if condition becomes worse
   Possible dryness of mouth or throat; using sugarless candy or gum, ice, or saliva substitute for relief; checking with physician or dentist if dryness of mouth continues for more than 2 weeks
For patients using cromolyn inhalation solution
» Not mixing cromolyn inhalation solution with ipratropium inhalation solution from the multiple-dose container for use in a nebulizer; mixing only with contents of single-dose vial of ipratropium inhalation solution, which is preservative-free

Side/adverse effects
   Signs of potential side effects, especially increased bronchospasm, difficulty in swallowing, acute eye pain, skin rash or hives, stomatitis, and swelling of tongue or lips

▲ For the Patient ▲

915360

ABOUT YOUR MEDICINE

Ipratropium (i-pra-TROE-pee-um) belongs to the group of medicines called bronchodilators (medicines that open up the bronchial tubes [air passages] of the lungs). It is taken by oral inhalation to control the symptoms of lung diseases, such as chronic bronchitis and emphysema. Ipratropium may also be used for other conditions as determined by your doctor.

If any of the information in this leaflet causes you special concern or if you want additional information about your medicine and its use, check with your doctor, nurse, or pharmacist. **Remember, keep this and all other medicines out of the reach of children and never share your medicines with others.**

BEFORE USING THIS MEDICINE

Tell your doctor, nurse, and pharmacist if you . . .
- are allergic to any medicine, either prescription or non-prescription (OTC);
- are pregnant or intend to become pregnant while using this medicine;
- are breast-feeding;
- are taking **any** other prescription or nonprescription (OTC) medicine;
- have any other medical problems.

PROPER USE OF THIS MEDICINE

Ipratropium usually comes with patient directions. Read them carefully before using this medicine.

For patients using ipratropium inhalation aerosol:
- If you are directed to use more than 1 inhalation of this medicine for each dose, allow 1 minute between the inhalations in order to receive the full effect of the medicine.

For patients using ipratropium inhalation solution:
- If you are using ipratropium inhalation solution in a nebulizer, make sure you understand exactly how to use it. If you have any questions about this, check with your doctor or pharmacist.

It is very important that you use ipratropium only as directed. Do not use more of it and do not use it more often than your doctor ordered. To do so may increase the chance of serious side effects.

Keep the spray or solution away from the eyes because it may cause irritation. Also, if the medicine gets in the eyes, it may cause blurred vision for a short time.

If you miss a dose of this medicine, use it as soon as possible. However, if it is almost time for your next dose, skip the missed dose and go back to your regular dosing schedule. Do not double doses.

PRECAUTIONS WHILE USING THIS MEDICINE

Check with your doctor at once if your symptoms do not improve within 30 minutes after using a dose of this medicine or if your condition gets worse.

For patients using ipratropium inhalation aerosol:

- If you are also using another bronchodilator inhalation aerosol, use the other bronchodilator inhalation aerosol first, then wait about 5 minutes before using this medicine, unless otherwise directed by your doctor. It is best not to use the two kinds of aerosols too close together, to lessen the chance of unwanted effects.

- If you are also using an adrenocorticoid inhalation aerosol or cromolyn inhalation aerosol, use the ipratropium inhalation aerosol first, then wait about 5 minutes before using the adrenocorticoid aerosol or cromolyn aerosol, unless otherwise directed by your doctor. It is best not to use the ipratropium aerosol and the adrenocorticoid or cromolyn aerosol too close together, to lessen the chance of unwanted effects.

For patients using ipratropium inhalation solution:

- **If you are also using cromolyn inhalation solution, do not mix this solution with the ipratropium inhalation solution for use in a nebulizer.** To do so will cause the solution to become cloudy and prevent the cromolyn from working as well as it should.

Ipratropium may cause dryness of the mouth or throat. For temporary relief of mouth dryness, use sugarless candy or gum, melt bits of ice in your mouth, or use a saliva substitute. However, if dry mouth continues for more than 2 weeks, check with your physician or dentist. Continuing dryness of the mouth may increase the chance of dental disease, including tooth decay, gum disease, and fungus infections.

POSSIBLE SIDE EFFECTS OF THIS MEDICINE
Side Effects That Should Be Reported To Your Doctor

> *Rare*—Skin rash or hives; ulcers or sores in mouth and on lips

Side Effects That Usually Do Not Require Medical Attention

These possible side effects may go away during treatment; however, if they continue or are bothersome, check with your doctor, nurse, or pharmacist.

> *More common*—Cough or dryness of mouth or throat; headache or dizziness; nervousness; stomach upset or nausea

> *Less common or rare*—Blurred vision or other changes in vision; difficult urination; metallic or unpleasant

taste; pounding heartbeat; stuffy nose; trembling; trouble in sleeping; unusual tiredness or weakness

Other side effects not listed above may also occur in some patients. If you notice any other effects, check with your doctor, nurse, or pharmacist.

IRON SUPPLEMENTS   Systemic

Including Ferrous Fumarate; Ferrous Gluconate; Ferrous Sulfate; Iron Dextran; Iron-Polysaccharide; Iron Sorbitol.

■For the Pharmacist■

In providing consultation, consider emphasizing the following selected information (» = major clinical significance):

Description of use
Description should include function in body, signs of deficiency

Importance of diet
Diet as treatment of choice; importance of diet
List of daily RDA for various age groups
Best dietary sources of iron

Before using this dietary supplement
» Conditions affecting use, especially:
Sensitivity to iron
Other medications, especially acetohydroxamic acid, dimercaprol, etidronate, or oral tetracyclines
Other medical problems, especially hemochromatosis, hemosiderosis, or other anemic conditions

Proper use of this dietary supplement
Taking on empty stomach 1 hour before or 2 hours after meals; or with food to lessen possibility of stomach upset
Taking with water or fruit juice, a full glass (240 mL) for adults, ½ glass (120 mL) for children
Following physician's directions if dietary supplement was prescribed
Following manufacturer's package directions on nonprescription (OTC) iron
For preventing, reducing, or removing iron stains on teeth:
Diluting liquid forms in water or fruit juice
Using drinking tube or straw
Placing dropper doses well back on tongue
Brushing teeth with baking soda or hydrogen peroxide 3%
» Proper dosing
Missed dose: Skipping missed dose; going back to regular schedule; not doubling doses
» Proper storage

Precautions while using this dietary supplement
Taking iron supplements 1 hour before or 2 hours after eating dairy products, eggs, coffee, tea, whole-grain breads and cereals, antacids, or calcium supplements
Not taking iron supplements orally if receiving iron by injection
Avoiding regular use of large amounts of iron supplements several times daily for more than 6 months unless approved by physician
Considering dietary iron as part of total daily intake
Extended-release dosage forms may not release iron properly; checking with physician if stools are not black during therapy
Keeping iron preparations out of the reach of children. Keeping syrup of ipecac readily available in case ordered for emergency
Keeping telephone numbers of poison control center, nearest hospital emergency room, and doctor readily available
» Suspected overdose: Immediately contacting physician, poison control center, or emergency room; following any instructions given

on phone; not delaying emergency treatment; taking container of iron medicine to emergency room

Side/adverse effects

Dietary supplement causes black stools which may be alarming to patient although medically insignificant; checking with physician if black stools occur with other symptoms of internal blood loss

Signs of potential side effects, especially abdominal pain or contact irritation in alimentary tract

▲ For the Patient ▲

912372

ABOUT YOUR DIETARY SUPPLEMENT

Iron is a mineral that the body needs to produce red blood cells. When the body does not get enough iron, it cannot produce the number of normal red blood cells needed to keep you in good health. This condition is called iron-deficiency (iron shortage) or iron-deficiency anemia.

Although many people in the U.S. get enough iron from their diet, some must take additional amounts to meet their needs. Only your doctor can determine if you have an iron deficiency, and if an iron supplement is necessary.

Lack of iron may lead to unusual tiredness, shortness of breath, a decrease in physical performance, learning problems in children, and may increase your chance of getting an infection. The best sources of absorbable iron are lean red meat, chicken, turkey, and fish.

If any of the information in this leaflet causes you special concern or if you want additional information about your dietary supplement and its use, check with your doctor, nurse, dietitian, or pharmacist. **Remember, keep this and all other medicines out of the reach of children and never share your medicines with others.**

BEFORE USING THIS DIETARY SUPPLEMENT

Tell your doctor, nurse, and pharmacist if you . . .
- are allergic to any medicine, either prescription or non-prescription (OTC);
- are pregnant or intend to become pregnant while using this medicine;
- are breast-feeding;
- are taking any other prescription or nonprescription (OTC) medicine, especially acetohydroxamic acid, dimercaprol, etidronate, or tetracyclines;
- have any other medical problems, especially blood disease.

PROPER USE OF THIS DIETARY SUPPLEMENT

After you start using this dietary supplement, continue to visit your doctor to see if you are benefiting from the iron. Some blood tests may be necessary.

Iron is best taken on an empty stomach, with water or fruit juice, about 1 hour before or 2 hours after meals. However, to lessen the possibility of stomach upset, iron may be taken with food or immediately after meals. If this is done, certain foods should not be taken at the same time as iron. These include cheese, eggs, milk, tea, coffee, spinach, whole-grain breads and cereals, bran, and yogurt.

If you miss a dose of this medicine, skip the missed dose and go back to your regular dosing schedule. Do not double doses.

PRECAUTIONS WHILE USING THIS DIETARY SUPPLEMENT

Do not take iron supplements and antacids or calcium supplements at the same time. It is best to space doses of these two products 1 to 2 hours apart.

Keep iron supplements out of the reach of children since overdose is very dangerous in children and may cause death. As few as 3 adult iron tablets can cause serious poisoning in small children. **If you think an overdose has been taken:**

- **Immediate medical attention is very important. Call your doctor, a poison control center, or the nearest hospital emergency room at once.**
- **Follow any instructions given to you.** If ipecac syrup has been ordered and given, do not delay going to the emergency room while waiting for the ipecac to empty the stomach. It may require 20 to 30 minutes to show results.
- **Go to the emergency room without delay, taking the container of iron medicine with you.** Early signs of iron overdose may not occur for up to 60 minutes or more after the overdose was taken. By this time emergency treatment should be obtained.

POSSIBLE SIDE EFFECTS OF THIS DIETARY SUPPLEMENT

Side Effects That Should Be Reported To Your Doctor

> *More common*—Abdominal or stomach pain or cramping

> *Less common or rare*—Chest or throat pain, especially when swallowing; stools with signs of blood

Early signs of iron poisoning include diarrhea (may contain blood), nausea, stomach pain (sharp), and severe vomiting (may contain blood).

Late signs of iron poisoning include bluish-colored lips, fingernails, and palms; convulsions (seizures); drowsiness; pale, clammy skin; unusual weakness; and weak and fast heartbeat.

Side Effects That Usually Do Not Require Medical Attention

These possible side effects may go away during treatment; however, if they continue or are bothersome, check with your doctor, nurse, or pharmacist.

More common—Constipation; diarrhea; nausea; vomiting

Less common—Dark urine; heartburn; staining of teeth (liquid dosage forms)

Stools commonly become dark green or black when iron preparations are taken by mouth. However, in rare cases, black stools of a sticky consistency may occur along with other symptoms such as red streaks in the stool, cramping, soreness, or sharp pains in the stomach or abdominal area. **Check with your doctor immediately** if these signs appear.

Other side effects not listed above may also occur in some patients. If you notice any other effects, check with your doctor, nurse, or pharmacist.

ISONIAZID   Systemic

■For the Pharmacist■

In providing consultation, consider emphasizing the following selected information (» = major clinical significance):

Before using this medication
» Conditions affecting use, especially:

    Hypersensitivity to isoniazid, ethionamide, pyrazinamide, niacin (nicotinic acid), or other chemically related medications

    Pregnancy—Isoniazid crosses the placenta; fetal serum concentrations may exceed maternal serum concentrations

    Breast-feeding—Isoniazid is distributed into breast milk

    Use in children—Children may be less susceptible to pyridoxine deficiency and hepatotoxicity than adults, unless they have pre-existing hepatic disease; newborn infants may have prolonged elimination

    Use in the elderly—Patients over the age of 50 have the highest incidence of hepatitis

    Other medicines, especially daily alcohol use, alfentanil, carbamazepine, disulfiram, other hepatotoxic medications, ketoconazole, phenytoin, or rifampin

    Other medical problems, especially alcoholism, active or in remission, or hepatic function impairment

Proper use of this medication

    Taking this medication with food or antacids, but not within 1 hour of aluminum-containing antacids, if gastrointestinal irritation occurs (oral only)

    Proper administration technique for oral liquids

» Compliance with full course of therapy, which may take 6 months to 2 years

» Taking pyridoxine concurrently to prevent or minimize symptoms of peripheral neuritis; not usually required in children if dietary intake is adequate

» Proper dosing

    Missed dose: Taking as soon as possible; not taking if almost time for next dose; not doubling doses

» Proper storage

Precautions while using this medication
» Regular visits to physician to check progress, as well as ophthalmologic examinations if signs of optic neuritis occur in either adults or children

    Checking with physician if vascular reactions occur following concurrent ingestion of cheese or fish with isoniazid

    Checking with physician if no improvement within 2 to 3 weeks

» Avoiding alcoholic beverages while taking this medication

» Need to report to physician promptly prodromal signs of hepatitis or peripheral neuritis

» Diabetics: False-positive reactions with copper sulfate urine glucose tests may occur

Side/adverse effects

    Hepatitis may be more likely to occur in patients over 50 years of age

    Signs of potential side effects, especially hepatitis, peripheral neuritis, blood dyscrasias, hypersensitivity, neurotoxicity, and optic neuritis

▲ For the Patient ▲

914163

ABOUT YOUR MEDICINE

Isoniazid (eye-soe-NYE-a-zid) is used to prevent or treat tuberculosis (TB). It may be given alone to prevent, or, in combination with other medicines, to treat TB. This medicine may also be used for other problems as determined by your doctor.

If you are being treated for active tuberculosis (TB): To help clear up your TB completely, you must keep taking this medicine for the full time of treatment, even if you begin to feel better. This is very important. It is also important that you do not miss any doses.

If any of the information in this leaflet causes you special concern or if you want additional information about your medicine and its use, check with your doctor, nurse, or pharmacist. **Remember, keep this and all other medicines out of the reach of children and never share your medicines with others.**

BEFORE USING THIS MEDICINE

This medicine may cause some serious side effects, including damage to the liver. Liver damage is more likely to occur in patients over 50 years of age. **You and your doctor should talk about the good this medicine will do, as well as the risks of taking it.**

Tell your doctor, nurse, and pharmacist if you . . .

- are allergic to any medicine, either prescription or non-prescription (OTC);
- are pregnant or intend to become pregnant while using this medicine;
- are breast-feeding;
- are taking **any** other prescription or nonprescription (OTC) medicine;
- have any other medical problems, especially alcohol abuse (or history of) or liver disease.

PROPER USE OF THIS MEDICINE

If isoniazid upsets your stomach, take it with food. Antacids may also help. However, do not take aluminum-containing antacids within 1 hour of taking isoniazid. They may keep this medicine from working properly.

To help clear up your tuberculosis (TB) completely, **it is very important that you keep taking this medicine for the full time of treatment** even if you begin to feel better after a few weeks. You may have to take it every day for as long as 6 months to 2 years. **It is important that you do not miss any doses.**

Your doctor may also want you to take pyridoxine (e.g., Hexa-Betalin, vitamin B_6) every day to help prevent or lessen some of the side effects of isoniazid. If it is needed, **it is** very important to take pyridoxine every day along with this medicine. Do not miss any doses.

If you do miss a dose of this medicine, take it as soon as possible. However, if it is almost time for your next dose, skip the missed dose and go back to your regular dosing schedule. Do not double doses.

PRECAUTIONS WHILE USING THIS MEDICINE

It is very important that your doctor check your progress at regular visits. Also, **check with your doctor immediately if blurred vision or loss of vision, with or without eye pain, occurs during treatment.** Your doctor may want you to have your eyes checked by an ophthalmologist (eye doctor).

If your symptoms do not improve within 2 to 3 weeks, or if they become worse, check with your doctor.

Liver problems may be more likely to occur if you drink alcoholic beverages regularly while you are taking isoniazid. Also, the regular use of alcohol may keep this medicine from working properly. **Therefore, you should strictly limit the amount of alcoholic beverages you drink while you are taking isoniazid.**

If isoniazid causes you to feel very tired or very weak, or causes clumsiness; unsteadiness; loss of appetite; nausea; numbness, tingling, burning, or pain in the hands and feet; or vomiting, check with your doctor immediately. These may be early warning signs of more serious liver or nerve problems that could develop later.

Diabetics—This medicine may cause false test results with some urine sugar tests. Check with your doctor before changing your diet or the dosage of your diabetes medicine.

POSSIBLE SIDE EFFECTS OF THIS MEDICINE
Side Effects That Should Be Reported To Your Doctor Immediately

> *More common*—Clumsiness or unsteadiness; dark urine; loss of appetite; nausea or vomiting; numbness, tingling, burning, or pain in hands and feet; unusual tiredness or weakness; yellow eyes or skin

> *Rare*—Blurred vision or loss of vision, with or without eye pain; convulsions (seizures); fever and sore throat; joint pain; mood or other mental changes; skin rash; unusual bleeding or bruising

Side Effects That Usually Do Not Require Medical Attention

These possible side effects may go away during treatment; however, if they continue or are bothersome, check with your doctor, nurse, or pharmacist.

> *More common*—Diarrhea; stomach pain

Other side effects not listed above may also occur in some patients. If you notice any other effects, check with your doctor, nurse, or pharmacist.

ISOTRETINOIN   Systemic

■ For the Pharmacist ■

In providing consultation, consider emphasizing the following selected information (» = major clinical significance):

Before using this medication
» Conditions affecting use, especially:

Sensitivity to isotretinoin, etretinate, tretinoin, or vitamin A derivatives

Pregnancy—Not taking isotretinoin during pregnancy, because it causes birth defects in humans. In addition, not taking if there is a chance that pregnancy may occur during treatment or within one month following treatment. Not taking isotretinoin unless an effective form of contraception (birth control) is used for at least 1 month before beginning treatment. Contraception must be continued during treatment and for one month after isotretinoin is stopped

Breast-feeding—Although it is not known whether isotretinoin passes into the breast milk, medication is not recommended during breast-feeding, because it may cause unwanted effects in nursing babies

Use in children—Use is not recommended, because children may be more sensitive to the effects of isotretinoin

Other medications, especially etretinate, tretinoin, Vitamin A, or tetracyclines

Proper use of this medication
» Importance of not taking more medication than the amount prescribed
» Proper dosing

Missed dose: Taking as soon as possible; not taking if almost time for next dose; not doubling doses
» Proper storage

Precautions while using this medication
Regular visits to physician to check progress during therapy
» Stopping medication immediately and checking with physician if pregnancy is suspected, since isotretinoin causes birth defects in humans
» Not donating blood to a blood bank during or for 30 days after therapy has been completed to prevent possibility of a pregnant patient receiving the blood
» Avoiding concurrent use of vitamin A and vitamin supplements containing vitamin A, unless prescribed by physician
» Not drinking, or at least reducing consumption of, alcoholic beverages, because of possible hypertriglyceridemia and consequent cardiovascular risks

Diabetics: May alter blood sugar concentrations
» Caution if decrease in night vision, which may be sudden, occurs; not driving, using machines, or doing other things that could be dangerous if unable to see well; checking with physician if this occurs

Possible dryness of eyes; may decrease tolerance to contact lenses during therapy and for up to about 2 weeks after discontinuation of therapy; checking with physician about using ocular lubricant to relieve dryness of eyes or if inflammation occurs

Possible photosensitivity; avoiding unprotected exposure to sunlight or use of sunlamp

Possible dryness of mouth and nose; for mouth dryness, using sugarless candy or gum, ice, or saliva substitute for relief; checking with physician or dentist if dry mouth continues for more than 2 weeks.

For patients with acne

Possibility that acne may appear to worsen during initial therapy; checking with physician if irritation or other symptoms of condition become severe

Side/adverse effects

Signs of potential side effects, especially bleeding or inflammation of gums; burning, redness, itching, or other sign of inflammation of eye; cataracts; corneal opacities; hepatitis; inflammatory bowel disease; mental depression; mood changes; optic neuritis; nosebleeds; pseudotumor cerebri; regional ileitis; scaling, redness, burning, pain, or other sign of inflammation of lips; skin infection; or skin rash

---

▲ For the Patient ▲

914174

ABOUT YOUR MEDICINE

Isotretinoin (eye-soe-TRET-i-noyn) is taken by mouth to treat severe, disfiguring cystic acne. It should be used only after other acne medicines have been tried and have failed to help the acne. Isotretinoin also may be used to treat other skin diseases as determined by your doctor.

Isotretinoin must not be used in women who are able to bear children unless other forms of treatment have been tried first and have failed. Isotretinoin must not be taken during pregnancy, because it causes birth defects in humans. If you are able to bear children, it is very important that you read, understand, and follow the pregnancy warnings for isotretinoin.

If any of the information in this leaflet causes you special concern or if you want additional information about your medicine and its use, check with your doctor, nurse, or pharmacist. **Remember, keep this and all other medicines out of the reach of children and never share your medicines with others.**

BEFORE USING THIS MEDICINE

Isotretinoin comes with patient information. It is very important that you read and understand this information. Be sure to ask your doctor about anything you do not understand.

Isotretinoin causes birth defects in humans. It must not be taken during pregnancy or if there is a chance that you may become pregnant during treatment or within one month following treatment. Isotretinoin must not be taken unless an effective form of contraception (birth control) is used for at least 1 month before the beginning of treatment. Contraception must be continued during the period of treatment, which is up to 20 weeks, and for 1 month after isotretinoin is stopped.

Be sure you have discussed this information with your doctor. In addition, you will be asked to sign an informed consent form stating that you understand the above information.

Tell your doctor, nurse, and pharmacist if you . . .
- are allergic to any medicine, either prescription or non-prescription (OTC);
- **are pregnant or may become pregnant while using this medicine;**
- are breast-feeding;
- are taking any other prescription or nonprescription (OTC) medicine, especially etretinate, tetracyclines, tretinoin, or vitamin A;
- have any other medical problems.

PROPER USE OF THIS MEDICINE

It is very important that you take isotretinoin only as directed. Do not take more of it, do not take it more often, and do not take it for a longer time than your doctor ordered. To do so may increase the chance of side effects.

If you miss a dose of this medicine, take it as soon as possible. However, if it is almost time for your next dose, skip the missed dose and go back to your regular dosing schedule. Do not double doses.

PRECAUTIONS WHILE USING THIS MEDICINE

Isotretinoin causes birth defects in humans if taken during pregnancy. Therefore, if you suspect that you may have become pregnant, stop taking this medicine immediately and check with your doctor.

Do not donate blood to a blood bank while you are taking isotretinoin or for 30 days after you stop taking it. This is to prevent the possibility of a pregnant patient receiving the blood.

Do not take vitamin A or any vitamin supplement containing vitamin A while taking this medicine, unless otherwise directed by your doctor.

Drinking too much alcohol while taking isotretinoin may increase the chance of unwanted effects on the heart and blood vessels. **It is best that you do not drink alcoholic beverages or that you at least reduce the amount you usually drink.**

In some patients, isotretinoin may cause a decrease in night vision. This decrease may occur suddenly. If it does occur, **do not drive, use machines, or do other jobs that require you to see well.** Also, check with your doctor.

POSSIBLE SIDE EFFECTS OF THIS MEDICINE
Side Effects That Should Be Reported To Your Doctor

More common—Burning, redness, itching, or other sign of eye inflammation; nosebleeds; scaling, redness, burning, pain, or other sign of inflammation of lips

Less common—Mental depression; skin infection or rash

Rare—Abdominal or stomach pain (severe); bleeding or inflammation of gums; blurred vision or other changes in vision; diarrhea (severe); headache (severe or continuing); mood changes; nausea and vomiting; pain or tenderness of eyes; rectal bleeding; yellow eyes or skin

Side Effects That Usually Do Not Require Medical Attention

These possible side effects may go away during treatment; however, if they continue or are bothersome, check with your doctor, nurse, or pharmacist.

More common—Dryness of mouth or nose; dryness or itching of skin

Other side effects not listed above may also occur in some patients. If you notice any other effects, check with your doctor, nurse, or pharmacist.

LEVODOPA   Systemic

■For the Pharmacist■

In providing consultation, consider emphasizing the following selected information (» = major clinical significance):

Before using this medication
» Conditions affecting use, especially:
   Sensitivity to levodopa
   Pregnancy—No studies in humans; depressed growth and malformations in animal studies
   Breast-feeding—Distributed into breast milk; may inhibit lactation
   Use in the elderly—Reduced tolerance to effects of levodopa; caution in resuming normal activity, especially in patients with osteoporosis
   Dental—Possible difficulty in retention of full dentures
   Other medications, especially haloperidol, hydantoin anticonvulsants, hydrocarbon inhalation anesthetics, phenothiazines, cocaine, MAO inhibitors, pyridoxine, and selegiline
   Other medical problems, especially severe cardiovascular disease, severe pulmonary diseases, glaucoma, melanoma (history of or suspected), peptic ulcer (history of), psychosis, renal function impairment, or urinary retention

Proper use of this medication
» Taking food shortly after taking medication to relieve gastric irritation; taking food before or concurrently may retard levodopa's effect
» Compliance with therapy; taking medication only as directed; not stopping medication unless ordered by physician
» Maximum effectiveness of medication may not occur for several weeks or months after therapy is initiated
» Proper dosing
   Missed dose: Taking as soon as possible; skipping dose if next scheduled dose is within 2 hours; not doubling doses
» Proper storage

Precautions while using this medication
   Caution if any kind of surgery (including dental surgery) or emergency treatment is required
   Diabetics: May interfere with urine tests for sugar and ketones
» Caution if drowsiness occurs
» Caution when getting up suddenly from lying or sitting position; dizziness and fainting may occur
» Avoiding foods or vitamin products containing pyridoxine (vitamin B_6); diminished levodopa effect when used with pyridoxine
» Caution in resuming normal physical activities when condition has improved, especially for geriatric patients
   Possibility of "on-off" phenomenon

Side/adverse effects
   Signs of potential side effects, especially difficult urination, duodenal ulcer, hemolytic anemia, hypertension, irregular heartbeat, mental depression, mood or mental changes, severe nausea or vomiting, orthostatic hypotension, spasm or closing of eyelids, uncontrolled movements of body
   Occasional darkening of urine or sweat may be alarming to patient although medically insignificant

---

▲ For the Patient ▲

912383

LEVODOPA/CARBIDOPA WITH LEVODOPA
(Oral): *Including Carbidopa with Levodopa; Levodopa.*

ABOUT YOUR MEDICINE

Levodopa (LEE-voe-doe-pa) is a medicine used alone or in combination with **carbidopa** (KAR-bi-doe-pa) to treat Parkinson's disease, sometimes referred to as shaking palsy or paralysis agitans.

If any of the information in this leaflet causes you special concern or if you want additional information about your medicine and its use, check with your doctor, nurse, or pharmacist. **Remember, keep this and all other medicines out of the reach of children and never share your medicines with others.**

BEFORE USING THIS MEDICINE

Tell your doctor, nurse, and pharmacist if you . . .
- are allergic to any medicine, either prescription or non-prescription (OTC);
- are pregnant or intend to become pregnant while using this medicine;
- are breast-feeding;
- are taking any other prescription or nonprescription (OTC) medicine, especially anticonvulsants, haloperidol, MAO inhibitors, phenothiazines, pyridoxine (vitamin B_6), or selegiline;
- have any other medical problems, especially asthma, bronchitis, emphysema, or other chronic lung disease; glaucoma; heart or blood vessel disease; kidney disease or difficult urination; mental illness; skin cancer; or stomach ulcer;
- use cocaine.

PROPER USE OF THIS MEDICINE

Take this medicine only as directed. Do not take more or less of it, do not take it more often, and do not stop taking it unless ordered by your doctor. Some people must take this medicine for several weeks before full benefit is received.

Your doctor may want you to take food shortly after taking this medicine (about 15 minutes after) to lessen possible stomach upset. If stomach upset is severe or continues, check with your doctor.

For patients taking carbidopa and levodopa extended-release tablets:
- Swallow the tablet whole without crushing or chewing, unless your doctor tells you not to. If your doctor tells you to, you may break the tablet in half.

If you miss a dose of this medicine, take it as soon as possible. However, if your next scheduled dose is within 2 hours, skip the missed dose and go back to your regular dosing schedule. Do not double doses.

PRECAUTIONS WHILE USING THIS MEDICINE

This medicine may cause some people to become drowsy or less alert than they are normally. **Make sure you know how you react to this medicine before you drive, use machines, or do other jobs that require you to be alert.**

Dizziness, lightheadedness, or fainting may occur, especially when you get up from a lying or sitting position. Getting up slowly may help.

Pyridoxine (vitamin B_6) has been found to reduce the effects of levodopa when taken alone (not in combination with carbidopa). If you are taking levodopa, do not take vitamin products containing vitamin B_6 unless prescribed. Also remember that certain foods contain large amounts of vitamin B_6.

As your condition improves and your body movements become easier, **be careful not to overdo physical activities. Injuries resulting from falls may occur.**

POSSIBLE SIDE EFFECTS OF THIS MEDICINE

Side Effects That Should Be Reported To Your Doctor

> *More common*—Mental depression; mood changes; unusual and uncontrolled movements of the upper body (such as the tongue, arms, head)

> *Less common (more common when levodopa is used alone)*—Difficult urination; dizziness or lightheadedness; irregular heartbeat; nausea and vomiting (severe or continuing); spasm or closing of eyelids

> *Rare*—High blood pressure; stomach pain; unusual tiredness or weakness

After taking this medicine for long periods of time, such as one to several years, some patients suddenly lose the ability to move. This may last from a few minutes to hours. The patient is then able to move as before until the condition unexpectedly occurs again. If you should have this problem, check with your doctor.

Side Effects That Usually Do Not Require Medical Attention

These possible side effects may go away during treatment; however, if they continue or are bothersome, check with your doctor, nurse, or pharmacist.

> *More common*—Anxiety

> *Less common*—Constipation or diarrhea; dryness of mouth

This medicine sometimes causes the urine and sweat to be darker than usual. The urine may at first be reddish, then turn to nearly black after being exposed to air. This effect is not important and is to be expected.

Other side effects not listed above may also occur in some patients. If you notice any other effects, check with your doctor, nurse, or pharmacist.

LINCOMYCIN   Systemic

■ For the Pharmacist ■

In providing consultation, consider emphasizing the following selected information (» = major clinical significance):

Before using this medication
» Conditions affecting use, especially:
   Hypersensitivity to lincomycin, clindamycin, or doxorubicin
   Pregnancy—Lincomycin crosses the placenta
   Breast-feeding—Lincomycin is distributed into breast milk
   Use in children—Lincomycin is not recommended in infants up to 1 month of age; lincomycin injection contains benzyl alcohol, which has been associated with a fatal gasping syndrome in premature infants
   Other medications, especially hydrocarbon inhalation anesthetics, neuromuscular blocking agents, antiperistaltic and adsorbent antidiarrheals, chloramphenicol, or erythromycins
   Other medical problems, especially a history of gastrointestinal disease, particularly ulcerative colitis, severe renal function impairment, or severe hepatic function impairment

Proper use of this medication
» Taking on an empty stomach with an 8 ounce glass of water
» Compliance with full course of therapy, especially in streptococcal infections
» Importance of not missing doses and taking at evenly spaced times
» Proper dosing
   Missed dose: Taking as soon as possible; not taking if almost time for next dose; not doubling doses
» Proper storage

Precautions while using this medication
   Regular visits to physician to check progress
   Checking with physician if no improvement within a few days
» For severe diarrhea, checking with physician before taking any antidiarrheals; for mild diarrhea, taking kaolin- or attapulgite-containing antidiarrheals at least 2 hours before or 3 to 4 hours after taking oral lincomycin; other antidiarrheals may worsen or prolong the diarrhea; checking with physician or pharmacist if mild diarrhea continues or worsens
   Caution if surgery with general anesthesia is required

Side/adverse effects
   Signs of potential side effects, especially hypersensitivity, neutropenia, thrombocytopenic purpura, and pseudomembranous colitis

▲ For the Patient ▲

914210

LINCOMYCINS (Oral): *Including Clindamycin; Lincomycin.*

ABOUT YOUR MEDICINE

Lincomycins (lin-koe-MYE-sins) belong to the general family of medicines called antibiotics. These medicines are used to treat infections. They will not work for colds, flu, or other virus infections.

If any of the information in this leaflet causes you special concern or if you want additional information about your medicine and its use, check with your doctor, nurse, or pharmacist. **Remember, keep this and all other medicines out of the reach of children and never share your medicines with others.**

BEFORE USING THIS MEDICINE

Tell your doctor, nurse, and pharmacist if you . . .
- are allergic to any medicine, either prescription or non-prescription (OTC);
- are pregnant or intend to become pregnant while using this medicine;
- are breast-feeding;
- are taking any other prescription or nonprescription (OTC) medicine, especially chloramphenicol, diarrhea medicine, or erythromycins;
- have any other medical problems, especially liver disease, or stomach or intestinal disease (history of) (especially colitis, including colitis caused by antibiotics, or enteritis).

PROPER USE OF THIS MEDICINE

If you are taking the capsule form of clindamycin, it should be taken with a full glass (8 ounces) of water or with meals to prevent irritation of the esophagus.

For patients taking lincomycin:
- Lincomycin is best taken with a full glass (8 ounces) of water on an empty stomach (either 1 hour before or 2 hours after meals).

To help clear up your infection completely, **keep taking this medicine for the full time of treatment** even if you begin to feel better after a few days. **If you have a "strep" infection, you should keep taking this medicine for at least 10 days. This is especially important in "strep" infections. Serious heart problems could develop later** if your infection is not cleared up completely. Also, if you stop taking this medicine too soon, your symptoms may return.

This medicine works best when there is a constant amount in the blood. **To help keep this amount constant, do not miss any doses. Also, it is best to take each dose at evenly spaced times day and night.**

If you do miss a dose of this medicine, take it as soon as possible. This will help to keep a constant amount of medicine in the blood. However, if it is almost time for your next dose, skip the missed dose and go back to your regular dosing schedule. Do not double doses.

PRECAUTIONS WHILE USING THIS MEDICINE

If your symptoms do not improve within a few days, or if they become worse, check with your doctor.

In some patients, lincomycins may cause diarrhea.

- Severe diarrhea may be a sign of a serious side effect. **Do not take any diarrhea medicine without first checking with your doctor.**
- For mild diarrhea, diarrhea medicine containing attapulgite (e.g., Kaopectate tablets, Diasorb) may be taken. However, attapulgite may keep lincomycins from being absorbed into the body. Therefore, these diarrhea medicines should be taken at least 2 hours before or 3 to 4 hours after you take lincomycins by mouth.

If you have any questions about this or if mild diarrhea continues or gets worse, check with your doctor, nurse, or pharmacist.

This medicine must not be given to other people or used for other infections unless you are otherwise directed by your doctor.

POSSIBLE SIDE EFFECTS OF THIS MEDICINE
Side Effects That Should Be Reported To Your Doctor Immediately

More common—Abdominal or stomach cramps and pain (severe); abdominal tenderness; diarrhea (watery and severe), which may also be bloody; fever

The above side effects may also occur up to several weeks after you stop taking this medicine.

Less common—Skin rash, redness, and itching; sore throat and fever; unusual bleeding or bruising

Side Effects That Usually Do Not Require Medical Attention

These possible side effects may go away during treatment; however, if they continue or are bothersome, check with your doctor, nurse, or pharmacist.

More common—Diarrhea (mild); nausea and vomiting; stomach pain

Other side effects not listed above may also occur in some patients. If you notice any other effects, check with your doctor, nurse, or pharmacist.

LINDANE   Topical

■ For the Pharmacist ■

In providing consultation, consider emphasizing the following selected information (» = major clinical significance):

Before using this medication
» Conditions affecting use, especially:
    Sensitivity to lindane
    Pregnancy—Lindane is absorbed through the skin and has the potential for causing toxic effects in the CNS of the fetus; not increasing the amount, frequency, or length of therapy that physician ordered; not being treated more than twice during a pregnancy
    Breast-feeding—Lindane is distributed into breast milk; another method of feeding infant should be used for 2 days after use of lindane
    Use in children—Caution is recommended, since infants and children are especially sensitive to the effects of lindane; in addition, use is not recommended in premature infants
    Use in the elderly—Absorption may be increased in the elderly because of increased permeability of their skin; elderly patients with a history of seizure activity may be especially sensitive to the CNS toxicity effects of lindane

Proper use of this medication
» Poison; importance of keeping away from mouth
» Importance of not using more lindane than the amount prescribed
» Avoiding contact with the eyes
» Not using on open wounds, such as cuts or sores on skin or scalp, to minimize systemic absorption
When applying lindane to another person: Wearing plastic disposable or rubber gloves to prevent systemic absorption, especially if you are pregnant or are breast-feeding
Proper administration:
    Reading patient directions carefully before using
If necessary, treating sexual partner or partners, especially, and all members of household, since infestation may spread to persons in close contact; checking with doctor if these persons have not been checked or if there are any questions
For cream or lotion dosage form
For scabies—
    Washing, rinsing, and drying skin well before using lindane if skin has any cream, lotion, ointment, or oil on it
    Drying skin well if warm bath or shower is taken before using lindane
    Applying enough lindane to dry skin to cover entire skin surface from neck down; rubbing in well
    Leaving lindane on skin for 8 hours
    Removing lindane by washing thoroughly
For shampoo dosage form
For lice—
    Shampooing, rinsing, and drying hair and scalp well before using lindane if hair or scalp has any cream, lotion, ointment, or oil-based product on it
» If applying shampoo in the shower or in the bathtub, making sure shampoo does not run down on other parts of body; also, not applying shampoo in a bathtub where shampoo may run into

bath water in which patient is sitting; this minimizes systemic absorption; when rinsing out the shampoo, thoroughly rinsing entire body to remove any shampoo that may have gotten on it

Applying enough to dry hair (1 ounce or less for short hair, 1½ ounces for medium length hair and 2 ounces or less for long hair) to thoroughly wet the hair and skin or scalp of affected and surrounding hairy areas

Rubbing thoroughly into hair and skin or scalp; allowing to remain in place for 4 minutes

Using just enough water to work up a good lather

Rinsing thoroughly; drying with clean towel

When hair is dry, combing with fine-toothed comb to remove any remaining nits or nit shells

» Not using as a regular shampoo
» Proper dosing
» Proper storage

Precautions while using this medication

To help prevent reinfestation or spreading of the infestation to other persons:

For scabies—Washing in very hot water or dry-cleaning all recently worn underwear and pajamas and used sheets, pillowcases, and towels

For lice—Washing in very hot water or dry-cleaning all recently worn clothing and used bed linens and towels

Side/adverse effects

Risk of systemic absorption greater in infants and children than in adults; use not recommended in premature neonates, because risk of systemic absorption greater than in older infants

Signs of potential side effects, especially skin irritation or rash not present before therapy or CNS toxicity

---

▲ For the Patient ▲

914221

ABOUT YOUR MEDICINE

Lindane (LIN-dane) is used to treat infestations of lice and scabies. Lindane cream and lotion are used to treat only scabies infestations. Lindane shampoo is used to treat only lice infestations.

If any of the information in this leaflet causes you special concern or if you want additional information about your medicine and its use, check with your doctor, nurse, or pharmacist. **Remember, keep this and all other medicines out of the reach of children and never share your medicines with others.**

BEFORE USING THIS MEDICINE

Tell your doctor, nurse, and pharmacist if you . . .

- are allergic to any medicine, either prescription or nonprescription (OTC);
- are pregnant or intend to become pregnant while using this medicine;
- are breast-feeding;
- are taking any other prescription or nonprescription (OTC) medicine;

• have any other medical problems.

PROPER USE OF THIS MEDICINE

Lindane is poisonous. Keep it away from the mouth because it is harmful and may be fatal if swallowed.

Use lindane only as directed. Do not use more of it, do not use it more often, and do not use it for a longer period of time than your doctor ordered. Do not use lindane on open wounds such as cuts or sores on the skin or scalp. To do so may increase the chance of absorption through the skin and the chance of lindane poisoning.

Keep lindane away from the eyes. If you should accidentally get some in your eyes, flush them thoroughly with water at once and contact your doctor.

When applying lindane to another person, you should wear plastic disposable or rubber gloves, especially if you are pregnant or are breast-feeding.

Your sexual partner or partners, especially, and all members of your household may need to be treated also, since the infestation may spread to persons in close contact. If these persons have not been checked for an infestation or if you have any questions about this, check with your doctor.

To use the cream or lotion form of lindane for scabies:
• If your skin has any cream, lotion, ointment, or oil on it, wash, rinse, and dry your skin well before applying lindane.
• Apply enough lindane to your dry skin to cover the entire skin surface from the neck down, including the soles of your feet, and rub in well.
• Leave lindane on for no more than 8 hours, then remove by washing thoroughly. Some manufacturers recommend leaving lindane on for 8 to 12 hours; however, USP medical experts recommend leaving it on for only 8 hours. If you have any questions about this, check with your doctor.

To use the shampoo form of lindane for lice:
• If your hair has any cream, lotion, ointment, or oil-based product on it, shampoo, rinse, and dry your hair and scalp well before applying lindane.
• If you apply this shampoo in the shower or in the bathtub, make sure the shampoo is not allowed to run down on other parts of your body. Also, do not apply this shampoo in a bathtub where the shampoo may run into the bath water in which you are sitting. To do so may increase the chance of absorption through the skin. When you rinse out the shampoo, be sure to thoroughly rinse your entire body.
• Apply enough shampoo to your dry hair (1 ounce or less for short hair, 1 and 1/2 ounces for medium length hair, and 2 ounces or less for long hair) to thoroughly wet the hair and skin or scalp of the affected and surrounding hairy areas.

- Thoroughly rub the shampoo into the hair and skin or scalp and allow to remain in place for 4 minutes. Then, use just enough water to work up a good lather.
- Rinse thoroughly and dry with a clean towel.
- When the hair is dry, comb with a fine-toothed comb to remove any remaining nits (eggs) or nit shells.
- **Do not use as a regular shampoo.**

PRECAUTIONS WHILE USING THIS MEDICINE

To help prevent reinfestation, all recently worn clothing and used bed linen and towels should be washed in very hot water or dry-cleaned.

POSSIBLE SIDE EFFECTS OF THIS MEDICINE

Side Effects That Should Be Reported To Your Doctor

    Rare—Skin irritation or rash not present before use of lindane

    Possible signs of lindane poisoning—Convulsions (seizures); dizziness, clumsiness, or unsteadiness; fast heartbeat; muscle cramps; nervousness, restlessness, or irritability; vomiting

Other side effects not listed above may also occur in some patients. If you notice any other effects, check with your doctor, nurse, or pharmacist.

After you stop using lindane, itching may occur and continue for 1 to several weeks. If this continues longer or is bothersome, check with your doctor.

LITHIUM   Systemic

■For the Pharmacist■

In providing consultation, consider emphasizing the following selected information (» = major clinical significance):

Before using this medication
» Conditions affecting use, especially:
    Sensitivity to lithium
    Pregnancy—Lithium crosses placenta; contraindicated in first trimester because of possible neonatal goiter and cardiovascular malformations; at delivery, hypotonia, lethargy, and cyanosis in newborns of mothers taking lithium at term
    Breast-feeding—Excreted in breast milk; may cause hypotonia, hypothermia, cyanosis, and ECG changes in some babies
    Use in children—May decrease bone formation or density
    Use in the elderly—Elderly more prone to develop CNS toxicity, hypothyroidism and goiter; lower doses and more frequent monitoring required
    Other medications, especially iodine-containing preparations, nonsteroidal anti-inflammatory drugs, chlorpromazine (and possibly other phenothiazines), diuretics, haloperidol, or molindone
    Other medical problems, especially history of leukemia, cardiovascular disease, epilepsy, parkinsonism, severe dehydration, renal insufficiency, urinary retention, or severe infections with prolonged sweating, vomiting, or diarrhea

Proper use of this medication
    Taking after a meal or snack to prevent laxative action and to decrease the severity of stomach upset, tremors, or weakness by slowing absorption rate
» Importance of adequate fluid (2.5 to 3 liters each day) and sodium intake
» Importance of not taking more medication than the amount prescribed
» Compliance with therapy; improvement in condition may require 1 to 3 weeks; importance of maintaining adequate blood levels even though symptoms improved
» Proper dosing
    Missed dose: Taking as soon as possible, unless within 4 hours (6 hours for extended-release tablets or slow-release capsules) of next scheduled dose; not doubling doses
» Proper storage
For extended-release or slow-release dosage form
    Swallowing tablet or capsule whole
    Not breaking, crushing, or chewing
For syrup dosage form
    Diluting dose with fruit juice or other flavored beverage before taking

Precautions while using this medication
» Regular visits to physician to check progress during therapy; importance of serum lithium monitoring
    Caution in drinking large amounts of coffee, tea, or colas because of diuretic effect
» Possible drowsiness or dizziness; caution if driving or doing jobs requiring alertness

» Caution during exercise, saunas, and hot weather
» Caution during illnesses that cause high fevers with profuse sweating, vomiting, or diarrhea
» Caution on self-imposed dieting
» Importance of patient and family knowing early symptoms of overdose or toxicity

For slow-release dosage form
» Not using interchangeably with any other dosage form

Side/adverse effects
» Early symptoms of lithium overdose or toxicity:
   Diarrhea
   Drowsiness
   Loss of appetite
   Muscle weakness
   Nausea or vomiting
   Slurred speech
   Trembling
   Side effects are more likely to occur in the elderly
   Signs of potential side effects, especially cardiovascular problems, leukocytosis, weight gain, blue color and pain in fingers and toes, coldness of arms and legs, pseudotumor cerebri, symptoms of hypothyroidism

---

▲ For the Patient ▲

913105

ABOUT YOUR MEDICINE

Lithium (LITH-ee-um) is used to treat the manic stage of bipolar disorder (manic-depressive illness). It may also help reduce the frequency and severity of depression in bipolar disorder. Lithium may also be used for other conditions as determined by your doctor.

It is important that you and your family understand the effects of lithium. These depend on your individual condition and response and the amount of lithium you use. You also must know when to contact your doctor if there are problems.

If any of the information in this leaflet causes you special concern or if you want additional information about your medicine and its use, check with your doctor, nurse, or pharmacist. **Remember, keep this and all other medicines out of the reach of children and never share your medicines with others.**

BEFORE USING THIS MEDICINE

Tell your doctor, nurse, and pharmacist if you . . .
• are allergic to any medicine, either prescription or non-prescription (OTC);
• are pregnant or intend to become pregnant while using this medicine;
• are breast-feeding;
• are taking **any** other prescription or nonprescription (OTC) medicine;

- have any other medical problems, especially epilepsy, heart disease, kidney disease, leukemia (history of), Parkinson's disease, problems with urination, severe infections, or severe water loss.

PROPER USE OF THIS MEDICINE

During treatment with lithium, drink 2 or 3 quarts of water or other fluids each day, and use a normal amount of salt, unless otherwise directed.

Take this medicine exactly as directed. Do not take more or less of it, do not take it more or less often, and do not take it for a longer time than your doctor ordered. To do so may increase the chance of unwanted effects. **Sometimes lithium must be taken for 1 to several weeks before you begin to feel better.**

In order for lithium to work properly, it must be taken every day in regularly spaced doses as ordered by your doctor. This is necessary to keep a constant amount of lithium in your blood. Do not miss any doses and do not stop taking the medicine even if you feel better.

If you do miss a dose, take it as soon as possible. However, if it is within 2 hours (6 hours for the long-acting tablets or capsules) of your next dose, skip the missed dose and go back to your regular schedule. Do not double doses.

PRECAUTIONS WHILE USING THIS MEDICINE

Your doctor should check your progress at regular visits to make sure that the medicine is working properly and that possible side effects are avoided. Laboratory tests may be necessary.

Lithium may not work properly if you drink large amounts of caffeine-containing coffee, tea, or colas.

Lithium may cause some people to become dizzy, drowsy, or less alert than they are normally. **Make sure you know how you react to this medicine before you drive, use machines, or do other jobs that require you to be alert.**

The loss of too much water and salt from your body may lead to serious side effects from lithium. **Use extra care in hot weather and during activities that cause you to sweat heavily, such as hot baths, saunas, or exercising. Also, check with your doctor before going on a diet to lose weight, or if you have an illness that causes sweating, vomiting, or diarrhea.**

POSSIBLE SIDE EFFECTS OF THIS MEDICINE
Side Effects That Should Be Reported To Your Doctor Immediately

Early signs of overdose or toxicity—Diarrhea; drowsiness; loss of appetite; muscle weakness; nausea or vomiting; slurred speech; trembling

>   *Late signs of overdose or toxicity*—Blurred vision; clum-
>   siness or unsteadiness; confusion; convulsions (sei-
>   zures); dizziness; trembling (severe); unusual increase
>   in amount of urine

Other Side Effects That Should Be Reported To Your Doctor

>   *Less common*—Fainting; fast, slow, or irregular heart-
>   beat; troubled breathing (especially during hard work
>   or exercise); unusual tiredness or weakness; weight gain

>   *Rare*—Blue color and pain in fingers and toes; cold arms
>   and legs; dizziness; eye pain; headache; unusual noises
>   in the ears; vision problems

>   *Signs of low thyroid function*—Dry, rough skin; hair loss;
>   hoarseness; mental depression; sensitivity to cold;
>   swelling of feet or lower legs; swelling of neck; unusual
>   excitement

Side Effects That Usually Do Not Require Medical Attention

These possible side effects may go away during treatment;
however, if they continue or are bothersome, check with your
doctor, nurse, or pharmacist.

>   *More common*—Increased frequency of urination or loss
>   of bladder control—more common in women, usually
>   beginning 2 to 7 years after start of treatment; in-
>   creased thirst; nausea (mild); trembling of hands
>   (slight)

Other side effects not listed above may also occur in some
patients. If you notice any other effects, check with your
doctor, nurse, or pharmacist.

LODOXAMIDE   Ophthalmic

■ For the Pharmacist ■

In providing consultation, consider emphasizing the following selected
information (» = major clinical significance):

Before using this medication
» Conditions affecting use, especially:
Sensitivity to lodoxamide
Use in children—Safety and efficacy have not been established
in children up to 2 years of age

Proper use of this medication
Proper administration technique; not touching applicator tip to any
surface; keeping container tightly closed
Compliance with therapy
» Proper dosing
Missed dose: Using as soon as possible
» Proper storage

Precautions while using this medication
» Checking with physician if symptoms do not improve or if condition
becomes worse

Side/adverse effects
Signs of potential side effects, especially blurred vision; foreign body
sensation; hyperemia; discomfort, pruritus, tearing or discharge,
or other eye irritation not present before therapy or becoming
worse during therapy; anterior chamber cells; blepharitis; che-
mosis; corneal abrasion; corneal erosion or ulcer, edema, mucus
from eye, or eye pain not present before therapy or becoming
worse during therapy; dizziness; headache; keratitis or keratopathy; or skin rash

▲ For the Patient ▲

919509

ABOUT YOUR MEDICINE

Lodoxamide (loe-DOX-a-mide) ophthalmic solution is used
in the eye to treat certain disorders of the eye caused by
allergies.

If any of the information in this leaflet causes you special
concern or if you want additional information about your
medicine and its use, check with your doctor, nurse, or pharmacist. **Remember, keep this and all other medicines out of
the reach of children and never share your medicines with
others.**

BEFORE USING THIS MEDICINE

Tell your doctor, nurse, and pharmacist if you . . .
* are allergic to any medicine, either prescription or nonprescription (OTC);
* are pregnant or intend to become pregnant while using
this medicine;
* are breast-feeding;

- are taking any other prescription or nonprescription (OTC) medicine;
- have any other medical problems.

PROPER USE OF THIS MEDICINE
To use the eye drops:

- First, wash your hands. Tilt the head back and, pressing your finger gently on the skin just beneath the lower eyelid, pull the lower eyelid away from the eye to make a space. Drop the medicine into this space. Let go of the eyelid and gently close the eyes. Do not blink. Keep the eyes closed for 1 or 2 minutes to allow the medicine to be absorbed by the eye.

- If you think you did not get the drop of medicine into your eye properly, use another drop.

- To keep the medicine as germ-free as possible, do not touch the applicator tip to any surface (including the eye). Also, keep the container tightly closed.

In order for this medicine to work properly, it must be used every day in regularly spaced doses as ordered by your doctor.

If you miss a dose of this medicine, apply it as soon as possible. Then go back to your regular dosing schedule.

PRECAUTIONS WHILE USING THIS MEDICINE
If your symptoms do not improve or if your condition becomes worse, check with your doctor.

POSSIBLE SIDE EFFECTS OF THIS MEDICINE
Side Effects That Should Be Reported To Your Doctor

Less common—Blurred vision; feeling of something in eye; itching, discomfort, redness, tearing, discharge or other eye or eyelid irritation (not present before using this medicine or becoming worse while using this medicine)

Rare—Dizziness, mucus from eye, eye pain, or swelling of eyelid (not present before you started using this medicine or becoming worse while you are using this medicine); headache; sensitivity of eyes to light; skin rash

Side Effects That Usually Do Not Require Medical Attention

These possible side effects may go away during treatment; however, if they continue or are bothersome, check with your doctor, nurse, or pharmacist.

More common—Burning or stinging (when medicine is applied)

Less common or rare—Aching eyes; crusting in corner of eye or on eyelid; drowsiness or sleepiness; dryness of nose or eyes; feeling of heat in eye; heat sensation on body; nausea or stomach discomfort; scales on eyelid or eyelash; sneezing; sticky feeling of eyes; tired eyes

Other side effects not listed above may also occur in some patients. If you notice any other effects, check with your doctor, nurse, or pharmacist.

LOPERAMIDE Oral-Local

■ For the Pharmacist ■

In providing consultation, consider emphasizing the following selected information (» = major clinical significance):

Before using this medication
» Conditions affecting use, especially:
    Sensitivity to loperamide
    Use in children—Risk of dehydration; variability in response to loperamide; increased susceptibility to CNS effects
    Use in the elderly—Risk of dehydration; variability in response to loperamide
    Other medical problems, especially diarrhea caused by antibiotics, severe colitis, or acute dysentery

Proper use of this medication
» Importance of not taking more medication than the amount prescribed
» Importance of maintaining adequate hydration and proper diet
    Missed dose: Not taking missed dose; not doubling doses
» Proper storage

Precautions while using this medication
    Regular visits to physician to check progress during prolonged therapy
» Consulting physician if diarrhea is not controlled within 48 hours and/or fever develops

Side/adverse effects
    Signs of potential side effects, especially allergic reaction or toxic megacolon

---

▲ For the Patient ▲

914243

ABOUT YOUR MEDICINE

Loperamide (loe-PER-a-mide) is a medicine used along with other measures to treat diarrhea.

Do not give antidiarrheals to young children (under 3 years of age) without first checking with their doctor. In older children and elderly persons with diarrhea, antidiarrheals may be used, but it is also very important that liquids be taken to replace the fluids lost by the body. If you have any questions about this, check with your doctor, nurse, or pharmacist.

If any of the information in this leaflet causes you special concern or if you want additional information about your medicine and its use, check with your doctor, nurse, or pharmacist. **Remember, keep this and all other medicines out of the reach of children and never share your medicines with others.**

BEFORE USING THIS MEDICINE

If you are taking this medicine without a prescription, carefully read and follow any precautions on the label. You should be especially careful if you . . .

- are allergic to any medicine, either prescription or nonprescription (OTC);
- are pregnant, intend to become pregnant, or are breast-feeding;
- are taking any other prescription or nonprescription (OTC) medicine, especially narcotic pain medicine;
- are taking an antibiotic, since the antibiotic may be the cause of the diarrhea;
- have any other medical problems, especially colitis (severe), or dysentery.

If you have any questions, check with your doctor, nurse, or pharmacist.

PROPER USE OF THIS MEDICINE

For safe and effective use of this medicine:

- **Follow your doctor's instructions if this medicine was prescribed.**
- Follow the manufacturer's package directions if you are treating yourself.

Importance of diet and fluids while treating diarrhea:

- **In addition to using medicine for diarrhea, it is very important that you replace the fluid lost by the body and follow a proper diet.** For the first 24 hours you should drink plenty of caffeine-free clear liquids, such as ginger ale, decaffeinated cola, decaffeinated tea, broth, and gelatin. During the next 24 hours you may eat bland foods, such as cooked cereals, bread, crackers, and applesauce.
- Check with your doctor as soon as possible if any of the following signs of too much fluid loss occur: decreased urination; dizziness and lightheadedness; dryness of mouth; increased thirst; wrinkled skin.

If you must take loperamide regularly and you miss a dose, skip the missed dose and go back to your regular dosing schedule. Do not double doses.

PRECAUTIONS WHILE USING THIS MEDICINE

Loperamide should not be used for more than two days, unless directed by your doctor. If you will be taking this medicine regularly for a long time, your doctor should check your progress at regular visits.

Check with your doctor if your diarrhea does not stop after two days or if you develop a fever.

POSSIBLE SIDE EFFECTS OF THIS MEDICINE

Side Effects That Should Be Reported To Your Doctor Immediately

When this medicine is used for short periods of time at low doses, side effects usually are rare. However, check with your doctor immediately if any of the following side effects are severe and occur suddenly, since they may be signs of a more severe and dangerous problem with your bowels:

> *Rare*—Bloating; constipation; loss of appetite; stomach pain (severe) with nausea and vomiting

Other Side Effects That Should Be Reported To Your Doctor

> *Rare*—Skin rash

Side Effects That Usually Do Not Require Medical Attention

These possible side effects may go away during treatment; however, if they continue or are bothersome, check with your doctor, nurse, or pharmacist.

> *Rare*—Drowsiness or dizziness; dryness of mouth

Other side effects not listed above may also occur in some patients. If you notice any other effects, check with your doctor, nurse, or pharmacist.

LORACARBEF   Systemic

■For the Pharmacist■

In providing consultation, consider emphasizing the following selected information (» = major clinical significance):

Before using this medication
» Conditions affecting use, especially:
    Allergy to penicillins or cephalosporins
    Other medications, especially probenecid
    Other medical problems, especially renal function impairment

Proper use of this medication
    Taking at least 1 hour before or 2 hours after meals
» Compliance with full course of therapy, especially in streptococcal infections
» Importance of not missing doses and taking at evenly spaced times
» Proper dosing
    Missed dose: Taking as soon as possible; not taking if almost time for next dose; not doubling doses
» Proper storage

Precautions while using this medication
    Checking with physician if no improvement within a few days
» May cause diarrhea—
    For severe diarrhea, checking with physician before taking any antidiarrheals
    For mild diarrhea, kaolin- or attapulgite-containing, but not other, antidiarrheals may be tried
    Checking with physician or pharmacist if mild diarrhea continues or worsens

Side/adverse effects
    Signs of potential side effects, especially hypersensitivity reactions

▲ For the Patient ▲

919327

ABOUT YOUR MEDICINE

Loracarbef (loe-ra-KAR-bef) is used to treat bacterial infections in many different parts of the body. This medicine will not work for colds, flu, or other virus infections.

If any of the information in this leaflet causes you special concern or if you want additional information about your medicine and its use, check with your doctor, nurse, or pharmacist. **Remember, keep this and all other medicines out of the reach of children and never share your medicines with others.**

BEFORE USING THIS MEDICINE

Tell your doctor, nurse, and pharmacist if you . . .
- are allergic to any medicine, either prescription or non-prescription (OTC);
- are pregnant or intend to become pregnant while using this medicine;

- are breast-feeding;
- are taking any other prescription or nonprescription (OTC) medicine, especially probenecid;
- have any other medical problems, especially kidney disease.

PROPER USE OF THIS MEDICINE

Loracarbef should be taken at least 1 hour before or at least 2 hours after meals.

To help clear up your infection completely, **keep taking loracarbef for the full time of treatment,** even if you begin to feel better after a few days. **If you have a "strep" infection, you should keep taking this medicine for at least 10 days. This is especially important in "strep" infections. Serious heart problems could develop later** if your infection is not cleared up completely. Also, if you stop taking this medicine too soon, your symptoms may return.

This medicine works best when there is a constant amount in the blood or urine. **To help keep the amount constant, do not miss any doses. Also, it is best to take the doses at evenly spaced times, day and night.** If this interferes with your sleep or other daily activities, or if you need help in planning the best times to take your medicine, check with your doctor, nurse, or pharmacist.

If you do miss a dose of this medicine, take it as soon as possible. This will help to keep a constant amount of medicine in the blood or urine. However, if it is almost time for your next dose, skip the missed dose and go back to your regular dosing schedule. Do not double doses.

PRECAUTIONS WHILE USING THIS MEDICINE

If your symptoms do not improve within a few days, or if they become worse, check with your doctor.

In some patients, loracarbef may cause diarrhea.
- Severe diarrhea may be a sign of a serious side effect. **Do not take any diarrhea medicine without first checking with your doctor.** Diarrhea medicines may make your diarrhea worse or last longer.
- For mild diarrhea, diarrhea medicine containing kaolin or attapulgite (e.g., Kaopectate tablets, Diasorb) may be taken. However, other kinds of diarrhea medicine should not be taken. They may make your diarrhea worse or last longer.
- If you have any questions about this or if mild diarrhea continues or gets worse, check with your doctor or pharmacist.

POSSIBLE SIDE EFFECTS OF THIS MEDICINE
Side Effects That Should Be Reported To Your Doctor

   More common—Itching; skin rash

Side Effects That Usually Do Not Require Medical Attention

These possible side effects may go away during treatment; however, if they continue or are bothersome, check with your doctor, nurse, or pharmacist.

> *More common*—Diarrhea; loss of appetite; nausea and vomiting; stomach pain

> *Rare*—Dizziness; drowsiness; headache; itching or discharge from the vagina; nervousness; trouble in sleeping

Other side effects not listed above may also occur in some patients. If you notice any other effects, check with your doctor, nurse, or pharmacist.

LOXAPINE   Systemic

■For the Pharmacist■

In providing consultation, consider emphasizing the following selected information (» = major clinical significance):

Before using this medication
» Conditions affecting use, especially:
Sensitivity to loxapine or amoxapine
Pregnancy—Studies in rats showed an increased number of fetal resorptions and decreased fetal weight
Use in elderly—Elderly patients are more likely to develop extrapyramidal, anticholinergic, hypotensive, and sedative effects; reduced dosage recommended
Dental—Loxapine-induced blood dyscrasias may result in infections, delayed healing, and bleeding; dry mouth may cause caries and candidiasis; increased motor activity of face, head, and neck may interfere with some dental procedures
Other medications, especially alcohol, other CNS depression–producing medications, other extrapyramidal reaction–producing medications, guanadrel, or guanethidine
Other medical problems, especially severe CNS depression, active alcoholism, or hepatic function impairment

Proper use of this medication
Taking with food, milk, or water to reduce stomach irritation
Measuring oral solution only with dropper provided by manufacturer
Mixing oral solution with orange or grapefruit juice just before each dose
» Compliance with therapy; not taking more or less medicine, nor taking more often, than directed
» Proper dosing
Missed dose: Taking as soon as possible; not taking if within 1 hour of next dose; return to regular dosing schedule; not doubling doses
» Proper storage

Precautions while using this medication
Regular visits to physician to check progress of therapy
» Checking with physician before discontinuing medication; gradual dosage reduction may be needed
» Avoiding use of alcoholic beverages or other CNS depressants during therapy
Avoiding use with antacids or antidiarrheal medication within 2 hours of taking loxapine
» Possible drowsiness; caution when driving, using machines, or doing other things requiring alertness while taking loxapine
Possible dizziness or lightheadedness; caution when getting up suddenly from a lying or sitting position
Possible skin photosensitivity; avoiding unprotected exposure to sun; using protective clothing; using a sun block product that includes protection against both UVA-caused photosensitivity reactions and UVB-caused sunburn reactions; avoiding use of sunlamp, tanning bed, or tanning booth
Possible dryness of the mouth: using sugarless gum or candy, ice, or saliva substitute for relief; checking with physician or dentist if dry mouth continues for more than 2 weeks

» Caution if any kind of surgery, dental treatment, or emergency
  treatment is required

Side/adverse effects

Side effects are more likely to occur in the elderly

Signs of potential side effects, especially tardive dyskinesia, akathisia, dystonias, parkinsonian effects, anticholinergic effects, allergic skin reactions, agranulocytosis, obstructive jaundice, neuroleptic malignant syndrome (NMS), constipation (severe)

» Stopping medication and notifying physician immediately if symptoms of NMS appear, especially muscle rigidity, fever, difficult
  or fast breathing, seizures, fast heartbeat, increased sweating,
  loss of bladder control, unusually pale skin, unusual tiredness or
  weakness

» Notifying physician immediately if early symptoms of tardive dyskinesia appear, such as fine worm-like movements of the tongue
  or other uncontrolled movements of the mouth, tongue, jaw, or
  arms and legs; dosage adjustment or discontinuation may be
  needed to prevent irreversibility

Possibility of withdrawal symptoms

▲ For the Patient ▲

914254

ABOUT YOUR MEDICINE

Loxapine (LOX-a-peen) is used to treat nervous, mental, and
emotional conditions.

If any of the information in this leaflet causes you special
concern or if you want additional information about your
medicine and its use, check with your doctor, nurse, or pharmacist. **Remember, keep this and all other medicines out of
the reach of children and never share your medicines with
others.**

BEFORE USING THIS MEDICINE

**Discuss with your doctor possible side effects of this medi-
cine.** Some may be serious and/or permanent. For example,
tardive dyskinesia (a movement disorder) may occur and
may not go away after you stop using the medicine.

Tell your doctor, nurse, and pharmacist if you . . .
  • are allergic to any medicine, either prescription or non-
    prescription (OTC);
  • are pregnant or intend to become pregnant while using
    this medicine;
  • are breast-feeding;
  • are taking **any** other prescription or nonprescription
    (OTC) medicine;
  • have any other medical problems, especially alcoholism
    or liver disease.

PROPER USE OF THIS MEDICINE

This medicine may be taken with food or a full glass
(8 ounces) of water or milk to reduce stomach irritation.
The liquid medicine must be mixed with orange juice or

grapefruit juice just before you take it to make it easier to take.

Do not take more of this medicine, do not take it more often, and do not take it for a longer time than your doctor ordered.

If you miss a dose of this medicine, take it as soon as possible. However, if it is within one hour of your next dose, skip the missed dose and go back to your regular dosing schedule. Do not double doses.

PRECAUTIONS WHILE USING THIS MEDICINE

Your doctor should check your progress at regular visits, especially during the first few months of treatment with this medicine.

This medicine will add to the effects of alcohol and other CNS depressants (medicines that slow down the nervous system). **Check with your doctor before taking any such depressants while you are taking this medicine.**

This medicine may cause some people to become drowsy or less alert than they are normally. Even if you take this medicine at bedtime, you may feel drowsy or less alert on arising. **Make sure you know how you react before you drive, use machines, or do other jobs that require you to be alert.**

Do not stop taking this medicine without first checking with your doctor. Your doctor may want you to reduce gradually the amount you are taking before stopping completely.

POSSIBLE SIDE EFFECTS OF THIS MEDICINE

Side Effects That Should Be Reported To Your Doctor Immediately

Stop taking loxapine and get emergency help immediately if any of the following side effects occur:

> *Rare*—Convulsions (seizures); difficult or fast breathing; fast or irregular heartbeat; fever (high); high or low blood pressure; increased sweating; loss of bladder control; muscle stiffness (severe); unusual tiredness or weakness; unusually pale skin

Check with your doctor immediately if any of the following side effects occur:

> *More common*—Lip smacking or puckering; puffing of cheeks; rapid or fine, worm-like movements of tongue; uncontrolled chewing movements; uncontrolled movements of arms or legs

Other Side Effects That Should Be Reported To Your Doctor

> *More common (with increase in dose)*—Difficulty in speaking or swallowing; loss of balance control; mask-like face; restlessness or desire to keep moving; shuffling walk; slowed movements; stiffness of arms and legs; trembling and shaking of hands

Less common—Constipation (severe); difficult urination; inability to move eyes; muscle spasms, especially of the neck and back; skin rash; twisting movements of the body

Rare—Increased blinking or spasms of eyelid; sore throat and fever; uncontrolled twisting movements of neck, trunk, arms, or legs; unusual bleeding or bruising; unusual face expressions or body positions; yellow eyes or skin

Side Effects That Usually Do Not Require Medical Attention

These possible side effects may go away during treatment; however, if they continue or are bothersome, check with your doctor, nurse, or pharmacist.

More common—Blurred vision; confusion; dizziness, lightheadedness, or fainting; drowsiness; dry mouth

Other side effects not listed above may also occur in some patients. If you notice any other effects, check with your doctor, nurse, or pharmacist.

After you stop taking this medicine, check with your doctor if any unusual effects occur, especially dizziness, nausea and vomiting, rapid or worm-like movements of the tongue, stomach upset or pain, trembling of fingers and hands, or uncontrolled chewing movements.

MAPROTILINE Systemic

■ For the Pharmacist ■

In providing consultation, consider emphasizing the following selected information (» = major clinical significance):

Before using this medication
» Conditions affecting use, especially:
  Sensitivity to maprotiline or tricyclic antidepressants
  Use in the elderly—Elderly patients may be more prone to develop anticholinergic, sedative, and hypotensive effects
  Dental—Dry mouth may cause caries, oral candidiasis, periodontal disease, and discomfort; rare blood dyscrasias may result in increased incidence of microbial infection, delayed healing, and gingival bleeding
  Other medications, especially alcohol or other CNS depression–producing medications, MAO inhibitors, or sympathomimetics
  Other medical problems, especially active alcoholism, asthma, bipolar disorder, blood disorders, cardiovascular disorders, glaucoma, hepatic function impairment, hyperthyroidism, increased intraocular pressure, schizophrenia, seizure disorders, or urinary retention

Proper use of this medication
» Compliance with therapy
» May require up to 2 to 3 weeks of therapy to obtain optimal antidepressant effects
» Proper dosing
  Missed dose: If dosing schedule is:
    More than one dose a day—Taking as soon as possible; if almost time for next dose, skipping missed dose; going back to regular dosing schedule; not doubling doses
    One dose a day at bedtime—Not taking missed dose following morning; checking with doctor
» Proper storage

Precautions while using this medication
  Regular visits to physician to check progress during therapy
» Avoiding the use of alcohol or other CNS depressants during maprotiline therapy
» Possible drowsiness; caution when driving, using machines, or doing other things requiring alertness
» Possible dizziness or lightheadedness; caution when getting up suddenly from a lying or sitting position
» Possible dryness of mouth; using sugarless gum or candy, ice, or saliva substitute for relief; checking with physician or dentist if dry mouth continues for more than 2 weeks
» Caution if any kind of surgery, dental treatment, or emergency treatment is required
» Checking with physician before discontinuing medication; gradual dosage reduction may be needed

Side/adverse effects
  Anticholinergic, sedative, and hypotensive effects more likely to occur in the elderly
  Precautions followed for 3 to 7 days after discontinuing medication
  Signs of potential side effects, especially skin rash, redness, swelling, or itching; severe constipation; convulsions; nausea or vomiting;

shakiness or trembling; unusual excitement; weight loss; agranulocytosis; anticholinergic effect; breast enlargement; confusion; hallucinations; hypotension; inappropriate secretion of milk; irregular heartbeat; jaundice; or swelling of testicles

---

▲ For the Patient ▲

914287

ABOUT YOUR MEDICINE

Maprotiline (ma-PROE-ti-leen) is used to relieve mental depression, including anxiety that sometimes occurs with depression.

If any of the information in this leaflet causes you special concern or if you want additional information about your medicine and its use, check with your doctor, nurse, or pharmacist. **Remember, keep this and all other medicines out of the reach of children and never share your medicines with others.**

BEFORE USING THIS MEDICINE

Tell your doctor, nurse, and pharmacist if you . . .
- are allergic to any medicine, either prescription or nonprescription (OTC);
- are pregnant or intend to become pregnant while using this medicine;
- are breast-feeding;
- compete in athletics;
- are taking **any** other prescription or nonprescription (OTC) medicine;
- have **any** other medical problems.

PROPER USE OF THIS MEDICINE

Take this medicine only as directed by your doctor in order to improve your condition as much as possible. **Sometimes this medicine must be taken for up to 2 or 3 weeks before you begin to feel better.**

If you miss a dose of this medicine and your dosing schedule is:
- More than one dose a day—Take the missed dose as soon as possible. Then go back to your regular dosing schedule. However, if it is almost time for your next dose, skip the missed dose and go back to your regular dosing schedule. Do not double doses.
- One dose a day at bedtime—Do not take the missed dose in the morning since it may cause disturbing side effects during waking hours. Instead, check with your doctor.

PRECAUTIONS WHILE USING THIS MEDICINE

It is very important that your doctor check your progress at regular visits. This will allow your dosage to be changed if necessary.

Do not stop taking this medicine without first checking with your doctor. Your doctor may want you to reduce gradually the amount you are taking before stopping completely. This will allow your body to adjust properly and reduce the possibility of unwanted effects.

Before having any kind of surgery or dental or emergency treatment, tell the physician or dentist in charge that you are using this medicine.

This medicine will add to the effects of alcohol and other CNS depressants (medicines that slow down the nervous system). **Check with your doctor before taking any such depressants while you are using this medicine.**

This medicine may cause blurred vision, especially during the first few weeks of treatment. It may also cause some people to become drowsy or less alert than they are normally. **Make sure you know how you react to this medicine before you drive, use machines, or do other jobs that require you to be alert or able to see well.**

Dizziness, lightheadedness, or fainting may occur, especially when you get up from a lying or sitting position. Getting up slowly may help. If this problem continues or gets worse, check with your doctor.

POSSIBLE SIDE EFFECTS OF THIS MEDICINE
Side Effects That Should Be Reported To Your Doctor

> *More common*—Skin rash, redness, swelling, or itching
>
> *Less common*—Constipation (severe); convulsions (seizures); nausea or vomiting; shakiness or trembling; unusual excitement
>
> *Rare*—Breast enlargement (in males and females); confusion (especially in the elderly); difficulty in urinating; fainting; hallucinations; inappropriate secretion of milk (in females); irregular heartbeat (pounding, racing, skipping); sore throat and fever; swelling of testicles; yellow eyes or skin

Side Effects That Usually Do Not Require Medical Attention

These possible side effects may go away during treatment; however, if they continue or are bothersome, check with your doctor, nurse, or pharmacist.

> *More common*—Blurred vision; decreased sexual ability; dizziness or lightheadedness (especially in the elderly); drowsiness; dryness of mouth; headache; increased or decreased sexual drive; tiredness or weakness

Other side effects not listed above may also occur in some patients. If you notice any other effects, check with your doctor, nurse, or pharmacist.

After you stop taking this medicine, your body will need time to adjust. This usually takes about 3 to 7 days. Continue to follow the precautions listed above during this time.

MECLIZINE   Systemic

■ For the Pharmacist ■

In providing consultation, consider emphasizing the following selected information (» = major clinical significance):

Before using this medication
» Conditions affecting use, especially:
  Sensitivity to meclizine
  Pregnancy—No adverse effects in human studies; animal studies have shown meclizine to cause cleft palate at doses above therapeutic range
  Breast-feeding—May be distributed into breast milk; may inhibit lactation due to anticholinergic effects
  Use in children—Possible increased susceptibility to anticholinergic side effects
  Use in the elderly—Possible increased susceptibility to anticholinergic side effects
  Other medications, especially other CNS depressants

Proper use of this medication
  Taking with food, water, or milk to minimize gastric irritation
  Not taking more medication than the amount recommended
  For motion sickness, taking at least 1 hour before traveling
» Proper dosing
  Missed dose (if on a regular dosing regimen): Taking as soon as possible; not taking if almost time for next dose; not doubling doses
» Proper storage

Precautions while using this medication
  Possible interference with skin tests using allergens; need to inform physician of using this medication
» Avoiding use of alcohol or other CNS depressants
» Caution if drowsiness occurs
  Possible dryness of mouth; using sugarless candy or gum or ice, or saliva substitute for relief

▲ For the Patient ▲

912394

MECLIZINE/BUCLIZINE/CYCLIZINE (Oral):
Including Meclizine; Buclizine; Cyclizine.

ABOUT YOUR MEDICINE

Meclizine (MEK-li-zeen), **buclizine** (BYOO-kli-zeen), and **cyclizine** (SYE-kli-zeen) are used to prevent and treat nausea, vomiting, and dizziness associated with motion sickness, and dizziness caused by other medical problems.

If any of the information in this leaflet causes you special concern or if you want additional information about your medicine and its use, check with your doctor, nurse, or pharmacist. **Remember, keep this and all other medicines out of the reach of children and never share your medicines with others.**

BEFORE USING THIS MEDICINE

If you are taking this medicine without a prescription, carefully read and follow any precautions on the label. You should be especially careful if you . . .

- are allergic to any medicine, either prescription or nonprescription (OTC);
- are pregnant, intend to become pregnant, or are breastfeeding;
- are taking any other prescription or nonprescription (OTC) medicine, especially other CNS depressants;
- have any other medical problems.

If you have any questions, check with your doctor, nurse, or pharmacist.

PROPER USE OF THIS MEDICINE

This medicine is used to relieve or prevent the symptoms of motion sickness or dizziness caused by other medical problems. Take it only as directed. Do not take more of it or take it more often than stated on the label or ordered by your doctor. To do so may increase the chance of side effects.

For patients taking this medicine for motion sickness:

—take buclizine or cyclizine at least 30 minutes before you begin to travel.
—take meclizine at least 1 hour before you begin to travel.

Take this medicine with food or a glass of water or milk to lessen stomach irritation, if necessary.

If you must take this medicine regularly and you miss a dose, take the missed dose as soon as possible. However, if it is almost time for your next dose, skip the missed dose and go back to your regular dosing schedule. Do not double doses.

PRECAUTIONS WHILE USING THIS MEDICINE

This medicine will add to the effects of alcohol and other CNS depressants (medicines that slow down the nervous system). **Check with your doctor before taking any such depressants while you are taking this medicine.**

This medicine may cause some people to become drowsy or less alert than they are normally. **Make sure you know how you react to this medicine before you drive, use machines, or do other jobs that require you to be alert.**

Buclizine, cyclizine, and meclizine may cause dryness of the mouth. For temporary relief use sugarless candy or gum, dissolve bits of ice in your mouth, or use a saliva substitute. However, if your mouth continues to feel dry for more than 2 weeks, check with your physician or dentist. Continuing dryness of the mouth may increase the chance of dental disease, including tooth decay, gum disease, and fungus infections.

POSSIBLE SIDE EFFECTS OF THIS MEDICINE
Side Effects That Usually Do Not Require Medical Attention

These possible side effects may go away during treatment; however, if they continue or are bothersome, check with your doctor, nurse, or pharmacist.

> *More common*—Drowsiness

> *Less common or rare*—Blurred vision; constipation; difficult or painful urination; dizziness; dryness of mouth, nose, and throat; fast heartbeat; headache; loss of appetite; nervousness, restlessness, or trouble in sleeping; skin rash; upset stomach

Other side effects not listed above may also occur in some patients. If you notice any other effects, check with your doctor, nurse, or pharmacist.

MEFLOQUINE   Systemic

■For the Pharmacist■

In providing consultation, consider emphasizing the following selected information (» = major clinical significance):

Before using this medication
» Conditions affecting use, especially:
      Allergies to mefloquine, quinidine, quinine, or related medications
      Pregnancy—Not recommended for use during pregnancy; however, the risk of maternal and fetal morbidity and mortality from malaria must be considered for women who are at high risk from falciparum malaria
      Breast-feeding—Distributed into breast milk in low concentrations
      Use in children—Not recommended for use in infants and children up to 2 years of age or less than 15 kg of body weight
      Other medications, especially beta-adrenergic blocking agents, calcium channel blocking agents, chloroquine, divalproex, quinidine, quinine, or valproic acid
      Other medical problems, especially a history of psychiatric disorders or heart block

Proper use of this medication
» Not giving to infants and children up to 2 years of age or less than 15 kg of body weight
   Taking with full glass (240 mL) of water and with food
» Proper storage
For suppression of malaria symptoms
   Starting medication 1 week before entering malarious area to ascertain response and allow time to substitute another medication if reactions occur
» Continuing medication while staying in area and for 4 weeks after leaving area
» Checking with physician immediately if fever or "flu-like" symptoms develop while traveling in, or within several months after departure from, endemic area
» Importance of not missing doses and taking medication on a regular schedule
» Proper dosing
   Missed dose: Taking as soon as possible; not taking if almost time for next dose; not doubling doses
For treatment of malaria
» Compliance with therapy

Precautions while using this medication
» Caution if visual disturbances, dizziness, lightheadedness, or hallucinations occur
   Mosquito-control measures to help prevent malaria:
      Sleeping under mosquito netting
      Wearing long-sleeved shirts or blouses and long trousers to protect arms and legs when mosquitoes are out
      Applying mosquito repellant to uncovered areas of skin when mosquitoes are out
      Using a pyrethrum-containing flying insect spray to kill mosquitoes

» Taking mefloquine at least 12 hours after the last dose of quinidine
or quinine
For treatment of malaria
Checking with physician if no improvement within a few days

Side/adverse effects
Signs of potential side effects, especially bradycardia and neuro-
psychiatric toxicity

▲ For the Patient ▲

917693

ABOUT YOUR MEDICINE

Mefloquine (ME-floe-kwin) is used to prevent or treat malaria.

If any of the information in this leaflet causes you special
concern or if you want additional information about your
medicine and its use, check with your doctor, nurse, or pharmacist. **Remember, keep this and all other medicines out of
the reach of children and never share your medicines with
others.**

BEFORE USING THIS MEDICINE

Tell your doctor, nurse, and pharmacist if you . . .
• are allergic to any medicine, either prescription or nonprescription (OTC);
• are pregnant or intend to become pregnant while using
this medicine;
• are breast-feeding;
• are taking any other prescription or nonprescription
(OTC) medicine, especially bepridil, beta-blockers,
chloroquine, diltiazem, divalproex, nicardipine, nifedipine, quinidine, quinine, valproic acid, or verapamil;
• have any other medical problems, especially heart block,
or a history of psychiatric (mental) disorders.

PROPER USE OF THIS MEDICINE

**Do not give this medicine to infants and children up to 2
years of age or to those weighing less than 15 kg (33 pounds).**

Mefloquine is best taken with a full glass (8 ounces) of water
and with food, unless otherwise directed by your doctor.

For patients taking mefloquine to prevent malaria:
• You should keep taking this medicine while you are in
the area and for 4 weeks after you leave the area. No
medicine will protect you completely from malaria.
However, to protect you as completely as possible, **it is
important that you keep taking this medicine for the full
time your doctor ordered.** Also, if fever or "flu-like"
symptoms develop during your travels or within 2 to 3
months after you leave the area, **check with your doctor
immediately.**

- This medicine works best when you take it on a regular schedule. **Do not miss any doses.** If you have any questions about this, check with your doctor, nurse, or pharmacist.
- **If you do miss a dose of this medicine,** take it as soon as possible. However, if it is almost time for your next dose, skip the missed dose and go back to your regular dosing schedule. Do not double doses.

For patients taking mefloquine to treat malaria:
- To help clear up your infection completely, **take this medicine exactly as directed by your doctor.**

PRECAUTIONS WHILE USING THIS MEDICINE

Mefloquine may cause vision problems. It may also cause some people to become dizzy or lightheaded or to have hallucinations. **Make sure you know how you react to this medicine before you drive, use machines, or do other jobs that require you to be alert.**

Malaria is spread by the bite of certain kinds of infected female mosquitoes. If you are living in, or will be traveling to, an area where there is a chance of getting malaria, the following mosquito-control measures will help to prevent infection:
- If possible, sleep under mosquito netting to avoid being bitten by malaria-carrying mosquitoes.
- Wear long-sleeved shirts or blouses and long trousers to protect your arms and legs, especially from dusk through dawn when mosquitoes are out.
- Apply mosquito repellant, preferably one containing DEET, to uncovered areas of the skin from dusk through dawn when mosquitoes are out.
- Use a pyrethrum-containing flying insect spray to kill mosquitoes in living and sleeping quarters during evening and nighttime hours.

If you are taking quinidine or quinine talk to your doctor before you take mefloquine. Mefloquine should be taken at least 12 hours after the last dose of quinidine or quinine.

For patients taking mefloquine to treat malaria:
- If your symptoms do not improve within a few days, or if they become worse, check with your doctor.

POSSIBLE SIDE EFFECTS OF THIS MEDICINE

Side Effects That Should Be Reported To Your Doctor Immediately

> *Rare*—Anxiety; confusion; convulsions; hallucinations; mental depression; mood or mental changes; restlessness; slow heartbeat

Side Effects That Usually Do Not Require Medical Attention

These possible side effects may go away during treatment; however, if they continue or are bothersome, check with your doctor, nurse, or pharmacist.

More common—Abdominal or stomach pain; diarrhea; difficulty concentrating; dizziness; headache; light-headedness; loss of appetite; nausea or vomiting; trouble in sleeping; visual changes

Other side effects not listed above may also occur in some patients. If you notice any other effects, check with your doctor, nurse, or pharmacist.

MEPROBAMATE   Systemic

■ For the Pharmacist ■

In providing consultation, consider emphasizing the following selected information (» = major clinical significance):

Before using this medication
» Conditions affecting use, especially:
> Sensitivity to meprobamate or other carbamate derivatives, such as carbromal, carisoprodol, mebutamate, or tybamate
>
> Pregnancy—Meprobamate crosses placenta; risk of congenital malformations may be increased when medication used during first trimester of pregnancy
>
> Breast-feeding—Excreted in breast milk in concentration of 2 to 4 times maternal plasma concentrations; use by nursing mothers may cause sedation in infant
>
> Use in the elderly—Elderly patients may be more sensitive to effects of meprobamate; lowest effective dose should be administered to avoid oversedation
>
> Dental—Prolonged use of meprobamate may decrease or inhibit salivary flow, which may contribute to development of caries, periodontal disease, oral candidiasis, and discomfort
>
> Other medications, especially alcohol or other CNS depression–producing medications
>
> Other medical problems, especially alcohol or drug abuse or dependence, or acute intermittent porphyria

Proper use of this medication
» Importance of not using more medication than the amount prescribed because of habit-forming potential
» Proper dosing
> Missed dose: Taking right away if remembered within an hour or so; not taking if remembered later; not doubling doses
» Proper storage

Precautions while using this medication
> Regular visits to physician to check progress during prolonged therapy
>
> Checking with physician before discontinuing medication after prolonged use; gradual dosage reduction may be necessary to avoid possibility of withdrawal symptoms
» Avoiding use of alcohol or other CNS depressants
> Caution if any laboratory tests required; possible interference with results of metyrapone or phentolamine tests
» Suspected overdose: Getting emergency help at once
» Caution if dizziness, lightheadedness, or drowsiness occurs
> Possible dryness of mouth; using sugarless gum or candy, ice, or saliva substitute for relief; checking with dentist if dry mouth continues for more than 2 weeks

Side/adverse effects
> Signs of potential side effects, especially allergic reaction; fast, pounding, or irregular heatbeat; intolerance to meprobamate; leukopenia; paradoxical reaction; and thrombocytopenia

▲ For the Patient ▲

914301

ABOUT YOUR MEDICINE

Meprobamate (me-proe-BA-mate) is used to relieve nervousness or tension. However, it should not be used for nervousness or tension caused by the stress of everyday life.

If any of the information in this leaflet causes you special concern or if you want additional information about your medicine and its use, check with your doctor, nurse, or pharmacist. **Remember, keep this and all other medicines out of the reach of children and never share your medicines with others.**

BEFORE USING THIS MEDICINE

Tell your doctor, nurse, and pharmacist if you . . .
* are allergic to any medicine, either prescription or nonprescription (OTC);
* are pregnant or intend to become pregnant while using this medicine;
* are breast-feeding;
* are taking any other prescription or nonprescription (OTC) medicine, especially CNS depressants;
* have any other medical problems, especially porphyria, or a history of drug abuse or dependence.

PROPER USE OF THIS MEDICINE

Take this medicine only as directed by your doctor. Do not take more of it, do not take it more often, and do not take it for a longer time than your doctor ordered. If too much is taken, it may become habit-forming.

If you miss a dose of this medicine, and remember within an hour or so of the missed dose, take it right away. But if you do not remember until later, skip the missed dose and go back to your regular dosing schedule. Do not double doses.

PRECAUTIONS WHILE USING THIS MEDICINE

If you will be taking this medicine regularly for a long time:
* Your doctor should check your progress at regular visits.
* Check with your doctor at least every 4 months to make sure you need to continue taking this medicine.

If you will be taking this medicine in large doses or for a long time, do not stop taking it without first checking with your doctor. Your doctor may want you to reduce gradually the amount you are taking before stopping completely.

This medicine will add to the effects of alcohol and other CNS depressants (medicines that slow down the nervous system, possibly causing drowsiness). **Check with your doctor before taking any such depressants while you are taking this medicine.**

If you think you or someone else may have taken an overdose, get emergency help at once. Taking an overdose of meprobamate or taking alcohol or other CNS depressants with meprobamate may lead to unconsciousness and possibly death. Some signs of an overdose are severe confusion, drowsiness, or weakness; shortness of breath or slow or troubled breathing; slurred speech; staggering; and slow heartbeat.

This medicine may cause some people to become dizzy, lightheaded, drowsy, or less alert than they are normally. Even if taken at bedtime, it may cause some people to feel drowsy or less alert on arising. **Make sure you know how you react to this medicine before you drive, use machines, or do other jobs that require you to be alert.**

POSSIBLE SIDE EFFECTS OF THIS MEDICINE
Side Effects That Should Be Reported To Your Doctor

   Less common—Skin rash, hives, or itching

   Rare—Confusion; fast, pounding, or irregular heartbeat; sore throat and fever; unusual bleeding or bruising; unusual excitement; wheezing, shortness of breath, or troubled breathing

Side Effects That Usually Do Not Require Medical Attention

These possible side effects may go away during treatment; however, if they continue or are bothersome, check with your doctor, nurse, or pharmacist.

   More common—Clumsiness or unsteadiness; drowsiness

Other side effects not listed above may also occur in some patients. If you notice any other effects, check with your doctor, nurse, or pharmacist.

After you stop using this medicine, your body may need time to adjust. If you took this medicine in high doses or for a long time, this may take about 2 days. During this time check with your doctor if you notice any unusual effects, especially clumsiness or unsteadiness; confusion; convulsions (seizures); hallucinations; increased dreaming; muscle twitching; nausea or vomiting; nervousness or restlessness; nightmares; trembling; trouble in sleeping.

METHENAMINE   Systemic

∎ For the Pharmacist ∎

In providing consultation, consider emphasizing the following selected information (» = major clinical significance):

Before using this medication
»   Conditions affecting use, especially:
    Hypersensitivity to methenamine
    Pregnancy—Methenamine crosses the placenta
    Breast-feeding—Methenamine is excreted in breast milk
    Other medications, especially urinary alkalinizers or thiazide
      diuretics
    Other medical problems, especially severe hepatic function impairment or severe renal function impairment

Proper use of this medication
»   Using phenaphthazine paper or other test and dietary measures to measure and appropriately adjust urine pH; importance of maintaining acidic urine (pH 5.5 or below)
   Taking after meals and at bedtime if nausea or gastrointestinal irritation occurs
   Proper administration technique for dry granules, oral liquids, and enteric-coated tablets
»   Compliance with full course of therapy
»   Proper dosing
   Missed dose: Taking as soon as possible; not taking if almost time for next dose; not doubling doses
»   Proper storage

Precautions while using this medication
   Checking with physician if no improvement within a few days

Side/adverse effects
   Signs of potential side effects, especially crystalluria, hematuria, and skin rash

▲ For the Patient ▲

914323

ABOUT YOUR MEDICINE

Methenamine (meth-EN-a-meen) belongs to the family of medicines called anti-infectives. It is used to help prevent and treat infections of the urinary tract.

If any of the information in this leaflet causes you special concern or if you want additional information about your medicine and its use, check with your doctor, nurse, or pharmacist. **Remember, keep this and all other medicines out of the reach of children and never share your medicines with others.**

BEFORE USING THIS MEDICINE

Tell your doctor, nurse, and pharmacist if you . . .
   • are allergic to any medicine, either prescription or nonprescription (OTC);

- are pregnant or intend to become pregnant while using this medicine;
- are breast-feeding;
- are taking any other prescription or nonprescription (OTC) medicine, especially thiazide diuretics (water pills) or urinary alkalizers (medicine that makes the urine less acid, such as acetazolamide, calcium- and/or magnesium-containing antacids, dichlorphenamide, methazolamide, potassium or sodium citrate and/or citric acid, or sodium bicarbonate [baking soda]);
- have any other medical problems, especially severe kidney or liver disease.

PROPER USE OF THIS MEDICINE

Before you start taking this medicine, check your urine with phenaphthazine paper or another test to see if it is acidic. **Your urine must be acidic (pH 5.5 or below) for this medicine to work properly.** If you have any questions about this, check with your doctor, nurse, or pharmacist.

The following changes in your diet may help make your urine more acid; however, check with your doctor first if you are on a special diet (for example, for diabetes). Avoid most fruits (especially citrus fruits and juices), milk and other dairy products, and other foods that make the urine less acid. Also, avoid antacids unless otherwise directed by your doctor. Eating more protein and foods such as cranberries (especially cranberry juice with vitamin C added), plums, or prunes may also help. If your urine is still not acid enough, check with your doctor.

If this medicine causes nausea or upset stomach, it may be taken after meals and at bedtime.

If you are taking the dry granule form of this medicine, dissolve the contents of each packet in 2 to 4 ounces of cold water immediately before taking. Stir well. Be sure to drink all the liquid to get the full dose of medicine.

If you are taking the oral liquid form of this medicine, use a specially marked measuring spoon or other device to measure each dose accurately. The average household teaspoon may not hold the right amount of liquid.

If you are taking the enteric-coated tablet form of this medicine, swallow the tablets whole. Do not break, crush, or take if chipped.

To help clear up your infection completely, **keep taking this medicine for the full time of treatment** even if you begin to feel better after a few days; **do not miss any doses.**

If you do miss a dose of this medicine, take it as soon as possible. However, if it is almost time for your next dose, skip the missed dose and go back to your regular dosing schedule. Do not double doses.

PRECAUTIONS WHILE USING THIS MEDICINE

If the symptoms of your infection do not improve within a few days, or if they become worse, check with your doctor.

This medicine must not be given to other people or used for other infections unless you are otherwise directed by your doctor.

POSSIBLE SIDE EFFECTS OF THIS MEDICINE

Side Effects That Should Be Reported To Your Doctor Immediately

    Less common—Skin rash

    Rare—Blood in urine; lower back pain; pain or burning while urinating

Side Effects That Usually Do Not Require Medical Attention

These possible side effects may go away during treatment; however, if they continue or are bothersome, check with your doctor, nurse, or pharmacist.

    Less common—Nausea and vomiting

Other side effects not listed above may also occur in some patients. If you notice any other effects, check with your doctor, nurse, or pharmacist.

METHOTREXATE—For Cancer   Systemic

■For the Pharmacist■

In providing consultation, consider emphasizing the following selected information (» = major clinical significance):

Before using this medication
» Conditions affecting use, especially:
    Sensitivity to methotrexate
    Pregnancy—Use not recommended because of mutagenic, teratogenic, and carcinogenic potential; advisability of using contraception; telling physician immediately if pregnancy is suspected
    Breast-feeding—Not recommended because of risk of serious side effects
    Pediatrics—Newborns and other infants may be more sensitive to effects
    Geriatrics—Side/adverse effects may be more frequent
    Other medications, especially alcohol or other hepatotoxic medications, probenecid, sulfinpyrazone, nonsteroidal anti-inflammatory drugs (NSAIDs), other bone marrow depressants, salicylates, or previous cytotoxic drug therapy or radiation therapy
    Other medical problems, especially chickenpox, herpes zoster, hepatic function impairment, renal function impairment, infection, oral mucositis, peptic ulcer, or ulcerative colitis

Proper use of this medication
» Importance of not taking more or less medication than the amount prescribed
    Caution in taking combination therapy; taking each medication at the right time
    Importance of ample fluid intake and subsequent increase in urine output to prevent nephrotoxicity and aid in excretion of uric acid
» Frequency of nausea and vomiting; importance of continuing medication despite stomach upset
    Checking with physician if vomiting occurs shortly after dose is taken
» Proper dosing
    Missed dose: Not taking at all; not doubling doses
» Proper storage

Precautions while using this medication
» Importance of close monitoring by physician
» Avoiding alcoholic beverages, which may increase hepatotoxicity
    Possible photosensitivity reactions; avoiding too much unprotected exposure to sun or overuse of sunlamp
» Avoiding salicylate-containing products and NSAIDs, which may increase toxicity
» Avoiding immunizations unless approved by physician; other persons in patient's household should avoid immunizations with oral poliovirus vaccine; avoiding other persons who have taken oral poliovirus vaccine or wearing a protective mask that covers nose and mouth
    Caution if bone marrow depression occurs:
» Avoiding exposure to persons with bacterial infections, especially during periods of low blood counts; checking with physician

immediately if fever or chills, cough or hoarseness, lower
back or side pain, or painful or difficult urination occurs

»   Checking with physician immediately if unusual bleeding or
bruising; black, tarry stools; blood in urine or stools; or pinpoint red spots on skin occur

Caution in use of regular toothbrush, dental floss, or toothpick;
physician, dentist, or nurse may suggest alternatives; checking with physician before having dental work done

Not touching eyes or inside of nose unless hands washed immediately before

Using caution to avoid accidental cuts with use of sharp objects
such as safety razor or fingernail or toenail cutters

Avoiding contact sports or other situations where bruising or
injury could occur

Side/adverse effects

May cause adverse effects such as blood problems; stomach, kidney,
or liver problems; loss of hair; or cancer; importance of discussing
possible effects with physician

Signs of potential side effects, especially gastrointestinal ulceration
and bleeding, enteritis, intestinal perforation, leukopenia, bacterial infection, septicemia, thrombocytopenia, ulcerative stomatitis, gingivitis, pharyngitis, renal failure, azotemia, hyperuricemia, severe nephropathy, severe acute methotrexate toxicity,
cutaneous vasculitis, reactivation of sunburn or reaction to ultraviolet light, hepatotoxicity, pneumonitis, pulmonary fibrosis,
and CNS effects

Physician or nurse can help in dealing with side effects

Possibility of hair loss; should return after treatment has ended

---

▲ For the Patient ▲

916384

ABOUT YOUR MEDICINE

Methotrexate (meth-o-TREX-ate) is used to treat some kinds
of cancer.

If any of the information in this leaflet causes you special
concern or if you want additional information about your
medicine and its use, check with your doctor, nurse, or pharmacist. **Remember, keep this and all other medicines out of
the reach of children and never share your medicines with
others.**

BEFORE USING THIS MEDICINE

Discuss with your doctor the possible side effects that may
be caused by this medicine. Some of them may be serious
and/or long-term.

Tell your doctor, nurse, and pharmacist if you . . .

- are allergic to any medicine, either prescription or nonprescription (OTC);
- are pregnant or intend to have children;
- are breast-feeding an infant;
- are taking **any** other prescription or nonprescription
(OTC) medicine;
- have any other medical problems, especially chickenpox
(including recent exposure), alcoholism, colitis, disease

of the immune system, herpes zoster (shingles), infection, kidney disease, mouth sores or inflammation, or stomach ulcer;
- have ever been treated with x-rays or cancer medicines.

PROPER USE OF THIS MEDICINE

Take this medicine only as directed by your doctor. Do not take more or less, and do not take it more often than ordered.

While you are using methotrexate, your doctor may want you to drink extra fluids so that you will pass more urine.

Methotrexate commonly causes nausea and vomiting. Ask your doctor, nurse, or pharmacist for ways to lessen these effects. If you vomit shortly after taking a dose, check with your doctor.

If you miss a dose of this medicine, do not take the missed dose at all and do not double the next one. Instead, go back to your regular dosing schedule and check with your doctor.

PRECAUTIONS WHILE USING THIS MEDICINE

It is very important that your doctor check your progress at regular visits.

Do not drink alcohol while using this medicine.

When you begin using methotrexate, avoid too much sun and do not use a sunlamp since you may become more sensitive than usual.

Do not take aspirin or other medicine for inflammation or pain without first checking with your doctor.

While you are taking methotrexate, and after you stop treatment, **do not have any immunizations (vaccinations) without your doctor's approval.**

Methotrexate can temporarily lower the number of white blood cells in your blood, increasing the chance of getting an infection. It can also lower the number of platelets, which are necessary for proper blood clotting. If this occurs:
- Avoid people with infections.
- Be careful when using a regular toothbrush, dental floss, or toothpick.
- Do not touch your eyes or the inside of your nose unless you have just washed your hands and have not touched anything else in the meantime.
- Be careful not to cut, bruise, or injure yourself.

POSSIBLE SIDE EFFECTS OF THIS MEDICINE

Side Effects That Should Be Reported To Your Doctor Immediately

> *More common*—Black, tarry stools; bloody vomit; diarrhea; reddening of skin; sores in mouth and on lips; stomach pain

> *Less common*—Blood in urine or stools; blurred vision; confusion; convulsions (seizures); cough or hoarseness;

fever or chills; lower back or side pain; painful or difficult urination; pinpoint red spots on skin; shortness of breath; swelling of feet or lower legs; unusual bleeding or bruising

Other Side Effects That Should Be Reported To Your Doctor

Less common—Back pain; dark urine; dizziness; drowsiness; headache; joint pain; unusual tiredness or weakness; yellow eyes or skin

Side Effects That Usually Do Not Require Medical Attention

These possible side effects may go away during treatment; however, if they continue or are bothersome, check with your doctor, nurse, or pharmacist.

More common—Loss of appetite; nausea or vomiting

This medicine may cause a temporary loss of hair in some people. After treatment with methotrexate has ended, normal hair growth should return.

Other side effects not listed above may also occur in some patients. If you notice any other effects, check with your doctor, nurse, or pharmacist.

After you stop methotrexate, check with your doctor as soon as possible if you notice back pain, blurred vision, confusion, convulsions, dizziness, drowsiness, fever, headache, or unusual tiredness or weakness.

METHOTREXATE—For Noncancerous Conditions Systemic

■ For the Pharmacist ■

In providing consultation, consider emphasizing the following selected information (» = major clinical significance):

Before using this medication
» Conditions affecting use, especially:
> Sensitivity to methotrexate
> Pregnancy—Use not recommended because of teratogenic, abortifacient, and carcinogenic potential; advisability of using contraception; telling physician immediately if pregnancy is suspected
> Breast-feeding—Not recommended because of risk of serious side effects
> Use in children—Newborns and other infants may be more sensitive to effects
> Use in the elderly—Side/adverse effects may be more frequent
> Other medications, especially alcohol or other hepatotoxic medications, nonsteroidal anti-inflammatory drugs (NSAIDs), other bone marrow depressants, probenecid, salicylates, or previous cytotoxic drug therapy or radiation therapy
> Other medical problems, especially hepatic function impairment, renal function impairment, chickenpox, herpes zoster, infection, oral mucositis, peptic ulcer, or ulcerative colitis

Proper use of this medication
» Importance of not taking more or less medication than the amount prescribed
» Frequency of nausea; importance of continuing medication despite stomach upset; checking with physician if vomiting occurs
> Checking with physician if vomiting occurs shortly after dose is taken
» Proper dosing
> Missed dose: Not taking at all; not doubling doses
» Proper storage

Precautions while using this medication
» Importance of close monitoring by the physician
» Avoiding alcoholic beverages, which may increase hepatotoxicity
> Possible photosensitivity reactions; avoiding too much unprotected exposure to sun or overuse of sunlamp
» Avoiding salicylate-containing products and NSAIDs, which may increase toxicity
» Avoiding immunizations unless approved by physician; other persons in patient's household should avoid immunizations with oral poliovirus vaccine; avoiding other persons who have taken oral poliovirus vaccine or wearing a protective mask that covers nose and mouth
> Caution if bone marrow depression occurs:
» Avoiding exposure to persons with bacterial infections, especially during periods of low blood counts; checking with physician immediately if fever or chills, cough or hoarseness, lower back or side pain, or painful or difficult urination occurs
» Checking with physician immediately if unusual bleeding or bruising; black, tarry stools; blood in urine or stools; or pinpoint red spots on skin occur

Caution in use of regular toothbrush, dental floss, or toothpick;
physician, dentist, or nurse may suggest alternatives; checking with physician before having dental work done

Not touching eyes or inside of nose unless hands washed immediately before

Using caution to avoid accidental cuts with use of sharp objects
such as safety razor or fingernail or toenail cutters

Avoiding contact sports or other situations where bruising or
injury could occur

Side/adverse effects

May cause adverse effects such as blood problems; stomach, kidney,
or liver problems; loss of hair; or cancer; importance of discussing
possible effects with physician

Signs of potential side effects, especially gastrointestinal ulceration
and bleeding, enteritis, intestinal perforation, leukopenia, bacterial infection, septicemia, thrombocytopenia, severe acute
methotrexate toxicity, cutaneous vasculitis, reactivation of sunburn or reaction to ultraviolet light, ulcerative stomatitis, gingivitis, pharyngitis, CNS effects, hepatotoxicity, pneumonitis,
and pulmonary fibrosis

Physician or nurse can help in dealing with side effects

Possibility of hair loss; should return after treatment has ended

---

▲ For the Patient ▲

916522

ABOUT YOUR MEDICINE

Methotrexate (meth-o-TREX-ate) is used to treat psoriasis
and rheumatoid arthritis. It may also be used for other conditions as determined by your doctor.

If any of the information in this leaflet causes you special
concern or if you want additional information about your
medicine and its use, check with your doctor, nurse, or pharmacist. **Remember, keep this and all other medicines out of
the reach of children and never share your medicines with
others.**

BEFORE USING THIS MEDICINE

Discuss with your doctor the possible side effects that may
be caused by this medicine. Some of them may be serious
and/or long-term.

Tell your doctor, nurse, and pharmacist if you . . .
- are allergic to any medicine, either prescription or nonprescription (OTC);
- are pregnant or intend to have children;
- are breast-feeding;
- are taking **any** other prescription or nonprescription
(OTC) medicine;
- have any other medical problems, especially chickenpox
(including recent exposure), alcohol abuse (or history
of), colitis, disease of the immune system, herpes zoster
(shingles), infection, kidney disease, liver disease, mouth
sores or inflammation, or stomach ulcer;
- have ever been treated with x-rays or cancer medicines.

PROPER USE OF THIS MEDICINE

Use this medicine only as directed by your doctor. Do not use more or less, and do not use it more often than ordered.

Methotrexate may cause nausea. Even if you begin to feel ill, **do not stop using this medicine without first checking with your doctor.** Ask your doctor, nurse, or pharmacist for ways to lessen this effect.

If you vomit shortly after using a dose, check with your doctor.

If you miss a dose of this medicine, do not use the missed dose at all and do not double the next one. Instead, go back to your regular dosing schedule and check with your doctor.

PRECAUTIONS WHILE USING THIS MEDICINE

It is very important that your doctor check your progress at regular visits.

Do not drink alcohol while using this medicine.

When you first begin using methotrexate, avoid too much sun and do not use a sunlamp since you may become more sensitive than usual. In case of a severe burn, check with your doctor. This is especially important if you are using this medicine for psoriasis because sunlight can make the psoriasis worse.

Do not take aspirin or other medicine for inflammation or pain without first checking with your doctor.

While you are using methotrexate, and for several weeks after you stop treatment, **do not have any immunizations (vaccinations) without your doctor's approval.**

POSSIBLE SIDE EFFECTS OF THIS MEDICINE

Side Effects That Should Be Reported To Your Doctor Immediately

> *Less common*—Diarrhea; reddening of skin; sores in mouth and on lips; stomach pain

> *Rare*—Black, tarry stools; blood in urine or stools; blurred vision; convulsions (seizures); cough or hoarseness; fever or chills; lower back or side pain; painful or difficult urination; pinpoint red spots on skin; shortness of breath; unusual bleeding or bruising

Other Side Effects That Should Be Reported To Your Doctor

> *Rare*—Back pain; dark urine; dizziness; drowsiness; headache; unusual tiredness or weakness; yellow eyes or skin

Side Effects That Usually Do Not Require Medical Attention

These possible side effects may go away during treatment; however, if they continue or are bothersome, check with your doctor, nurse, or pharmacist.

Less common or rare—Acne; boils; loss of appetite; nausea or vomiting; pale skin; skin rash or itching

This medicine may cause a temporary loss of hair in some people. After treatment with methotrexate has ended, normal hair growth should return.

Other side effects not listed above may also occur in some patients. If you notice any other effects, check with your doctor, nurse, or pharmacist.

METHOXSALEN   Systemic

■ For the Pharmacist ■

In providing consultation, consider emphasizing the following selected information (» = major clinical significance):

Before using this medication
» Conditions affecting use, especially:
     Sensitivity to methoxsalen
     Diet—Avoiding eating furocoumarin-containing foods (limes, figs, parsley, parsnips, mustard, carrots, celery)
     Other medical problems, especially acute lupus erythematosus; albinism; aphakia; cataracts; hydroa; leukoderma of infectious origin; porphyria; xeroderma pigmentosum; history of skin cancer; history of having taken arsenicals; history of having received x-rays, cytotoxic therapy, or coal tar and ultraviolet light B (UVB) therapy
     Not using for suntanning purposes

Proper use of this medication
     Usually comes with patient instructions; reading carefully before using medication
» May take 6 to 8 weeks to work; importance of not increasing the dosage of medication or exposure to ultraviolet light because of the risk of serious burns
     The hard capsule dosage form may be taken with food or milk (the soft capsule dosage form may be taken with low fat food or low fat milk) to reduce gastrointestinal irritation
» Proper dosing
     Late or missed dose: Notifying physician for rescheduling of light treatment
» Proper storage

Precautions while using this medication
     Importance of regular visits to physician to have progress checked, including eye examinations
» Protecting skin from sunlight, even through window glass or on cloudy days, for at least 24 hours before and 8 hours following treatment; protecting lips with sun block lipstick that has a skin protection factor (SPF) of at least 15
     Possibility of continued skin sensitivity to sunlight because of medication; using extra precautions for at least 48 hours following each treatment; not sunbathing anytime during course of treatment
» Wearing special sunglasses during daylight hours (even in indirect light, such as through window glass or on cloudy days) for 24 hours following each dose of medication
» Possibility of dry skin or itching; checking with physician before treating
» Possible long-term effects (cataracts, premature skin aging, carcinogenesis)

Side/adverse effects
     Slight reddening of skin 24 to 48 hours after treatment is normal response to therapy
     There is an increased risk of developing skin cancer. The body should be examined regularly and the physician shown skin sores that do not heal, new skin growths, and skin growths that have changed in appearance or feel

Premature aging of the skin may occur as a result of prolonged
PUVA therapy. This effect is permanent and is similar to the
results of excessive exposure to sunlight
Signs of potential side effects, especially blistering and peeling of
skin; reddened, sore skin; swelling, especially in feet or lower
legs
Note: Some side effects are more likely to occur in children.

▲ For the Patient ▲

917649

ABOUT YOUR MEDICINE

Methoxsalen (meth-OX-a-len) belongs to the group of medicines called psoralens. It is used with ultraviolet light (found
in sunlight and some special lamps) in a treatment called
PUVA to treat vitiligo, a disease in which skin color is lost,
and psoriasis, a skin condition associated with red, scaly
patches. Methoxsalen may also be used for other conditions
as determined by your doctor.

If any of the information in this leaflet causes you special
concern or if you want additional information about your
medicine and its use, check with your doctor, nurse, or pharmacist. **Remember, keep this and all other medicines out of
the reach of children and never share your medicines with
others.**

BEFORE USING THIS MEDICINE

Tell your doctor, nurse, and pharmacist if you . . .
- are allergic to any medicine, either prescription or nonprescription (OTC);
- are pregnant or intend to become pregnant while using
this medicine;
- are breast-feeding;
- are taking any other prescription or nonprescription
(OTC) medicine;
- have any other medical problems, especially cataracts
or loss of the lens of the eye, lupus erythematosus, porphyria, skin cancer (history of), or other skin conditions;
- have recently been treated with x-rays or cancer medicines.

PROPER USE OF THIS MEDICINE

Methoxsalen usually comes with patient directions. Read
them carefully.

This medicine may take 6 to 8 weeks to really help your
condition. **Do not increase the amount of methoxsalen you
are taking or spend extra time in the sunlight or under an
ultraviolet lamp.** This will not make the medicine act any
more quickly and may result in a serious burn.

**If you are late in taking, or miss taking, a dose of this med-
icine,** notify your doctor so your light treatment can be re-
scheduled. Remember that exposure to sunlight or ultraviolet light must take place a certain number of hours **after**

you take the medicine or it will not work. If taking the hard gelatin capsules, this is 2 to 4 hours. If taking the soft gelatin capsules, this is 1 and 1/2 to 2 hours.

PRECAUTIONS WHILE USING THIS MEDICINE

Your doctor should check your progress at regular visits to make sure this medicine is working and that it does not cause unwanted effects. Eye examinations should be included.

This medicine increases the sensitivity of your skin and lips to sunlight. Therefore, **exposure to the sun, even through window glass or on a cloudy day, could cause a serious burn**. If you must go out during the daylight hours:

- **Before each treatment, cover all your skin for at least 24 hours** by wearing protective clothing and a wide-brimmed hat. In addition, **protect your lips with a special sun block lipstick that has a protection factor of at least 15**. Check with your doctor before using sun block products on other parts of your body before a treatment.
- **After each treatment, cover your skin for at least 8 hours** by wearing protective clothing. In addition, use a sun block product that has a protection factor of at least 15 on your lips and on those areas of your body that are not covered.

For 24 hours after you take each dose of methoxsalen, your eyes should be protected during daylight hours with special wraparound sunglasses that totally block or absorb ultraviolet light (ordinary sunglasses are not adequate). This is to prevent cataracts. These glasses should be worn even in indirect light, such as light coming through window glass or on a cloudy day.

This medicine may cause your skin to become dry or itchy. **However, check with your doctor before applying anything to your skin.**

POSSIBLE SIDE EFFECTS OF THIS MEDICINE

Side Effects That Should Be Reported To Your Doctor Immediately

Blistering and peeling of skin; reddened, sore skin; swelling (especially of feet or lower legs)

Side Effects That Usually Do Not Require Medical Attention

These possible side effects may go away during treatment; however, if they continue or are bothersome, check with your doctor, nurse, or pharmacist.

More common—Itching of skin; nausea

Less common—Dizziness; headache; leg cramps; mental depression; nervousness; skin rash; trouble in sleeping

Treatment with this medicine usually causes a slight reddening of your skin 24 to 48 hours after the treatment. This is an expected effect. However, check with your doctor right away if your skin becomes sore and red or blistered.

There is an increased risk of skin cancer after use of methoxsalen. Check your body regularly and show your doctor any skin sores that do not heal, new skin growths, and skin growths that have changed in the way they look or feel.

Premature aging of the skin may occur as a result of prolonged methoxsalen therapy. This effect is permanent.

Other side effects not listed above may also occur in some patients. If you notice any other effects, check with your doctor, nurse, or pharmacist.

METHOXSALEN Topical

■For the Pharmacist■

In providing consultation, consider emphasizing the following selected information (**»** = major clinical significance):

Before using this medication
» Conditions affecting use, especially:
    Sensitivity to methoxsalen
    Carcinogenicity—Possibility of increased risk of squamous cell carcinoma, especially in patients with predisposing risk factors such as fair skin and those with increased sensitivity to sunlight
    Diet—Avoiding eating furocoumarin-containing foods (limes, figs, parsley, parsnips, mustard, carrots, celery)
    Use in children—Not recommended for use in children up to 12 years of age
    Other medical problems, especially acute lupus erythematosus; albinism; hydroa; leukoderma of infectious origin; polymorphic light eruptions; porphyria; xeroderma pigmentosum; history of skin cancer; history of having taken arsenicals; history of having received x-rays, cytotoxic therapy, or coal tar and ultraviolet light B (UVB) therapy

Proper use of this medication
    Using medication only under the direct supervision of the physician
» Proper dosing

Precautions while using this medication
    Importance of regular visits to physician for treatments and to have progress checked
» Protecting skin from sunlight, even through window glass or on a cloudy day, for at least 12 to 48 hours following treatment; washing treated areas after light treatment
    Possibility of continued skin sensitivity to sunlight because of medication; using extra precautions for at least 72 hours following each treatment; not sunbathing anytime during course of treatment
» Possibility of dry skin or itching; checking with physician before treating

Side/adverse effects
    There is an increased risk of developing skin cancer when treated with systemic methoxsalen. The possibility of increased risk may exist also with topical methoxsalen. The treated areas should be examined regularly and the physician shown skin sores that do not heal, new skin growths, and skin growths that have changed in appearance or feel.
    Premature aging of the skin may occur as a result of prolonged treatment with systemic methoxsalen. The possibility of risk may exist also with topical methoxsalen. This effect is permanent and is similar to the results of excessive exposure to sunlight.
    Signs of potential side effects, especially symptoms of overdose or overexposure to ultraviolet light

---

▲ For the Patient ▲

917650

ABOUT YOUR MEDICINE

Methoxsalen (meth-OX-a-len) belongs to the group of medicines called psoralens. It is used with ultraviolet light (found in sunlight and some special lamps) in a treatment called psoralen plus ultraviolet light A (PUVA) to treat vitiligo, a disease in which skin color is lost. Methoxsalen may also be used for other conditions as determined by your doctor.

If any of the information in this leaflet causes you special concern or if you want additional information about your medicine and its use, check with your doctor, nurse, or pharmacist. **Remember, keep this and all other medicines out of the reach of children and never share your medicines with others.**

BEFORE USING THIS MEDICINE

Tell your doctor, nurse, and pharmacist if you . . .
- are allergic to any medicine, either prescription or nonprescription (OTC);
- are pregnant or intend to become pregnant while using this medicine;
- are breast-feeding;
- are taking any other prescription or nonprescription (OTC) medicine;
- have any other medical problems, especially lupus erythematosus or porphyria;
- have recently been treated with x-rays or cancer medicines.

PROPER USE OF THIS MEDICINE

Use this medicine only under the direct supervision of your doctor.

After UVA exposure, wash the treated area of skin with soap and water. Then use a sunscreen or wear protective clothing to protect the area.

PRECAUTIONS WHILE USING THIS MEDICINE

It is important that you visit your doctor as directed for treatments and to have your progress checked.

This medicine increases the sensitivity of the treated areas of your skin to sunlight. Therefore, **exposure to the sun, even through window glass or on a cloudy day, could cause a serious burn.** After each light treatment, thoroughly wash the treated areas of your skin. Also, if you must go out during daylight hours, cover the treated areas of your skin for at least 12 to 48 hours following treatment by wearing protective clothing or a sun block product that has a skin protection factor (SPF) of at least 15. Some patients may require a product with a higher SPF number, especially if they have a fair complexion. If you have any questions about this, check with your doctor or pharmacist.

The treated areas of your skin may continue to be sensitive to sunlight for some time after treatment with this medicine. Use extra caution for at least 72 hours following each treatment if you plan to spend any time in the sun. In addition, do not sunbathe anytime during your course of treatment with methoxsalen.

This medicine may cause your skin to become dry or itchy. **However, check with your doctor before applying anything to your skin to treat this problem.**

POSSIBLE SIDE EFFECTS OF THIS MEDICINE
Side Effects That Should Be Reported To Your Doctor Immediately

> Blistering and peeling of skin; reddened, sore skin; swelling, especially of the feet or lower legs

There is an increased risk of skin cancer after use of methoxsalen. Check the treated areas of your body regularly and show your doctor any skin sores that do not heal, new skin growths, and skin growths that have changed in the way they look or feel.

Premature aging of the skin may occur as a result of prolonged methoxsalen therapy. This effect is permanent.

Other side effects not listed above may also occur in some patients. If you notice any other effects, check with your doctor, nurse, or pharmacist.

METHYLDOPA   Systemic

■ For the Pharmacist ■

In providing consultation, consider emphasizing the following selected information (» = major clinical significance):

Before using this medication
» Conditions affecting use, especially:
  Sensitivity to methyldopa
  Breast-feeding—Distributed into breast milk
  Use in the elderly—Increased sensitivity to hypotensive and sedative effects
  Other medications, especially MAO inhibitors
  Other medical problems, especially active hepatic disease, history of hepatic disease associated with methyldopa, history of autoimmune hemolytic anemia, or pheochromocytoma

Proper use of this medication
  Possible need for control of weight and diet, especially sodium intake
» Patient may not experience symptoms of hypertension; importance of taking medication even if feeling well
» Does not cure, but helps control hypertension; possible need for lifelong therapy; checking with physician before discontinuing medication; serious consequences of untreated hypertension
  Getting into habit of taking at same time each day to help increase compliance
» Proper dosing
  Missed dose: Taking as soon as possible; not taking if almost time for next dose; not doubling doses
» Proper storage

Precautions while using this medication
  Regular visits to physician to check progress
» Not using other medications, especially nonprescription sympathomimetics, unless ordered by physician
» Reporting fever to physician
  Caution if any kind of surgery (including dental surgery) or emergency treatment is required
» Caution when driving or doing things requiring alertness, because of possible drowsiness
  Caution when getting up suddenly from a lying or sitting position
  Possible dryness of mouth; using sugarless candy or gum, ice, or saliva substitute for relief; checking with physician or dentist if dry mouth continues for more than 2 weeks
  Caution if any laboratory tests required; possible interference with test results

Side/adverse effects
  Signs of potential side effects, especially edema, drug fever, mental status changes, colitis, hemolytic anemia, cholestasis, hepatitis, leukopenia, granulocytopenia, myocarditis, pancreatitis, SLE-like syndrome, and thrombocytopenia

▲ For the Patient ▲

912408

ABOUT YOUR MEDICINE

Methyldopa (meth-ill-DOE-pa) belongs to the general class of medicines called antihypertensives. It is used to treat high blood pressure (hypertension).

If any of the information in this leaflet causes you special concern or if you want additional information about your medicine and its use, check with your doctor, nurse, or pharmacist. **Remember, keep this and all other medicines out of the reach of children and never share your medicines with others.**

BEFORE USING THIS MEDICINE

Tell your doctor, nurse, and pharmacist if you . . .
- are allergic to any medicine, either prescription or non-prescription (OTC);
- are pregnant or intend to become pregnant while using this medicine;
- are breast-feeding;
- are taking any other prescription or nonprescription (OTC) medicine, especially MAO inhibitors or medicines for appetite control, asthma, colds, cough, hay fever, or sinus;
- have any other medical problems, especially liver disease or pheochromocytoma (PCC).

PROPER USE OF THIS MEDICINE

This medicine will not cure your high blood pressure but it does help control it. You must continue to take it—even if you feel well—if you expect to keep your blood pressure down. **You may have to take high blood pressure medicine for the rest of your life.**

If you miss a dose of this medicine, take it as soon as possible. However, if it is almost time for your next dose, skip the missed dose and go back to your regular dosing schedule. Do not double doses.

PRECAUTIONS WHILE USING THIS MEDICINE

It is important that your doctor check your progress at regular visits while you are taking this medicine.

If you have a fever and there seems to be no reason for it, check with your doctor immediately. This is especially important the first few weeks you take methyldopa.

Methyldopa may cause some people to become drowsy or less alert than they are normally. **Make sure you know how you react to this medicine before you drive, use machines, or do other jobs that require you to be alert.**

Tell the doctor in charge that you are taking this medicine before you have any medical tests. The results of some tests may be affected by this medicine.

POSSIBLE SIDE EFFECTS OF THIS MEDICINE

Side Effects That Should Be Reported To Your Doctor Immediately

> *Less common*—Fever shortly after starting to take this medicine

Other Side Effects That Should Be Reported To Your Doctor

> *More common*—Swelling of feet or lower legs

> *Less common*—Mental depression or anxiety; nightmares or unusually vivid dreams

> *Rare*—Continuing tiredness or weakness after having taken this medicine for several weeks; dark or amber urine; fever, chills, troubled breathing, and fast heartbeat; general feeling of discomfort, illness, or weakness; joint pain; pale stools; severe or continuing diarrhea or stomach cramps; severe stomach pain with nausea and vomiting; skin rash or itching; yellow eyes or skin

Side Effects That Usually Do Not Require Medical Attention

These possible side effects may go away during treatment; however, if they continue or are bothersome, check with your doctor, nurse, or pharmacist.

> *More common*—Drowsiness; dryness of mouth; headache

> *Less common*—Decreased sexual ability or interest in sex; dizziness or lightheadedness when getting up from a lying or sitting position; nausea or vomiting; numbness, tingling, pain or weakness in hands or feet; slow heartbeat; stuffy nose; swelling of breasts or unusual milk production

Other side effects not listed above may also occur in some patients. If you notice any other effects, check with your doctor, nurse, or pharmacist.

METHYLERGONOVINE   Systemic

■For the Pharmacist■

In providing consultation, consider emphasizing the following selected information (» = major clinical significance):

Before using this medication
» Conditions affecting use, especially:
> Allergies or sensitivity to methylergonovine or other ergot alkaloids
> Pregnancy—Should not be used prior to delivery or delivery of the placenta
> Breast-feeding—Ergot alkaloids are excreted in breast milk
> Other medical problems, especially cardiac or vascular disease, hepatic function impairment, severe hypertension or history of hypertension, renal function impairment, and sepsis

Proper use of this medication
» Importance of not using more medication or using for longer than prescribed; risk of ergotism and gangrene with prolonged use
» Proper dosing
> Missed dose: Not taking missed dose; not doubling doses
» Proper storage

Precautions while using this medication
> Notifying physician if infection develops, since infection may cause increased sensitivity to medication

Side/adverse effects
> Signs of potential side effects, especially allergic reaction, coronary vasospasm or other cardiovascular complications, dyspnea, severe hypertension, or peripheral vasospasm

▲ For the Patient ▲

913808

ERGONOVINE/METHYLERGONOVINE (Oral):
Including Ergonovine; Methylergonovine.

ABOUT YOUR MEDICINE

Ergonovine (er-goe-NOE-veen) and **methylergonovine** (meth-ill-er-goe-NOE-veen) belong to the group of medicines known as ergot alkaloids. These medicines are usually given to stop heavy bleeding that sometimes occurs after the birth of a baby. Ergonovine and methylergonovine may also be used for other conditions as determined by your doctor.

If any of the information in this leaflet causes you special concern or if you want additional information about your medicine and its use, check with your doctor, nurse, or pharmacist. **Remember, keep this and all other medicines out of the reach of children and never share your medicines with others.**

BEFORE USING THIS MEDICINE

Tell your doctor, nurse, and pharmacist if you . . .
- are allergic to any medicine, either prescription or non-prescription (OTC);
- are pregnant or intend to become pregnant while using this medicine;
- are breast-feeding;
- are taking any other prescription or nonprescription (OTC) medicine, especially bromocriptine, nitrates or other medicines for angina, or other ergot alkaloids;
- have any other medical problems, especially angina (chest pain), blood vessel disease, high blood pressure, infection, kidney disease, liver disease, Raynaud's phenomenon, or stroke (history of).

PROPER USE OF THIS MEDICINE

Take this medicine only as directed by your doctor. Do not take more of it, do not take it more often, and do not take it for a longer time than your doctor ordered. If too much is taken or if it is taken for a longer time than your doctor ordered, it may cause serious effects.

If you miss a dose of this medicine, do not take the missed dose at all and do not double the next one. Instead, go back to your regular dosing schedule.

PRECAUTIONS WHILE USING THIS MEDICINE

If you have an infection or illness of any kind, check with your doctor before taking this medicine, since you may be more sensitive to the effects of it.

POSSIBLE SIDE EFFECTS OF THIS MEDICINE

Side Effects That Should Be Reported To Your Doctor Immediately

>   *Less common*—Chest pain

>   *Rare*—Blurred vision; convulsions (seizures); crushing chest pain; headache (sudden and severe); irregular heartbeat; unexplained shortness of breath

Other Side Effects That Should Be Reported To Your Doctor

>   *Less common*—Slow heartbeat

>   *Rare*—Itching of skin; pain in arms, legs, or lower back; pale or cold hands or feet; weakness in legs

>   *With long-term use*—Dry, shriveled-looking skin on hands, lower legs, or feet; false feeling of insects crawling on the skin; pain and redness in an arm or leg; paralysis of one side of the body

Side Effects That Usually Do Not Require Medical Attention

These possible side effects may go away during treatment; however, if they continue or are bothersome, check with your doctor, nurse, or pharmacist.

> *More common*—Cramping of the uterus; nausea; vomiting

Other side effects not listed above may also occur in some patients. If you notice any other effects, check with your doctor, nurse, or pharmacist.

METHYLPHENIDATE   Systemic

■For the Pharmacist■

In providing consultation, consider emphasizing the following selected information (» = major clinical significance):

Before using this medication
» Conditions affecting use, especially:
    Sensitivity to methylphenidate
    Use in children—In attention-deficit hyperactivity disorder (ADHD), usually discontinued after puberty; drug-free periods recommended during treatment; monitoring of height and weight recommended; children more likely to develop stomach pain, trouble in sleeping, and loss of appetite and weight
    Other medications, especially other CNS stimulation–producing medications, MAO inhibitors, or pimozide
    Other medical problems, especially severe anxiety, tension, or agitation; severe depression; glaucoma; hypertension; motor tics; or Tourette's syndrome

Proper use of this medication
    Taking on an empty stomach about 30 to 45 minutes before meals
    Proper administration for extended-release dosage form: Swallowing whole; not breaking, crushing, or chewing
    Taking the last dose (not including extended-release tablets) for each day before 6 p.m. to minimize the possibility of insomnia
» Importance of not using more medication than the amount prescribed because of possible habit-forming potential
    Not increasing dose if medication seems less effective after a few weeks; checking with physician
» Proper dosing
    Missed dose: Taking as soon as possible; taking any remaining doses for that day at regularly spaced intervals; not doubling doses
» Proper storage

Precautions while using this medication
    Regular visits to physician to check progress during therapy
» Checking with physician before discontinuing medication after long-term and high-dose therapy; gradual dosage reduction may be necessary to avoid possibility of withdrawal symptoms
» Suspected psychological or physical dependence; checking with physician

Side/adverse effects
    Possibility of withdrawal effects
    Signs of potential side effects, especially cardiovascular effects, excessive CNS stimulation, hypersensitivity reaction, anemia, blurred vision, convulsions, leukopenia, toxic psychosis, or weight loss

---

▲ For the Patient ▲

913127

ABOUT YOUR MEDICINE

Methylphenidate (meth-ill-FEN-i-date) belongs to the group of medicines called central nervous system (CNS) stimulants. It is used to treat attention-deficit hyperactivity disorder (ADHD). It is also used in the treatment of narcolepsy (uncontrolled desire for sleep or sudden attacks of deep sleep).

If any of the information in this leaflet causes you special concern or if you want additional information about your medicine and its use, check with your doctor, nurse, or pharmacist. **Remember, keep this and all other medicines out of the reach of children and never share your medicines with others.**

BEFORE USING THIS MEDICINE

Tell your doctor, nurse, and pharmacist if you . . .
- are allergic to any medicine, either prescription or non-prescription (OTC);
- are pregnant or intend to become pregnant while using this medicine;
- are breast-feeding;
- are taking any other prescription or nonprescription (OTC) medicine, especially MAO inhibitors, other CNS stimulants, or pimozide;
- have any other medical problems, especially Gilles de la Tourette's syndrome (or any other tics), glaucoma, high blood pressure, or severe anxiety, tension, or depression;
- are now using or have used cocaine.

PROPER USE OF THIS MEDICINE

Take this medicine only as directed by your doctor. Do not take more of it, do not take it more often, and do not take it for a longer time than your doctor ordered. If too much is taken, it may become habit-forming.

Take this medicine about 30 to 45 minutes before meals to help it work better.

To help prevent trouble in sleeping, take the last dose of this medicine for each day before 6 p.m. unless otherwise directed by your doctor.

If you think this medicine is not working as well after you have taken it for several weeks, **do not increase the dose.** Instead, check with your doctor.

If you miss a dose of this medicine, take it as soon as possible. Then take any remaining doses for that day at regularly spaced intervals. Do not double doses.

PRECAUTIONS WHILE USING THIS MEDICINE

Your doctor should check your progress at regular visits to make sure that this medicine does not cause unwanted effects.

If you will be taking this medicine in large doses for a long period of time, **do not stop taking it without first checking with your doctor.** Your doctor may want you to reduce gradually the amount you are taking before stopping completely.

If you have been using this medicine for a long time and you think you may have become mentally or physically dependent on it, check with your doctor. Some signs of dependence on methylphenidate are:

—a strong desire or need to continue taking the medicine.

—a need to increase the dose to receive the effects of the medicine.

—withdrawal side effects (for example, mental depression, unusual behavior, or unusual tiredness or weakness) occurring after the medicine is stopped.

POSSIBLE SIDE EFFECTS OF THIS MEDICINE
Side Effects That Should Be Reported To Your Doctor

More common—Fast heartbeat

Less common—Bruising; chest pain; fever; joint pain; skin rash or hives; uncontrolled movements of the body

Rare—Blurred vision or any change in vision; convulsions (seizures); sore throat and fever; unusual tiredness or weakness

With long-term use—Mood or mental changes; weight loss

Side Effects That Usually Do Not Require Medical Attention

These possible side effects may go away during treatment; however, if they continue or are bothersome, check with your doctor, nurse, or pharmacist.

More common—Loss of appetite; nervousness; trouble in sleeping

Less common—Dizziness; drowsiness; headache; nausea; stomach pain

Some of the above side effects, such as loss of appetite, stomach pain, trouble in sleeping, and weight loss are more likely to occur in children, who are usually more sensitive to the effects of methylphenidate.

Other side effects not listed above may also occur in some patients. If you notice any other effects, check with your doctor, nurse, or pharmacist.

After you stop using this medicine, your body may need time to adjust. The length of time this takes depends on the amount of medicine you were using and how long you used it. During this period of time check with your doctor if you notice any unusual effects, especially severe mental depression, unusual behavior, or unusual tiredness or weakness.

METHYPRYLON   Systemic

■ For the Pharmacist ■

In providing consultation, consider emphasizing the following selected information (» = major clinical significance):

Before using this medication
» Conditions affecting use, especially:
    Sensitivity to methyprylon
    Use in the elderly—Elderly patients may be more sensitive to effects of methyprylon
    Other medications, especially alcohol or other CNS depression-producing medications
    Other medical problems, especially history of drug abuse or dependence

Proper use of this medication
» Importance of not using more medication than the amount prescribed because of habit-forming potential
» Proper storage

Precautions while using this medication
    Regular visits to physician to check progress during prolonged therapy
    Checking with physician before discontinuing medication after prolonged use; gradual dosage reduction may be necessary to avoid possibility of withdrawal symptoms
» Avoiding use of alcohol or other CNS depressants
» Suspected overdose: Getting emergency help at once
» Caution if dizziness or daytime drowsiness occurs

Side/adverse effects
    Signs of potential side effects, especially allergic reaction, unexplained fever, mental depression, neutropenia, paradoxical reaction, and thrombocytopenia
    Side/adverse effects more likely to occur in elderly patients, who may be more sensitive to effects of methyprylon

▲ For the Patient ▲

914356

ABOUT YOUR MEDICINE

Methyprylon (meth-i-PRYE-lon) is used to treat insomnia (trouble in sleeping). However, it has generally been replaced by other medicines for the treatment of insomnia. If methyprylon is used regularly (for example, every day) to help produce sleep, it may not be effective for more than 1 week.

If any of the information in this leaflet causes you special concern or if you want additional information about your medicine and its use, check with your doctor, nurse, or pharmacist. **Remember, keep this and all other medicines out of the reach of children and never share your medicines with others.**

BEFORE USING THIS MEDICINE
Tell your doctor, nurse, and pharmacist if you . . .
- are allergic to any medicine, either prescription or non-prescription (OTC);
- are pregnant or intend to become pregnant while using this medicine;
- are breast-feeding;
- are taking any other prescription or nonprescription (OTC) medicine, especially CNS depressants;
- have any other medical problems, especially a history of drug abuse or dependence.

PROPER USE OF THIS MEDICINE
Take this medicine only as directed by your doctor. Do not take more of it, do not take it more often, and do not take it for a longer time than your doctor ordered. If too much is taken, it may become habit-forming.

PRECAUTIONS WHILE USING THIS MEDICINE
If you will be taking this medicine regularly for a long time:
- Your doctor should check your progress at regular visits.
- Do not stop taking it without first checking with your doctor. Your doctor may want you to reduce gradually the amount you are taking before stopping completely.

This medicine will add to the effects of alcohol and other CNS depressants (medicines that slow down the nervous system). **Check with your doctor before taking any such depressants while you are taking this medicine.**

If you think you or someone else may have taken an overdose, get emergency help at once. Taking an overdose of methyprylon or taking alcohol or other CNS depressants with methyprylon may lead to unconsciousness and possibly death. Some signs of an overdose are confusion, fast heartbeat, severe weakness, shortness of breath or slow or troubled breathing, and staggering.

This medicine may cause some people to become dizzy, drowsy, or less alert than they are normally. Even if taken at bedtime, it may cause some people to feel drowsy or less alert on arising. **Make sure you know how you react to this medicine before you drive, use machines, or do other jobs that require you to be alert.**

POSSIBLE SIDE EFFECTS OF THIS MEDICINE
Side Effects That Should Be Reported To Your Doctor

Less common—Skin rash; unusual excitement

Rare—Fever (unexplained); mental depression; ulcers or sores in mouth or throat (continuing); unusual bleeding or bruising

Side Effects That Usually Do Not Require Medical Attention

These possible side effects may go away during treatment; however, if they continue or are bothersome, check with your doctor, nurse, or pharmacist.

> *More common*—Dizziness; drowsiness (daytime); headache

Other side effects not listed above may also occur in some patients. If you notice any other effects, check with your doctor, nurse, or pharmacist.

After you stop using this medicine, your body may need time to adjust. The length of time this takes depends on the amount of medicine you were using and how long you used it. During this time check with your doctor if you notice any unusual effects, especially confusion; convulsions (seizures); hallucinations; increased dreaming; increased sweating; nausea or vomiting; nightmares; restlessness or nervousness; stomach cramps; trembling; trouble in sleeping; or unusual weakness.

METHYSERGIDE   Systemic

■For the Pharmacist■

In providing consultation, consider emphasizing the following selected information (» = major clinical significance):

Before using this medication
» Conditions affecting use, especially:
 Sensitivity to ergot derivatives
 Breast-feeding—Ergot alkaloids inhibit lactation; also, they are excreted in breast milk and may cause ergotism in the infant
 Use in children—Use is not recommended, because of the hazards associated with long-term use of methysergide
 Use in the elderly—Increased risk of hypothermia and other adverse effects associated with peripheral vasoconstriction
 Other medical problems, especially cardiovascular disease, hepatic function impairment, hypertension, peripheral vascular disease, severe pruritus (especially when associated with hepatic disease), severe infection, pulmonary disease, rheumatoid arthritis, valvular heart disease, and renal function impairment

Proper use of this medication
» Importance of not using more medication than the amount prescribed; risk of ergotism and gangrene with overdosage
» Taking with meals or milk to reduce gastrointestinal irritation
 Missed dose: Not taking at all; not doubling doses
» Proper dosing
» Proper storage

Precautions while using this medication
» Checking with physician before discontinuing medication; withdrawal headache may occur
» Not taking for longer than 6 months at a time
» Caution in driving or doing jobs requiring alertness because of possible dizziness, lightheadedness, or drowsiness
 Caution when getting up suddenly from a lying or sitting position
 Avoiding alcohol, which aggravates headache
 Avoiding smoking since nicotine constricts blood vessels
 Avoiding exposure to excessive cold, which may aggravate peripheral vasoconstriction
 Notifying physician if infection develops, since infection may cause increased sensitivity to medication

Side/adverse effects
 Signs of potential side effects, especially CNS stimulation, fibrosis, ischemia, peripheral edema, and leukopenia

▲ For the Patient ▲

914367

ABOUT YOUR MEDICINE

Methysergide (meth-i-SER-jide) belongs to the group of medicines known as ergot alkaloids. It is used to prevent migraine headaches and some kinds of throbbing headaches. It is not used to treat an attack once it has started.

If any of the information in this leaflet causes you special concern or if you want additional information about your medicine and its use, check with your doctor, nurse, or pharmacist. **Remember, keep this and all other medicines out of the reach of children and never share your medicines with others.**

BEFORE USING THIS MEDICINE

Tell your doctor, nurse, and pharmacist if you . . .
- are allergic to any medicine, either prescription or nonprescription (OTC);
- are pregnant or intend to become pregnant while using this medicine;
- are breast-feeding;
- are taking any other prescription or nonprescription (OTC) medicine;
- have any other medical problems, especially arthritis, heart or blood vessel disease, high blood pressure, infection, itching (severe), or kidney, liver, or lung disease;
- smoke;
- use cocaine.

PROPER USE OF THIS MEDICINE

Take methysergide only as directed by your doctor. If the amount you are to take does not prevent your headaches from occurring as often as before, do not take more than your doctor ordered. Instead, check with your doctor. Taking too much of this medicine or taking it too frequently may cause serious effects such as nausea and vomiting; cold, painful hands or feet; or even gangrene.

If methysergide upsets your stomach, it may be taken with meals or milk. If stomach upset continues or is severe, check with your doctor.

If you miss a dose of this medicine, skip the missed dose and go back to your regular dosing schedule. Do not double doses.

PRECAUTIONS WHILE USING THIS MEDICINE

If you have been taking methysergide regularly, **do not stop taking it without first checking with your doctor.** Your doctor may want you to reduce gradually the amount you are using before stopping completely. If you stop taking it suddenly, your headaches may return or worsen.

Your doctor will tell you how long you should take this medicine. Usually it is not taken for longer than 6 months at a time. **If your doctor tells you to stop taking the medicine for a while, do not continue to take it.** If your body does not get a rest from the medicine, it can have harmful effects.

Methysergide may cause some people to become dizzy, lightheaded, drowsy, or less alert than they are normally. Even if taken at bedtime, it may cause some people to feel drowsy or less alert on arising. **Make sure you know how you react**

to this medicine before you drive, use machines, or do other jobs that require you to be alert.

POSSIBLE SIDE EFFECTS OF THIS MEDICINE

Side Effects That Should Be Reported To Your Doctor Immediately

Chest pain or tightness in chest; difficult or painful urination; dizziness (severe); fever; increase or decrease (large) in amount of urine; leg cramps; pain in arms, legs, groin, lower back or side; pale or cold hands or feet; shortness of breath or difficult breathing; swelling of hands, ankles, feet or lower legs

Other Side Effects That Should Be Reported To Your Doctor

More common—Abdominal or stomach pain; itching; numbness and tingling of fingers, toes, or face; weakness in legs

Less common or rare—Changes in vision; clumsiness or unsteadiness; excitement or difficulty in thinking; fast or slow heartbeat; feeling of being outside the body; fever with or without chills, general feeling of discomfort or illness, headache, and sore throat; hallucinations; loss of appetite or weight loss; mental depression; nightmares; raised red spots on skin; redness or flushing of face; skin rash

Side Effects That Usually Do Not Require Medical Attention

These possible side effects may go away during treatment; however, if they continue or are bothersome, check with your doctor, nurse, or pharmacist.

More common—Diarrhea; dizziness or lightheadedness; drowsiness; nausea or vomiting

Other side effects not listed above may also occur in some patients. If you notice any other effects, check with your doctor, nurse, or pharmacist.

After you stop using this medicine, your body may need time to adjust. The length of time this takes depends on the amount of medicine you were using and how long you used it. During this time check with your doctor if your headaches begin again or worsen.

METOCLOPRAMIDE   Systemic

■For the Pharmacist■

In providing consultation, consider emphasizing the following selected information (» = major clinical significance):

Before using this medication
» Conditions affecting use, especially:

Sensitivity to metoclopramide, procaine, or procainamide

Breast-feeding—Distributed into breast milk

Use in children—Extrapyramidal effects more likely; increased risk of methemoglobinemia in premature and full-term infants

Use in the elderly—Extrapyramidal effects more likely

Other medications, especially alcohol and CNS depressants

Other medical problems, especially epilepsy; gastrointestinal bleeding, mechanical obstruction, or perforation; or severe renal function impairment

Proper use of this medication
» Taking 30 minutes before meals and at bedtime (for oral dosage forms)
» Not taking more medication than the amount prescribed
» Proper dosing

Missed dose: Using as soon as possible; not using if almost time for next dose
» Proper storage

Precautions while using this medication
» Avoiding use of alcohol or other CNS depressants
» Caution if drowsiness occurs

Side/adverse effects
Signs of potential side effects, especially agranulocytosis, extrapyramidal effects, and tardive dyskinesia

▲ For the Patient ▲

914378

ABOUT YOUR MEDICINE

Metoclopramide (met-oh-KLOE-pra-mide) is a medicine that increases the movements or contractions of the stomach and intestines. When taken by mouth, metoclopramide is used to treat the symptoms of a certain type of stomach problem called diabetic gastroparesis. It relieves symptoms such as nausea, vomiting, continued feeling of fullness after meals, and loss of appetite. Metoclopramide is also used to treat symptoms such as heartburn caused by a backward flow of gastric acid into the esophagus. Metoclopramide may also be used for other conditions as determined by your doctor.

If any of the information in this leaflet causes you special concern or if you want additional information about your medicine and its use, check with your doctor, nurse, or pharmacist. **Remember, keep this and all other medicines out of**

the reach of children and never share your medicines with others.

BEFORE USING THIS MEDICINE

Tell your doctor, nurse, and pharmacist if you . . .

- are allergic to any medicine, either prescription or non-prescription (OTC);
- are pregnant or intend to become pregnant while using this medicine;
- are breast-feeding;
- are taking any other prescription or nonprescription (OTC) medicine;
- have any other medical problems, especially abdominal or stomach bleeding, epilepsy, intestinal blockage, pheo-chromocytoma (PCC), or severe kidney disease.

PROPER USE OF THIS MEDICINE

Take this medicine 30 minutes before meals and at bedtime, unless otherwise directed by your doctor.

Take metoclopramide only as directed. Do not take more of it, do not take it more often, and do not take it for a longer period of time than your doctor ordered. To do so may increase the chance of side effects.

If you miss a dose of this medicine, take it as soon as possible. However, if it is almost time for your next dose, skip the missed dose and go back to your regular dosing schedule. Do not double doses.

PRECAUTIONS WHILE USING THIS MEDICINE

This medicine will add to the effects of alcohol and other CNS depressants (medicines that slow down the nervous system). **Check with your doctor before taking any such depressants while you are using this medicine.**

This medicine may cause some people to become dizzy, light-headed, drowsy, or less alert than they are normally. **Make sure you know how you react to this medicine before you drive, use machines, or do other jobs that require you to be alert.**

POSSIBLE SIDE EFFECTS OF THIS MEDICINE
Side Effects That Should Be Reported To Your Doctor

Rare—Chills; difficulty in speaking or swallowing; dizziness or fainting; fast or irregular heartbeat; fever; general feeling of tiredness or weakness; headache (severe or continuing); increase in blood pressure; lip smacking or puckering; loss of balance control; mask-like face; rapid or worm-like movements of tongue; shuffling walk; sore throat; stiffness of arms or legs; trembling and shaking of hands and fingers; uncontrolled chewing movements; uncontrolled movements of arms and legs

With high doses (may occur within minutes of receiving a dose of metoclopramide and last for 2 to 24 hours)— Aching or discomfort in lower legs; panic-like sensation; sensation of crawling in legs; unusual nervousness, restlessness, or irritability

Possible signs of overdose (may also occur rarely with usual doses, especially in children and young adults)— Confusion; drowsiness (severe)

Side Effects That Usually Do Not Require Medical Attention

These possible side effects may go away during treatment; however, if they continue or are bothersome, check with your doctor, nurse, or pharmacist.

More common—Diarrhea (with high doses); drowsiness; restlessness

Other side effects not listed above may also occur in some patients. If you notice any other effects, check with your doctor, nurse, or pharmacist.

METRONIDAZOLE Systemic

■ For the Pharmacist ■

In providing consultation, consider emphasizing the following selected information (» = major clinical significance):

Before using this medication
» Conditions affecting use, especially:
  Hypersensitivity to metronidazole
  Pregnancy—Metronidazole crosses the placenta; use is not recommended during the first trimester of pregnancy
  Breast-feeding—Metronidazole is distributed into breast milk; metronidazole is not recommended during breast-feeding
  Dental—Metronidazole may cause dry mouth, an unpleasant or sharp metallic taste, and alteration of taste sensation
  Other medications, especially alcohol, coumarin- or indandione-derivative anticoagulants, or disulfiram
  Other medical problems, especially active organic disease of the CNS, a history of blood dyscrasias, or severe hepatic function impairment

Proper use of this medication
  Taking with meals or a snack to minimize gastrointestinal irritation
» Compliance with full course of therapy
» Importance of not missing doses and taking at evenly spaced times
» Proper dosing
  Missed dose: Taking as soon as possible; not taking if almost time for next dose; not doubling doses
» Proper storage

Precautions while using this medication
  Follow-up visit to physician after treatment for giardiasis to ensure that infection has been eradicated.
  Checking with physician if no improvement within a few days
» Avoiding use of alcoholic beverages or other alcohol-containing preparations while taking and for at least 1 day after discontinuing this medication
  Possible dryness of mouth; using sugarless candy or gum, ice, or saliva substitute for relief; checking with dentist if dry mouth continues for more than 2 weeks
» Caution if dizziness or lightheadedness occurs
  Prevention of reinfection in trichomoniasis; possible need for concurrent treatment of male sexual partner and use of a condom

Side/adverse effects
  Signs of potential side effects, especially CNS toxicity, hypersensitivity, leukopenia, pancreatitis, seizures, peripheral neuropathy, vaginal candidiasis, and thrombophlebitis
  Dark urine may be alarming to patient although medically insignificant

▲ For the Patient ▲

912420

ABOUT YOUR MEDICINE

Metronidazole (me-troe-NI-da-zole) is used to treat infections. It may also be used for other problems as determined by your doctor. It will not work for colds, flu, or other virus infections.

If any of the information in this leaflet causes you special concern or if you want additional information about your medicine and its use, check with your doctor, nurse, or pharmacist. **Remember, keep this and all other medicines out of the reach of children and never share your medicines with others.**

BEFORE USING THIS MEDICINE

Tell your doctor, nurse, and pharmacist if you . . .
- are allergic to any medicine, either prescription or nonprescription (OTC);
- are pregnant or intend to become pregnant while using this medicine;
- are breast-feeding;
- are taking any other prescription or nonprescription (OTC) medicine, especially anticoagulants (blood thinners) or disulfiram;
- have any other medical problems, especially blood disease or a history of blood disease; central nervous system (CNS) disease, including epilepsy; or severe liver disease.

PROPER USE OF THIS MEDICINE

If this medicine upsets your stomach, it may be taken with meals or a snack. If stomach upset continues, check with your doctor.

To help clear up your infection completely, **keep taking this medicine for the full time of treatment** even if you begin to feel better after a few days; **do not miss any doses.**

If you do miss a dose of this medicine, take it as soon as possible. This will help to keep a constant amount of medicine in the blood. However, if it is almost time for your next dose, skip the missed dose and go back to your regular dosing schedule. Do not double doses.

PRECAUTIONS WHILE USING THIS MEDICINE

If your symptoms do not improve within a few days, or if they become worse, check with your doctor.

Drinking alcoholic beverages while taking this medicine may cause stomach pain, nausea, vomiting, headache, or flushing or redness of the face. Other alcohol-containing preparations (for example, elixirs, cough syrups, tonics) may also cause problems. Therefore, **you should not drink alcoholic beverages or use other alcohol-containing preparations while taking this medicine and for at least one day after stopping it.**

This medicine may cause some people to become dizzy or lightheaded. **Make sure you know how you react to this medicine before you drive, use machines, or do other jobs that require you to be alert.** If these reactions are especially bothersome, check with your doctor.

This medicine must not be given to other people or used for other infections unless you are otherwise directed by your doctor.

POSSIBLE SIDE EFFECTS OF THIS MEDICINE
Side Effects That Should Be Reported To Your Doctor Immediately

> *Less common*—Numbness, tingling, pain, or weakness in hands or feet

> *Rare*—Convulsions (seizures)

Other Side Effects That Should Be Reported To Your Doctor

> *Less common*—Any vaginal irritation, discharge, or dryness not present before use of this medicine; clumsiness or unsteadiness; mood or other mental changes; skin rash, hives, redness, or itching; sore throat and fever; stomach and back pain (severe)

Side Effects That Usually Do Not Require Medical Attention

These possible side effects may go away during treatment; however, if they continue or are bothersome, check with your doctor, nurse, or pharmacist.

> *More common*—Diarrhea; dizziness or lightheadedness; headache; loss of appetite; nausea; stomach pain or cramps; vomiting

In some patients metronidazole may cause dark urine. This is only temporary and will go away when you stop taking this medicine.

Other side effects not listed above may also occur in some patients. If you notice any other effects, check with your doctor, nurse, or pharmacist.

METRONIDAZOLE   Topical

■For the Pharmacist■

In providing consultation, consider emphasizing the following selected information (》 = major clinical significance):

Before using this medication
》 Conditions affecting use, especially:
 Sensitivity to topical metronidazole or to methyl- and propyl-parabens
 Pregnancy—Absorbed metronidazole crosses the placenta and enters fetal circulation rapidly

Proper use of this medication
》 Not using medication in or near the eyes; tearing may occur
 Washing eyes out immediately with large amounts of cool tap water if medication gets into eyes; checking with physician if eyes continue to burn or are painful
 Before applying, thoroughly washing affected area(s) with a mild, nonirritating cleanser, rinsing well, and gently patting dry
 To use:
  After washing affected area(s), applying medication with fingertips; washing medication off hands afterward
》 Importance of applying medication to entire affected area
》 Compliance with full course of therapy, which may take 9 weeks or longer
》 Proper dosing
 Missed dose: Applying as soon as possible; not applying if almost time for next dose
》 Proper storage

Precautions while using this medication
 Checking with physician if no improvement within 3 weeks; may take up to 9 weeks before full therapeutic benefit is seen
 Possibility of stinging or burning of the skin after application; checking with physician if irritation continues
 Using only "oil-free" cosmetics to avoid worsening rosacea

▲ For the Patient ▲

917274

ABOUT YOUR MEDICINE

Topical **metronidazole** (me-troe-NI-da-zole) is applied to the skin in adults to help control rosacea (roe-ZAY-she-ah), also known as acne rosacea and "adult acne." This medicine helps to reduce the redness of the skin and the number of pimples, usually found on the face, in patients with rosacea.

If any of the information in this leaflet causes you special concern or if you want additional information about your medicine and its use, check with your doctor, nurse, or pharmacist. **Remember, keep this and all other medicines out of the reach of children and never share your medicines with others.**

BEFORE USING THIS MEDICINE

Tell your doctor, nurse, and pharmacist if you . . .

- are allergic to any medicine, either prescription or non-prescription (OTC);
- are pregnant or intend to become pregnant while using this medicine;
- are breast-feeding;
- are taking any other prescription or nonprescription (OTC) medicine;
- have any other medical problems

PROPER USE OF THIS MEDICINE

Do not use this medicine in or near the eyes. Watering of the eyes may occur when the medicine is used too close to the eyes.

If this medicine does get into your eyes, wash them out immediately, but carefully, with large amounts of cool tap water. If your eyes still burn or are painful, check with your doctor.

Before applying this medicine, thoroughly wash the affected area(s) with a mild, nonirritating cleanser, rinse well, and gently pat dry.

To use:

- After washing the affected area(s), apply this medicine with your fingertips.
- Apply and rub in a thin film of medicine, using enough to cover the affected area(s) lightly. **You should apply the medicine to the whole area usually affected by rosacea, not just to the pimples themselves.**
- Wash the medicine off your hands.

To help keep your rosacea under control, **keep using this medicine for the full time of treatment.** You may have to continue using this medicine every day for 9 weeks or longer. **Do not miss any doses.**

If you do miss a dose of this medicine, apply it as soon as possible. However, if it is almost time for your next dose, skip the missed dose and go back to your regular dosing schedule.

PRECAUTIONS WHILE USING THIS MEDICINE

If your rosacea does not improve within 3 weeks, or if it becomes worse, check with your doctor. However, treatment of rosacea may take up to 9 weeks or longer before you see full improvement.

Stinging or burning of the skin may be expected after this medicine is applied. These effects may last up to a few minutes or more. If irritation continues, check with your doctor. You may have to use the medicine less often or stop using it altogether. Follow your doctor's directions.

You may continue to use cosmetics (make-up) while you are using this medicine for rosacea. However, it is best to use only "oil-free" cosmetics. Also, it is best not to use cosmetics too heavily or too often. They may make your rosacea worse. If you have any questions about this, check with your doctor.

POSSIBLE SIDE EFFECTS OF THIS MEDICINE
Side Effects That Usually Do Not Require Medical Attention

These possible side effects may go away during treatment; however, if they continue or are bothersome, check with your doctor, nurse, or pharmacist.

> *Less common*—Dry skin; redness or other sign of skin irritation not present before use of this medicine; stinging or burning of the skin; watering of eyes

Other side effects not listed above may also occur in some patients. If you notice any other effects, check with your doctor, nurse, or pharmacist.

METRONIDAZOLE   Vaginal

■For the Pharmacist■

In providing consultation, consider emphasizing the following selected
information (» = major clinical significance):

Before using this medication
» Conditions affecting use, especially:
  Sensitivity to metronidazole
  Pregnancy—Metronidazole crosses the placenta; use cautiously
    during pregnancy, possibly withholding its use in the first
    trimester
  Breast-feeding—Metronidazole is distributed into breast milk
    and is not recommended during breast-feeding
  Other medications, especially alcohol, coumarin- or indandione-
    derivative anticoagulants, or disulfiram
  Other medical problems, especially epilepsy or other neurologic
    disease or severe hepatic function impairment

Proper use of this medication
  Washing hands immediately before and after vaginal administration
  Avoiding getting medication into the eyes; washing with large amounts
    of cool tap water immediately if medication does get into eyes;
    checking with physician if eyes continue to be painful
  Reading patient directions carefully before use
  Proper administration technique:
    Following directions regarding filling the applicator, insertion
    technique, and cleaning the applicator after each use
    For cream or gel dosage forms
    Puncturing metal tamper-resistant seal on tube with top of cap
    For insert dosage form
    Placing insert into the applicator, immersing exposed insert in
      tap water for a few seconds before vaginal insertion to fa-
      cilitate disintegration
» Compliance with full course of therapy, even during menstruation
» Proper dosing
  Missed dose: Inserting as soon as possible; not inserting if almost
    time for next dose
» Proper storage

Precautions while using this medication
  Checking with physician if no improvement within a few days
  Follow-up visit to physician after treatment for bacterial vaginosis
    to ensure that infection has been eradicated
» Avoiding use of alcoholic beverages or other alcohol-containing prep-
    arations while using and for at least 1 day after discontinuing
    this medication
» Caution if dizziness or lightheadedness occurs
  Protecting clothing because of possible soiling with vaginal metro-
    nidazole; avoiding use of tampons
» Using hygienic measures to cure infection and prevent reinfection,
    e.g., wearing freshly washed cotton panties instead of synthetic
    panties
» Sexual abstinence is recommended during treatment to prevent cross-
    infection, reinfection, or dilution of the dose

For trichomoniasis:
» Using condoms to prevent reinfection with trichomoniasis after treatment; possible need for concurrent treatment of male partner for trichomoniasis

Side/adverse effects
Signs of potential side effects, especially candida cervicitis or vaginitis, abdominal cramping or pain, burning or irritation of penis of sexual partner, increased frequency of urination, vulvitis, altered taste sensation, CNS effects, dryness of mouth, furry tongue, gastrointestinal disturbances, loss of appetite

Dark urine may be alarming to patient although medically insignificant

Possibility of vaginal candidiasis occurring after medication has been discontinued

---

▲ For the Patient ▲

919575

ABOUT YOUR MEDICINE

Metronidazole (me-troe-NI-da-zole) is used to treat certain vaginal infections. This medicine will not work for vaginal fungus or yeast infections.

If any of the information in this leaflet causes you special concern or if you want additional information about your medicine and its use, check with your doctor, nurse, or pharmacist. **Remember, keep this and all other medicines out of the reach of children and never share your medicines with others.**

BEFORE USING THIS MEDICINE

Tell your doctor, nurse, and pharmacist if you . . .
- are allergic to any medicine, either prescription or non-prescription (OTC);
- are pregnant or intend to become pregnant while using this medicine;
- are breast-feeding;
- are taking any other prescription or nonprescription (OTC) medicine, especially alcohol or alcohol-containing medicines, anticoagulants (blood thinners), or disulfiram;
- have any other medical problems, especially central nervous system (CNS) disease, including epilepsy; liver disease (severe); or low white blood cell count (or history of).

PROPER USE OF THIS MEDICINE
Wash your hands before and after using the medicine.

Vaginal metronidazole products usually come with patient directions. Read them carefully before using this medicine.

To help you clear up your infection completely, **it is very important that you keep using this medicine for the full time of treatment,** even if your symptoms begin to clear up after a few days. If you stop using this medicine too soon, your symptoms may return. **Do not miss any doses. Also, continue using this medicine even if your menstrual period starts during treatment.**

If you do miss a dose of this medicine, use it as soon as possible. However, if it is almost time for your next dose, skip the missed dose and go back to your regular dosing schedule.

PRECAUTIONS WHILE USING THIS MEDICINE

If your symptoms do not improve within a few days, or if they become worse, check with your doctor.

Do not drink alcoholic beverages or use other alcohol-containing preparations while using this medicine and for at least one day after stopping it.

This medicine may cause some people to become dizzy or lightheaded. **Make sure you know how you react to this medicine before you drive, use machines, or do anything else that requires you to be alert or clearheaded.** If these reactions are especially bothersome, check with your doctor.

Vaginal medicines usually leak out of the vagina during treatment. To keep the medicine from getting on your clothing, wear a minipad or sanitary napkin. **Do not use tampons** since they may soak up the medicine.

To help clear up your infection completely and to help make sure it does not return, good health habits are also required.

- Wear cotton panties (or panties or pantyhose with cotton crotches) instead of synthetic (for example, nylon or rayon) panties.
- Wear only freshly washed panties daily.

Do not have sexual intercourse while you are using this medicine. Having sexual intercourse may reduce the strength of the medicine.

Many vaginal infections (for example, trichomoniasis) are spread by having sexual intercourse. You can give the infection to your sexual partner, and he can give the infection back to you later. Your partner may also need to be treated for some infections. **Until you are sure that the infection is completely cleared up after your treatment with this medicine, your partner should wear a condom during sexual intercourse.** If you have any questions about this, check with your doctor, nurse, or pharmacist.

POSSIBLE SIDE EFFECTS OF THIS MEDICINE
Side Effects That Should Be Reported To Your Doctor

More common—Itching in the vagina; pain during sexual intercourse; thick, white vaginal discharge with or without odor

Less common—Abdominal or stomach cramping or pain; burning or irritation of penis of sexual partner; burning on urination or need to urinate more often; itching, stinging, or redness of the genital area

Metronidazole may cause your urine to become dark. This is harmless and will go away when you stop using this medicine.

Other side effects not listed above may also occur in some patients. If you notice any other effects, check with your doctor, nurse, or pharmacist.

After you stop using this medicine, your body may need time to adjust. The length of time this takes depends on the amount of medicine you were using and how long you used it. During this time check with your doctor if you notice any vaginal or genital irritation or itching; pain during intercourse; or thick, white discharge not present before treatment, with or without odor.

MEXILETINE   Systemic

■ For the Pharmacist ■

In providing consultation, consider emphasizing the following selected information (» = major clinical significance):

Before using this medication
» Conditions affecting use, especially:
Sensitivity to amide-type anesthetics
Pregnancy—Increased incidence of fetal resorptions in animals
Breast-feeding—Distributed into breast milk
Medical problems, especially atrioventricular (AV) block, pre-existing 2nd or 3rd degree, without pacemaker or cardiogenic shock

Proper use of this medication
» Compliance with therapy; taking as directed even if feeling well
Taking with food, milk, or an antacid to reduce stomach upset
» Importance of not missing doses and taking at evenly spaced intervals
» Proper dosing
Missed dose: Taking as soon as possible if remembered within 4 hours; not taking if remembered later; not doubling doses
» Proper storage

Precautions while using the medication
Regular visits to physician to check progress
Carrying medical identification card or bracelet
» Caution if any kind of surgery (including dental surgery) or emergency treatment is required
» Caution when driving or doing things requiring alertness, because of possible dizziness

Side/adverse effects
Signs of adverse effects, especially chest pain, premature ventricular contractions, shortness of breath, leukopenia, agranulocytosis, thrombocytopenia, and seizures

▲ For the Patient ▲

913036

ANTIARRHYTHMICS, TYPE I (Oral): *Including Disopyramide; Encainide; Flecainide; Mexiletine; Moricizine; Procainamide; Propafenone; Quinidine; Tocainide.*

ABOUT YOUR MEDICINE

Type I antiarrhythmics are used to correct irregular heartbeats to a normal rhythm and to slow an overactive heart.

There is a chance that these medicines may cause new heart rhythm problems when they are used. Usually this effect is rare and mild. However, some of these medicines are more likely than others to cause this effect. For example, encainide and flecainide have been shown to cause severe problems in some patients, and so they are only used to treat serious heart rhythm problems. Discuss this possible effect with your doctor.

If any of the information in this leaflet causes you special concern or if you want additional information about your medicine and its use, check with your doctor, nurse, or pharmacist. **Remember, keep this and all other medicines out of the reach of children and never share your medicines with others.**

BEFORE USING THIS MEDICINE
Tell your doctor, nurse, and pharmacist if you
- are allergic to any medicine, either prescription or non-prescription (OTC);
- are pregnant or intend to become pregnant while using this medicine;
- are breast-feeding;
- are taking **any** other prescription or nonprescription (OTC) medicine;
- have **any** other medical problems.

PROPER USE OF THIS MEDICINE
Take this medicine exactly as directed by your doctor, even though you may feel well. Do not take more medicine than ordered.

For patients taking the extended-release capsules or tablets:
- Swallow whole without breaking, crushing, or chewing.

It is best to take each dose at evenly spaced times day and night.

For patients taking mexiletine:
- To lessen the possibility of stomach upset, this medicine should be taken with food or immediately after meals or with milk or an antacid.

If you miss a dose of this medicine, take it as soon as possible. However, if you do not remember until it is almost time for the next dose, skip the missed dose and go back to your regular dosing schedule. Do not double doses.

PRECAUTIONS WHILE USING THIS MEDICINE
It is important that your doctor check your progress at regular visits to make sure the medicine is working properly to help your heart.

Do not suddenly stop taking this medicine without first checking with your doctor. Stopping it suddenly may cause a serious change in heart activity.

Dizziness or lightheadedness or blurred vision may occur. **Make sure you know how you react to this medicine before you drive, use machines, or do other jobs that require you to be alert and able to see well.**

For patients taking disopyramide:
- **If signs of hypoglycemia (low blood sugar) such as chills, hunger, nausea, nervousness, or sweating appear, eat or**

drink a food containing sugar and call your doctor right away.

- **Use extra care not to become overheated during exercise or hot weather,** since this medicine will often make you sweat less and could possibly result in heatstroke.

POSSIBLE SIDE EFFECTS OF THIS MEDICINE

Side Effects That Should Be Reported To Your Doctor Immediately

For quinidine only, especially after the first dose or first few doses—Breathing difficulty; changes in vision; dizziness, lightheadedness, or fainting; fever; severe headache; ringing in ears; skin rash

Other Side Effects That Should Be Reported To Your Doctor

For all antiarrhythmics—Chest pain; fast or irregular heartbeat; fever or chills; shortness of breath or painful breathing; skin rash or itching; unusual bleeding or bruising

For disopyramide (in addition to above)—Difficult urination; swelling of feet or lower legs

For encainide, flecainide, moricizine, and propafenone (in addition to above)—Swelling of feet or lower legs; trembling or shaking

Side Effects That Usually Do Not Require Medical Attention

These possible side effects may go away during treatment; however, if they continue or are bothersome, check with your doctor, nurse, or pharmacist.

For all antiarrhythmics—Blurred or double vision; dizziness or lightheadedness

For disopyramide (in addition to above)—Dry mouth and throat

For flecainide (in addition to above)—Seeing spots

For mexiletine (in addition to above)—Heartburn; nausea and vomiting; nervousness; trembling or shaking of hands; unsteadiness or trouble walking

For procainamide (in addition to above)—Diarrhea; loss of appetite

For propafenone (in addition to above)—Change in taste

For quinidine (in addition to above)—Bitter taste; diarrhea; flushing of skin with itching; loss of appetite; nausea or vomiting; stomach pain or cramps

For tocainide (in addition to above)—Loss of appetite; nausea

Other side effects not listed above may also occur in some patients. If you notice any other effects, check with your doctor, nurse, or pharmacist.

MINOXIDIL   Systemic

■ For the Pharmacist ■

In providing consultation, consider emphasizing the following selected information (» = major clinical significance):

Before using this medication
» Conditions affecting use, especially:
    Sensitivity to minoxidil
    Pregnancy—Decreased conception and increased resorption in animals; hypertrichosis reported in newborns
    Breast-feeding—Passes into breast milk
    Other medications, especially guanethidine or nitrates
    Other medical problems, especially congestive heart failure, coronary insufficiency, pericardial effusion, pheochromocytoma, or renal function impairment

Proper use of this medication
    Possible need for control of weight and diet, especially sodium intake
» Patient may not experience symptoms of hypertension; importance of taking medication even if feeling well
» Does not cure, but helps control hypertension; possible need for lifelong therapy; serious consequences of untreated hypertension
    Getting into the habit of taking at same time each day to help increase compliance
    Caution in taking combination therapy; taking each drug at the right time
» Proper dosing
    Missed dose: Taking as soon as remembered if within a few hours; not taking if forgotten until next day; not doubling doses
» Proper storage

Precautions while using this medication
    Regular visits to physician to check progress
» Checking resting pulse as directed; checking with physician if an increase of 20 or more beats per minute above normal occurs
» Checking weight daily; weight gain of 2 to 3 lb (approximately 1 kg) in adults is normal and is usually lost with continued treatment; checking with physician if rapid weight gain of more than 5 lb (2 lb in children) or signs of fluid retention occur
» Not taking other medications, especially nonprescription sympathomimetics, unless discussed with physician

Side/adverse effects
    Probability of hypertrichosis, which is reversible when medication is withdrawn
    Signs of potential side effects, especially sodium and water retention, reflex sympathetic activation, angina, pericarditis, allergic reaction, Stevens-Johnson syndrome, paresthesia, and pulmonary hypertension

▲ For the Patient ▲

914403

ABOUT YOUR MEDICINE
Minoxidil (mi-NOX-i-dill) belongs to the general class of medicines called antihypertensives. It is used to treat high blood pressure (hypertension).

Minoxidil is being applied to the scalp in liquid form by some balding men to stimulate hair growth. However, improper use of liquids made from minoxidil tablets can result in minoxidil being absorbed into the body, where it may cause unwanted effects on the heart and blood vessels.

If any of the information in this leaflet causes you special concern or if you want additional information about your medicine and its use, check with your doctor, nurse, or pharmacist. **Remember, keep this and all other medicines out of the reach of children and never share your medicines with others.**

BEFORE USING THIS MEDICINE

Tell your doctor, nurse, and pharmacist if you . . .

- are allergic to any medicine, either prescription or non-prescription (OTC);
- are pregnant or intend to become pregnant while using this medicine;
- are breast-feeding;
- are taking any other prescription or nonprescription (OTC) medicine, especially nitrates (medicine for angina) or other antihypertensives;
- have any other medical problems, especially angina (chest pain), heart or blood vessel disease, kidney disease, or pheochromocytoma.

PROPER USE OF THIS MEDICINE

Importance of diet—When prescribing medicine for your condition, your doctor may also prescribe a personal diet for you. Such a diet may be low in sodium (salt). Medicine is usually more effective when such a diet is properly followed.

Many patients who have high blood pressure will not notice any signs of the problem. In fact, many may feel normal. It is very important that you **take your medicine exactly as directed** and that you keep your doctor's appointments even if you feel well.

This medicine will not cure your high blood pressure but it does help control it. You must continue to take it—even if you feel well—if you expect to keep your blood pressure down. **You may have to take high blood pressure medicine for the rest of your life.**

If you miss a dose of this medicine and remember within a few hours, take it when you remember. However, if you do not remember until the next day, skip the missed dose and go back to your regular schedule. Do not double doses.

PRECAUTIONS WHILE USING THIS MEDICINE

Ask your doctor about checking your pulse rate before and after taking minoxidil. Then, while you are taking this medicine, **check your pulse regularly while you are resting.** If it increases by 20 beats or more a minute, check with your doctor right away.

While you are taking minoxidil, **weigh yourself every day.** A weight gain of 2 to 3 pounds (about 1 kg) in an adult is normal and should be lost with continued treatment. However, if you suddenly gain 5 pounds (2 kg) or more (for a child, 2 pounds [1 kg] or more) or if you notice swelling of your feet or lower legs, check with your doctor right away.

Do not take other medicines unless they have been discussed with your doctor. This especially includes over-the-counter (nonprescription) medicines for appetite control, asthma, colds, cough, hay fever, or sinus problems.

POSSIBLE SIDE EFFECTS OF THIS MEDICINE

Side Effects That Should Be Reported To Your Doctor Immediately

> *More common*—Fast or irregular heartbeat; rapid weight gain of more than 5 pounds (2 pounds in children)

> *Less common*—Chest pain; shortness of breath

Other Side Effects That Should Be Reported To Your Doctor

> *More common*—Bloating; flushing or redness of skin; swelling of feet or lower legs

> *Less common*—Numbness or tingling of hands, feet, or face

> *Rare*—Skin rash and itching

Side Effects That Usually Do Not Require Medical Attention

These possible side effects may go away during treatment; however, if they continue or are bothersome, check with your doctor, nurse, or pharmacist.

> *More common*—Increase in hair growth, usually on face, arms, and back

This medicine causes a temporary increase in hair growth in most people. Hair may grow longer and darker in both men and women. This may first be noticed on the face several weeks after you start taking minoxidil. Later, new hair growth may be noticed on the back, arms, legs, and scalp. Talk to your doctor about shaving or using a hair remover during this time. After treatment with minoxidil has ended, the hair will stop growing, although it may take several months for the new hair growth to go away.

Other side effects not listed above may also occur in some patients. If you notice any other effects, check with your doctor, nurse, or pharmacist.

MINOXIDIL   Topical

■For the Pharmacist■

In providing consultation, consider emphasizing the following selected information (» = major clinical significance):

Before using this medication
» Conditions affecting use, especially:
    Sensitivity to minoxidil
    Pregnancy—Animal studies have shown problems during pregnancy, but not birth defects
    Breast-feeding—Not recommended, since medication may cause problems in nursing babies
    Other medications, especially topical corticosteroids, petrolatum, or retinoids

Proper use of this medication
    Reading patient instructions carefully
» Not using more medication or more frequently than prescribed; not applying to other parts of body; risk of adverse systemic effects with excessive use
» Not using other skin products on treated skin
    Proper administration technique:
    Shampooing hair each morning, before first daily application; applying to affected area of dry scalp, beginning at the center of the balding area
    Method of application depends on applicator used (pump spray, extended tip, or rub-on assembly)
    Washing hands immediately after application to remove any medication that may be on them
    Not using hairdryer to speed drying
    Not going to bed until at least 30 minutes after application, to minimize transfer onto pillowcase
    Checking with physician before applying to abraded, irritated, or sunburned scalp
» Avoiding contact with eyes, nose, or mouth; flushing area with large amounts of cool tap water if accidental contact occurs; avoiding inhalation of pump spray
» Proper dosing
    Missed dose: Using as soon as remembered if within a few hours; not using if almost time for next dose; not doubling amount used
» Proper storage

Precautions while using this medication
    Regular visits to physician to check progress
    Telling physician if itching, burning, or redness occur after application; if reaction is severe, washing minoxidil off and checking with physician before using again

Side/adverse effects
    Signs of potential side effects, especially dermatitis, allergic reaction, burning of scalp, folliculitis, increased alopecia, dizziness, eczema, lightheadedness, headache, sexual dysfunction, visual disturbances (including decreased visual acuity), and systemic absorption (chest pain, fast or irregular heartbeat, hypotension, neuritis, sodium and water retention, and vasodilation)

▲ For the Patient ▲

916726

ABOUT YOUR MEDICINE

Minoxidil (mi-NOX-i-dill) applied to the scalp is used to stimulate hair growth in men and women with a certain type of baldness. Minoxidil may also be used for other conditions as determined by your doctor.

If hair growth is going to occur with the use of minoxidil, it usually occurs after the medicine has been used for about 4 months and lasts only as long as the medicine continues to be used. The new hair will be lost within a few months after minoxidil treatment is stopped.

If any of the information in this leaflet causes you special concern or if you want additional information about your medicine and its use, check with your doctor, nurse, or pharmacist. **Remember, keep this and all other medicines out of the reach of children and never share your medicines with others.**

BEFORE USING THIS MEDICINE

Tell your doctor, nurse, and pharmacist if you . . .
- are allergic to any medicine, either prescription or non-prescription (OTC);
- are pregnant or intend to become pregnant while using this medicine;
- are breast-feeding;
- are taking any other prescription or nonprescription (OTC) medicine, especially minoxidil taken by mouth, or are using any medicine on your scalp, especially corticosteroids (cortisone-like medicine), petrolatum, or tretinoin;
- have any other medical problems.

PROPER USE OF THIS MEDICINE

This medicine usually comes with patient instructions. It is important that you read the instructions carefully.

It is very important that you use this medicine only as directed. Do not use more of it, do not use it more often than your doctor ordered, and do not apply it to other parts of your body. Such use may increase the chance of the medicine being absorbed through the skin. Absorption into the body may affect the heart and blood vessels and cause unwanted effects.

Do not use any other skin product on the same skin area on which you use minoxidil.

To apply minoxidil solution:
- Shampoo your hair each morning before applying minoxidil. Make sure your hair and scalp are completely dry before applying this medicine.

- Apply the amount prescribed to the area of the scalp being treated, beginning in the center of the area. Follow your doctor's instructions on how to apply the solution, using the applicator provided.

- Immediately after using this medicine, wash your hands to remove any medicine that may be on them.

- Do not use a hairdryer to dry the scalp after you apply minoxidil solution. Blowing with a hairdryer on the scalp may make the treatment less effective.

- If you are using this medicine at bedtime, do not go to bed until at least 30 minutes after you use it. This will help prevent the medicine from rubbing off on the pillowcase.

If your scalp becomes abraded, irritated, or sunburned, check with your doctor before applying minoxidil.

Keep this medicine away from the eyes, nose, and mouth. If you should accidentally get some in your eyes, nose, or mouth, flush the area thoroughly with cool tap water. If you are using the pump spray, be careful not to breathe in the spray.

If you miss a dose of this medicine, go back to your regular dosing schedule. Do not double doses.

PRECAUTIONS WHILE USING THIS MEDICINE

It is important that your doctor check your progress at regular visits to make sure that this medicine is working properly and to check for unwanted effects.

Tell your doctor if you notice itching, redness, or burning of your scalp after you apply minoxidil. If the itching, redness, or burning is severe, wash the medicine off and check with your doctor before using it again.

POSSIBLE SIDE EFFECTS OF THIS MEDICINE
Side Effects That Should Be Reported To Your Doctor

Less common—Itching or skin rash

Rare—Blurred vision or other change in vision; burning of scalp; decrease in sexual ability or desire; dizziness; increased hair loss; lightheadedness; soreness at root of hair; swelling of face

Signs of too much medicine being absorbed into the body—Rare—Chest pain; fast or irregular heartbeat; flushing; headache; numbness or tingling of hands, feet, or face; swelling of face, hands, feet, or lower legs; weight gain (rapid)

Side Effects That Usually Do Not Require Medical Attention

These possible side effects may go away during treatment; however, if they continue or are bothersome, check with your doctor, nurse, or pharmacist.

Less common—Dry or flaking skin; reddened skin

Other side effects not listed above may also occur in some
patients. If you notice any other effects, check with your
doctor, nurse, or pharmacist.

MISOPROSTOL   Systemic

■ For the Pharmacist ■

In providing consultation, consider emphasizing the following selected information (» = major clinical significance):

Before using this medication
» Conditions affecting use, especially:
   Sensitivity to prostaglandins or prostaglandin analogs
   Pregnancy—Contraindicated during pregnancy because of risk of miscarriage; patients of childbearing potential must take measures to assure they are not pregnant prior to therapy and to prevent pregnancy during therapy
   Breast-feeding—Not recommended because of possibility of causing diarrhea in nursing infant

Proper use of this medication
   Taking with or after meals and at bedtime
» Proper dosing
   Missed dose: Taking as soon as possible; not taking if almost time for next dose; not doubling doses
» Proper storage
For use in the treatment of duodenal ulcer
   Taking antacids for relief of ulcer pain; not taking magnesium-containing antacids
   Compliance with full course of therapy and keeping appointments for check-ups
» Not taking for more than 4 weeks unless otherwise directed by physician

Precautions while using this medication
   Stopping medication and checking with physician immediately if pregnancy is suspected
   Consulting physician if diarrhea develops and continues for more than a week

Side/adverse effects
   Signs of potential side effects, especially continuing and severe diarrhea

▲ For the Patient ▲

916657

ABOUT YOUR MEDICINE

Misoprostol (mye-soe-PROST-ole) is taken to prevent stomach ulcers in patients taking anti-inflammatory drugs, including aspirin. Misoprostol may also be used for other conditions as determined by your doctor.

If any of the information in this leaflet causes you special concern or if you want additional information about your medicine and its use, check with your doctor, nurse, or pharmacist. **Remember, keep this and all other medicines out of the reach of children and never share your medicines with others.**

BEFORE USING THIS MEDICINE

Tell your doctor, nurse, and pharmacist if you . . .
- are allergic to any medicine, either prescription or non-prescription (OTC);
- are pregnant or intend to become pregnant while using this medicine;
- are breast-feeding;
- are taking any other prescription or nonprescription (OTC) medicine;
- have any other medical problems.

PROPER USE OF THIS MEDICINE

Misoprostol is best taken with or after meals and at bedtime, unless otherwise directed by your doctor.

Antacids may be taken with misoprostol, if needed, to help relieve stomach pain, unless you are otherwise directed by your doctor. However, do not take magnesium-containing antacids, since they may worsen the diarrhea that is sometimes caused by misoprostol.

Take this medicine for the full time of treatment, even if you begin to feel better. Also, it is important that you keep your appointments with your doctor so that he or she will be better able to tell you when to stop taking this medicine.

If you miss a dose of this medicine, take it as soon as possible. However, if it is almost time for your next dose, skip the missed dose and go back to your regular dosing schedule. Do not double doses.

PRECAUTIONS WHILE USING THIS MEDICINE

Misoprostol may cause miscarriage if taken during pregnancy. Therefore, if you suspect that you may have become pregnant, stop taking this medicine immediately and check with your doctor.

This medicine may cause diarrhea in some people. The diarrhea will usually disappear within a few days as your body adjusts to the medicine. However, check with your doctor if the diarrhea is severe and/or does not stop after a week. Your doctor may need to lower the dose of misoprostol you are taking.

POSSIBLE SIDE EFFECTS OF THIS MEDICINE

Side Effects That Usually Do Not Require Medical Attention

These possible side effects may go away during treatment; however, if they continue or are bothersome, check with your doctor, nurse, or pharmacist.

> *More common*—Abdominal or stomach pain (mild); diarrhea

> *Less common or rare*—Bleeding from vagina; constipation; cramps in lower abdomen or stomach area; gas; headache; nausea and/or vomiting

Other side effects not listed above may also occur in some patients. If you notice any other effects, check with your doctor, nurse, or pharmacist.

MOLINDONE   Systemic

■For the Pharmacist■

In providing consultation, consider emphasizing the following selected information (» = major clinical significance):

Before using this medication
» Conditions affecting use, especially:
  Sensitivity to molindone or other antipsychotic medications
  Pregnancy—Studies in mice have shown a slight increase in resorptions
  Use in the elderly—Elderly patients are more likely to develop extrapyramidal, anticholinergic, hypotensive, and sedative effects; reduced dosage recommended
  Dental—Dry mouth may cause caries, candidiasis, periodontal disease, and discomfort; increased motor activity of face, head, and neck may interfere with some dental procedures
  Other medications, especially alcohol, other CNS depression–producing medications, other extrapyramidal reaction–producing medications, or lithium
  Other medical problems, especially severe drug-induced CNS depression

Proper use of this medication
  Taking with food or a full glass (8 ounces) of water or milk to reduce gastric irritation
  Taking liquid form of medicine undiluted or mixed with water, milk, fruit juice, or carbonated beverage
» Compliance with therapy: importance of not taking more or less medication than the amount prescribed
» May require several weeks of therapy to obtain optimal effects
» Proper dosing
  Missed dose: Taking as soon as possible; not taking if within 2 hours of next scheduled dose; resuming regular schedule; not doubling doses
» Proper storage

Precautions while using this medication
  Regular visits to physician to check progress of therapy
» Checking with physician before discontinuing medication; gradual dosage reduction may be needed
» Avoiding use of antacids or antidiarrheal medication within 2 hours of taking molindone
» Avoiding use of alcoholic beverages or other CNS depressants during therapy
  Avoiding the use of over-the-counter medications for colds or allergies, to prevent increased anticholinergic effects and risk of heat stroke
» Possible drowsiness; caution when driving, using machinery, or doing other things that require alertness
» Possible dizziness or lightheadedness; caution when getting up suddenly from a lying or sitting position
» Possible heat stroke: caution during exercise, hot weather, or hot baths or saunas
  Possible dryness of mouth; using sugarless gum or candy, ice, or saliva substitute for relief; checking with physician or dentist if dry mouth continues for more than 2 weeks

Side/adverse effects

» Stopping medication and notifying physician immediately if symptoms of neuroleptic malignant syndrome (NMS) appear

» Notifying physician as soon as possible if early signs of tardive dyskinesia appear

Possibility of withdrawal emergent dyskinesia

Signs of potential side effects, especially akathisia, dystonias, parkinsonism, tardive dyskinesia, mental depression, allergic reaction, heat stroke, cholestatic jaundice or hepatitis, neuroleptic malignant syndrome (NMS), or tardive dystonia

---

▲ For the Patient ▲

915698

ABOUT YOUR MEDICINE

Molindone (moe-LIN-done) is used to treat nervous, mental, and emotional conditions.

If any of the information in this leaflet causes you special concern or if you want additional information about your medicine and its use, check with your doctor, nurse, or pharmacist. **Remember, keep this and all other medicines out of the reach of children and never share your medicines with others.**

BEFORE USING THIS MEDICINE

Discuss with your doctor possible side effects of this medicine. Some may be serious and/or permanent. For example, tardive dyskinesia (a movement disorder) may occur and may not go away after you stop using the medicine.

Tell your doctor, nurse, and pharmacist if you . . .

- are allergic to any medicine, either prescription or nonprescription (OTC);
- are pregnant or intend to become pregnant while using this medicine;
- are breast-feeding;
- are taking **any** other prescription or nonprescription (OTC) medicine;
- have any other medical problems.

PROPER USE OF THIS MEDICINE

Molindone should be taken with food or a full glass of water or milk.

Take this medicine only as directed. Do not take more of it, do not take it more often, and do not take it for a longer time than ordered. **Sometimes this medicine must be taken for several weeks before its full effect is reached.**

If you miss a dose of this medicine, take it as soon as possible. However, if it is within 2 hours of your next dose, skip the missed dose and go back to your regular dosing schedule. Do not double doses.

PRECAUTIONS WHILE USING THIS MEDICINE

Your doctor should check your progress at regular visits.

Do not stop taking this medicine without first checking with your doctor. Your doctor may want you to reduce gradually the amount you are taking.

Do not take molindone within 1 or 2 hours of taking antacids or medicine for diarrhea.

This medicine will add to the effects of alcohol and other CNS depressants (medicines that slow down the nervous system). **Check with your doctor before taking any such depressants while you are using this medicine.**

Molindone may cause some people to become drowsy or less alert than they are normally. **Make sure you know how you react to this medicine before you drive, use machines, or do other jobs that require you to be alert.**

Dizziness or lightheadedness may occur, especially when you get up from a lying or sitting position. Getting up slowly may help.

This medicine will often make you sweat less, causing your body temperature to rise. **Use extra care not to become overheated during exercise, hot baths or saunas, or hot weather while you are taking this medicine.** Overheating may make you feel dizzy or faint and can result in heatstroke.

POSSIBLE SIDE EFFECTS OF THIS MEDICINE

Side Effects That Should Be Reported To Your Doctor Immediately

Stop taking this medicine and get emergency help immediately if any of the following side effects occur:

 Rare—Convulsions (seizures); difficult or fast breathing; fast heartbeat or irregular pulse; fever (high); high or low (irregular) blood pressure; increased sweating; loss of bladder control; muscle stiffness (severe); unusual tiredness or weakness; unusually pale skin

Other Side Effects That Should Be Reported To Your Doctor

 More common—Difficulty in talking or swallowing; inability to move eyes; lip smacking or puckering; loss of balance control; mask-like face; muscle spasms, especially of the neck and back; puffing of cheeks; rapid or worm-like movements of the tongue; restlessness or need to keep moving (severe); shuffling walk; stiff arms and legs; trembling and shaking of hands; twisting movements of body; uncontrolled movements of arms and legs; unusual chewing movements

 Less common or rare—Confusion; hot, dry skin, or lack of sweating; mental depression; muscle weakness; skin rash; yellow eyes or skin

Side Effects That Usually Do Not Require Medical Attention

These possible side effects may go away during treatment; however, if they continue or are bothersome, check with your doctor, nurse, or pharmacist.

> *More common*—Blurred vision; constipation; decreased sweating; difficult urination; dizziness or lightheadedness, especially when getting up suddenly; drowsiness; dry mouth; headache; nausea; stuffy nose

Some side effects may occur after you have stopped taking this medicine. Check with your doctor as soon as possible if you notice uncontrolled chewing movements, lip smacking or puckering, puffing of cheeks, rapid or worm-like movements of tongue, or uncontrolled movements of arms and legs.

Other side effects not listed above may also occur in some patients. If you notice any other effects, check with your doctor, nurse, or pharmacist.

MORICIZINE Systemic

■ For the Pharmacist ■

In providing consultation, consider emphasizing the following selected
information (» = major clinical significance):

Before using this medication
» Conditions affecting use, especially:
 Sensitivity to moricizine
 Other medical problems, especially second or third degree atrioventricular (AV) block, right bundle branch block associated
 with a left hemiblock, cardiogenic shock, or sick sinus syndrome

Proper use of this medication
» Compliance with therapy; taking as directed even if feeling well
» Importance of not missing doses and taking at evenly spaced inter-
 vals
» Proper dosing
 Missed dose: Taking as soon as possible if remembered within 4
 hours; not taking if remembered later; not doubling doses
» Proper storage

Precautions while using this medication
 Regular visits to physician to check progress
 Carrying medical identification card or bracelet
» Caution if any kind of surgery (including dental surgery) or emer-
 gency treatment is required
 Caution when driving or doing things requiring alertness because of
 possible dizziness

Side/adverse effects
 Signs of potential side effects, especially chest pain, congestive heart
 failure, ventricular tachyarrhythmias, and drug fever

▲ For the Patient ▲

913036

ANTIARRHYTHMICS, TYPE I (Oral): *Including
Disopyramide; Encainide; Flecainide; Mexiletine;
Moricizine; Procainamide; Propafenone; Quinidine;
Tocainide.*

ABOUT YOUR MEDICINE

Type I antiarrhythmics are used to correct irregular heartbeats to a normal rhythm and to slow an overactive heart.

There is a chance that these medicines may cause new heart
rhythm problems when they are used. Usually this effect is
rare and mild. However, some of these medicines are more
likely than others to cause this effect. For example, encainide
and flecainide have been shown to cause severe problems in
some patients, and so they are only used to treat serious
heart rhythm problems. Discuss this possible effect with
your doctor.

If any of the information in this leaflet causes you special concern or if you want additional information about your medicine and its use, check with your doctor, nurse, or pharmacist. **Remember, keep this and all other medicines out of the reach of children and never share your medicines with others.**

BEFORE USING THIS MEDICINE

Tell your doctor, nurse, and pharmacist if you . . .
- are allergic to any medicine, either prescription or non-prescription (OTC);
- are pregnant or intend to become pregnant while using this medicine;
- are breast-feeding;
- are taking **any** other prescription or nonprescription (OTC) medicine;
- have **any** other medical problems.

PROPER USE OF THIS MEDICINE

Take this medicine exactly as directed by your doctor, even though you may feel well. Do not take more medicine than ordered.

For patients taking the extended-release capsules or tablets:
- Swallow whole without breaking, crushing, or chewing.

It is best to take each dose at evenly spaced times day and night.

For patients taking mexiletine:
- To lessen the possibility of stomach upset, this medicine should be taken with food or immediately after meals or with milk or an antacid.

If you miss a dose of this medicine, take it as soon as possible. However, if you do not remember until it is almost time for the next dose, skip the missed dose and go back to your regular dosing schedule. Do not double doses.

PRECAUTIONS WHILE USING THIS MEDICINE

It is important that your doctor check your progress at regular visits to make sure the medicine is working properly to help your heart.

Do not suddenly stop taking this medicine without first checking with your doctor. Stopping it suddenly may cause a serious change in heart activity.

Dizziness or lightheadedness or blurred vision may occur. **Make sure you know how you react to this medicine before you drive, use machines, or do other jobs that require you to be alert and able to see well.**

For patients taking disopyramide:
- **If signs of hypoglycemia (low blood sugar) such as chills, hunger, nausea, nervousness, or sweating appear, eat or drink a food containing sugar and call your doctor right away.**

• **Use extra care not to become overheated during exercise or hot weather,** since this medicine will often make you sweat less and could possibly result in heatstroke.

POSSIBLE SIDE EFFECTS OF THIS MEDICINE
Side Effects That Should Be Reported To Your Doctor Immediately

> *For quinidine only, especially after the first dose or first few doses*—Breathing difficulty; changes in vision; dizziness, lightheadedness, or fainting; fever; severe headache; ringing in ears; skin rash

Other Side Effects That Should Be Reported To Your Doctor

> *For all antiarrhythmics*—Chest pain; fast or irregular heartbeat; fever or chills; shortness of breath or painful breathing; skin rash or itching; unusual bleeding or bruising

> *For disopyramide (in addition to above)*—Difficult urination; swelling of feet or lower legs

> *For encainide, flecainide, moricizine, and propafenone (in addition to above)*—Swelling of feet or lower legs; trembling or shaking

Side Effects That Usually Do Not Require Medical Attention

These possible side effects may go away during treatment; however, if they continue or are bothersome, check with your doctor, nurse, or pharmacist.

> *For all antiarrhythmics*—Blurred or double vision; dizziness or lightheadedness

> *For disopyramide (in addition to above)*—Dry mouth and throat

> *For flecainide (in addition to above)*—Seeing spots

> *For mexiletine (in addition to above)*—Heartburn; nausea and vomiting; nervousness; trembling or shaking of hands; unsteadiness or trouble walking

> *For procainamide (in addition to above)*—Diarrhea; loss of appetite

> *For propafenone (in addition to above)*—Change in taste

> *For quinidine (in addition to above)*—Bitter taste; diarrhea; flushing of skin with itching; loss of appetite; nausea or vomiting; stomach pain or cramps

> *For tocainide (in addition to above)*—Loss of appetite; nausea

Other side effects not listed above may also occur in some patients. If you notice any other effects, check with your doctor, nurse, or pharmacist.

MUPIROCIN Topical

■ For the Pharmacist ■

In providing consultation, consider emphasizing the following selected information (» = major clinical significance):

Proper use of this medication
» Not for ophthalmic use
  To use:
      Before applying, washing affected area(s) with soap and water and drying thoroughly; applying small amount and rubbing in gently
      After applying, covering treated area(s) with gauze dressing if desired
» Compliance with full course of therapy
» Proper dosing
  Missed dose: Applying as soon as possible; not applying if almost time for next dose
» Proper storage

Precautions while using this medication
  Checking with physician or pharmacist if no improvement within 3 to 5 days

▲ For the Patient ▲

916680

ABOUT YOUR MEDICINE

Mupirocin (myoo-PEER-oh-sin) is used to treat bacterial infections. It is applied to the skin to treat impetigo. It may also be used for other bacterial skin infections as determined by your doctor.

If any of the information in this leaflet causes you special concern or if you want additional information about your medicine and its use, check with your doctor, nurse, or pharmacist. **Remember, keep this and all other medicines out of the reach of children and never share your medicines with others.**

BEFORE USING THIS MEDICINE

Tell your doctor, nurse, and pharmacist if you . . .
- are allergic to any medicine, either prescription or non-prescription (OTC);
- are pregnant or intend to become pregnant while using this medicine;
- are breast-feeding;
- are taking any other prescription or nonprescription (OTC) medicine;
- have any other medical problems.

PROPER USE OF THIS MEDICINE
Do not use this medicine in the eyes.

To use:

- Before applying this medicine, wash the affected area with soap and water, and dry thoroughly. Then apply a small amount to the affected area and rub in gently.

- After applying this medicine, the treated area may be covered with a gauze dressing if desired.

To help clear up your skin infection completely, keep using mupirocin for the full time of treatment, even if your symptoms have disappeared. **Do not miss any doses.**

If you do miss a dose of this medicine, apply it as soon as possible. However, if it is almost time for your next dose, skip the missed dose and go back to your regular dosing schedule.

PRECAUTIONS WHILE USING THIS MEDICINE
If your skin infection does not improve within 3 to 5 days, or if it becomes worse, check with your doctor or pharmacist.

POSSIBLE SIDE EFFECTS OF THIS MEDICINE
Side Effects That Usually Do Not Require Medical Attention

These possible side effects may go away during treatment; however, if they continue or are bothersome, check with your doctor, nurse, or pharmacist.

> *Less common*—Dry skin; skin burning, itching, pain, rash, redness, stinging, or swelling

Other side effects not listed above may also occur in some patients. If you notice any other effects, check with your doctor, nurse, or pharmacist.

NABILONE   Systemic

■For the Pharmacist■

In providing consultation, consider emphasizing the following selected
information (» = major clinical significance):

Before using this medication
» Conditions affecting use, especially:
  Sensitivity to nabilone or other marijuana products
  Pregnancy—No studies in humans; increased risk of fetal re-
    sorptions and stillbirths in animal studies with doses many
    times the usual human dose
  Breast-feeding—Use not recommended; although not known if
    distributed into breast milk, possibility exists
  Use in the elderly—Increased sensitivity to cardiac effects and
    orthostatic hypotension; caution recommended because of
    psychoactive effects and potential for dependence
  Other medications, especially CNS depressants
  Other medical problems, especially manic depression and schizo-
    phrenia

Proper use of this medication
» Importance of not taking more medication than the amount pre-
    scribed because of danger of overdose
» Proper dosing
» Missed dose: Taking as soon as possible; not taking if almost time
    for next dose; not doubling doses
» Proper storage

Precautions while using this medication
» Avoiding use of alcohol or other CNS depressants during therapy
» Suspected overdose: Getting emergency help at once
» Caution if dizziness, drowsiness, lightheadedness, or false sense of
    well-being occurs
  Caution when getting up suddenly from a lying or sitting position
  Possible dryness of mouth; using sugarless candy or gum, ice, or
    saliva substitute for relief

Side/adverse effects
  Signs of potential side effects, especially psychiatric effects, diffi-
    culty in breathing, hypotension, tachycardia, hypertension, and
    unusual tiredness or weakness

▲ For the Patient ▲

915701

ABOUT YOUR MEDICINE

Nabilone (NAB-i-lone) is chemically related to marijuana.
It is used to prevent the nausea and vomiting that may occur
after treatment with cancer medicines. It is used only when
other kinds of medicine for nausea and vomiting do not work.

If any of the information in this leaflet causes you special
concern or if you want additional information about your
medicine and its use, check with your doctor, nurse, or pharmacist. **Remember, keep this and all other medicines out of**

the reach of children and never share your medicines with others.

BEFORE USING THIS MEDICINE

Tell your doctor, nurse, and pharmacist if you . . .
- are allergic to any medicine, either prescription or non-prescription (OTC);
- are pregnant or intend to become pregnant while using this medicine;
- are breast-feeding;
- are taking any other prescription or nonprescription (OTC) medicine, especially central nervous system (CNS) depressants or tricyclic antidepressants;
- have any other medical problems, especially manic depression or schizophrenia.

PROPER USE OF THIS MEDICINE

Take this medicine only as directed by your doctor. Do not take more of it, do not take it more often, and do not take it for a longer time than your doctor ordered. If too much is taken, it may lead to other medical problems because of an overdose.

If you miss a dose of this medicine, take it as soon as you remember. However, if it is almost time for your next dose, skip the missed dose and go back to your regular dosing schedule. **Do not double doses.**

PRECAUTIONS WHILE USING THIS MEDICINE

Nabilone will add to the effects of alcohol and other CNS depressants (medicines that slow down the nervous system). **Check with your doctor before taking any such depressants while you are taking this medicine.**

If you think you or someone else may have taken an overdose, get emergency help at once. Taking an overdose of this medicine or taking alcohol or CNS depressants with this medicine may cause severe mental effects. Symptoms of overdose include changes in mood; confusion; difficulty in breathing; dizziness (severe) or fainting; hallucinations; increase in blood pressure; mental depression; nervousness or anxiety; fast, slow, irregular, or pounding heartbeat; and unusual tiredness or weakness (severe).

This medicine may cause some people to become drowsy, dizzy, or lightheaded, or to feel a false sense of well-being. **Make sure you know how you react to this medicine before you drive, use machines, or do other jobs that require you to be alert and clearheaded.**

Dizziness, lightheadedness, or fainting may occur, especially when you get up suddenly from a lying or sitting position. Getting up slowly may help lessen this problem.

Nabilone may cause dryness of the mouth. For temporary relief, use sugarless candy or gum, melt bits of ice in your mouth, or use a saliva substitute.

POSSIBLE SIDE EFFECTS OF THIS MEDICINE
Side Effects That Should Be Reported To Your Doctor Immediately

> *Signs of overdose*—Changes in mood; confusion; difficulty in breathing; dizziness (severe) or fainting; fast, slow, irregular, or pounding heartbeat; hallucinations; increase in blood pressure; mental depression; nervousness or anxiety; unusual tiredness or weakness (severe)

Side Effects That Usually Do Not Require Medical Attention

These possible side effects may go away during treatment; however, if they continue or are bothersome, check with your doctor, nurse, or pharmacist.

> *More common*—Clumsiness or unsteadiness; difficulty concentrating; drowsiness; dry mouth; false sense of well-being; headache

> *Less common or rare*—Blurred vision or any changes in vision; dizziness or lightheadedness, especially when getting up from a lying or sitting position—more common with high doses; loss of appetite; muscle pain or weakness

Other side effects not listed above may also occur in some patients. If you notice any other effects, check with your doctor, nurse, or pharmacist.

NALIDIXIC ACID   Systemic

■For the Pharmacist■

In providing consultation, consider emphasizing the following selected
information (》 = major clinical significance):

Before using this medication
》 Conditions affecting use, especially:
> Hypersensitivity to nalidixic acid or other quinolone derivatives
> (cinoxacin, fluoroquinolones)
> Pregnancy—Nalidixic acid crosses the placenta and is not rec-
> ommended during pregnancy
> Breast-feeding—Nalidixic acid is excreted in breast milk
> Use in children—Nalidixic acid is not recommended in infants
> up to 3 months of age since it has been found to cause ar-
> thropathy in young animals
> Other medications, especially coumarin- and indandione-deriv-
> ative anticoagulants
> Other medical problems, especially a history of seizure disorders
> or severe hepatic impairment

Proper use of this medication
》 Not giving to infants up to 3 months of age; has caused arthropathy
in immature animals
> Taking on an empty stomach, or with food or milk if gastrointestinal
> irritation occurs
> Proper administration technique for oral liquids
》 Compliance with full course of therapy
》 Proper dosing
> Missed dose: Taking as soon as possible; not taking if almost time
> for next dose; not doubling doses
》 Proper storage

Precautions while using this medication
> Regular visits to physician to check progress if therapy lasts longer
> than 2 weeks
> Checking with physician if no improvement within 2 days
》 Caution if blurred vision or other vision problems, dizziness, or
drowsiness occurs
》 Possible skin photosensitivity; avoiding unprotected exposure to sun;
using protective clothing; using a sun block product that includes
protection against both UVA-caused photosensitivity reactions
and UVB-caused sunburn reactions; avoiding use of sunlamp,
tanning bed, or tanning booth
》 Diabetics: False-positive reactions with copper sulfate urine glucose
tests may occur

Side/adverse effects
> Signs of potential side effects, especially visual disturbances, blood
> dyscrasias, cholestatic jaundice, CNS toxicity, and hypersensi-
> tivity

▲ For the Patient ▲

919189

ABOUT YOUR MEDICINE

Nalidixic (nal-i-DIX-ik) **acid** is used to treat infections of the urinary tract. It may also be used for other problems as determined by your doctor.

If any of the information in this leaflet causes you special concern or if you want additional information about your medicine and its use, check with your doctor, nurse, or pharmacist. **Remember, keep this and all other medicines out of the reach of children and never share your medicines with others.**

BEFORE USING THIS MEDICINE

Tell your doctor, nurse, and pharmacist if you . . .
* are allergic to any medicine, either prescription or non-prescription (OTC);
* are pregnant or intend to become pregnant while using this medicine;
* are breast-feeding;
* are taking any other prescription or nonprescription (OTC) medicine, especially anticoagulants (blood thinners);
* have any other medical problems, especially liver disease or a history of convulsive disorders (seizures, epilepsy).

PROPER USE OF THIS MEDICINE

Do not give this medicine to infants or children unless otherwise directed by your doctor. It has been shown to cause bone problems in young animals.

Nalidixic acid is best taken with a full glass (8 ounces) of water on an empty stomach (either 1 hour before or 2 hours after meals). However, if this medicine causes nausea or upset stomach, it may be taken with food or milk.

For patients taking the oral liquid form of this medicine:
* Use a specially marked measuring spoon or other device to measure each dose accurately. The average household teaspoon may not hold the right amount of liquid.

To help clear up your infection completely, **keep taking this medicine for the full time of treatment,** even if you begin to feel better after a few days. **Do not miss any doses.**

If you do miss a dose of this medicine, take it as soon as possible. However, if it is almost time for your next dose, skip the missed dose and go back to your regular dosing schedule. Do not double doses.

PRECAUTIONS WHILE USING THIS MEDICINE

If you will be taking this medicine for more than 2 weeks, your doctor should check your progress at regular visits.

If your symptoms do not improve within 2 days, or if they become worse, check with your doctor.

This medicine may cause blurred vision or other vision problems. It may also cause some people to become dizzy, drowsy, or less alert than they are normally. **Make sure you know how you react to this medicine before you drive, use machines, or do other jobs that could be dangerous if you are dizzy or are not alert or able to see well.**

Nalidixic acid may cause your skin to be more sensitive to sunlight than it is normally. When you first begin taking this medicine, avoid too much sun and do not use a sunlamp until you see how you react to the sun, especially if you tend to burn easily. **If you have a severe reaction, check with your doctor.**

For diabetic patients—**This medicine may cause false test results with some urine glucose (sugar) tests.** Check with your doctor before changing your diet or the dosage of your diabetes medicine.

POSSIBLE SIDE EFFECTS OF THIS MEDICINE
Side Effects That Should Be Reported To Your Doctor Immediately

> *More common*—Blurred or decreased vision; change in color vision; double vision; halos around lights; over-bright appearance of lights

> *Rare*—Bulging of fontanel (soft spot) on top of head of an infant; convulsions (seizures); dark or amber urine; hallucinations; headache (severe); mood or other mental changes; pale skin; pale stools; skin rash and itching; sore throat and fever; stomach pain (severe); unusual bleeding or bruising; unusual tiredness or weakness; yellow eyes or skin

Side Effects That Usually Do Not Require Medical Attention

These possible side effects may go away during treatment; however, if they continue or are bothersome, check with your doctor, nurse, or pharmacist.

> *More common*—Diarrhea; dizziness; drowsiness; headache; nausea or vomiting; stomach pain

> *Less common*—Increased sensitivity of skin to sunlight

Other side effects not listed above may also occur in some patients. If you notice any other effects, check with your doctor, nurse, or pharmacist.

NALTREXONE   Systemic

■For the Pharmacist■

In providing consultation, consider emphasizing the following selected
  information (» = major clinical significance):

Before using this medication
» Conditions affecting use, especially:
> Allergic reaction to naltrexone, history of
> Other medications, especially opioids
> Other medical problems, especially hepatitis or other hepatic
> disease

Proper use of this medication
» Importance of taking each dose as scheduled
» Proper dosing
> Missed dose: If dosing schedule is—
>> One tablet every day: Taking as soon as possible; not taking if
>> not remembered until next day; not doubling next day's dose
>> One tablet every weekday and two tablets on Saturday:
>>> If weekday dose missed—Following missed dose directions
>>> as for one tablet every day
>>> If Saturday dose missed—Taking two tablets as soon as pos-
>>> sible if remembered same day or taking one tablet if not
>>> remembered until Sunday, then returning to regular dos-
>>> ing schedule on Monday
>> Two tablets every other day:
>>> Taking two tablets as soon as remembered, skipping a day,
>>> then continuing every other day; or
>>> Taking two tablets as soon as possible if remembered same
>>> day or taking one tablet if not remembered until next
>>> day, then returning to regular dosing schedule
>> Two tablets on Monday and Wednesday and three tablets on
>> Friday:
>>> If Monday or Wednesday dose missed—Taking two tablets
>>> as soon as possible if remembered same day or taking one
>>> tablet if not remembered until next day, then returning
>>> to regular dosing schedule
>>> If Friday dose missed—Taking three tablets as soon as pos-
>>> sible if remembered same day; taking two tablets if not
>>> remembered until Saturday or one tablet if not remem-
>>> bered until Sunday; returning to regular dosing schedule
>>> on Monday
>> Three tablets every three days:
>>> Taking three tablets as soon as remembered, skipping two
>>> days, then continuing every three days; or
>>> Taking three tablets as soon as possible if remembered same
>>> day; taking two tablets if not remembered until next day
>>> or one tablet if not remembered until following day, then
>>> returning to regular dosing schedule
» Proper storage

Precautions while using this medication
» Regular visits to physician or clinic; blood tests may be needed to
  detect possible hepatotoxicity

» Importance of compliance with other treatments, including attending counseling sessions and/or support group meetings; naltrexone intended only as an aid to other forms of therapy in discouraging return to opioid use

» Not attempting to overcome effects of medication by taking large doses of opioids; such attempts may lead to coma or death

» Not using opioid medications to relieve pain, diarrhea, or cough because medication also prevents therapeutic effects of opioids

» Never sharing medication with friends, including those dependent on opioids

» Notifying all physicians, dentists, and pharmacists of use of medication

» Carrying identification card indicating use of medication

Side/adverse effects

Signs of potential side effects, especially aching, burning, or swollen eyes; blurred vision; CNS effects; earache; edema; fever; gastrointestinal ulceration; nosebleeds; phlebitis; ringing or buzzing in ears; shortness of breath; skin rash or itching; swollen glands; and uncomfortable or frequent urination

---

▲ For the Patient ▲

917230

ABOUT YOUR MEDICINE

Naltrexone (nal-TREX-zone) is used to help narcotic addicts who have stopped taking narcotics to stay drug-free. The medicine is not a cure for addiction. It is used as part of an overall program that may include counseling, attending support group meetings, and other treatment recommended by your doctor.

If any of the information in this leaflet causes you special concern or if you want additional information about your medicine and its use, check with your doctor, nurse, or pharmacist. **Remember, keep this and all other medicines out of the reach of children and never share your medicines with others.**

BEFORE USING THIS MEDICINE

Tell your doctor, nurse, and pharmacist if you . . .

- are allergic to any medicine, either prescription or non-prescription (OTC);
- are pregnant or intend to become pregnant while using this medicine;
- are breast-feeding;
- are taking any other prescription or nonprescription (OTC) medicine;
- have any other medical problems, especially hepatitis or other liver disease;
- think that you still may be having withdrawal symptoms.

PROPER USE OF THIS MEDICINE

Take naltrexone regularly as ordered by your doctor. It may be helpful to have someone else, such as a family member, doctor, or nurse, give you each dose as scheduled.

If you miss a dose of this medicine, and you are using:

- One tablet every day—Take the missed dose as soon as possible. However, if you do not remember until the next day, skip the missed dose and go back to your regular dosing schedule. Do not double the next day's dose.

- Other dosing schedules—Check with your doctor, nurse, or pharmacist.

PRECAUTIONS WHILE USING THIS MEDICINE

It is very important that your doctor check your progress at regular visits. Your doctor may want to do certain blood tests to see if the medicine is causing unwanted effects.

Remember that use of naltrexone is only part of your treatment. **Be sure that you follow all of your doctor's orders, including seeing your therapist and/or attending support group meetings on a regular basis.**

Do not try to overcome the effects of naltrexone by taking very large amounts of narcotics. To do so may cause coma or death.

Naltrexone also blocks the useful effects of narcotics. **Always use a non-narcotic medicine to treat pain, diarrhea, or cough.** If you have any questions about the proper medicine to use, check with your doctor, nurse, or pharmacist.

Never share this medicine with anyone else. This is especially important if the other person is using narcotics because naltrexone will cause withdrawal symptoms.

Tell all medical doctors, dentists, and pharmacists you go to that you are taking naltrexone.

It is recommended that you carry identification stating that you are taking naltrexone. Identification cards may be available from your doctor.

POSSIBLE SIDE EFFECTS OF THIS MEDICINE
Side Effects That Should Be Reported To Your Doctor

More common—Skin rash

Rare—Abdominal or stomach pain (severe); blurred vision or aching, burning, or swollen eyes; confusion; discomfort while urinating and/or frequent urination; earache; fever; hallucinations; increased blood pressure; itching; mental depression or other mood or mental changes; nosebleeds (unexplained); pain, tenderness, or color changes in legs or feet; ringing or buzzing in ears; shortness of breath; swelling of face, feet, or lower legs; swollen glands; weight gain

Side Effects That Usually Do Not Require Medical Attention

These possible side effects may go away during treatment; however, if they continue or are bothersome, check with your doctor, nurse, or pharmacist.

More common—Abdominal or stomach cramping or pain (mild or moderate); anxiety, nervousness, restlessness, and/or trouble in sleeping; headache; joint or muscle pain; nausea or vomiting; unusual tiredness

Less common or rare—Chills; constipation; cough, hoarseness, runny or stuffy nose, sinus problems, sneezing, and/or sore throat; diarrhea; dizziness; fast or pounding heartbeat; increased thirst; irritability; loss of appetite; sexual problems in males

Other side effects not listed above, possibly including withdrawal symptoms, may also occur in some patients. If you notice any other effects, check with your doctor, nurse, or pharmacist.

NICOTINE   Systemic

Including Nicotine (Oral); Nicotine (Transdermal).

■ For the Pharmacist ■

In providing consultation, consider emphasizing the following selected information (» = major clinical significance):

Before using this medication
» Conditions affecting use, especially:

Pregnancy—Not recommended during pregnancy; spontaneous abortions have been reported; use only if the likelihood of smoking cessation justifies the potential risk in pregnant patients who continue to smoke

Breast-feeding—Distributed into breast milk

Use in children—Small amounts of nicotine can cause serious harm in children

Dental—Chewing gum may cause severe occlusive stress resulting in damage to teeth, dentures, or dental work

Other medications, especially insulin, propoxyphene, propranolol, or xanthine-derivative bronchodilators (except dyphylline)

Other medical problems, especially severe angina pectoris, life-threatening cardiac arrhythmias, postmyocardial infarction state

Proper use of this medication
» Proper administration of the chewing gum:

Reading patient instructions carefully before using

Participating in a supervised stop-smoking program

Using gum only when there is an urge to smoke

Chewing gum slowly and intermittently for 30 minutes

Not chewing too fast, not chewing more than one piece of gum at a time, and not chewing one piece too soon after another, to avoid adverse effects or overdose

» Compliance with chewing gum therapy:

Reducing number of pieces chewed each day over a 2- to 3-month period

Importance of carrying gum at all times during therapy

Using hard sugarless candy between doses of gum to help alleviate mucosal discomfort

» Proper administration of the transdermal systems:

Reading patient instructions carefully before using

Participating in a supervised stop-smoking program

Keeping patch in sealed pouch until ready to apply to skin

Not trimming or cutting patch

Applying to clean, dry skin area on upper arm or torso free of oil, hair, scars, cuts, burns, or irritation

Pressing the patch firmly in place with palm for about 10 seconds; making sure there is good contact, especially around edges

Keeping patch in place even during showering, bathing, or swimming; replacing systems that have fallen off

Washing hands with plain water after handling patches; soap will enhance transdermal absorption of nicotine

Alternating application sites

Folding used patches in half with adhesive sides together, and replacing in protective pouch or aluminum foil; disposing of patch carefully, out of reach of children or pets

Getting into the habit of changing patch at the same time each
day to help increase compliance
» Proper dosing
» Proper storage

Precautions while using this medication
» Regular visits to physician to check progress in smoking cessation
» Not smoking during treatment with nicotine replacement products
» Not using nicotine replacement products during pregnancy
» Prevention of accidental ingestion of nicotine replacement products
by children or pets to prevent poisoning
For the chewing gum only
» Not chewing more than 30 2-mg pieces, or 15 4-mg pieces of gum
a day
» Not using gum for longer than 6 months to avoid physical depen-
dence
» Discontinuing use and consulting physician or dentist if excessive
sticking to dental work occurs; gum may damage dental work
or dentures
For the transdermal systems only
» Calling physician and not applying new patch if evidence of allergic
reaction; knowing that allergic reaction to nicotine patch could
cause reaction to use of cigarettes or other products containing
nicotine
» Not using patches for longer than 20 weeks

Side/adverse effects
Signs of potential side effects, especially injury to mouth, teeth, or
dental work (with gum only); irregular heartbeat; or hypersensitivity reaction (with transdermal systems only)

▲ For the Patient ▲

914491

NICOTINE (Oral)

ABOUT YOUR MEDICINE

Nicotine (NIK-o-teen) in a flavored chewing gum is used to
help you stop smoking. It is used for up to 12 to 20 weeks
as part of a supervised stop-smoking program. These programs may include education, counseling, and psychological
support. It is best to use nicotine gum while taking part in
such a program.

If any of the information in this leaflet causes you special
concern or if you want additional information about your
medicine and its use, check with your doctor, nurse, or pharmacist. **Remember, keep this and all other medicines out of
the reach of children and never share your medicines with
others.**

BEFORE USING THIS MEDICINE
Tell your doctor, nurse, and pharmacist if you . . .
• are allergic to any medicine, either prescription or nonprescription (OTC);
• are pregnant or intend to become pregnant while using
this medicine;
• are breast-feeding;

- are taking any other prescription or nonprescription (OTC) medicine, especially asthma medicines (such as aminophylline, oxtriphylline, and theophylline), insulin, propoxyphene, or propranolol;
- have any other medical problems, especially heart or blood vessel disease, or temporomandibular joint (TMJ) disorder.

PROPER USE OF THIS MEDICINE

Nicotine gum usually comes with patient directions. **Read the directions carefully before using this medicine.**

When you feel the urge to smoke, chew one piece of gum very slowly until you taste it or feel a slight tingling in your mouth. Stop chewing and place ("park") the chewing gum tablet between your cheek and gum until the taste or tingling is almost gone. Then chew slowly until you taste it again. Continue chewing and stopping ("parking") in this way for about 30 minutes in order to get the full dose of nicotine.

Do not chew too fast, do not chew more than one piece at a time, and do not chew a piece of gum too soon after another. To do so may cause unwanted side effects, increased belching, or an overdose.

Use nicotine gum exactly as directed by your doctor. Remember that it is also important to participate in a stop-smoking program during treatment. To do so may make it easier for you to stop smoking.

As your urge to smoke becomes less frequent, **gradually reduce the number of pieces of gum you chew each day** until you are chewing one or two pieces a day. This may be possible within 2 to 3 months.

Carry nicotine gum with you at all times in case you feel the sudden urge to smoke. One cigarette may be enough to start you on the smoking habit again.

Using hard sugarless candy between doses of gum may help relieve the discomfort in your mouth.

PRECAUTIONS WHILE USING THIS MEDICINE

Your doctor should check your progress at regular visits to make sure nicotine gum is working properly and that possible side effects are avoided.

Do not chew more than 30 2-mg pieces, or 15 4-mg pieces of gum a day. Chewing too many pieces may be harmful. **Also, do not smoke during treatment with nicotine gum** because of the risk of nicotine overdose.

Nicotine should not be used during pregnancy. If there is a possibility you might become pregnant, you may want to use some type of birth control. If you think you may have become pregnant, stop taking this medicine immediately and check with your doctor.

Nicotine gum must be kept out of reach of children and pets.
If a child chews or swallows one or more pieces of nicotine
gum, contact your doctor or poison control center at once.

Do not use nicotine gum for longer than 6 months. To do so
may result in physical dependence on the nicotine.

**If the gum sticks to your dental work, stop using it and check
with your physician or dentist.** Dentures or other dental work
may be damaged because nicotine gum is stickier and harder
to chew than ordinary gum.

POSSIBLE SIDE EFFECTS OF THIS MEDICINE
Side Effects That Should Be Reported To Your Doctor

    More common—Injury to mouth, teeth, or dental work

    Rare—Irregular heartbeat

*Side Effects That Usually Do Not Require Medical
Attention*

These possible side effects may go away during treatment;
however, if they continue or are bothersome, check with your
doctor, nurse, or pharmacist.

    More common—Belching; fast heartbeat; headache
    (mild); increased appetite; increased watering of mouth
    (mild); jaw muscle ache; sore mouth or throat

Other side effects not listed above may also occur in some
patients. If you notice any other effects, check with your
doctor, nurse, or pharmacist.

▲ For the Patient ▲

918368

NICOTINE (Transdermal)

ABOUT YOUR MEDICINE
Nicotine (NIK-o-teen) in a skin patch is used to help you
stop smoking. It is used for up to 12 to 20 weeks as part of
a supervised stop-smoking program. These programs may
include education, counseling, and psychological support. It
is best to use nicotine patches while taking part in such a
program.

If any of the information in this leaflet causes you special
concern or if you want additional information about your
medicine and its use, check with your doctor, nurse, or pharmacist. **Remember, keep this and all other medicines out of
the reach of children and never share your medicines with
others.**

BEFORE USING THIS MEDICINE
Tell your doctor, nurse, and pharmacist if you . . .
    • are allergic to any medicine, either prescription or non-
      prescription (OTC);

- are pregnant or intend to become pregnant while using this medicine;
- are breast-feeding;
- are taking any other prescription or nonprescription (OTC) medicine, especially asthma medicines (such as aminophylline, oxtriphylline, and theophylline), insulin, propoxyphene, or propranolol;
- have any other medical problems, especially heart or blood vessel disease.

PROPER USE OF THIS MEDICINE

Use this medicine exactly as directed by your doctor. It will work only if applied correctly. **This medicine usually comes with patient instructions. Read them carefully before using this product.**

Do not remove the patch from its pouch until you are ready to put it on.

Apply the patch to a clean, dry area of skin on your upper arm, chest, or back. Choose an area that is not very oily, has little or no hair, and is free of scars, cuts, burns, or any other skin irritations.

Press the patch firmly in place with the palm of your hand for about 10 seconds. Make sure there is good contact with your skin, especially around the edges of the patch.

The patch should stay in place even when you are showering, bathing, or swimming. Apply a new patch if one falls off.

Rinse your hands with plain water without soap after you have finished applying the patch to your skin. Nicotine on your hands could get into your eyes and nose and cause stinging, redness, or more serious problems.

After 16 or 24 hours, depending on which product you are using, remove the patch. Choose a different place on your skin to apply the next patch. Do not put a new patch in the same place for at least one week. Do not leave the patch on for more than 24 hours.

After removing a used patch, fold the patch in half with the sticky sides together. Place the folded, used patch in its protective pouch or in aluminum foil. Be sure to dispose of it out of the reach of children and pets.

PRECAUTIONS WHILE USING THIS MEDICINE

Your doctor should check your progress at regular visits to make sure nicotine patches are working properly and that possible side effects are avoided.

Do not smoke during treatment with nicotine patches because of the risk of nicotine overdose.

Nicotine patches must be kept out of the reach of children and pets. Even used nicotine patches contain enough nicotine to cause problems in children. If a child handles a patch that is out of the sealed pouch, take it away from the child and contact your doctor or poison control center at once.

Nicotine should not be used during pregnancy. If there is a possibility you might become pregnant, you may want to use some type of birth control. If you think you may have become pregnant, stop using this medicine immediately and check with your doctor.

Mild itching, burning, or tingling may occur when the patch is first applied, and should go away within an hour. After a patch is removed, the skin underneath it may be somewhat red. It should not remain red for more than a day. **If you get a skin rash from the patch, or if the skin becomes swollen or very red, call your doctor.** Do not put on a new patch. If you become allergic to the nicotine in the patch, you could get sick from using cigarettes.

Do not use nicotine patches for longer than 12 to 20 weeks (depending on the product) if you have stopped smoking.

POSSIBLE SIDE EFFECTS OF THIS MEDICINE
Side Effects That Should Be Reported To Your Doctor

> *Rare*—Hives, itching, rash, redness, or swelling; irregular heartbeat

Side Effects That Usually Do Not Require Medical Attention

These possible side effects may go away during treatment; however, if they continue or are bothersome, check with your doctor, nurse, or pharmacist.

> *More common*—Fast heartbeat; headache (mild); increased appetite; redness, itching, or burning at site of application—usually stops within an hour

Other side effects not listed above may also occur in some patients. If you notice any other effects, check with your doctor, nurse, or pharmacist.

NITRATES Systemic

Including Erithrityl Tetranitrate (Oral); Erithrityl Tetranitrate (Sublingual); Isosorbide Dinitrate (Oral); Isosorbide Dinitrate (Sublingual); Isosorbide Mononitrate (Oral); Nitroglycerin (Oral); Nitroglycerin (Sublingual); Nitroglycerin (Topical); Pentaerythritol Tetranitrate (Oral).

■For the Pharmacist■

In providing consultation, consider emphasizing the following selected information (» = major clinical significance):

Before using this medication
» Conditions affecting use, especially:
  Sensitivity to nitrates or nitrites
  Use in the elderly—May be more sensitive to the hypotensive effects
  Other medications, especially alcohol, antihypertensives, or other vasodilators
  Other medical problems, especially:
  For all nitrates
  Severe anemia, cerebral hemorrhage or head trauma, glaucoma, hyperthyroidism, or recent myocardial infarction
  For nitroglycerin injection only (in addition to the above)
  Hypovolemia, pericardial tamponade, or constrictive pericarditis

Proper use of this medication
» Compliance with therapy
» Reading patient instructions carefully
  Proper administration
  For regular tablets
  Taking with full glass of water on empty stomach
  For extended-release capsule or tablet
  Taking with full glass of water on empty stomach
» Not breaking, crushing, or chewing before swallowing
  For buccal dosage form
  Placing under upper lip (above incisors) against gum or between cheek and upper gum; placing between upper lip (above incisors) and gum if food or drink to be taken within 3 to 5 hours; patients with dentures may place anywhere between cheek and gum
  Touching with tongue or drinking hot liquids may increase rate of dissolution
  Bedtime use not recommended because of risk of aspiration
  Replacing tablet if inadvertently swallowed
  Not using chewing tobacco while tablet in place
» Not chewing or crushing, or swallowing tablet whole
  For chewable tablet
  Chewing well and holding in mouth for approximately 2 minutes
  For lingual aerosol
  Removing plastic cover; not shaking container
  Holding container vertically and spraying onto or under tongue; not inhaling spray
  Closing mouth after each spray; not swallowing immediately
  For sublingual tablet
  Placing under the tongue; avoiding eating, drinking, smoking, or using chewing tobacco while tablet is dissolving

»   Not chewing or crushing, or swallowing tablet whole
    For ointment
        Cleansing skin before applying; measuring; using applicator;
            spreading evenly over same size of skin area in each appli-
            cation; not rubbing into skin; applying to skin free of hair in
            different areas; proper application of occlusive dressing, if
            ordered
    For transdermal dosage form
        Not trimming or cutting patch; applying to clean, dry skin free
            of hair, scars, cuts, or irritation (after removal of previous
            system); replacing systems that have loosened or fallen off;
            alternating application sites
For use in treating acute angina attacks
»   Sitting down and using medication at first sign of angina attack;
            caution if dizziness or faintness occurs
        Remaining calm until medicine has opportunity to work
»   Relief usually occurs within 5 minutes—
        Dose may be repeated if pain not relieved in 5 to 10 minutes;
            calling physician or going to emergency room if angina pain
            not relieved by 3 doses in 15 minutes
        Not repeating dose; using sublingual nitroglycerin and calling
            physician or going to emergency room if angina pain not
            relieved in 15 minutes
For use in preventing angina
»   Does not relieve angina attacks but rather prevents them (exceptions
            are chewable and sublingual isosorbide dinitrate)
        Using 5 to 10 minutes prior to anticipated stress to prevent attack
        Missed dose:
    For oral extended-release
        Taking/using as soon as possible unless next scheduled dose is
            within 6 hours
        Returning to regular dosing schedule; not doubling doses
    For all other nitrates
        Taking/using as soon as possible unless next scheduled dose is
            within 2 hours
        Returning to regular dosing schedule; not doubling doses
»   Proper storage
        Protecting from freezing
        Not puncturing, breaking, or burning aerosol container
        Storing in cool place, tightly closed
        Lack of reliability of flushing or headache as test of potency
For sublingual nitroglycerin
»   Keeping in original glass, screw-cap bottle (unless using special ni-
            troglycerin container) with cotton plug removed; avoiding han-
            dling tablets; capping quickly and tightly after each use; not
            storing in same container as other medications; not carrying close
            to body or in auto glove compartment; not storing in refrigerator
            or bathroom medicine cabinet

Precautions while using this medication
»   Checking with physician before discontinuing medication; gradual
            dosage reduction may be needed
»   Caution when getting up suddenly from a lying or sitting position
»   Caution in using alcohol, while standing for long periods or exer-
            cising, and during hot weather because of enhanced orthostatic
            hypotensive effects
»   Headache as a common effect; should decrease with continuing
            therapy; checking with physician if continuing or severe

For isosorbide dinitrate and pentaerythritol tetranitrate
    Notifying physician if undigested extended-release tablets are found
        in stools (for isosorbide dinitrate and pentaerythritol tetranitrate
        only)

Side/adverse effects
    Signs of potential side effects, especially blurred vision, dryness of
        mouth, severe or prolonged headache, and skin rash

▲ For the Patient ▲

912485

NITRATES (Oral) *Including Erythrityl Tetranitrate;*
Isosorbide Dinitrate; Isosorbide Mononitrate;
Nitroglycerin; Pentaerythritol Tetranitrate.

ABOUT YOUR MEDICINE

Nitrates improve the supply of blood and oxygen to the heart.
When taken by mouth and swallowed, these medicines are
used to reduce the number of angina (chest pain) attacks.
Nitrates may also be used for other conditions as determined
by your doctor.

If any of the information in this leaflet causes you special
concern or if you want additional information about your
medicine and its use, check with your doctor, nurse, or pharmacist. **Remember, keep this and all other medicines out of
the reach of children and never share your medicines with
others.**

BEFORE USING THIS MEDICINE

Tell your doctor, nurse, and pharmacist if you . . .
- are allergic to any medicine, either prescription or nonprescription (OTC);
- are pregnant or intend to become pregnant while using
  this medicine;
- are breast-feeding;
- are taking any other prescription or nonprescription
  (OTC) medicine, especially high blood pressure medicine or other heart medicine;
- have any other medical problems, especially severe anemia; glaucoma; overactive thyroid; or a recent heart
  attack, stroke, or head injury.

PROPER USE OF THIS MEDICINE

Take this medicine exactly as directed by your doctor. It will
work only if taken correctly.

**This form of nitrate is used to reduce the number of angina
attacks. In most cases, it will not relieve an attack that has
already started,** because it works too slowly. Check with your
doctor if you need a fast-acting medicine to relieve the pain
of an angina attack.

**Take this medicine with a full glass (8 ounces) of water on
an empty stomach.** If taken either 1 hour before or 2 hours
after meals, it will start working sooner.

Extended-release capsules and tablets are not to be broken, crushed, or chewed before they are swallowed. If broken up, they will not release the medicine properly.

If you are taking this medicine regularly and you miss a dose, take it as soon as possible. However, if your next scheduled dose is within 2 hours (or within 6 hours for extended-release capsules or tablets), skip the missed dose and go back to your regular dosing schedule. Do not double doses.

PRECAUTIONS WHILE USING THIS MEDICINE

If you have been using this medicine regularly for several weeks or more, do not suddenly stop using it. Stopping suddenly may bring on attacks of angina. Check with your doctor for the best way to reduce gradually the amount you are taking before stopping completely.

Dizziness, lightheadedness, or faintness may occur, especially when you get up quickly from a lying or sitting position. Getting up slowly may help. **Be careful to limit the amount of alcohol you drink and during exercise, hot weather, or if standing for a long time.**

After taking a dose of this medicine you may get a headache that lasts for a short time. This is a common side effect, which should become less noticeable after you have taken the medicine for a while. If this effect continues or if the headaches are severe, check with your doctor.

POSSIBLE SIDE EFFECTS OF THIS MEDICINE
Side Effects That Should Be Reported To Your Doctor

> *Rare*—Blurred vision; dryness of mouth; headache (severe or prolonged); skin rash

Side Effects That Usually Do Not Require Medical Attention

These possible side effects may go away during treatment; however, if they continue or are bothersome, check with your doctor, nurse, or pharmacist.

> *More common*—Dizziness, lightheadedness, or fainting when standing up; fast pulse; flushing of face and neck; headache; nausea or vomiting; restlessness

Other side effects not listed above may also occur in some patients. If you notice any other effects, check with your doctor, nurse, or pharmacist.

▲ For the Patient ▲
912860

NITRATES (Sublingual): *Including Erythrityl Tetranitrate; Isosorbide Dinitrate; Nitroglycerin.*

ABOUT YOUR MEDICINE

Nitrates improve the supply of blood and oxygen to the heart. Sublingual nitroglycerin and isosorbide dinitrate are used either to relieve the pain of angina (chest pain) attacks or to reduce the number of such attacks. Sublingual erythrityl tetranitrate is used only to reduce the number of angina attacks.

If any of the information in this leaflet causes you special concern or if you want additional information about your medicine and its use, check with your doctor, nurse, or pharmacist. **Remember, keep this and all other medicines out of the reach of children and never share your medicines with others.**

BEFORE USING THIS MEDICINE

Tell your doctor, nurse, and pharmacist if you . . .
- are allergic to any medicine, either prescription or nonprescription (OTC);
- are pregnant or intend to become pregnant while using this medicine;
- are breast-feeding;
- are taking any other prescription or nonprescription (OTC) medicine, especially high blood pressure medicine or other heart medicine;
- have any other medical problems, especially severe anemia; glaucoma; overactive thyroid; or a recent heart attack, stroke, or head injury.

PROPER USE OF THIS MEDICINE

Make sure you understand the proper way to use this medicine. Follow your doctor's instructions. **Sublingual tablets should not be chewed, crushed, or swallowed.** Do not eat, drink, smoke, or use chewing tobacco while a tablet is dissolving.

For patients using nitroglycerin or isosorbide dinitrate to relieve the pain of an angina attack:
- When you begin to feel an attack of angina starting (chest pains or a tightness or squeezing in the chest), sit down. Then place a tablet under your tongue and let it dissolve. Do not chew or swallow the tablet. If you become dizzy or feel faint while sitting, take several deep breaths and bend forward with your head between your knees.
- This medicine usually gives relief in 1 to 5 minutes. However, if the pain is not relieved, dissolve a second tablet under the tongue. If the pain continues for another 5 minutes, a third tablet may be used. **If you still have chest pains after a total of 3 tablets in a 15-minute period, contact your doctor or go to a hospital emergency room without delay.**

For patients using erythrityl tetranitrate or isosorbide dinitrate regularly to prevent angina attacks: If you miss a dose of this medicine, use it as soon as possible. However, if the next scheduled dose is within 2 hours, skip the missed dose and go back to your regular dosing schedule. Do not double doses.

For patients using nitroglycerin tablets: It is important to store nitroglycerin properly in order for it to keep its strength. Carefully follow any directions for storage that are on the bottle.

PRECAUTIONS WHILE USING THIS MEDICINE

If you have been using this medicine regularly for several weeks, do not suddenly stop using it. Stopping suddenly may bring on attacks of angina. Check with your doctor for the best way to reduce gradually the amount you are taking before stopping completely.

Dizziness, lightheadedness, or faintness may occur, especially when you get up quickly from a lying or sitting position. Getting up slowly may help. **Be careful to limit the amount of alcohol you drink and during exercise, hot weather, or if standing for a long time.**

After using a dose of this medicine you may get a headache that lasts for a short time. This is a common side effect, which should become less noticeable after you have used the medicine for a while. If this effect continues, or if the headaches are severe, check with your doctor.

POSSIBLE SIDE EFFECTS OF THIS MEDICINE
Side Effects That Should Be Reported To Your Doctor

    Rare—Blurred vision; dryness of mouth; headache (severe or prolonged); skin rash

Side Effects That Usually Do Not Require Medical Attention

These possible side effects may go away during treatment; however, if they continue or are bothersome, check with your doctor, nurse, or pharmacist.

    More common—Dizziness or lightheadedness when standing up; fast pulse; flushing of face and neck; headache; nausea or vomiting; restlessness

Other side effects not listed above may also occur in some patients. If you notice any other effects, check with your doctor, nurse, or pharmacist.

▲ For the Patient ▲
913138

NITROGLYERIN (Topical): *Including Nitroglycerin Ointment; Nitroglycerin Transdermal System.*

ABOUT YOUR MEDICINE
Nitroglycerin (nye-troe-GLI-ser-in) is used to treat the symptoms of angina (chest pain). When applied to the skin, nitroglycerin is used to reduce the number of angina attacks. It is available either as an ointment or a transdermal (stick-on) patch.

Topical nitroglycerin may also be used for other conditions as determined by your doctor.

If any of the information in this leaflet causes you special concern or if you want additional information about your medicine and its use, check with your doctor, nurse, or pharmacist. **Remember, keep this and all other medicines out of the reach of children and never share your medicines with others.**

BEFORE USING THIS MEDICINE

Tell your doctor, nurse, and pharmacist if you . . .

- are allergic to any medicine, either prescription or non-prescription (OTC);
- are pregnant or intend to become pregnant while using this medicine;
- are breast-feeding;
- are taking any other prescription or nonprescription (OTC) medicine, especially high blood pressure medicine or other heart medicine;
- have any other medical problems, especially anemia (severe), glaucoma, or overactive thyroid, or if you have recently had a heart attack, stroke, or head injury.

PROPER USE OF THIS MEDICINE

Use nitroglycerin exactly as directed by your doctor. It will work only if applied correctly.

The ointment and transdermal forms of nitroglycerin are used to reduce the number of angina attacks. They will not relieve an attack that has already started because they work too slowly. Check with your doctor if you need a fast-acting medicine to relieve the pain of an angina attack.

This medicine comes with patient instructions. Read them carefully and follow the directions for applying the ointment or stick-on patch. If you have any questions, check with your doctor or pharmacist.

If you miss a dose of this medicine, apply it as soon as possible (unless you are using the ointment and the next scheduled dose is within 2 hours). Then go back to your regular dosing schedule. Do not increase the amount used.

PRECAUTIONS WHILE USING THIS MEDICINE

If you have been using nitroglycerin regularly for several weeks or more, do not suddenly stop using it. Stopping suddenly may bring on attacks of angina. Check with your doctor for the best way to reduce gradually the amount you are using before stopping completely.

Dizziness, lightheadedness, or faintness may occur, especially when you get up quickly from a lying or sitting position. Getting up slowly may help. **Be careful to limit the amount of alcohol you drink and during exercise, hot weather, or if standing for a long time.**

After using a dose of this medicine you may get a headache that lasts for a short time. This is a common side effect, which should become less noticeable after you have used the medicine for a while. If this effect continues, or if the headaches are severe, check with your doctor.

POSSIBLE SIDE EFFECTS OF THIS MEDICINE
Side Effects That Should Be Reported To Your Doctor

> *Rare*—Blurred vision; dryness of mouth; headache (severe or prolonged)

Side Effects That Usually Do Not Require Medical Attention

These possible side effects may go away during treatment; however, if they continue or are bothersome, check with your doctor, nurse, or pharmacist.

> *More common*—Dizziness or lightheadedness when standing up; fast pulse; flushing of face and neck; headache; nausea or vomiting; restlessness

> *Less common*—Sore, reddened skin

Other side effects not listed above may also occur in some patients. If you notice any other effects, check with your doctor, nurse, or pharmacist.

NITROFURANTOIN   Systemic

■For the Pharmacist■

In providing consultation, consider emphasizing the following selected information (» = major clinical significance):

Before using this medication
» Conditions affecting use, especially:
  Hypersensitivity to nitrofurans
  Pregnancy—Nitrofurantoin is contraindicated at term and during labor and delivery because of the possibility of hemolytic anemia in the fetus
  Breast-feeding—Not recommended since hemolytic anemia may occur in G6PD-deficient infants
  Use in children—Nitrofurantoin is contraindicated in infants up to 1 month of age because of the possibility of hemolytic anemia
  Use in the elderly—Side effects, such as acute pneumonitis and peripheral polyneuropathy, may occur more frequently in elderly patients
  Other medications, especially other hemolytics, other neurotoxic medications, probenecid, or sulfinpyrazone
  Other medical problems, especially G6PD deficiency, peripheral neuropathy, pulmonary disease, or renal function impairment

Proper use of this medication
» Not giving to infants up to 1 month of age
  Taking with food or milk
  Proper administration technique for oral liquid:
    Shaking well before each dose
    Using a specially marked measuring spoon or other device
    May be mixed with water, milk, fruit juices, or infants' formulas
  Proper administration technique for extended-release tablets: Swallowing tablet whole; not breaking, crushing, or chewing before swallowing
» Compliance with full course of therapy
» Proper dosage
  Missed dose: Taking as soon as possible; not taking if almost time for next dose; not doubling doses
» Proper storage

Precautions while using this medication
  Regular visits to physician to check progress if on long-term therapy
  Checking with physician if no improvement within a few days
» Diabetics: False-positive reactions with copper sulfate urine glucose tests may occur

Side/adverse effects
  Rust-yellow to brown discoloration of urine may be alarming to patient although medically insignificant
  Signs of potential side effects, especially hemolytic anemia, jaundice, neurotoxicity, pneumonitis, and polyneuropathy

▲ For the Patient ▲

912496

ABOUT YOUR MEDICINE

Nitrofurantoin (nye-troe-fyoor-AN-toyn) belongs to the general family of medicines called anti-infectives. It is used to treat infections of the urinary tract caused by bacteria. It may also be used for other conditions as determined by your doctor.

If any of the information in this leaflet causes you special concern or if you want additional information about your medicine and its use, check with your doctor, nurse, or pharmacist. **Remember, keep this and all other medicines out of the reach of children and never share your medicines with others.**

BEFORE USING THIS MEDICINE

Tell your doctor, nurse, and pharmacist if you . . .
- are allergic to any medicine, either prescription or non-prescription (OTC);
- are pregnant or intend to become pregnant while using this medicine;
- are breast-feeding;
- are taking **any** other prescription or nonprescription (OTC) medicine;
- have any other medical problems, especially glucose-6-phosphate dehydrogenase (G6PD) deficiency, kidney disease (other than infection), lung disease, or nerve damage.

PROPER USE OF THIS MEDICINE

Do not give this medicine to infants up to 1 month of age.

Nitrofurantoin is best taken with food or milk. This may lessen stomach upset and help your body absorb the medicine better.

For patients taking the oral liquid form of this medicine:
- Shake the oral liquid forcefully before each dose to help make it pour more smoothly and to be sure the medicine is evenly mixed.
- Use a specially marked measuring spoon or other device to measure each dose accurately. The average household teaspoon may not hold the right amount of liquid.
- Nitrofurantoin may be mixed with water, milk, fruit juice, or infants' formulas. If it is mixed with other liquids, take the medicine immediately after mixing. Be sure to drink all the liquid in order to get the full dose of medicine.

For patients taking the extended-release capsule form of this medicine:
- Swallow the capsule whole.
- Do not open, crush, or chew the capsules before swallowing them.

To help clear up your infection completely, **keep taking this medicine for the full time of treatment** even if you begin to feel better after a few days; **do not miss any doses**.

If you do miss a dose of this medicine, take it as soon as possible. However, if it is almost time for your next dose, skip the missed dose and go back to your regular dosing schedule. Do not double doses.

PRECAUTIONS WHILE USING THIS MEDICINE

It is important that your doctor check your progress at regular visits if you will be taking this medicine for a long time.

If your symptoms do not improve within a few days, or if they become worse, check with your doctor.

Diabetics—This medicine may cause false test results with some urine sugar tests. Check with your doctor before changing your diet or the dosage of your diabetes medicine.

This medicine must not be given to other people or used for other infections unless you are otherwise directed by your doctor.

POSSIBLE SIDE EFFECTS OF THIS MEDICINE

Side Effects That Should Be Reported To Your Doctor Immediately

> *More common*—Chest pain; chills; cough; fever; troubled breathing

> *Less common*—Dizziness; drowsiness; headache; numbness, tingling, or burning of face or mouth; pale skin; sore throat and fever; unusual muscle weakness; unusual tiredness or weakness

> *Rare*—Itching; joint pain; skin rash; yellow eyes or skin

Side Effects That Usually Do Not Require Medical Attention

These possible side effects may go away during treatment; however, if they continue or are bothersome, check with your doctor, nurse, or pharmacist.

> *More common*—Abdominal or stomach pain or upset; diarrhea; loss of appetite; nausea or vomiting

Nitrofurantoin may cause the urine to become rust-yellow to brown. This side effect does not require medical attention.

Other side effects not listed above may also occur in some patients. If you notice any other effects, check with your doctor, nurse, or pharmacist.

NONSTEROIDAL ANTI-INFLAMMATORY DRUGS Systemic

Including Diclofenac; Diflunisal; Etodolac; Fenoprofen; Floctafenine; Flurbiprofen; Ibuprofen; Indomethacin; Ketoprofen; Meclofenamate; Mefenamic Acid; Nabumetone; Naproxen; Oxaprozin; Phenylbutazone; Piroxicam; Sulindac; Tenoxicam; Tiaprofenic Acid; Tolmetin.

■ For the Pharmacist ■

In providing consultation, consider emphasizing the following selected information (» = major clinical significance):

Before using this medication
» Conditions affecting use, especially:
  Allergies to aspirin or any of the nonsteroidal anti-inflammatory drugs (NSAIDs)
  Pregnancy—Use of an NSAID during second half of pregnancy not recommended because of potential adverse effect on fetal blood flow and possible prolongation of pregnancy, dystocia, and difficult and/or delayed delivery
  Breast-feeding—
    For indomethacin: Has caused convulsions in a nursing infant
    For meclofenamate and piroxicam: These NSAIDs have caused adverse effects in animal studies
    For phenylbutazone: May cause blood dyscrasias or other adverse effects in the infant
  Use in children—
    For indomethacin: Because of toxicity, should be used with caution and only in patients unresponsive to less toxic NSAIDs
    For naproxen: Skin rash more common in pediatric patients
    For phenylbutazone: Because of toxicity, not recommended in children < 15 years of age
  Use in the elderly—Increased risk of toxicity; initial dosage should be reduced and patients carefully monitored
  Other medications, especially—
    For all NSAIDs: Anticoagulants, aspirin, cephalosporins that may induce hypoprothrombinemia, cyclosporine, lithium, methotrexate, plicamycin, probenecid, triamterene, and valproic acid
    For indomethacin (in addition to those applying to all NSAIDs): Zidovudine
    For phenylbutazone (in addition to those applying to all NSAIDs): Digitalis, penicillamine, and phenytoin
    For buffered phenylbutazone (in addition to those applying to all NSAIDs and to phenylbutazone): Ciprofloxacin, enoxacin, itraconazole, ketoconazole, lomefloxacin, norfloxacin, ofloxacin, and oral tetracyclines
    For tiaprofenic acid (in addition to those applying to all NSAIDs): Phenytoin
  Other medical problems, especially—
    For all NSAIDs: Blood dyscrasias, bone marrow depression, cardiac or cardiopulmonary disease or predisposition to, clotting defects, hepatic disease, peptic ulcer or other inflammatory or ulcerative gastrointestinal tract disease or predisposition to, renal disease or predisposition to, and stomatitis

For indomethacin (in addition to those applying to all NSAIDs): Epilepsy, mental illness, and parkinsonism

For phenylbutazone (in addition to those applying to all NSAIDs): Polymyalgia rheumatica and temporal arteritis

For sulindac (in addition to those applying to all NSAIDs): Renal calculus or history of

For rectal dosage forms (in addition to those applying to oral use of the NSAIDs with rectal dosage forms): Anal or rectal bleeding, hemorrhoids, inflammatory lesions of anus or rectum, and proctitis or recent history of

Proper use of this medication

For all NSAIDs

» Not taking more medication than prescribed or recommended on OTC package label

» For use in arthritis—Compliance with therapy; noticeable improvement in condition usually requires a few days to a week of treatment (but up to 2 weeks, and sometimes even longer, in severe cases) and maximum effectiveness may require several weeks of treatment

» Proper dosing

Missed dose (scheduled dosing): If dosing schedule is—

Once or twice a day: Taking as soon as possible if remembered within one or two hours after dose should have been taken; skipping dose if not remembered until later

More than twice a day: Taking as soon as possible; not taking if almost time for next dose; not doubling doses

» Proper storage

For all capsule and tablet dosage forms

Taking with a full glass of water and not lying down for 15 to 30 minutes after taking

For indomethacin, mefenamic acid, phenylbutazone, and piroxicam

» Taking oral dosage forms with meals or antacids (a magnesium- and aluminum-containing antacid may be preferred) to reduce gastrointestinal irritation

For flurbiprofen extended-release tablets, nabumetone, and naproxen extended-release tablets

Taking with food or antacids (a magnesium- and aluminum-containing antacid may be preferred) to reduce gastrointestinal irritation; taking with food also increases absorption

For immediate-release and extended-release oral dosage forms of NSAIDs not listed above

Taking with food or antacids (a magnesium- and aluminum-containing antacid may be preferred) to reduce gastrointestinal irritation, although when used for acute conditions (e.g., pain, gout, fever, or dysmenorrhea) the first 1 or 2 doses may be taken on an empty stomach to speed the onset of action

For oral suspensions

Not mixing suspension with an antacid or other liquid prior to use

For delayed-release (enteric-coated) or extended-release dosage forms, diflunisal tablets, and all phenylbutazone tablet formulations

Swallowing whole; not breaking, chewing or crushing before swallowing

For all suppository dosage forms

Proper administration technique

For indomethacin suppositories

Retaining in rectum for 1 full hour to ensure maximum absorption

For nonprescription use of ibuprofen or naproxen

» Reading patient information sheet provided in package

For phenylbutazone
» Taking for prescribed indications only; not taking to relieve other aches and pains

For mefenamic acid
» Not taking longer than 7 days at a time unless otherwise directed by physician

Precautions while using this medication
» Regular visits to physician during prolonged therapy
» Possibility that use of alcohol may increase the risk of ulceration and, with phenylbutazone, depressant effects

Not taking 2 or more NSAIDs, including ketorolac, concurrently, and not taking acetaminophen or aspirin or other salicylates for more than a few days while receiving NSAID therapy, unless concurrent use is prescribed by, and patient remains under the care of, a physician or dentist

Caution if any surgery is required because of possible enhanced bleeding (although may be less of a problem with diclofenac, diflunisal, meclofenamate, mefenamic acid, and nabumetone)

Caution if confusion, dizziness or lightheadedness, drowsiness, or vision problems occur
» Possibility of photosensitivity

Possibility of gastrointestinal ulceration and bleeding
» Notifying physician immediately if influenza-like symptoms (chills, fever, or muscle aches and pains) occur shortly prior to or together with a skin rash; rarely, these symptoms may indicate a serious reaction to the medication

Possibility of anaphylaxis

For buffered phenylbutazone
» Not taking within:
  —6 hours before or 2 hours after ciprofloxacin or lomefloxacin
  —8 hours before or 2 hours after enoxacin
  —2 hours after itraconazole
  —3 hours before or after ketoconazole
  —2 hours before or after norfloxacin or ofloxacin
  —1 to 3 hours before or after an oral tetracycline

For mefenamic acid
  Discontinuing use and checking with physician if severe diarrhea occurs

For nonprescription use of ibuprofen or naproxen
  Checking with health care professional if symptoms do not improve or if they worsen, if using for fever and fever lasts more than 3 days or returns, or if painful area is red or swollen

Side/adverse effects
» Stopping medication and obtaining emergency treatment if symptoms of any of the following occur:
  For all NSAIDs
  Anaphylaxis, angioedema, or bronchospasm
» Stopping medication and checking with physician immediately if symptoms of the following occur:
  For all NSAIDs
  Spitting up blood, unexplained nosebleeds, chest pain, convulsions, fainting, gastrointestinal ulceration or bleeding, and blood dyscrasias
  For mefenamic acid (in addition to those applying to all NSAIDs)
  Diarrhea
  For phenylbutazone (in addition to those applying to all NSAIDs)
  Edema

Signs and symptoms of other potential side effects, especially:
For all NSAIDs
Dysarthria, hallucinations, aseptic meningitis, migraine, mood or mental changes, peripheral neuropathy, syncope, or other central nervous system effects; dermatitis (allergic or exfoliative), Stevens-Johnson syndrome, or other dermatologic effects; colitis, dysphagia, esophagitis, gastritis, gastroenteritis, or other digestive system effects; crystalluria, urinary tract irritation or infection, or other genitourinary effects; anemia or hypocoagulation; hepatitis; angiitis, fever, allergic rhinitis, or other hypersensitivity reactions not listed previously; loosening or splitting of fingernails; lymphadenopathy; vision problems, conjunctivitis, or other ocular effects; stomatitis, glossitis, or other oral/perioral effects; hearing problems or tinnitus; pancreatitis; and edema, hyperkalemia, polyuria, renal impairment or failure, or other renal effects
For indomethacin (in addition to those applying to all NSAIDs)
Headache (severe), especially in the morning
Possibility that the following may occur many days or weeks after medication is discontinued:
For phenylbutazone
Blood dyscrasias

▲ For the Patient ▲

912088

ABOUT YOUR MEDICINE

Anti-inflammatory analgesics (also called nonsteroidal anti-inflammatory drugs [NSAIDs]) are used to relieve some of the symptoms caused by arthritis (rheumatism), such as inflammation, swelling, stiffness, and joint pain. Some are also used to relieve bursitis, gout, menstrual cramps, sprains, strains, or tendinitis, and as analgesics in relieving other kinds of pain. They may also be used for other conditions as determined by your doctor.

If any of the information in this leaflet causes you special concern or if you want additional information about your medicine and its use, check with your doctor, nurse, or pharmacist. **Remember, keep this and all other medicines out of the reach of children and never share your medicines with others.**

BEFORE USING THIS MEDICINE

If you are taking this medicine without a prescription, carefully read and follow any precautions on the label. You should be especially careful if you . . .
- are allergic to any medicine, either prescription or nonprescription (OTC);
- are pregnant, intend to become pregnant, or are breast-feeding;
- are taking **any** other prescription or nonprescription (OTC) medicine;
- have **any** other medical problems.

If you have any questions, check with your doctor, nurse, or pharmacist.

PROPER USE OF THIS MEDICINE
Always take this medicine with food or antacids. Also, always take it with a full glass (8 ounces) of water.

Do not take more of this medicine, do not take it more often, and do not take it for a longer time than directed.

When used for arthritis, this medicine must be taken regularly as ordered.

If you are taking this medicine regularly and you miss a dose, take it as soon as possible. However, if it is almost time for your next dose, skip the missed dose and go back to your regular schedule. Do not double doses.

PRECAUTIONS WHILE USING THIS MEDICINE
It is important to have regular check-ups with your doctor if you are taking this medicine regularly. Serious side effects, such as ulcers or bleeding, can occur without warning.

Do not take other anti-inflammatories, including aspirin, regularly or drink alcoholic beverages while taking this medicine, unless otherwise directed by your doctor.

This medicine may cause some people to become drowsy, dizzy, or less alert than they are normally. **Make sure you know how you react before you drive, use machines, or do other jobs that require you to be alert.**

POSSIBLE SIDE EFFECTS OF THIS MEDICINE
Stop taking this medicine and check with your doctor immediately if you notice severe abdominal or stomach pain, cramping, or burning; bloody or black, tarry stools; chest pain; convulsions (seizures); fainting; large, hive-like swellings on face, eyelids, mouth, lips, or tongue; severe and continuing nausea, heartburn, or indigestion; shortness of breath, troubled breathing, wheezing, or tightness in chest or fast or irregular breathing; sore throat, fever, and chills; spitting blood; sudden decrease in amount of urine; vomiting blood or material that looks like coffee grounds; or unusual bleeding or bruising.

Other Side Effects That Should Be Reported To Your Doctor

More common—Headache (for indomethacin); skin rash

Less common or rare—Bleeding or crusting sores on lips; bloody or cloudy urine or any problems with urination; burning feeling in throat, chest, or stomach; confusion or forgetfulness; cough or hoarseness; diarrhea (severe); fast, pounding, or irregular heartbeat; hallucinations; headache (severe) with stiff neck; hearing problems or change in hearing; hives, itching, or other skin problems; increased or unusually high blood pressure; mental depression or other mood changes; muscle cramps, pain, or weakness, or uncontrollable muscle movements; nosebleeds; numbness, tingling, pain, or weakness in hands or feet; pain in lower back or side (severe); painful or swollen glands; pain or redness in eyes; pinpoint red spots on skin; ringing or buzzing in ears; sore throat and fever; sores, ulcers, or white spots in mouth; spitting blood; swelling of face, fingers, hands, feet, or lower legs; swelling or tenderness in upper stomach; unusual thirst; unusual tiredness or weakness; weight gain (rapid); vision problems; yellow eyes or skin

Side Effects That Usually Do Not Require Medical Attention

These possible side effects may go away during treatment; however, if they continue or are bothersome, check with your doctor, nurse, or pharmacist.

> *More common*—Bloated feeling or gas; diarrhea, mild nausea, or vomiting; dizziness, lightheadedness, or drowsiness; headache; mild heartburn, indigestion, or stomach pain or cramps

Other side effects not listed above may also occur in some patients. If you notice any other effects, check with your doctor, nurse, or pharmacist.

NORFLOXACIN Ophthalmic

■ For the Pharmacist ■

In providing consultation, consider emphasizing the following selected
   information (» = major clinical significance):

Before using this medication
» Conditions affecting use, especially:
       Sensitivity to norfloxacin or other quinolone derivatives
       Pregnancy—Ophthalmic norfloxacin is not recommended during
          pregnancy, because it is not known whether it can cause
          arthropathy in immature animals as can systemic norfloxacin
       Breast-feeding—Ophthalmic norfloxacin is not recommended,
          because it is not known whether it can cause arthropathy in
          immature animals as can systemic norfloxacin
       Use in children—Ophthalmic norfloxacin is not recommended
          in infants, because it is not known whether it can cause ar-
          thropathy in immature animals as can systemic norfloxacin

Proper use of this medication
       Proper administration technique
» Proper dosage
» Compliance with full course of therapy
       Missed dose: Applying as soon as possible; not applying if almost
          time for next dose
» Proper storage

Precautions while using this medication
       Checking with physician if no improvement within a few days
       Possible photophobic reactions; wearing sunglasses and avoiding pro-
          longed exposure to bright light

Side/adverse effects
       Signs of potential side effects, especially skin rash or other sign of
          hypersensitivity

▲ For the Patient ▲

919860

ABOUT YOUR MEDICINE

Norfloxacin (nor-FLOX-a-sin) is an antibiotic. The ophthalmic preparation is used to treat infections of the eye.

If any of the information in this leaflet causes you special
concern or if you want additional information about your
medicine and its use, check with your doctor, nurse, or pharmacist. **Remember, keep this and all other medicines out of
the reach of children and never share your medicines with
others.**

BEFORE USING THIS MEDICINE

Tell your doctor, nurse, and pharmacist if you . . .
   • are allergic to any medicine, either prescription or non-
      prescription (OTC);
   • are pregnant or intend to become pregnant while using
      this medicine;

- are breast-feeding;
- are taking any other prescription or nonprescription (OTC) medicine;
- have any other medical problems.

PROPER USE OF THIS MEDICINE

To use:

- First, wash your hands. Tilt the head back and, pressing your finger gently on the skin just beneath the lower eyelid, pull the lower eyelid away from the eye to make a space. Drop the medicine into the space. Let go of the eyelid and gently close the eyes. Do not blink. Keep the eyes closed for 1 or 2 minutes to allow the medicine to come into contact with the infection.
- If you think you did not get the drop of medicine into your eye properly, use another drop.
- To keep the medicine as germ-free as possible, do not touch the applicator tip to any surface (including the eye). Also, keep the container tightly closed.

To help clear up your infection completely, **keep using this medicine for the full time of treatment,** even if your symptoms begin to clear up after a few days. If you stop using this medicine too soon, your symptoms may return. **Do not miss any doses.**

If you do miss a dose of this medicine, use it as soon as possible. However, if it is almost time for your next dose, skip the missed dose and go back to your regular dosing schedule.

PRECAUTIONS WHILE USING THIS MEDICINE

If your symptoms do not improve within a few days, or if they become worse, check with your doctor.

This medicine may cause your eyes to become more sensitive to light than they are normally. Wearing sunglasses and avoiding too much exposure to bright light may help lessen the discomfort.

POSSIBLE SIDE EFFECTS OF THIS MEDICINE

Side Effects That Should Be Reported To Your Doctor Immediately

Rare—Skin rash or other sign of allergic reaction

Side Effects That Usually Do Not Require Medical Attention

These possible side effects may go away during treatment; however, if they continue or are bothersome, check with your doctor, nurse, or pharmacist.

More common—Burning or other eye discomfort

Less common—Bitter taste following use in the eye; increased sensitivity of eye to light; redness of the lining of the eyelids; swelling of the membrane covering the white part of the eye

Other side effects not listed above may also occur in some patients. If you notice any other effects, check with your doctor, nurse, or pharmacist.

OFLOXACIN   Ophthalmic

■For the Pharmacist■

In providing consultation, consider emphasizing the following selected
  information (» = major clinical significance):

Before using this medication
» Conditions affecting use, especially:
    Sensitivity to ofloxacin or other fluoroquinolones or their deriv-
      atives
    Pregnancy—Studies using ophthalmic ofloxacin have not been
      done; however, studies in animals given very high doses of
      systemic ofloxacin have shown fetotoxicity
    Breast-feeding—Oral ofloxacin is distributed into breast milk;
      it is not known whether ophthalmic ofloxacin is distributed
      into breast milk
    Use in children—Safety and efficacy have not been established
      in infants up to 1 year of age

Proper use of this medication
    Proper administration technique
» Compliance with full course of therapy
» Proper dosing
    Missed dose: Applying as soon as possible; not applying if almost
      time for next dose
» Proper storage

Precautions while using this medication
    Checking with physician if no improvement within 7 days
    Possible photophobic reactions; wearing sunglasses and avoiding pro-
      longed exposure to bright light

Side/adverse effects
    Signs of potential side effects, especially dizziness

▲ For the Patient ▲

919553

ABOUT YOUR MEDICINE

Ofloxacin (oh-FLOKS-a-sin) is an antibiotic used to treat
bacterial infections of the eye.

If any of the information in this leaflet causes you special
concern or if you want additional information about your
medicine and its use, check with your doctor, nurse, or pharmacist. **Remember, keep this and all other medicines out of
the reach of children and never share your medicines with
others.**

BEFORE USING THIS MEDICINE

Tell your doctor, nurse, and pharmacist if you . . .
  • are allergic to any medicine, either prescription or non-
    prescription (OTC);
  • are pregnant or intend to become pregnant while using
    this medicine;
  • are breast-feeding;

- are taking any other prescription or nonprescription (OTC) medicine;
- have any other medical problems.

PROPER USE OF THIS MEDICINE

To use:
- First, wash your hands. Tilt the head back and, pressing your finger gently on the skin just beneath the lower eyelid, pull the lower eyelid away from the eye to make a space. Drop the medicine into this space. Let go of the eyelid and gently close the eyes. Do not blink. Keep the eyes closed for 1 or 2 minutes to allow the medicine to come into contact with the infection.
- If you think you did not get the drop of medicine into your eyes properly, use another drop.
- To keep the medicine as germ-free as possible, do not touch the applicator tip to any surface (including the eye). Also, keep the container tightly closed.

To help clear up your eye infection completely, **keep using ophthalmic ofloxacin for the full time of treatment,** even if your symptoms have disappeared. **Do not miss any doses.**

If you do miss a dose of this medicine, use it as soon as possible. However, if it is almost time for your next dose, skip the missed dose and go back to your regular dosing schedule.

PRECAUTIONS WHILE USING THIS MEDICINE

If your eye infection does not improve within 7 days, or if it becomes worse, check with your doctor.

This medicine may cause your eyes to become more sensitive to light than they are normally. Wearing sunglasses and avoiding too much exposure to bright light may help lessen the discomfort.

POSSIBLE SIDE EFFECTS OF THIS MEDICINE

Side Effects That Should Be Reported To Your Doctor

    Rare—Dizziness

Side Effects That Usually Do Not Require Medical Attention

These possible side effects may go away during treatment; however, if they continue or are bothersome, check with your doctor, nurse, or pharmacist.

    More common—Burning of eye

    Less common—Increased sensitivity of eye to light; stinging, redness, itching, tearing, or dryness of eye

Other side effects not listed above may also occur in some patients. If you notice any other effects, check with your doctor, nurse, or pharmacist.

OLSALAZINE   Oral-Local

■For the Pharmacist■

In providing consultation, consider emphasizing the following selected
  information (**»** = major clinical significance):

Before using this medication
» Conditions affecting use, especially:
        Sensitivity to olsalazine, mesalamine, or salicylates
        Other medical problems, especially renal function impairment

Proper use of this medication
    Taking with food to lessen gastrointestinal irritation
» Compliance with full course of therapy
» Proper dosing
    Missed dose: Taking as soon as possible; not taking if almost time
        for next dose; not doubling doses
» Proper storage

Precautions while using this medication
» Regular visits to physician to check blood counts in patients on long-
        term therapy

Side/adverse effects
    Signs of potential side effects, especially blood dyscrasias, exacer-
        bation of ulcerative colitis, and hepatitis

▲ For the Patient ▲

917784

ABOUT YOUR MEDICINE

Olsalazine (ole-SAL-a-zeen) is used in patients who have had
ulcerative colitis to prevent the condition from occurring
again.

If any of the information in this leaflet causes you special
concern or if you want additional information about your
medicine and its use, check with your doctor, nurse, or pharmacist. **Remember, keep this and all other medicines out of
the reach of children and never share your medicines with
others.**

BEFORE USING THIS MEDICINE
Tell your doctor, nurse, and pharmacist if you . . .
  • are allergic to any medicine, either prescription or non-
     prescription (OTC);
  • are pregnant or intend to become pregnant while using
     this medicine;
  • are breast-feeding;
  • are taking any other prescription or nonprescription
     (OTC) medicine;
  • have any other medical problems.

PROPER USE OF THIS MEDICINE

Olsalazine is best taken with food, to lessen stomach upset and diarrhea. If stomach or intestinal problems continue or are bothersome, check with your doctor.

Keep taking this medicine for the full time of treatment, even if you begin to feel better after a few days. **Do not miss any doses.**

If you do miss a dose of this medicine, take it as soon as possible. However, if it is almost time for your next dose, skip the missed dose and go back to your regular dosing schedule. Do not double doses.

PRECAUTIONS WHILE USING THIS MEDICINE

It is very important that your doctor check your progress at regular visits, especially if you will be taking this medicine for a long time. Olsalazine may cause blood problems.

POSSIBLE SIDE EFFECTS OF THIS MEDICINE

Side Effects That Should Be Reported To Your Doctor

   Rare—Bloody diarrhea; fever; pale skin; skin rash; sore throat; unusual bleeding or bruising; unusual tiredness or weakness; yellow eyes or skin

Side Effects That Usually Do Not Require Medical Attention

These possible side effects may go away during treatment; however, if they continue or are bothersome, check with your doctor, nurse, or pharmacist.

   More common—Abdominal or stomach pain or upset; diarrhea; loss of appetite; nausea or vomiting

   Less common—Aching joints and muscles; acne; anxiety or depression; drowsiness or dizziness; headache; insomnia

Other side effects not listed above may also occur in some patients. If you notice any other effects, check with your doctor, nurse, or pharmacist.

OMEPRAZOLE   Systemic

■ For the Pharmacist ■

In providing consultation, consider emphasizing the following selected
information (» = major clinical significance):

Before using this medication
» Conditions affecting use, especially:
  Sensitivity to omeprazole
  Breast feeding—May be distributed into breast milk; may cause
    potentially serious adverse effects in nursing infants
  Other medical problems, especially chronic hepatic disease or
    history of
  Other medications, especially anticoagulants, diazepam, or
    phenytoin

Proper use of this medication
  Taking medication immediately before a meal, preferably the morn-
    ing meal
  May take antacids for relief of pain, unless otherwise instructed by
    physician
  Swallowing capsule whole; not crushing, breaking, chewing, or open-
    ing the capsule
» Compliance with full course of therapy
» Proper dosing
  Missed dose: Taking as soon as possible; not taking if almost time
    for next dose; not doubling doses
» Proper storage

Precautions while using this medication
  Checking with physician if condition does not improve or worsens

Side/adverse effects
  Signs of potential side effects, especially hematologic abnormalities,
    hematuria, proteinuria, and urinary tract infection

▲ For the Patient ▲

917117

ABOUT YOUR MEDICINE

Omeprazole (o-MEP-ra-zole) is used to treat certain conditions in which there is too much acid in the stomach. It is
used to treat duodenal ulcers and gastroesophageal reflux
disease, a condition in which the acid in the stomach washes
back up into the esophagus. Omeprazole is also used to treat
Zollinger-Ellison disease, a condition in which the stomach
produces too much acid. It may also be used for other conditions as determined by your doctor.

If any of the information in this leaflet causes you special
concern or if you want additional information about your
medicine and its use, check with your doctor, nurse, or pharmacist. **Remember, keep this and all other medicines out of
the reach of children and never share your medicines with
others.**

BEFORE USING THIS MEDICINE
Tell your doctor, nurse, and pharmacist if you . . .

- are allergic to any medicine, either prescription or non-prescription (OTC);
- are pregnant or intend to become pregnant while using this medicine;
- are breast-feeding;
- are taking any other prescription or nonprescription (OTC) medicine, especially anticoagulants, diazepam, or phenytoin;
- have any other medical problems, especially liver disease.

PROPER USE OF THIS MEDICINE
Take omeprazole immediately before a meal, preferably in the morning.

It may take several days before this medicine begins to relieve stomach pain. To help relieve this pain, antacids may be taken with omeprazole, unless your doctor has told you not to use them.

Swallow the capsule whole. Do not crush, break, chew, or open the capsule.

Take this medicine for the full time of treatment, even if you begin to feel better. Also, keep your appointments with your doctor for check-ups so that your doctor will be better able to tell you when to stop taking this medicine.

If you miss a dose of this medicine, take it as soon as possible. However, if it is almost time for your next dose, skip the missed dose and go back to your regular dosing schedule. Do not double doses.

PRECAUTIONS WHILE USING THIS MEDICINE
If your condition does not improve, or if it becomes worse, check with your doctor.

POSSIBLE SIDE EFFECTS OF THIS MEDICINE
Side Effects That Should Be Reported To Your Doctor

> *Rare*—Bloody or cloudy urine; continuing ulcers or sores in mouth; difficult, burning, or painful urination; frequent urge to urinate; sore throat and fever; unusual bleeding or bruising; unusual tiredness or weakness

Side Effects That Usually Do Not Require Medical Attention

These possible side effects may go away during treatment; however, if they continue or are bothersome, check with your doctor, nurse, or pharmacist.

> *More common*—Abdominal or stomach pain

> *Less common*—Chest pain; constipation; diarrhea or loose stools; dizziness; gas; headache; heartburn; muscle pain;

nausea and vomiting; skin rash or itching; unusual drowsiness; unusual tiredness

Other side effects not listed above may also occur in some patients. If you notice any other effects, check with your doctor, nurse, or pharmacist.

OPIOID (NARCOTIC) ANALGESICS Systemic

Including Butorphanol; Codeine; Hydrocodone; Hydromorphone; Levorphanol; Meperidine; Methadone; Morphine; Nalbuphine; Opium; Oxycodone; Oxymorphone; Pentazocine; Pentazocine and Naloxone; Propoxyphene.

■ For the Pharmacist ■

In providing consultation, consider emphasizing the following selected information (» = major clinical significance):

Before using this medication
» Conditions affecting use, especially:
    Sensitivity to the opioid considered for use, history of
    Pregnancy—Opioids cross the placenta; regular use by pregnant women may cause physical dependence in the fetus and withdrawal symptoms in the neonate
    Breast-feeding—Butorphanol, codeine, meperidine, methadone, morphine, and propoxyphene are known to be excreted in breast milk; high-dose methadone may cause dependence in nursing infants
    Use in children—Children up to 2 years of age are more susceptible to the effects of opioids, especially respiratory depression; also, children may be more likely to experience paradoxical CNS excitation during therapy
    Use in the elderly—Geriatric patients are more susceptible to the effects of opioids, especially respiratory depression
    Dental—May cause dryness of mouth, which can lead to caries, periodontal disease, oral candidiasis, and discomfort
    Other medical problems, especially diarrhea caused by antibiotics or poisoning, asthma or other respiratory problems, and severe inflammatory bowel disease
    Other medications, especially alcohol or other CNS depressants, monoamine oxidase inhibitors, naltrexone, rifampin, and zidovudine

Proper use of this medication
    Proper administration of:
»   Injections (if dispensed to the patient for home use)
»   Meperidine syrup—Mixing with ½ glass (4 ounces) of water to lessen numbing effect in mouth and throat
»   Methadone oral concentrate—Diluting with water to at least 1 ounce before taking, unless premixed at a methadone treatment center
»   Methadone dispersible tablets—Must be dissolved in water or fruit juice before taking
    Morphine oral liquid—May be mixed with fruit juice to improve taste
»   Morphine extended-release tablets—Swallowing tablets whole; not breaking, crushing, or chewing
    Suppository dosage forms—proper administration technique
    Proper administration of opium tincture:
    Medication may be diluted in water, which will cause it to turn milky
    Taking with food or meals if gastrointestinal irritation occurs

» Importance of not taking more medication than the amount prescribed because of danger of overdose and habit-forming potential

» Not increasing dose if medication is less effective after a few weeks; checking with physician

» Missed dose (if on scheduled dosing): Taking as soon as possible; not taking if almost time for next dose; not doubling doses

» Proper storage

Precautions while using this medication

Regular visits to physician to check progress during long-term therapy

» Avoiding use of alcoholic beverages or other CNS depressants during therapy, unless prescribed or otherwise approved by physician

» Caution if dizziness, drowsiness, lightheadedness, or false sense of well-being occurs

» Caution when getting up suddenly from a lying or sitting position

Lying down if nausea or vomiting, or dizziness or lightheadedness occurs

Need to inform physician or dentist of use of medication if any kind of surgery (including dental surgery) or emergency treatment is required

Possible dryness of mouth; using sugarless gum or candy, ice, or saliva substitute for relief; checking with dentist if dry mouth continues for more than 2 weeks

» Checking with physician before discontinuing medication after prolonged use of high doses; gradual dosage reduction may be necessary to avoid withdrawal symptoms

» Suspected overdose: Getting emergency help at once

For opium tincture when used as antidiarrheal only

» Consulting physician if diarrhea continues and/or fever develops

Side/adverse effects

Signs of potential side effects, especially respiratory depression or impairment; allergic reactions; confusion, convulsions, hallucinations, mental depression, or other signs of CNS toxicity; hepatotoxicity; hypertension; and paradoxical CNS excitation, especially in children

---

▲ For the Patient ▲

912441

ABOUT YOUR MEDICINE

Narcotic analgesics (nar-KOT-ik an-al-JEE-zicks) are medicines used to relieve pain. Codeine and hydrocodone are also used to relieve coughing. Methadone is also used to help some people control their dependence on heroin or other narcotics. Narcotic analgesics may also be used for other purposes as determined by your doctor.

If any of the information in this leaflet causes you special concern or if you want additional information about your medicine and its use, check with your doctor, nurse, or pharmacist. **Remember, keep this and all other medicines out of the reach of children and never share your medicines with others.**

BEFORE USING THIS MEDICINE

Tell your doctor, nurse, and pharmacist if you . . .

- are allergic to any medicine, either prescription or non-prescription (OTC);
- are pregnant or intend to become pregnant while using this medicine;
- are breast-feeding;
- are taking any other prescription or nonprescription (OTC) medicine, especially carbamazepine, CNS depressants, MAO inhibitors, rifampin, or zidovudine;
- have any other medical problems, especially asthma, chronic lung disease, or colitis.

PROPER USE OF THIS MEDICINE

Take this medicine only as directed by your medical doctor or dentist. Do not take more of it and do not take it more often or for a longer period of time than directed. If too much is taken, the medicine may become habit-forming or lead to medical problems because of an overdose.

If you must take this medicine regularly and you miss a dose, take it as soon as you remember. However, if it is almost time for your next dose, skip the missed dose and go back to your regular schedule. **Do not double doses.**

PRECAUTIONS WHILE USING THIS MEDICINE

Narcotic analgesics will add to the effects of alcohol and other CNS depressants (medicines that slow down the nervous system). **Check with your doctor before taking any such depressants while you are using this medicine.**

This medicine may cause some people to become drowsy, dizzy, or lightheaded, or to feel a false sense of well-being. **Make sure you know how you react to this medicine before you drive, use machines, or do other jobs that require you to be alert and clearheaded.**

If you have been taking this medicine regularly for several weeks or more, **do not suddenly stop taking it without first checking with your doctor.** Your doctor may want you to reduce your dose gradually.

If you think an overdose has been taken, get emergency help at once. Taking an overdose or taking alcohol or CNS depressants with this medicine may lead to unconsciousness or death. Signs of overdose include confusion; seizures; severe nervousness or restlessness, dizziness, drowsiness, or weakness; and unusually slow or troubled breathing.

POSSIBLE SIDE EFFECTS OF THIS MEDICINE
Side Effects That Should Be Reported To Your Doctor

> *Less common or rare*—Feelings of unreality; hallucinations; hives, itching, or skin rash; increased sweating; mental depression or other mood changes; redness or flushing of face; ringing or buzzing in ears; shortness

of breath or wheezing; swelling of face; trembling or uncontrolled muscle movements; unusual excitement or restlessness, especially in children; unusually fast or pounding heartbeat

If you are taking propoxyphene, you should also tell your doctor if you notice darkening of your urine, pale stools, or yellow eyes or skin.

Side Effects That Usually Do Not Require Medical Attention

These possible side effects may go away during treatment; however, if they continue or are bothersome, check with your doctor, nurse, or pharmacist.

> *More common*—Dizziness; drowsiness; feeling faint; lightheadedness; nausea or vomiting

Other side effects not listed above may also occur in some patients. If you notice any other effects, check with your doctor, nurse, or pharmacist.

After you stop using this medicine, your body may need time to adjust. **Check with your doctor if you notice any unusual effects,** especially body aches; diarrhea; fever; gooseflesh; large pupils of eyes; loss of appetite; nausea or vomiting; nervousness or restlessness; runny nose; sneezing; shivering or trembling; stomach cramps; trouble in sleeping; unusual sweating, yawning, or irritability; unusually fast heartbeat; or weakness.

OPIOID (NARCOTIC) ANALGESICS AND ACETAMINOPHEN Systemic

Including Acetaminophen and Codeine; Acetaminophen, Codeine, and Caffeine; Dihydrocodeine and Acetaminophen; Dihydrocodeine, Acetaminophen, and Caffeine; Hydrocodone and Acetaminophen; Meperidine and Acetaminophen; Oxycodone and Acetaminophen; Pentazocine and Acetaminophen; Propoxyphene and Acetaminophen.

■ For the Pharmacist ■

In providing consultation, consider emphasizing the following selected information (» = major clinical significance):

Before using this medication
» Conditions affecting use, especially:

Sensitivity to acetaminophen or to opioid analgesic considered for use, history of

Pregnancy—Acetaminophen and opioid analgesics cross the placenta; regular use of opioids by pregnant women may cause physical dependence in the fetus and withdrawal symptoms in the neonate

Breast-feeding—Acetaminophen, codeine, meperidine, and propoxyphene are excreted in breast milk

Use in children—Children up to 2 years of age are more susceptible to the effects of opioids, especially respiratory depression; also, children may be more likely to experience paradoxical CNS excitation during therapy

Use in the elderly—Geriatric patients are more susceptible to the effects of opioids, especially respiratory depression

Other medications, especially alcohol or other CNS depressants, monoamine oxidase inhibitors, tricyclic antidepressants, zidovudine, and naltrexone

Other medical problems, especially alcoholism (active or in remission), diarrhea caused by antibiotics or poisoning, asthma or other respiratory problems, hepatic disease, viral hepatitis, and severe inflammatory bowel disease

Proper use of this medication
» Importance of not taking more medication than the amount prescribed because of danger of overdose and habit-forming potential of opioid analgesics; also, acetaminophen may cause liver damage with long-term or high-dose use
» Not increasing dose if medication is less effective after a few weeks; checking with physician
» Missed dose (if on scheduled dosing): Taking as soon as possible; not taking if almost time for next dose; not doubling doses
» Proper storage

Precautions while using this medication
Regular visits to physician to check progress during long-term or high-dose therapy
» Caution if other medications containing opioid analgesics or acetaminophen are used
» Avoiding use of alcohol or other central nervous system (CNS) depressants during therapy unless prescribed or otherwise approved by physician

Possibility that drinking large amounts of alcohol may increase risk of liver damage with acetaminophen

Not regularly taking aspirin or other salicylates or other nonsteroidal anti-inflammatory analgesics concurrently, unless directed by physician or dentist

» Caution if dizziness, drowsiness, lightheadedness, or false sense of well-being occurs

Caution when getting up suddenly from a lying or sitting position

Lying down if nausea or vomiting, or dizziness or lightheadedness occurs

Caution if any kind of surgery (including dental surgery) or emergency treatment is required

Possible dryness of mouth; using sugarless gum or candy, ice, or saliva substitute for relief; checking with dentist if dry mouth continues for more than 2 weeks

» Checking with physician before discontinuing medication after prolonged use of high doses; gradual dosage reduction may be necessary to avoid withdrawal symptoms

» Suspected overdose: Getting emergency help at once

Side/adverse effects

Signs of potential side effects, especially respiratory depression or impairment; allergic reactions; confusion, convulsions, hallucinations, mental depression, or other signs of CNS toxicity; agranulocytosis; hepatotoxicity; hypertension; paradoxical CNS excitation, especially in children; renal function impairment; and thrombocytopenia

---

▲ For the Patient ▲

912452

ABOUT YOUR MEDICINE

Combination medicines containing **narcotic analgesics** (nar-KOT-ik an-al-JEE-zicks) and **acetaminophen** (a-seat-a-MIN-oh-fen) are used to relieve pain.

If any of the information in this leaflet causes you special concern or if you want additional information about your medicine and its use, check with your doctor, nurse, or pharmacist. **Remember, keep this and all other medicines out of the reach of children and never share your medicines with others.**

BEFORE USING THIS MEDICINE

Tell your doctor, nurse, and pharmacist if you . . .

- are allergic to any medicine, either prescription or nonprescription (OTC);
- are pregnant or intend to become pregnant while using this medicine;
- are breast-feeding;
- are taking any other prescription or nonprescription (OTC) medicine, especially carbamazepine, CNS depressants, MAO inhibitors, or naltrexone;
- have any other medical problems, especially colitis; emphysema, asthma, or chronic lung disease; heart disease; or hepatitis or other liver disease.

PROPER USE OF THIS MEDICINE

Take this medicine only as directed by your medical doctor or dentist. Do not take more of it and do not take it more often or for a longer period of time than ordered. If too much of a narcotic analgesic is taken, it may become habit-forming or lead to medical problems because of an overdose.

If you must take this medicine regularly and you miss a dose, take it as soon as possible. However, if it is almost time for your next dose, skip the missed dose and go back to your regular dosing schedule. **Do not double doses.**

PRECAUTIONS WHILE USING THIS MEDICINE

Check the labels of all nonprescription (OTC) and prescription medicines you now take. If any contain acetaminophen or a narcotic, be especially careful, since taking them while taking this medicine may lead to overdose.

This medicine will add to the effects of alcohol and other CNS depressants (medicines that slow down the nervous system). **Check with your doctor before taking any such depressants while you are using this medicine.**

This medicine may cause some people to become drowsy, dizzy, or lightheaded, or to feel a false sense of well-being. **Make sure you know how you react to this medicine before you drive, use machines, or do other jobs that require you to be alert and clearheaded.**

If you have been taking this medicine regularly for several weeks, **do not suddenly stop using it without checking with your doctor.** Your doctor may want you to reduce gradually the amount you are taking before stopping completely.

If you think you or someone else may have taken an overdose, get emergency help at once. Taking an overdose or taking alcohol or CNS depressants with this medicine may lead to unconsciousness or death. Signs of overdose include confusion; convulsions (seizures); severe nervousness or restlessness, dizziness, drowsiness, or weakness; or unusually slow or troubled breathing.

POSSIBLE SIDE EFFECTS OF THIS MEDICINE
Side Effects That Should Be Reported To Your Doctor

Less common or rare—Black, tarry stools; bloody or cloudy urine; confusion; difficult or painful urination; fast, slow, or pounding heartbeat; frequent urge to urinate; hallucinations; irregular breathing; mental depression; pale stools; pinpoint red spots on skin; ringing or buzzing in ears; shortness of breath or troubled breathing; skin rash, hives, or itching; sore throat and fever; sudden decrease in amount of urine; swelling of face; trembling or uncontrolled muscle movements; unusual bleeding or bruising; unusual excitement, especially in children; yellow eyes or skin

Side Effects That Usually Do Not Require Medical Attention

These possible side effects may go away during treatment; however, if they continue or are bothersome, check with your doctor, nurse, or pharmacist.

> *More common*—Dizziness or lightheadedness; drowsiness; feeling faint; nausea or vomiting; unusual tiredness or weakness

Other side effects not listed above may also occur in some patients. If you notice any other effects, check with your doctor, nurse, or pharmacist.

After you stop using this medicine, your body may need time to adjust. This may take several days or more. **Check with your doctor if you notice any unusual effects,** especially body aches; diarrhea; gooseflesh; nausea or vomiting; shivering or trembling; stomach cramps; fever, runny nose, or sneezing; unusual sweating, nervousness, restlessness or irritability; unusually fast heartbeat; or weakness.

OPIOID (NARCOTIC) ANALGESICS AND ASPIRIN Systemic

Including Aspirin and Codeine; Aspirin, Codeine, and Caffeine; Aspirin, Caffeine, and Dihydrocodeine; Aspirin and Dihydrocodeine; Buffered Aspirin, Codeine, and Caffeine; Hydrocodone and Aspirin; Hydrocodone, Aspirin, and Caffeine; Oxycodone and Aspirin; Pentazocine and Aspirin; Propoxyphene and Aspirin; Propoxyphene, Aspirin, and Caffeine.

■ For the Pharmacist ■

In providing consultation, consider emphasizing the following selected information (» = major clinical significance):

Before using this medication

» Conditions affecting use, especially:

Sensitivity to the opioid considered for use, to aspirin, or to nonsteroidal anti-inflammatory drugs (NSAIDs), history of

Pregnancy—Aspirin and opioid analgesics cross the placenta; high-dose chronic use or abuse of aspirin in the third trimester may be hazardous to the mother as well as the fetus and/or neonate, causing heart problems in fetus or neonate and/or bleeding in mother, fetus, or neonate; high-dose chronic use or abuse may also prolong and complicate labor and delivery; also, regular use of opioids by pregnant women may cause physical dependence in the fetus and withdrawal symptoms in the neonate; not taking aspirin during the third trimester unless prescribed by physician

Breast-feeding—Aspirin, codeine, and propoxyphene are excreted in breast milk

Use in children and teenagers—Checking with physician before giving to children or teenagers with symptoms of acute febrile illness, especially influenza or varicella, because of the risk of Reye's syndrome; also, increased susceptibility to aspirin toxicity in children, especially with fever and dehydration; also, children up to 2 years of age are more susceptible to the effects of opioids, especially respiratory depression; in addition, children may be more likely to experience opioid-induced paradoxical CNS excitation during therapy

Use in the elderly—Increased risk of aspirin toxicity and of opioid-induced adverse effects, especially respiratory depression

Other medications, especially alcohol or other CNS depressants, anticoagulants, antidiabetic agents (oral), those cephalosporins that may cause hypoprothrombinemia, methotrexate, monoamine oxidase inhibitors, moxalactam, naltrexone, NSAIDs, platelet aggregation inhibitors, plicamycin, probenecid, sulfinpyrazone, urinary alkalizers, valproic acid, vancomycin, and zidovudine

Other medical problems, especially coagulation or platelet function disorders, diarrhea caused by antibiotics or poisoning, asthma or other respiratory problems, and gastrointestinal problems such as ulceration or erosive gastritis (especially a bleeding ulcer) or other severe inflammatory bowel disease

Proper use of this medication
» Taking with food or a full glass (240 mL) of water to minimize stomach irritation
» Not taking medication if it has a strong vinegar-like odor
» Importance of not taking more medication than the amount prescribed because of danger of overdose of aspirin or opioid analgesics and habit-forming potential of opioid analgesics
» Not increasing dose if medication seems less effective after a few weeks; checking with physician instead
» Missed dose (if on scheduled dosing): Taking as soon as possible; not taking if almost time for next dose; not doubling doses
» Proper storage

Precautions while using this medication
Regular visits to physician to check progress during long-term therapy
» Caution if other medications containing aspirin or other salicylates or opioid analgesics are used
» Avoiding use of alcohol or other central nervous system (CNS) depressants during therapy unless prescribed or otherwise approved by physician; also, alcohol consumption may increase risk of aspirin-induced stomach problems
Not taking acetaminophen or ibuprofen or other nonsteroidal antiinflammatory analgesics concurrently for more than a few days unless directed by physician or dentist
» Caution if dizziness, drowsiness, lightheadedness, or false sense of well-being occurs
Caution when getting up suddenly from a lying or sitting position
Lying down if nausea or vomiting, or dizziness or lightheadedness occurs
Need to inform physician or dentist of use of medication if any kind of surgery (including dental surgery) or emergency treatment is required
Caution if any kind of surgery is required; aspirin should be discontinued 5 days prior to surgery unless otherwise directed by physician or dentist
Not taking a tetracycline antibiotic within 1 to 2 hours of buffered formulations
Diabetics: Aspirin may cause false urine sugar test results with prolonged use of 8 or more 325-mg (5-grain), or 4 or more 650-mg (10-grain), doses per day
Possible dryness of mouth; using sugarless gum or candy, ice, or saliva substitute for relief; checking with dentist if dry mouth continues for more than 2 weeks
» Checking with physician before discontinuing medication after prolonged use of high doses; gradual dosage reduction may be necessary to avoid withdrawal symptoms
» Suspected overdose: Getting emergency help at once

Side/adverse effects
Signs of potential side effects, especially respiratory depression or impairment; allergic reactions; confusion, convulsions, hallucinations, mental depression, or other signs of CNS toxicity; gastrointestinal toxicity; hepatotoxicity; hypertension, and paradoxical CNS excitation, especially in children

▲ For the Patient ▲

912463

ABOUT YOUR MEDICINE

Combination medicines containing **narcotic analgesics** (nar-KOT-ik an-al-JEE-zicks) and **aspirin** (AS-pir-in) are used to relieve pain.

If any of the information in this leaflet causes you special concern or if you want additional information about your medicine and its use, check with your doctor, nurse, or pharmacist. **Remember, keep this and all other medicines out of the reach of children and never share your medicines with others.**

BEFORE USING THIS MEDICINE

Do not give a medicine containing aspirin to a child or teenager with flu or chickenpox without first discussing its use with your child's doctor.

Tell your doctor, nurse, and pharmacist if you . . .
- are allergic to any medicine, either prescription or nonprescription (OTC);
- are pregnant or intend to become pregnant while using this medicine;
- are breast-feeding;
- are taking any other prescription or nonprescription (OTC) medicine;
- have any other medical problems, especially asthma, allergies, and nasal polyps (history of); chronic lung disease; colitis; hemophilia or other bleeding problems; kidney disease; or stomach ulcer or other stomach problems.

PROPER USE OF THIS MEDICINE

Take this medicine with food and a full glass (8 ounces) of water as directed. Do not take more or for a longer time than ordered.

Do not take this medicine if it has a strong vinegar-like odor. This odor means the aspirin in it is breaking down.

If you must take this medicine regularly and you miss a dose, take it as soon as possible. However, if it is almost time for your next dose, skip the missed dose and go back to your regular dosing schedule. **Do not double doses.**

PRECAUTIONS WHILE USING THIS MEDICINE

Check the labels of all over-the-counter (OTC) and prescription medicines you now take. If any contain a narcotic or a salicylate, be especially careful, since taking them while taking this medicine may lead to overdose.

This medicine will add to the effects of alcohol and other CNS depressants. **Check with your physician or dentist before taking any such depressants while you are using this medicine.**

This medicine may cause some people to become drowsy, dizzy, or lightheaded, or to feel a false sense of well-being. **Make sure you know how you react before you drive, use machines, or do jobs that require you to be alert.**

If you have been taking this medicine regularly for several weeks, **do not suddenly stop using it without checking with your doctor.** Your doctor may want you to reduce gradually the amount you are taking before stopping completely.

If you think an overdose has been taken, get emergency help at once. Taking an overdose or taking alcohol or CNS depressants with this medicine may lead to unconsciousness or death. Signs of overdose include hearing loss; ringing in the ear; hallucinations; severe confusion, excitement, nervousness, restlessness, dizziness, drowsiness, or weakness; shortness of breath or troubled breathing; or convulsions (seizures).

POSSIBLE SIDE EFFECTS OF THIS MEDICINE
Side Effects That Should Be Reported To Your Doctor

> *Less common or rare*—Bloody or black tarry stools; dark or bloody urine; fast, slow, or pounding heartbeat; increased sweating (more common with hydrocodone); mental depression; pale stools; redness or flushing of face (more common with hydrocodone); skin rash, hives, or itching; swelling of face; tightness in chest or wheezing; trembling or uncontrolled muscle movements; unusual excitement; unusual tiredness or weakness; vomiting of blood or material that looks like coffee grounds; yellow eyes or skin

Side Effects That Usually Do Not Require Medical Attention

These effects may go away during treatment or if you lie down; however, if they continue or are bothersome, check with your doctor, nurse, or pharmacist.

> *More common*—Dizziness or lightheadedness; drowsiness; feeling faint; heartburn or indigestion; nausea or vomiting; stomach pain (mild)

Other side effects not listed above may also occur in some patients. If you notice any other effects, check with your doctor, nurse, or pharmacist.

After you stop using this medicine, your body may need time to adjust. **Check with your doctor if you notice any unusual effects,** especially body aches; diarrhea; gooseflesh; nausea or vomiting; shivering or trembling; stomach cramps; fever, runny nose, or sneezing; increased sweating; nervousness, restlessness, irritability, or weakness.

OXICONAZOLE Topical

■ For the Pharmacist ■

In providing consultation, consider emphasizing the following selected information (» = major clinical significance):

Before using this medication
» Conditions affecting use, especially:
    Sensitivity to oxiconazole
    Breast-feeding—Distributed into breast milk

Proper use of this medication
    Applying sufficient medication to cover affected and surrounding areas, and rubbing in gently
» Avoiding contact with the eyes; not using in vagina
» Compliance with full course of therapy; fungal infections may require prolonged therapy
» Proper dosing
    Missed dose: Applying as soon as possible; not applying if almost time for next dose
» Proper storage

Precautions while using this medication
    Checking with physician if no improvement occurs within 2 to 4 weeks
» Using hygienic measures to cure infection and prevent reinfection:
    For tinea cruris
        Avoiding underwear that is tight-fitting or made from synthetic materials; wearing loose-fitting cotton underwear instead
        Using a bland, absorbent powder or an antifungal powder on the skin; using the powder between administration times for oxiconazole
    For tinea pedis
        Carefully drying feet, especially between toes, after bathing
        Avoiding socks made from wool or synthetic materials; wearing clean, cotton socks and changing them each day or more often if feet perspire excessively
        Wearing sandals or well-ventilated shoes
        Using bland, absorbent powder or an antifungal powder between toes, on feet, and in socks and shoes 1 or 2 times a day; using the powder between administration times for oxiconazole

Side/adverse effects
    Signs of potential side effects, especially hypersensitivity

▲ For the Patient ▲

913783

ANTIFUNGALS (Topical): *Including Carbol-Fuchsin; Ciclopirox; Clioquinol; Clotrimazole; Econazole; Haloprogin; Ketoconazole; Miconazole; Nystatin; Oxiconazole; Sulconazole; Tolnaftate; Undecylenic Acid, Compound.*

ABOUT YOUR MEDICINE

Topical antifungal medicines are used to treat infections caused by a fungus, such as ringworm or athlete's foot. Not all antifungal medicines will work for all infections. Therefore, do not use this medicine for any other infection unless you have checked with your doctor. Some of these medicines may also be used for other infections as determined by your doctor.

If any of the information in this leaflet causes you special concern or if you want additional information about your medicine and its use, check with your doctor, nurse, or pharmacist. **Remember, keep this and all other medicines out of the reach of children and never share your medicines with others.**

BEFORE USING THIS MEDICINE

Tell your doctor, nurse, and pharmacist if you . . .
  * are allergic to any medicine, either prescription or non-prescription (OTC);
  * are pregnant or intend to become pregnant while using this medicine;
  * are breast-feeding;
  * are taking any other prescription or nonprescription (OTC) medicine;
  * have any other medical problems.

PROPER USE OF THIS MEDICINE

Keep this medicine away from the eyes. Also, do not use it in the vagina.

If you are treating an infant or a child with eczema, do not use carbol-fuchsin more than once a day.

For patients using the cream, ointment, lotion, or solution form of this medicine: Apply enough medicine to cover the affected and surrounding skin areas and rub in gently.

To use the aerosol form of this medicine: Shake well before using. From a distance of about 6 inches, spray the medicine on the affected areas. If used on the feet, spray it between the toes and in socks and shoes. Do not inhale the medicine, and do not use near heat, near open flame, or while smoking.

Do not apply an airtight covering (such as kitchen plastic wrap) **over this medicine** unless directed to do so. To do so may irritate the skin.

For products containing carbol-fuchsin: Carbol-fuchsin is a poison if swallowed. Use only on the affected areas as directed. Do not swallow the medicine.

To help clear up your infection completely, it is very important that you keep using your medicine for the full time of treatment even if your symptoms begin to clear up after a few days. You may have to continue using this medicine every day for several weeks or more. **Do not miss any doses.**

If you do miss a dose of this medicine, apply it as soon as possible. However, if it is almost time for your next dose, skip the missed dose and go back to your regular dosing schedule.

PRECAUTIONS WHILE USING THIS MEDICINE

If your skin problem does not improve within two to four weeks (one week if using carbol-fuchsin), or if it becomes worse, check with your doctor.

To help clear up your infection completely and to help make sure it does not return, good health habits are also required. The following measures will help reduce chafing and irritation and will keep the area cool and dry:

- For patients who have ringworm of the groin or body: Dry yourself carefully after bathing. Wear loose-fitting, cotton underwear and clothing. Try to keep moisture from building up on affected areas. Use a bland, absorbent powder (for example, talcum powder) or a nonprescription antifungal powder on the skin. It is best to apply the powder in between the times you apply any other antifungal medicine.
- For patients who have ringworm of the foot: After bathing, carefully dry the feet, especially between the toes. Wear clean, cotton socks and change them daily or more often if the feet sweat freely. It is best to wear sandals or well-ventilated shoes. Use a bland, absorbent powder or a nonprescription antifungal powder between the toes, on the feet, and in socks and shoes freely once or twice a day. It is best to apply the powder in between the times you apply any other antifungal medicine.

For patients using carbol-fuchsin or clioquinol: This medicine may stain clothing, skin, hair, and nails. Avoid getting it on your clothing since bleaching may not remove the stain.

POSSIBLE SIDE EFFECTS OF THIS MEDICINE
Side Effects That Should Be Reported To Your Doctor

   Rare—Skin rash, hives, peeling, burning, itching, redness, swelling, blistering, oozing, or other irritation not present before use of this medicine

When you apply the solution form of this medicine, a mild temporary stinging may be expected.

Other side effects not listed above may also occur in some patients. If you notice any other effects, check with your doctor, nurse, or pharmacist.

OXYBUTYNIN Systemic

■For the Pharmacist■

In providing consultation, consider emphasizing the following selected information (» = major clinical significance):

Before using this medication
» Conditions affecting use, especially:
  Sensitivity to oxybutynin
  Use in the elderly—Increased sensitivity to anticholinergic effects
  Dental—Possible development of dental problems because of decreased salivary flow
  Other medications, especially other anticholinergics
  Other medical problems, especially cardiac diseases, glaucoma, hemorrhage, hiatal hernia, intestinal atony, myasthenia gravis, paralytic ileus, prostatic hypertrophy, obstruction in gastrointestinal or urinary tract, tachycardia, ulcerative colitis, urinary retention

Proper use of this medication
  Taking medication on an empty stomach with water, or with food or milk to reduce gastric irritation
» Importance of not taking more medication than the amount prescribed
» Proper dosing
  Missed dose: Taking as soon as possible; if almost time for next dose, not taking at all; not doubling doses
» Proper storage

Precautions while using this medication
» Avoiding use of alcohol or other CNS depressants
  Possible increased sensitivity of eyes to light
» Caution if drowsiness or blurred vision occurs
» Caution during exercise and hot weather; overheating may result in heat stroke
  Possible dryness of mouth, nose, and throat; using sugarless gum or candy, ice, or saliva substitute for relief of dry mouth; checking with physician or dentist if dry mouth continues for more than 2 weeks

Side/adverse effects
  Signs of potential side effects, especially allergic reaction or increased intraocular pressure

▲ For the Patient ▲

914629

ABOUT YOUR MEDICINE

Oxybutynin (ox-i-BYOO-ti-nin) belongs to the group of medicines called antispasmodics. It helps decrease muscle spasms of the bladder and the frequent urge to urinate caused by these spasms.

If any of the information in this leaflet causes you special concern or if you want additional information about your

medicine and its use, check with your doctor, nurse, or pharmacist. **Remember, keep this and all other medicines out of the reach of children and never share your medicines with others.**

BEFORE USING THIS MEDICINE

Tell your doctor, nurse, and pharmacist if you . . .
- are allergic to any medicine, either prescription or non-prescription (OTC);
- are pregnant or intend to become pregnant while using this medicine;
- are breast-feeding;
- are taking any other prescription or nonprescription (OTC) medicine, especially amantadine, other anticholinergics (medicines to help reduce stomach acid and for abdominal or stomach spasms or cramps), antidepressants, antidyskinetics, antihistamines, antipsychotics, buclizine, carbamazepine, cyclizine, cyclobenzaprine, disopyramide, flavoxate, ipratropium, meclizine, methylphenidate, orphenadrine, procainamide, promethazine, quinidine, or trimeprazine;
- have any other medical problems, especially bleeding (severe), colitis (severe), enlarged prostate, glaucoma, heart disease, intestinal blockage or other intestinal or stomach problems, myasthenia gravis, problems with urination, or urinary tract blockage.

PROPER USE OF THIS MEDICINE

This medicine is usually taken with water on an empty stomach. However, your doctor may want you to take it with food or milk to lessen stomach upset.

Take this medicine only as directed. Do not take more of it, do not take it more often, and do not take it for a longer time than your doctor ordered. To do so may increase the chance of side effects.

If you miss a dose of this medicine, take it as soon as possible. However, if it is almost time for your next dose, skip the missed dose and go back to your regular dosing schedule. Do not double doses.

PRECAUTIONS WHILE USING THIS MEDICINE

This medicine will add to the effects of alcohol and other CNS depressants (medicines that slow down the nervous system, possibly causing drowsiness). **Check with your doctor before taking any such depressants while you are using this medicine.**

This medicine may cause your eyes to become more sensitive to light than they are normally. Wearing sunglasses and avoiding too much exposure to bright light may help lessen the discomfort.

This medicine may cause some people to become drowsy or have blurred vision. **Make sure you know how you react to** this medicine before you drive, use machines, or do other jobs that require you to be alert or to see well.

Oxybutynin may make you sweat less, causing your body temperature to increase. **Use extra care not to become overheated during exercise or hot weather while you are taking this medicine,** since overheating may result in heatstroke. Also, hot baths or saunas may make you feel dizzy or faint while you are taking this medicine.

Your mouth, nose, and throat may feel very dry while you are taking this medicine. For temporary relief of mouth dryness, use sugarless candy or gum, melt bits of ice in your mouth, or use a saliva substitute. However, if your mouth continues to feel dry for more than 2 weeks, check with your medical doctor or dentist. Continuing dryness of the mouth may increase the chance of dental disease, including tooth decay, gum disease, and fungal infections.

POSSIBLE SIDE EFFECTS OF THIS MEDICINE
Side Effects That Should Be Reported To Your Doctor

   Rare—Eye pain; skin rash or hives

Side Effects That Usually Do Not Require Medical Attention

These possible side effects may go away during treatment; however, if they continue or are bothersome, check with your doctor, nurse, or pharmacist.

   More common—Constipation; decreased sweating; drowsiness; dryness of mouth, nose, and throat

   Less common or rare—Blurred vision; decreased flow of breast milk; decreased sexual ability; difficult urination; difficulty in swallowing; headache; increased sensitivity of eyes to light; nausea or vomiting; trouble in sleeping; unusual tiredness or weakness

Other side effects not listed above may also occur in some patients. If you notice any other effects, check with your doctor, nurse, or pharmacist.

PAROXETINE   Systemic

■For the Pharmacist■

In providing consultation, consider emphasizing the following selected
information (》 = major clinical significance):

Before using this medication
》 Conditions affecting use, especially:
  Sensitivity to paroxetine
  Pregnancy—Studies in rats using higher than the maximum hu-
   man mg/kg doses have shown increased pre-and post-im-
   plantation losses and decreased viability of pups; clinical sig-
   nificance is unknown
  Breast-feeding—Distributed into breast milk
  Dental—Decreased salivary flow may contribute to caries, per-
   iodontal disease, candidiasis, and discomfort
  Other medications, especially monoamine oxidase (MAO) in-
   hibitors, tryptophan, and warfarin

Proper use of this medication
》 Compliance with therapy; not taking more or less medicine than
  prescribed
》 Up to 4 weeks or more of therapy may be required before antide-
  pressant effects are achieved
》 Proper dosing
  Missed dose: Taking as soon as possible; continuing on regular sched-
   ule with next dose; not doubling doses
》 Proper storage

Precautions while using this medication
  Regular visits to physician to check progress of therapy
  Checking with physician before discontinuing medication
》 Avoiding use of alcoholic beverages; not taking other CNS depressants unless prescribed by physician
》 Possible blurred vision, drowsiness, impairment of judgment, thinking, or motor skills; caution when driving or doing jobs requiring
  alertness
》 Possible dizziness or lightheadedness; caution when getting up suddenly from a lying or sitting position
》 Possible dryness of mouth; using sugarless gum or candy, ice, or
  saliva substitute for relief; checking with physician or dentist if
  dry mouth continues for more than 2 weeks

Side/adverse effects
  Possibility of withdrawal symptoms
  Signs of potential side effects, especially agitation; myalgia, myasthenia, or myopathy; orthostatic hypotension; rash; extrapyramidal symptoms; hyponatremia; mania or hypomania; serotonin
  syndrome

▲ For the Patient ▲

919316

ABOUT YOUR MEDICINE

Paroxetine (pa-ROX-uh-teen) is used to treat mental depression.

If any of the information in this leaflet causes you special concern or if you want additional information about your medicine and its use, check with your doctor, nurse, or pharmacist. **Remember, keep this and all other medicines out of the reach of children and never share your medicines with others.**

BEFORE USING THIS MEDICINE

Tell your doctor, nurse, and pharmacist if you . . .
- are allergic to any medicine, either prescription or non-prescription (OTC);
- are pregnant or intend to become pregnant while using this medicine;
- are breast-feeding;
- are taking any other prescription or nonprescription (OTC) medicine, especially MAO inhibitors, tryptophan, or warfarin (a blood thinner);
- have any other medical problems.

PROPER USE OF THIS MEDICINE

Take this medicine only as directed by your doctor, to benefit your condition as much as possible. Do not take more of it, do not take it more often, and do not take it for a longer time than your doctor ordered.

You may have to take paroxetine for up to 4 weeks or longer before you begin to feel better.

Paroxetine may be taken with or without food. Take it as directed.

If you miss a dose of this medicine, take it as soon as possible. However, if it is almost time for your next dose, skip the missed dose and go back to your regular dosing schedule. Do not double doses.

PRECAUTIONS WHILE USING THIS MEDICINE

It is important that your doctor check your progress at regular visits, to allow for changes in your dose and to help lessen any side effects.

Do not stop taking this medicine without first checking with your doctor. Your doctor may want you to gradually reduce the amount you are taking before stopping completely. This is to decrease the chance of side effects.

This medicine may add to the effects of alcohol and other CNS depressants (medicines that slow down the nervous system). **Check with your doctor before taking any such depressants while you are using this medicine.**

This medicine may cause some people to become drowsy or have blurred vision. **Make sure you know how you react to paroxetine before you drive, use machines, or do other jobs that could be dangerous if you are not alert or able to see clearly.**

Dizziness, lightheadedness, or fainting may occur, especially when you get up from a lying or sitting position. Getting up

slowly may help. If this problem continues or gets worse, check with your doctor.

This medicine may cause dryness of the mouth. For temporary relief, use sugarless gum or candy, melt bits of ice in your mouth, or use a saliva substitute. However, if your mouth continues to feel dry for more than 2 weeks, check with your physician or dentist. Continuing dryness of the mouth may increase the chance of dental disease, including tooth decay, gum disease, and fungus infections.

POSSIBLE SIDE EFFECTS OF THIS MEDICINE
Side Effects That Should Be Reported To Your Doctor

Less common—Agitation; lightheadedness or fainting; muscle pain or weakness; rash

Rare—Diarrhea; difficulty in speaking; drowsiness; dryness of mouth; fever; inability to move eyes; increased sweating; increased thirst; lack of energy; loss of or decrease in body movements; mood or behavior changes; overactive reflexes; racing heartbeat; restlessness; shivering or shaking; sudden or unusual body or face movements; talking, feeling, and acting with excitement and activity you cannot control

Signs of overdose—Drowsiness (severe); dryness of mouth (severe); irritability; large pupils; nausea (severe); racing heartbeat; tremor (severe); vomiting (severe)

Side Effects That Usually Do Not Require Medical Attention

These possible side effects may go away during treatment; however, if they continue or are bothersome, check with your doctor, nurse, or pharmacist.

More common—Constipation; decreased sexual ability; dizziness; headache; nausea; problems in urinating; tremor; trouble in sleeping; unusual tiredness or weakness; vomiting

Less common—Anxiety or nervousness; blurred vision; change in your sense of taste; decreased or increased appetite; decreased sexual desire; fast or irregular heartbeat; tingling, burning, or prickly sensations; weight loss or gain

Other side effects not listed above may also occur in some patients. If you notice any other effects, check with your doctor, nurse, or pharmacist.

After you stop using this medicine, your body may need time to adjust. During this time, check with your doctor if you notice any unusual effects.

PEMOLINE   Systemic

■ For the Pharmacist ■

In providing consultation, consider emphasizing the following selected information (» = major clinical significance):

Before using this medication
» Conditions affecting use, especially:
  Sensitivity to pemoline
  Pregnancy—Animal studies have shown an increase in stillbirths and reduced postnatal survival rate
  Use in children—Inhibition of growth reported with CNS stimulants, but data inconclusive; drug-free periods recommended; symptoms of behavior disturbance and thought disorder exacerbated in psychotic children
  Other medical problems, especially hepatic function impairment; Tourette's disorder; psychosis; or renal function impairment

Proper use of this medication
  Proper administration of chewable tablet: Tablet must be chewed
» May require 3 to 4 weeks of therapy to obtain optimal effects
» Importance of not taking more medication than the amount prescribed because of possible habit-forming potential
» Proper dosing
  Missed dose: Taking as soon as possible; if remembered the next day, skipping missed dose; continuing on schedule; not doubling doses
» Proper storage

Precautions while using this medication
  Regular visits to physician to check progress during therapy
  Checking with physician before discontinuing medication after long-term and high-dose therapy; gradual dosage reduction may be necessary to avoid possibility of withdrawal symptoms
» Caution if dizziness occurs
» Suspected physical or psychological dependence; checking with physician

Side/adverse effects
  Signs of potential side effects, especially jaundice

▲ For the Patient ▲

914684

ABOUT THIS MEDICINE

Pemoline (PEM-oh-leen) belongs to the group of medicines called central nervous system (CNS) stimulants. It is used to treat children with attention-deficit hyperactivity disorder (ADHD).

If any of the information in this leaflet causes you special concern or if you want additional information about this medicine and its use, check with the child's doctor, nurse, or pharmacist. **Remember, keep this and all other medicines out of the reach of children and never share medicines with others.**

BEFORE USING THIS MEDICINE

Discuss with the child's doctor the possible side effects of this medicine. Pemoline, when used for a long time, has been reported to slow the growth rate in children. Some doctors recommend drug-free periods during treatment with pemoline. Pemoline may also cause unwanted effects on behavior in children with severe emotional problems.

Tell the doctor, nurse, and pharmacist if the child . . .
- is allergic to any medicine, either prescription or non-prescription (OTC);
- is taking any other prescription or nonprescription (OTC) medicine;
- has any other medical problems, especially Gilles de la Tourette's disorder or other tics, kidney or liver disease, or emotional or mental illness.

Also tell the doctor if a teenage child is pregnant or breast-feeding.

PROPER USE OF THIS MEDICINE

If the child is taking the chewable tablet form of this medicine, these tablets must be chewed before swallowing. The child should not swallow them whole.

Sometimes this medicine must be taken for 3 to 4 weeks before improvement is noticed.

The child must take this medicine only as directed. He or she should not take more of it, should not take it more often, and should not take it for a longer time than ordered. If too much is taken, it may become habit-forming.

If the child misses a dose of this medicine, he or she should take it as soon as possible. Then go back to the regular dosing schedule. If you do not remember the missed dose until the next day, the child should skip it and go back to the regular dosing schedule. Do not double doses.

PRECAUTIONS WHILE USING THIS MEDICINE

The doctor should check the child's progress at regular visits to make sure that this medicine does not cause unwanted effects.

If pemoline will be taken in large doses for a long time, the child should not stop taking it unless you first check with the child's doctor. He or she may want to reduce gradually the amount being taken before stopping it completely.

This medicine may cause some children to become dizzy or less alert than they are normally. **Make sure you know how the child reacts to this medicine before he or she rides a bicycle or does other things that require the child to be alert.**

If the child has been using this medicine for a long time and you think he or she may have become mentally or physically dependent on it, check with the child's doctor. Some signs of dependence on pemoline are:
—a strong desire or need to continue taking the medicine.

—a need to increase the dose to receive the effects of the medicine.

—withdrawal side effects (for example, mental depression, unusual behavior, or unusual tiredness or weakness) occurring after the medicine is stopped.

POSSIBLE SIDE EFFECTS OF THIS MEDICINE
Side Effects That Should Be Reported To The Child's Doctor

Rare—Yellow eyes or skin

Side Effects That Usually Do Not Require Medical Attention

These possible side effects may go away during treatment; however, if they continue or are bothersome, check with the child's doctor, nurse, or pharmacist.

More common—Loss of appetite; trouble in sleeping; weight loss

Other side effects not listed above may also occur in some patients. If you notice any other effects, check with the child's doctor, nurse, or pharmacist.

After the child stops using this medicine, the child's body may need time to adjust. The length of time this takes depends on the amount of medicine that was being used and how long the child used it. During this time check with the child's doctor if you notice any unusual effects, especially mental depression (severe), unusual behavior, or unusual tiredness or weakness.

PENICILLAMINE   Systemic

■For the Pharmacist■

In providing consultation, consider emphasizing the following selected information (» = major clinical significance):

Before using this medication
» Conditions affecting use, especially:

Sensitivity to penicillamine or penicillin, history of

Pregnancy—Has been reported to cause birth defects in humans

Use in the elderly—Increased risk of hematologic toxicity

Other medications, especially gold compounds and phenylbutazone

Other medical problems, especially a history of penicillamine-induced agranulocytosis or aplastic anemia

Proper use of this medication
For patients with cystinuria

Importance of high fluid intake, especially at night

Possible need for low-methionine diet

For patients with rheumatoid arthritis

Taking medication on an empty stomach

Improvement in condition may require 2 to 3 months of therapy

For patients with Wilson's disease

Taking medication on an empty stomach

Possible need for low-copper diet

Improvement in condition may require 1 to 3 months of therapy

For patients with lead poisoning

Taking medication on an empty stomach

For all patients
» Compliance with therapy; checking with physician before discontinuing medication since interruption of therapy may cause sensitivity reactions when therapy is reinstituted
» Proper dosing

Missed dose: If dosing schedule is—

Once a day: Taking as soon as possible; not taking if not remembered until next day; not doubling doses

Two times a day: Taking as soon as possible; not taking if almost time for next dose; not doubling doses

More than two times a day: Taking if remembered within an hour; not taking if not remembered until later; not doubling doses
» Proper storage

Precautions while using this medication
Regular visits to physician to check progress during therapy

Caution if any kind of surgery (including dental surgery) is required because of the effects of penicillamine on collagen and elastin

Avoiding concurrent use of iron-containing medications

Side/adverse effects
Signs of potential side effects, especially allergic reactions, stomatitis, blood dyscrasias, glomerulopathy, obstructive bronchiolitis, exfoliative dermatitis, Goodpasture's syndrome, jaundice, myasthenia gravis syndrome, toxic epidermal necrolysis, optic neuritis, pancreatitis, peptic ulcer reactivation, ringing or buzzing in ears, and SLE-like syndrome

▲ For the Patient ▲

914695

ABOUT YOUR MEDICINE

Penicillamine (pen-i-SILL-a-meen) is used in the treatment of medical problems such as Wilson's disease (too much copper in the body) and rheumatoid arthritis. Also, it is used to prevent kidney stones. Penicillamine may also be used for other conditions as determined by your doctor.

If any of the information in this leaflet causes you special concern or if you want additional information about your medicine and its use, check with your doctor, nurse, or pharmacist. **Remember, keep this and all other medicines out of the reach of children and never share your medicines with others.**

BEFORE USING THIS MEDICINE

Tell your doctor, nurse, and pharmacist if you . . .
- are allergic to any medicine, either prescription or non-prescription (OTC);
- are pregnant or intend to become pregnant while using this medicine;
- are breast-feeding;
- are taking any other prescription or nonprescription (OTC) medicine, especially gold compounds;
- have **any** other medical problems.

PROPER USE OF THIS MEDICINE

Take this medicine regularly as directed. Do not stop taking it without first checking with your doctor.

For patients taking this medicine **to prevent kidney stones**:
- You should drink 2 full glasses (8 ounces each) of water at bedtime and another 2 full glasses (8 ounces each) during the night.
- It is very important that you follow any special instructions, including diet.

For patients taking this medicine **for rheumatoid arthritis**:
- Take this medicine on an empty stomach (at least 1 hour before or 2 hours after meals) and at least 1 hour before or after any other food, milk, or medicine.
- After you begin taking this medicine, 2 or 3 months may pass before you feel its effects. It is very important that you keep taking the medicine, even if you do not feel better, in order to give it time to work.

For patients taking this medicine **for Wilson's disease**:
- Take this medicine on an empty stomach (at least 1/2 to 1 hour before meals or 2 hours after meals).
- It is very important that you follow any special instructions, including diet.
- After you begin taking this medicine, 1 to 3 months may pass before you notice any improvement in your condition.

If you miss a dose of this medicine and your schedule is:
- One dose a day—Take the missed dose as soon as possible. But if you do not remember the missed dose until the next day, skip the missed dose and go back to your regular dosing schedule. Do not double the next day's dose.
- Two doses a day—Take the missed dose as soon as possible. However, if it is almost time for your next dose, skip the missed dose and go back to your regular dosing schedule. Do not double doses.
- More than two doses a day—If you remember within an hour or so of the missed dose, take it right away. But if you do not remember until later, skip the missed dose and go back to your regular schedule. Do not double doses.

PRECAUTIONS WHILE USING THIS MEDICINE
Your doctor should check your progress at regular visits to make sure that this medicine does not cause unwanted effects.

POSSIBLE SIDE EFFECTS OF THIS MEDICINE
Side Effects That Should Be Reported To Your Doctor

More common—Fever; joint pain; skin rash, hives, or itching; swollen and/or painful glands; ulcers, sores, or white spots on lips or in mouth

Less common—Bloody, dark, or cloudy urine; shortness of breath, troubled breathing, tightness in chest, or wheezing; sore throat and fever with or without chills; swelling of face, feet, or lower legs; unusual bleeding or bruising; unusual tiredness or weakness; weight gain

Rare—Abdominal or stomach pain (severe); blisters on skin; chest pain; coughing; difficulty in breathing, chewing, talking, or swallowing; eye pain; general feeling of body discomfort; pale stools; redness, tenderness, itching, burning, or peeling of skin; red or irritated eyes; red, thickened, or scaly skin; ringing or buzzing in ears; spitting up blood; unexplained coughing, wheezing, or shortness of breath; unusual muscle weakness; vision problems; yellow eyes or skin

Side Effects That Usually Do Not Require Medical Attention

These possible side effects may go away during treatment; however, if they continue or are bothersome, check with your doctor, nurse, or pharmacist.

More common—Diarrhea; loss of appetite; loss of taste; nausea or vomiting; stomach pain (mild)

Other side effects not listed above may also occur in some patients. If you notice any other effects, check with your doctor, nurse, or pharmacist.

PENICILLINS   Systemic

*Including Amoxicillin; Amoxicillin and Clavulanate;
Ampicillin; Bacampicillin; Carbenicillin; Cloxacillin;
Cyclacillin; Dicloxacillin; Flucloxacillin; Methicillin;
Mezlocillin; Nafcillin; Oxacillin; Penicillin G; Penicillin V;
Piperacillin; Pivampicillin; Pivmecillinam; Ticarcillin.*

■For the Pharmacist■

In providing consultation, consider emphasizing the following selected
information (» = major clinical significance):

Before using this medication
» Conditions affecting use, especially:
>> Allergy to penicillins, cephalosporins, or cephamycins
>> Pregnancy—Penicillins cross the placenta
>> Breast-feeding—Penicillins are distributed into breast milk
>> Use in children—Neonates and young infants may have reduced
elimination of renally eliminated penicillins due to incompletely developed renal function
>> Other medications, especially aminoglycosides; angiotensin-converting enzyme inhibitors; cholestyramine; colestipol;
coumarin- or indandione-derivative anticoagulants; estrogen-containing oral contraceptives; heparin; methotrexate;
nonsteroidal anti-inflammatory drugs (NSAIDs), especially
aspirin; other platelet aggregation inhibitors; other potassium-containing medications; potassium-sparing diuretics;
potassium supplements; probenecid; sulfinpyrazone; or
thrombolytic agents
>> Other medical problems, especially a history of bleeding disorders; congestive heart failure; cystic fibrosis; active or history
of gastrointestinal disease, especially antibiotic-associated
colitis; infectious mononucleosis; or renal function impairment

Proper use of this medication
Taking on an empty stomach (for ampicillin, bacampicillin oral suspension, carbenicillin; cloxacillin, dicloxacillin, flucloxacillin,
nafcillin, oxacillin, penicillin G)
Taking on a full or empty stomach (for amoxicillin, bacampicillin
tablets, penicillin V, pivampicillin, pivmecillinam)
Taking amoxicillin suspension straight or mixed with formulas, milk,
fruit juice, water, ginger ale, or other cold drinks; taking immediately after mixing; drinking full dose
Not drinking acidic fruit juices or other acidic beverages within 1
hour of taking oral penicillin G
Proper administration technique for oral liquids and/or pediatric
drops
Not using after expiration date
» Compliance with full course of therapy, especially in streptococcal
infections
» Importance of not missing doses and taking at evenly spaced times
» Proper dosing
Missed dose: Taking as soon as possible; not taking if almost time
for next dose; not doubling doses
» Proper storage

Precautions while using this medication
Checking with physician if no improvement within a few days
» For severe diarrhea, checking with physician before taking any antidiarrheals; for mild diarrhea, kaolin- or attapulgite-containing
   antidiarrheals may be used, but antiperistaltic antidiarrheals
   should be avoided; checking with physician or pharmacist if mild
   diarrhea continues or worsens
» Possibly using an alternate or additional method of contraception if
   taking estrogen-containing oral contraceptives concurrently, especially with ampicillin, amoxicillin, or penicillin V
» Diabetics: False-positive reactions with copper sulfate urine glucose
   tests may occur
   Possible interference with diagnostic tests

Side/adverse effects
Signs of potential side effects, especially allergic reactions, hepatotoxicity, interstitial nephritis, leukopenia or neutropenia, mental disturbances, pain at site of injection, platelet dysfunction or
thrombocytopenia, *Clostidium difficile* colitis, and seizures

---

▲ For the Patient ▲

912510

ABOUT YOUR MEDICINE

Penicillins (pen-i-SILL-ins) are used to treat infections caused
by bacteria. They will not work for colds, flu, or other virus
infections. Some penicillins are also used to prevent "strep"
infections in patients with a history of rheumatic heart disease.

If any of the information in this leaflet causes you special
concern or if you want additional information about your
medicine and its use, check with your doctor, nurse, or pharmacist. **Remember, keep this and all other medicines out of
the reach of children and never share your medicines with
others.**

BEFORE USING THIS MEDICINE

Tell your doctor, nurse, and pharmacist if you . . .
• are allergic to any medicine, either prescription or nonprescription (OTC);
• are pregnant or intend to become pregnant while using
  this medicine;
• are breast-feeding;
• are taking any other prescription or nonprescription
  (OTC) medicine, especially birth control pills containing estrogen, cholestyramine, colestipol, or probenecid;
• have any other medical problems, especially infectious
  mononucleosis ("mono") or history of stomach or intestinal disease, such as colitis, including colitis caused by
  antibiotics, or enteritis.

PROPER USE OF THIS MEDICINE

Most penicillins are best taken with a full glass (8 ounces)
of water on an empty stomach; however, some are best taken

with a snack or meal. Follow your doctor's or pharmacist's directions on how to take your medicine.

If you are taking penicillin G, do not take acidic fruit juices (for example, orange or grapefruit juice) or other acidic beverages within 1 hour of the time you take penicillin G. To do so may keep the medicine from working properly.

Keep taking this medicine for the full time of treatment even if you begin to feel better after a few days; **do not miss any doses. This is especially important if you have a "strep" infection since serious heart problems could develop later** if your infection is not cleared up completely.

If you do miss a dose of this medicine, take it as soon as possible. However, if it is almost time for your next dose, skip the missed dose and go back to your regular dosing schedule. Do not double doses.

PRECAUTIONS WHILE USING THIS MEDICINE
If your symptoms do not improve within a few days, or if they become worse, check with your doctor.

In some patients, penicillins may cause diarrhea. Severe diarrhea may be a sign of a serious side effect. **Do not take any diarrhea medicine without first checking with your doctor.**

Oral contraceptives (birth control pills) containing estrogen may not work properly if you take them while you are taking ampicillin, bacampicillin, or penicillin V. Unplanned pregnancies may occur. Use a different or additional means of birth control while taking any of these penicillins.

Diabetics—Some penicillins may cause false test results with some urine sugar tests. Check with your doctor before changing your diet or the dosage of your diabetes medicine.

This medicine must not be given to other people or used for other infections unless you are otherwise directed by your doctor.

POSSIBLE SIDE EFFECTS OF THIS MEDICINE
Side Effects That Should Be Reported To Your Doctor Immediately

Stop taking this medicine and get emergency help immediately if you notice:

> *Rare (may be less common with some penicillins)*—Difficulty in breathing; lightheadedness; skin rash, hives, itching, or wheezing

Other Side Effects That Should Be Reported To Your Doctor Immediately

> *Rare (may be more common with some penicillins)*—Abdominal bloating; blood in urine; convulsions (seizures); decreased amount of urine; diarrhea (watery and severe) which may also be bloody; fever; joint pain;

sore throat and fever; stomach or abdominal cramps and pain (severe); unusual bleeding or bruising

Some of the above side effects may occur up to several weeks after you stop taking this medicine.

Side Effects That Usually Do Not Require Medical Attention

These possible side effects may go away during treatment; however, if they continue or are bothersome, check with your doctor, nurse, or pharmacist.

>   *More common (may be less common with some penicillins)*—Diarrhea (mild); nausea or vomiting; sore mouth or tongue

Other side effects not listed above may also occur in some patients. If you notice any other effects, check with your doctor, nurse, or pharmacist.

PENTOXIFYLLINE   Systemic

■For the Pharmacist■

In providing consultation, consider emphasizing the following selected information (» = major clinical significance):

Before using this medication
» Conditions affecting use, especially:
  Sensitivity to pentoxifylline or other methylxanthines
  Breast-feeding—Passes into breast milk; breast-feeding may be inadvisable on the basis of tumorigenic effects in animal studies
  Use in the elderly—Increased risk of side effects because of decreased clearance
  Other medical problems, especially hepatic or renal function impairment or any condition in which there is a risk of bleeding

Proper use of this medication
  Swallowing whole without crushing, breaking, or chewing
» Taking with meals and/or antacids to reduce gastrointestinal irritation
» Proper dosing
  Missed dose: Taking as soon as possible; not taking if almost time for next dose; not doubling doses
» Proper storage

Precautions while using this medication
  Checking with physician before discontinuing medication; pentoxifylline may take several weeks to work
  Avoiding smoking (nicotine constricts blood vessels)

Side/adverse effects
  Signs of potential side effects, especially arrhythmias and chest pain

▲ For the Patient ▲

915202

ABOUT YOUR MEDICINE

Pentoxifylline (pen-tox-IF-i-lin) improves the flow of blood through blood vessels. It is used to reduce leg pain caused by poor blood circulation. Pentoxifylline makes it possible to walk farther before having to rest because of leg cramps.

If any of the information in this leaflet causes you special concern or if you want additional information about your medicine and its use, check with your doctor, nurse, or pharmacist. **Remember, keep this and all other medicines out of the reach of children and never share your medicines with others.**

BEFORE USING THIS MEDICINE

Tell your doctor, nurse, and pharmacist if you . . .
  • are allergic to any medicine, either prescription or nonprescription (OTC);

- are pregnant or intend to become pregnant while using this medicine;
- are breast-feeding;
- are taking any other prescription or nonprescription (OTC) medicine;
- have any other medical problems, especially any condition in which there is a risk of bleeding (e.g., recent stroke), or kidney or liver disease.

PROPER USE OF THIS MEDICINE

Swallow the tablet whole. Do not crush, break, or chew it before swallowing.

Pentoxifylline should be taken with meals to lessen the chance of stomach upset. Taking an antacid with the medicine may also help.

If you miss a dose of this medicine, take it as soon as possible. However, if it is almost time for your next dose, skip the missed dose and go back to your regular dosing schedule. Do not double doses.

PRECAUTIONS WHILE USING THIS MEDICINE

It may take several weeks for this medicine to work. If you feel that pentoxifylline is not working, do not stop taking it on your own. Instead, check with your doctor.

Smoking tobacco may worsen your condition since nicotine may further narrow your blood vessels. Therefore, it is best to avoid smoking.

POSSIBLE SIDE EFFECTS OF THIS MEDICINE
Side Effects That Should Be Reported To Your Doctor

   Rare—Chest pain; irregular heartbeat

Side Effects That Usually Do Not Require Medical Attention

These possible side effects may go away during treatment; however, if they continue or are bothersome, check with your doctor, nurse, or pharmacist.

   Less common—Dizziness; headache; nausea or vomiting; stomach discomfort

Other side effects not listed above may also occur in some patients. If you notice any other effects, check with your doctor, nurse, or pharmacist.

PERGOLIDE   Systemic

■ For the Pharmacist ■

In providing consultation, consider emphasizing the following selected
information (» = major clinical significance):

Before using this medication
» Conditions affecting use, especially:
Sensitivity to pergolide or other ergot alkaloids
Breast-feeding—May prevent lactation in mothers who intend
to breast-feed
Dental—Reduced salivary flow may contribute to dental prob-
lems

Proper use of this medication
Taking with meals to reduce gastric effects
» Proper dosing
Missed dose: Taking as soon as possible; not taking if almost time
for next dose; not doubling doses
» Proper storage

Precautions while using this medication
Regular visits to physician to check progress
» Caution when driving or doing jobs requiring alertness, because of
possible drowsiness or dizziness
Dizziness may be more likely to occur after initial doses; taking first
dose at bedtime or while lying down; getting up slowly from
sitting or lying position
Possible dryness of mouth; using sugarless gum or candy, ice, or
saliva substitute for relief; checking with physician or dentist if
dry mouth continues for more than 2 weeks
Checking with physician before reducing dosage or discontinuing
medication

Side/adverse effects
Signs of potential side effects, especially CNS effects, urinary tract
infection, hypertension, cerebrovascular hemorrhage, and myocardial infarction

▲ For the Patient ▲

917810

ABOUT YOUR MEDICINE

Pergolide (PER-go-lide) belongs to the group of medicines
known as ergot alkaloids. It is used with levodopa or with
carbidopa and levodopa combination to treat people who
have Parkinson's disease.

If any of the information in this leaflet causes you special
concern or if you want additional information about your
medicine and its use, check with your doctor, nurse, or pharmacist. **Remember, keep this and all other medicines out of
the reach of children and never share your medicines with
others.**

BEFORE USING THIS MEDICINE

Tell your doctor, nurse, and pharmacist if you . . .
- are allergic to any medicine, either prescription or non-prescription (OTC);
- are pregnant or intend to become pregnant while using this medicine;
- are breast-feeding;
- are taking any other prescription or nonprescription (OTC) medicine;
- have any other medical problems.

PROPER USE OF THIS MEDICINE

If pergolide upsets your stomach, it may be taken with meals. If stomach upset continues, check with your doctor.

If you miss a dose of this medicine, take it as soon as you remember it. However, if it is almost time for your next dose, skip the missed dose and go back to your regular dosing schedule. Do not double doses.

PRECAUTIONS WHILE USING THIS MEDICINE

It is important that your doctor check your progress at regular visits, to make sure that this medicine is working and to check for unwanted effects.

This medicine may cause some people to become drowsy, dizzy, or less alert than they are normally. **Make sure you know how you react to this medicine before you drive, use machines, or do other jobs that require you to be alert.**

Dizziness, lightheadedness, or fainting may occur after the first doses of pergolide, especially when you get up from a lying or sitting position. Getting up slowly may help. Taking the first dose at bedtime or when you are able to lie down may also lessen problems. If the problem continues or gets worse, check with your doctor.

Pergolide may cause dryness of the mouth. For temporary relief, use sugarless candy or gum, melt bits of ice in your mouth, or use a saliva substitute. However, if your mouth continues to feel dry for more than 2 weeks, check with your medical doctor or dentist. Continuing dryness of the mouth may increase the chance of dental disease, including tooth decay, gum disease, and fungus infections.

It may take several weeks for pergolide to work. Do not stop taking this medicine or reduce the amount you are taking without first checking with your doctor.

POSSIBLE SIDE EFFECTS OF THIS MEDICINE
Side Effects That Should Be Reported To Your Doctor Immediately

> *Rare*—Chest pain (severe); convulsions (seizures); fainting; fast heartbeat; headache (severe or continuing); increased sweating; nausea and vomiting (continuing

or severe); nervousness; unexplained shortness of breath; vision changes, such as blurred vision or temporary blindness; weakness (sudden)

Other Side Effects That Should Be Reported To Your Doctor

More common—Confusion; hallucinations; pain or burning while urinating; uncontrolled movements of the body, such as the face, tongue, arms, hands, head, and upper body

Less common—High blood pressure

Side Effects That Usually Do Not Require Medical Attention

These possible side effects may go away during treatment; however, if they continue or are bothersome, check with your doctor, nurse, or pharmacist.

More common—Abdominal or stomach pain; constipation; dizziness or lightheadedness, especially when getting up from a lying or sitting position; drowsiness; lower back pain; nausea; runny nose; weakness

Less common—Chills; diarrhea; dryness of mouth; loss of appetite; swelling of the face; vomiting

Other side effects not listed above may also occur in some patients. If you notice any other effects, check with your doctor, nurse, or pharmacist.

PHENAZOPYRIDINE   Systemic

■ For the Pharmacist ■

In providing consultation, consider emphasizing the following selected
information (» = major clinical significance):

Before using this medication
» Conditions affecting use, especially:
   Allergic reaction to phenazopyridine, history of
   Other medical problems, especially glucose-6-phosphate dehy-
      drogenase (G6PD) deficiency

Proper use of this medication
   Taking with or following food (a meal or a snack) to reduce gastric
      upset
» Not using any saved portion of medication in the future unless
   authorized by physician
» Proper dosing
   Missed dose: Taking as soon as possible; not taking if almost time
      for next dose; not doubling doses
» Proper storage

Precautions while using this medication
» Informing physician if symptoms worsen
» Medication causes urine to turn reddish orange and may stain cloth-
   ing
   Not wearing soft contact lenses during therapy because of possible
      permanent staining
   Diabetics: May cause false urine sugar and urine ketone test results
   Possible interference with laboratory test results; notifying person
      in charge that medication is being used

Side/adverse effects
   Signs of potential side effects, especially allergic dermatitis, aseptic
      meningitis, hemolytic anemia, hepatotoxicity, methemoglobi-
      nemia, and renal impairment or failure

▲ For the Patient ▲

912532

ABOUT YOUR MEDICINE

Phenazopyridine (fen-az-oh-PEER-i-deen) is a medicine used
to relieve the pain, burning, and discomfort caused by infection or irritation of the urinary tract. It is not an antibiotic
and will not cure the infection itself.

If any of the information in this leaflet causes you special
concern or if you want additional information about your
medicine and its use, check with your doctor, nurse, or pharmacist. **Remember, keep this and all other medicines out of
the reach of children and never share your medicines with
others.**

BEFORE USING THIS MEDICINE

Tell your doctor, nurse, and pharmacist if you . . .
   • are allergic to any medicine, either prescription or non-
      prescription (OTC);

- are pregnant or intend to become pregnant while using this medicine;
- are breast-feeding;
- are taking any other prescription or nonprescription (OTC) medicine;
- have any other medical problems, especially glucose-6-phosphate dehydrogenase (G6PD) deficiency.

PROPER USE OF THIS MEDICINE

Phenazopyridine is best taken with food or after eating a meal or a snack to lessen stomach upset.

Do not use any leftover medicine for future urinary tract problems without first checking with your doctor. An infection may require additional medicine.

If you miss a dose of this medicine, take it as soon as possible. However, if it is almost time for your next dose, skip the missed dose and go back to your regular dosing schedule. Do not double doses.

PRECAUTIONS WHILE USING THIS MEDICINE

Check with your doctor if symptoms such as bloody urine, difficult or painful urination, frequent urge to urinate, or sudden decrease in the amount of urine appear or become worse while you are taking this medicine.

Phenazopyridine causes the urine to turn reddish orange. This is to be expected while you are using it. This effect is harmless and will go away after you stop taking the medicine. Also, the medicine may stain clothing.

For patients who wear soft contact lenses:
- It is best not to wear soft contact lenses while being treated with this medicine. Phenazopyridine may cause discoloration or staining of contact lenses. It may not be possible to remove the stain.

Before you have any medical tests, tell the person in charge that you are taking this medicine. The results of some tests may be affected by this medicine.

POSSIBLE SIDE EFFECTS OF THIS MEDICINE

Side Effects That Should Be Reported To Your Doctor

Blue or blue-purple color of skin; fever and confusion; shortness of breath, tightness in chest, wheezing, or troubled breathing; skin rash; sudden decrease in the amount of urine; swelling of face, fingers, feet, or lower legs; unusual tiredness or weakness; yellow eyes or skin

Side Effects That Usually Do Not Require Medical Attention

These possible side effects may go away during treatment; however, if they continue or are bothersome, check with your doctor, nurse, or pharmacist.

Less common or rare—Dizziness; headache; indigestion; stomach cramps or pain

Other side effects not listed above may also occur in some patients. If you notice any other effects, check with your doctor, nurse, or pharmacist.

PHENOTHIAZINES   Systemic

Including Acetophenazine; Chlorpromazine; Fluphenazine;
Mesoridazine; Methotrimeprazine; Pericyazine;
Perphenazine; Pipotiazine; Prochlorperazine; Promazine;
Thiopropazate; Thioproperazine; Thioridazine;
Trifluoperazine; Triflupromazine.

■ For the Pharmacist ■

In providing consultation, consider emphasizing the following selected
information (**》** = major clinical significance):

Before using this medication
》 Conditions affecting use, especially:
   Sensitivity to any phenothiazine
   Pregnancy—Not recommended for use during pregnancy be-
      cause of reports of jaundice, hypo- or hyperreflexia, and ex-
      trapyramidal symptoms in neonates
   Breast-feeding—Distributed into breast milk; may cause drows-
      iness, dystonias, and tardive dyskinesia in the baby
   Use in children—Children, especially those with acute illnesses,
      are more prone to extrapyramidal symptoms
   Use in the elderly—Elderly patients are more likely to develop
      extrapyramidal, anticholinergic, hypotensive, and sedative
      effects; reduced dosage recommended
   Dental—Phenothiazine-induced blood dyscrasias may result in
      infections, delayed healing, and bleeding; dry mouth may
      cause caries and candidiasis; increased motor activity of face,
      head, and neck may interfere with some dental procedures
   Other medications, especially alcohol, other CNS depression–
      producing medications, tricyclic antidepressants, antithyroid
      agents, epinephrine, other hypotension-producing medica-
      tions, other extrapyramidal-producing medications, levodopa,
      lithium, or metrizamide
   Other medical problems, especially cardiovascular disease, se-
      vere CNS depression, active alcoholism, blood dyscrasias,
      liver disease, or Reye's syndrome

Proper use of this medication
   Proper administration of this medication:
   For oral dosage forms
      Taking with food, milk, or water to reduce stomach irritation
》   Diluting medication that comes in dropper bottle with recom-
         mended beverages prior to use
      Swallowing the extended-release dosage form whole
   For rectal dosage forms
      Chilling suppository if too soft to insert
      How to insert suppository
》 Compliance with therapy; not taking more or less medication than
      prescribed
》 Several weeks of therapy may be required to produce desired effects
      in treatment of nervous, mental, or emotional conditions
》 Proper dosing
   Missed dose: When dosing schedule is—
      One dose a day: Taking as soon as possible unless almost time
         for next dose, then going back to regular dosing schedule;
         not doubling doses

More than one dose a day: Taking as soon as possible if within an hour or so of missed dose; skipping missed dose if not remembered until later; going back to regular dosing schedule; not doubling doses

» Proper storage

Precautions while using this medication

Regular visits to physician to check progress of therapy

» Checking with physician before discontinuing medication; gradual dosage reduction may be needed

Avoiding use of antacids or antidiarrheal medication within 2 hours of taking phenothiazine

» Avoiding use of alcoholic beverages or other CNS depressants during therapy

Avoiding the use of over-the-counter medications for colds or allergies, to prevent increased anticholinergic effects and risk of heat stroke

Caution if any laboratory tests required; possible interference with ECG readings, and with gonadorelin, immunologic urine pregnancy, metyrapone, and urine bilirubin test results

» Caution if any kind of surgery, dental treatment, or emergency treatment is required; telling physician or dentist in charge about phenothiazine because of possible drug interactions or blood dyscrasias

» Possible drowsiness or blurred vision; caution when driving, using machines, or doing other things requiring alertness or accurate vision

» Possible dizziness or lightheadedness (orthostatic hypotension); caution when getting up suddenly from a lying or sitting position

» Possible heat stroke: Caution during exercise, hot weather, or when taking hot baths

Possible hypothermia: Caution during prolonged exposure to cold

» Possible dryness of mouth; using sugarless gum or candy, ice, or saliva substitute for relief; checking with physician or dentist if dry mouth continues for more than 2 weeks

» Possible skin photosensitivity; avoiding unprotected exposure to sun; using protective clothing; using a sun block product that includes protection against both UVA-caused photosensitivity reactions and UVB-caused sunburn reactions; avoiding use of sunlamp, tanning bed, or tanning booth

» Possible eye photosensitivity; wearing sunglasses that block ultraviolet light

» Avoiding spilling liquid dosage form on skin or clothing; may cause skin irritation

» Observing precautions for up to 12 weeks with long-acting parenteral forms

Side/adverse effects

Side effects more likely to occur in the elderly

Signs of potential side effects, especially tardive dyskinesia, dystonias, parkinsonian effects, anticholinergic effects, blurred vision, possible pigmentary retinopathy, allergic skin reactions, photosensitivity, agranulocytosis, cholestatic jaundice, heat stroke, neuroleptic malignant syndrome, priapism, melanosis, dryness of mouth, orthostatic hypotension, or akathisia

» Stopping medication and notifying physician immediately if symptoms of neuroleptic malignant syndrome (NMS) appear, especially muscle rigidity, fever, difficult or fast breathing, seizures, fast heartbeat, increased sweating, loss of bladder control, unusually pale skin, unusual tiredness or weakness

» Notifying physician immediately if early symptoms of tardive dyskinesia appear, such as fine worm-like movements of the tongue or other uncontrolled movements of the mouth, tongue, jaw, or arms and legs; dosage adjustment or discontinuation may be needed to prevent irreversibility
Possibility of withdrawal symptoms

▲ For the Patient ▲

912554

ABOUT YOUR MEDICINE

Phenothiazines (fee-noe-THYE-a-zeens) are used to treat nervous, mental, and emotional disorders. Some are used also to control anxiety or agitation in certain patients, severe nausea and vomiting, severe hiccups, and moderate to severe pain. Chlorpromazine is also used in the treatment of certain types of porphyria, and with other medicines in the treatment of tetanus. Phenothiazines may also be used for other conditions as determined by your doctor.

If any of the information in this leaflet causes you special concern or if you want additional information about your medicine and its use, check with your doctor, nurse, or pharmacist. **Remember, keep this and all other medicines out of the reach of children and never share your medicines with others.**

BEFORE USING THIS MEDICINE

Discuss with your doctor possible side effects of this medicine. Some may be serious and/or permanent. For example, tardive dyskinesia (a movement disorder) may occur and may not go away after you stop using the medicine.

Tell your doctor, nurse, and pharmacist if you . . .
• are allergic to any medicine, either prescription or nonprescription (OTC);
• are pregnant or intend to become pregnant while using this medicine;
• are breast-feeding;
• are taking **any** other prescription or nonprescription (OTC) medicine;
• have **any** other medical problems.

PROPER USE OF THIS MEDICINE

Phenothiazines may be taken with food or a full glass (8 ounces) of water or milk to reduce stomach irritation.

If you miss a dose of this medicine, take it as soon as possible. However, if it is almost time for your next dose, skip the missed dose. Do not double doses.

PRECAUTIONS WHILE USING THIS MEDICINE

Do not stop taking this medicine without first checking with your doctor. Your doctor may want you to reduce gradually the amount you are taking.

This medicine will add to the effects of alcohol and other CNS depressants (medicines that slow down the nervous system). **Check with your doctor before taking any such depressants while you are taking this medicine.**

This medicine may cause changes in vision or cause some people to become drowsy or less alert than they are normally. **Make sure you know how you react before you drive or do jobs that require you to be alert and to see well.**

Dizziness, lightheadedness, or fainting may occur, especially when getting up from a lying or sitting position. Getting up slowly may help.

This medicine may make you sweat less, causing your body temperature to rise. **Do not become overheated during exercise or hot weather, since overheating may result in heat stroke.**

Before having any kind of surgery or dental or emergency treatment, tell the physician or dentist in charge that you are using this medicine.

Some people who take this medicine may become more sensitive to sunlight. Stay out of direct sunlight and protect yourself from getting too much sun.

POSSIBLE SIDE EFFECTS OF THIS MEDICINE
Side Effects That Should Be Reported To Your Doctor Immediately

Stop taking this medicine and check with your doctor or get emergency help immediately if any of the following side effects occur:

Rare—Convulsions (seizures); fast or irregular heartbeat; high fever; high or low blood pressure; increased sweating; loss of bladder control; muscle stiffness (severe); troubled breathing; unusually pale skin; unusual tiredness

Other Side Effects That Should Be Reported To Your Doctor

More common—Blurred vision or difficulty in seeing at night; difficulty in talking or swallowing; fainting; inability to move eyes; lip smacking or puckering; loss of balance control; mask-like face; muscle spasms of face, neck, or back; puffing of cheeks; restlessness; shuffling walk or stiff arms and legs; tic-like, twitching, or twisting movements; trembling of hands; uncontrolled chewing or tongue movements; uncontrolled movements or weakness of arms or legs

Less common—Difficulty in urinating; skin rash; sunburn (severe)

Rare—Abdominal or stomach pains; aching muscles and joints; confusion; fever and chills; hot, dry skin or lack of sweating; muscle weakness; nausea, vomiting, or diarrhea; painful, inappropriate penile erection (continuing); skin itching (severe) or discoloration (tan or blue-gray); sore throat and fever; unusual bleeding or bruising; yellow eyes or skin

Side Effects That Usually Do Not Require Medical Attention

These possible side effects may go away during treatment; however, if they continue or are bothersome, check with your doctor, nurse, or pharmacist.

More common—Constipation; decreased sweating; drowsiness; dryness of mouth; lightheadedness or dizziness; stuffy nose

Other side effects not listed above may also occur in some patients. If you notice any other effects, check with your doctor, nurse, or pharmacist.

After you stop using this medicine, your body may need time to adjust. Check with your doctor if you notice any of the above side effects.

PHENYLPROPANOLAMINE   Systemic

■For the Pharmacist■

In providing consultation, consider emphasizing the following selected information (» = major clinical significance):

Before using this medication
» Conditions affecting use, especially:
>> Sensitivity to phenylpropanolamine or other sympathomimetics
>> Pregnancy—Psychiatric side effects more likely in postpartum women
>> Use in children—Psychiatric side effects more likely in children up to 6 years of age; not recommended for use as appetite suppressant in children up to 12 years of age; in adolescents between 12 and 18 years of age, use for appetite suppression recommended only with doctor's supervision
>> Other medications, especially beta-adrenergic blocking agents, CNS stimulation–producing medications, other sympathomimetics, digitalis glycosides, monoamine oxidase (MAO) inhibitors, or rauwolfia alkaloids
>> Other medical problems, especially severe coronary artery disease, other cardiovascular disorders, or hypertension

Proper use of this medication
Proper administration of extended-release dosage forms: swallowing whole; not breaking, crushing, or chewing; taking with a full glass of water; taking around 10 am if taking only one dose of medication a day
» Importance of not taking more medication than the amount recommended or for a longer period of time than directed
Taking the last dose of medication a few hours before bedtime to minimize the possibility of insomnia
» Proper dosing
» Proper storage
For decongestant use only
Missed dose: Taking as soon as possible; not taking within 2 hours (12 hours for extended-release dosage forms) of next scheduled dose; not doubling doses
For appetite suppressant use only
Not taking for longer than a few weeks without physician's permission

Precautions while using this medication
Not drinking large amounts of caffeine-containing coffee, tea, or colas
» Caution if dizziness occurs; not driving, using machines, or doing anything else that requires alertness while taking medication
For decongestant use only
» Checking with physician if cold symptoms do not improve within 7 days or if fever is present

Side/adverse effects
Signs of potential side effects, especially severe headache, increased blood pressure, painful or difficult urination, or tightness in chest

---

▲ For the Patient ▲

914709

ABOUT YOUR MEDICINE

Phenylpropanolamine (fen-ill-proe-pa-NOLE-a-meen), commonly known as PPA, is used as a nasal decongestant or as an appetite suppressant.

If any of the information in this leaflet causes you special concern or if you want additional information about your medicine and its use, check with your doctor, nurse, or pharmacist. **Remember, keep this and all other medicines out of the reach of children and never share your medicines with others.**

BEFORE USING THIS MEDICINE

If you are taking this medicine without a prescription, carefully read and follow any precautions on the label. You should be especially careful if you . . .

- are allergic to any medicine, either prescription or non-prescription (OTC);
- are pregnant, intend to become pregnant, or are breast-feeding;
- compete in athletics;
- are taking **any** other prescription or nonprescription (OTC) medicine;
- have any other medical problems, especially heart or blood vessel disease (including a history of heart attack or stroke), or high blood pressure;

If you have any questions, check with your doctor, nurse, or pharmacist.

PROPER USE OF THIS MEDICINE

For patients taking an extended-release form of this medicine:

- Swallow the capsule or tablet whole. Do not crush, break, or chew before swallowing.
- Take with a full glass (at least 8 ounces) of water.
- If taking only one dose of this medicine a day, take it in the morning around 10 a.m.

Take phenylpropanolamine (PPA) only as directed. Do not take more of it, do not take it more often, and do not take it for a longer time than directed. To do so may increase the chance of side effects.

For patients taking this medicine as an appetite suppressant:
- Do not take this medicine for longer than a few weeks without your doctor's permission.

If PPA causes trouble in sleeping, take the last dose for each day a few hours before bedtime. If you are taking an extended-release form of this medicine, take your daily dose at least 12 hours before bedtime.

Phenylpropanolamine should not be used for weight control in children under the age of 12 years. Children 12 to 18 years old should not take phenylpropanolamine for weight control unless its use is ordered and supervised by their doctor.

For patients taking phenylpropanolamine for nasal congestion:

* **If you miss a dose,** take it as soon as possible. However, if it is within 2 hours (or 12 hours for extended-release forms) of your next dose, skip the missed dose and go back to your regular dosing schedule. Do not double doses.

PRECAUTIONS WHILE USING THIS MEDICINE

This medicine may cause some people to become dizzy. **Make sure you know how you react to this medicine before you drive or use machines or do anything else that could be dangerous if you are dizzy or not alert.**

If you are taking this medicine for nasal congestion and cold symptoms do not improve within 7 days or if you also have a high fever, check with your doctor. These signs may mean that you have other medical problems.

POSSIBLE SIDE EFFECTS OF THIS MEDICINE

Side Effects That Should Be Reported To Your Doctor

> *Rare*—Headache (severe); increased blood pressure; painful or difficult urination; tightness in chest

> *Early signs of overdose*—Abdominal or stomach pain; fast, pounding, or irregular heartbeat; headache (severe); increased sweating not caused by exercise; nausea and vomiting (severe); nervousness or restlessness (severe)

Side Effects That Usually Do Not Require Medical Attention

These possible side effects may go away during treatment; however, if they continue or are bothersome, check with your doctor, nurse, or pharmacist.

> *Less common (more common with high doses)*—Dizziness; dryness of nose or mouth; headache (mild); nausea (mild); nervousness or restlessness (mild); trouble in sleeping; unusual feeling of well-being

Other side effects not listed above may also occur in some patients. If you notice any other effects, check with your doctor, nurse, or pharmacist.

PHYSOSTIGMINE   Ophthalmic

■For the Pharmacist■

In providing consultation, consider emphasizing the following selected information (» = major clinical significance):

Before using this medication
» Conditions affecting use, especially:
   Sensitivity to physostigmine
   Other medical problems, especially active uveitis

Proper use of this medication
   Not using solution if it becomes discolored
   Proper administration technique
   Washing hands immediately after application to remove any medication that may be on them
» Importance of not using more medication than the amount prescribed
» Proper dosing
   Missed dose: If dosing schedule is—
      One dose a day: Applying as soon as possible; not applying if not remembered until next day; applying next regularly scheduled dose
      More than one dose a day: Applying as soon as possible; not applying if almost time for next dose; applying next dose at regularly scheduled time
   Preventing contamination:
   For solution dosage form
      Not touching applicator tip to any surface; keeping container tightly closed
   For ointment dosage form
      Not touching applicator tip to any surface; wiping tip of ointment tube with clean tissue; keeping tube tightly closed
» Proper storage

Precautions while using this medication
   Regular visits to physician to check eye pressure during therapy
» Caution if blurred vision or change in near or distant vision occurs, especially at night

Side/adverse effects
   Signs of potential side effects, especially systemic absorption

▲ For the Patient ▲

912849

GLAUCOMA EYE MEDICINE—SHORT-ACTING CHOLINERGIC: *Including Carbachol; Physostigmine; Pilocarpine.*

ABOUT YOUR MEDICINE

Short-acting cholinergic (ko-lin-ER-jik) **glaucoma eye medicines** are used in the eye to treat certain kinds of glaucoma and other eye conditions.

If any of the information in this leaflet causes you special concern or if you want additional information about your

medicine and its use, check with your doctor, nurse, or pharmacist. **Remember, keep this and all other medicines out of the reach of children and never share your medicines with others.**

BEFORE USING THIS MEDICINE

Tell your doctor, nurse, and pharmacist if you . . .
- are allergic to any medicine, either prescription or non-prescription (OTC);
- are pregnant or intend to become pregnant while using this medicine;
- are breast-feeding;
- are taking **any** other prescription or nonprescription (OTC) medicine;
- have any other medical problems, especially other eye disease or problems.

PROPER USE OF THIS MEDICINE

Use this medicine only as directed. Do not use more of it and do not use it more often than your doctor ordered. To do so may increase the chance of too much medicine being absorbed into the body and the chance of side effects.

To use the ophthalmic solution (eye drops) form of this medicine:
- First, wash your hands. Tilt the head back and, pressing your finger gently on the skin just beneath the lower eyelid, pull the lower eyelid away from the eye to make a space. Drop the medicine into this space. Let go of the eyelid and gently close the eyes. Do not blink. Keep the eyes closed and apply pressure to the inner corner of the eye with your finger for 1 or 2 minutes to allow the medicine to be absorbed by the eye.
- Wash hands to remove any medicine that may be on them.
- Do not use solution if it is discolored.

To use the ophthalmic ointment (eye ointment) or the eye gel form of this medicine:
- First, wash your hands. Pull lower eyelid away from eye to form a pouch. Squeeze a thin strip of ointment or gel into the pouch. A 1-cm (approximately 1/3-inch) strip of ointment or a 1 and 1/2-cm (approximately 1/2-inch) strip of gel is usually enough unless otherwise directed by your doctor. Close eyes and keep them closed for 1 or 2 minutes.
- Wash hands to remove any medicine that may be on them.
- Wipe the tip of the tube with a clean tissue.

To use the eye system form of this medicine:
- This medicine usually comes with patient directions. Read them carefully.
- If you think a medicine unit may be damaged, do not use it.

- If the unit seems to be releasing too much medicine into your eye, remove it and replace with a new unit.
- Insert the unit at bedtime, unless otherwise directed by your doctor.

To keep the medicine as germ-free as possible, do not touch the applicator tip to any surface (including the eye) and keep the container tightly closed.

If you miss a dose of this medicine, apply the missed dose as soon as possible. However, if it is almost time for your next dose, skip the missed dose and go back to your regular dosing schedule. Do not double doses.

PRECAUTIONS WHILE USING THIS MEDICINE

Your doctor should check your eye pressure at regular visits.

For a short time after you apply this medicine, your vision may be blurred or there may be a change in your near or distant vision, especially at night. **Make sure your vision is clear before you drive, use machines, or do other jobs that require you to see well.**

POSSIBLE SIDE EFFECTS OF THIS MEDICINE
Side Effects That Should Be Reported To Your Doctor

Signs of too much medicine being absorbed into the body—Flushing or redness of face; frequent urge to urinate; increased sweating; loss of bladder control; muscle tremors or weakness; nausea, vomiting, or diarrhea; shortness of breath, troubled breathing, wheezing, or tightness in chest; slow or irregular heartbeat; stomach cramps or pain; unusual tiredness or weakness; watering of mouth

Side Effects That Usually Do Not Require Medical Attention

These possible side effects may go away during treatment; however, if they continue or are bothersome, check with your doctor, nurse, or pharmacist.

More common—Blurred vision; change in near or distant vision; eye pain

Less common—Burning, redness, stinging, watering, or other eye irritation; headache or browache; twitching of eyelids

Other side effects not listed above may also occur in some patients. If you notice any other effects, check with your doctor, nurse, or pharmacist.

PILOCARPINE   Ophthalmic

■ For the Pharmacist ■

In providing consultation, consider emphasizing the following selected
   information (» = major clinical significance):

Before using this medication
» Conditions affecting use, especially:
      Sensitivity to pilocarpine
      Other medical problems, especially acute iritis or other condi-
         tions in which pupillary constriction is undesirable

Proper use of this medication
   Proper administration technique
   Washing hands immediately after application to remove any med-
      ication that may be on them
» Importance of not using more medication than the amount pre-
      scribed
» Proper dosing
   Missed dose:
      For gel dosage form—Applying as soon as possible; not applying
         if not remembered until next day; applying next dose at reg-
         ularly scheduled time
      For solution dosage form—Applying as soon as possible; not
         applying if almost time for next dose; applying next dose at
         regularly scheduled time
      For eye system dosage form—Replacing as soon as possible;
         inserting next eye system at regularly scheduled time
» Proper storage
For gel or solution dosage forms
   Preventing contamination: Not touching applicator tip to any sur-
      face; keeping container tightly closed
For ocular system dosage form
   Reading patient instructions carefully before using
   Not using if damaged
   Removing and replacing with new unit if too much medicine is being
      released

Precautions while using this medication
   Regular visits to physician to check eye pressure during therapy
» Caution if blurred vision or change in near or far vision occurs,
      especially at night

Side/adverse effects
   Signs of potential side effects, especially symptoms of systemic ab-
      sorption or eye pain

▲ For the Patient ▲

912849

**GLAUCOMA EYE MEDICINE—SHORT-ACTING
CHOLINERGIC:** *Including Carbachol; Physostigmine;
Pilocarpine.*

ABOUT YOUR MEDICINE

Short-acting cholinergic (ko-lin-ER-jik) **glaucoma eye medicines** are used in the eye to treat certain kinds of glaucoma and other eye conditions.

If any of the information in this leaflet causes you special concern or if you want additional information about your medicine and its use, check with your doctor, nurse, or pharmacist. **Remember, keep this and all other medicines out of the reach of children and never share your medicines with others.**

BEFORE USING THIS MEDICINE

Tell your doctor, nurse, and pharmacist if you . . .
- are allergic to any medicine, either prescription or non-prescription (OTC);
- are pregnant or intend to become pregnant while using this medicine;
- are breast-feeding;
- are taking **any** other prescription or nonprescription (OTC) medicine;
- have any other medical problems, especially other eye disease or problems.

PROPER USE OF THIS MEDICINE

Use this medicine only as directed. Do not use more of it and do not use it more often than your doctor ordered. To do so may increase the chance of too much medicine being absorbed into the body and the chance of side effects.

To use the ophthalmic solution (eye drops) form of this medicine:
- First, wash your hands. Tilt the head back and, pressing your finger gently on the skin just beneath the lower eyelid, pull the lower eyelid away from the eye to make a space. Drop the medicine into this space. Let go of the eyelid and gently close the eyes. Do not blink. Keep the eyes closed and apply pressure to the inner corner of the eye with your finger for 1 or 2 minutes to allow the medicine to be absorbed by the eye.
- Wash hands to remove any medicine that may be on them.
- Do not use solution if it is discolored.

To use the ophthalmic ointment (eye ointment) or the eye gel form of this medicine:
- First, wash your hands. Pull lower eyelid away from eye to form a pouch. Squeeze a thin strip of ointment or gel into the pouch. A 1-cm (approximately 1/3-inch) strip of ointment or a 1 and 1/2-cm (approximately 1/2-inch) strip of gel is usually enough unless otherwise directed by your doctor. Close eyes and keep them closed for 1 or 2 minutes.

- Wash hands to remove any medicine that may be on them.
- Wipe the tip of the tube with a clean tissue.

To use the eye system form of this medicine:
- This medicine usually comes with patient directions. Read them carefully.
- If you think a medicine unit may be damaged, do not use it.
- If the unit seems to be releasing too much medicine into your eye, remove it and replace with a new unit.
- Insert the unit at bedtime, unless otherwise directed by your doctor.

To keep the medicine as germ-free as possible, do not touch the applicator tip to any surface (including the eye) and keep the container tightly closed.

If you miss a dose of this medicine, apply the missed dose as soon as possible. However, if it is almost time for your next dose, skip the missed dose and go back to your regular dosing schedule. Do not double doses.

PRECAUTIONS WHILE USING THIS MEDICINE
Your doctor should check your eye pressure at regular visits.

For a short time after you apply this medicine, your vision may be blurred or there may be a change in your near or distant vision, especially at night. **Make sure your vision is clear before you drive, use machines, or do other jobs that require you to see well.**

POSSIBLE SIDE EFFECTS OF THIS MEDICINE
Side Effects That Should Be Reported To Your Doctor

Signs of too much medicine being absorbed into the body—Flushing or redness of face; frequent urge to urinate; increased sweating; loss of bladder control; muscle tremors or weakness; nausea, vomiting, or diarrhea; shortness of breath, troubled breathing, wheezing, or tightness in chest; slow or irregular heartbeat; stomach cramps or pain; unusual tiredness or weakness; watering of mouth

Side Effects That Usually Do Not Require Medical Attention

These possible side effects may go away during treatment; however, if they continue or are bothersome, check with your doctor, nurse, or pharmacist.

More common—Blurred vision; change in near or distant vision; eye pain

Less common—Burning, redness, stinging, watering, or other eye irritation; headache or browache; twitching of eyelids

Other side effects not listed above may also occur in some patients. If you notice any other effects, check with your doctor, nurse, or pharmacist.

PIMOZIDE Systemic

■For the Pharmacist■

In providing consultation, consider emphasizing the following selected information (》 = major clinical significance):

Before using this medication
》 Conditions affecting use, especially:
  Sensitivity to pimozide or other neuroleptic agents
  Pregnancy—Animal studies have shown fewer pregnancies; retarded fetal development; maternal toxicity; mortality; decreased weight gain; embryotoxicity; increased resorptions
  Use in children—Not recommended for any condition other than Tourette's syndrome; therapy should be initiated gradually in patients up to 12 years of age; children are more sensitive to effects of pimozide
  Use in the elderly—Elderly patients are more likely to develop extrapyramidal, anticholinergic, hypotensive, and sedative effects; reduced dosage recommended
  Dental—Pimozide-induced blood dyscrasias may result in infections, delayed healing, and bleeding; dry mouth may cause caries, candidiasis, periodontal disease, and discomfort; increased motor activity of face, head, and neck may interfere with some dental procedures
  Other medications, especially alcohol, other CNS depression–producing medications, amphetamines, methylphenidate, pemoline, tricyclic antidepressants, disopyramide, maprotiline, phenothiazines, other extrapyramidal reaction–producing medications, procainamide, quinidine, or anticholinergics
  Other medical problems, especially cardiac arrhythmias, tics other than those caused by Tourette's disorder, severe CNS depression, history of breast cancer, or hypokalemia

Proper use of this medication
》 Importance of not taking more medication than the amount prescribed
》 Proper dosing
  Missed dose: Taking as soon as possible; taking any remaining doses for that day at regularly spaced intervals; not doubling doses
》 Proper storage

Precautions while using this medication
  Regular visits to physician to check progress of therapy
》 Checking with physician before discontinuing medication; gradual dosage reduction may be needed
》 Avoiding use of alcoholic beverages or other CNS depressants during therapy
》 Possible drowsiness, blurred vision, or muscle stiffness; caution when driving, using machinery, or doing other things requiring alertness, clear vision, and good muscle control
  Possible dizziness or lightheadedness; avoiding getting up suddenly from a sitting or lying position
》 Caution if any kind of surgery, dental treatment, or emergency surgery is required
  Possible dryness of mouth; using sugarless gum or candy, ice, or saliva substitute for relief; checking with physician or dentist if dry mouth continues for more than 2 weeks

Side/adverse effects

Side effects more likely in children and elderly or debilitated patients

» Stopping medication and notifying physician immediately if symptoms of neuroleptic malignant syndrome (NMS) appear

» Notifying physician as soon as possible if early symptoms of tardive dyskinesia appear

Possibility of withdrawal symptoms

Signs of potential side effects, especially akathisia, ventricular arrhythmias, parkinsonism, mood or behavior changes, dystonic reactions, tardive dyskinesia or dystonia, blood dyscrasias, obstructive jaundice, or NMS

▲ For the Patient ▲

915440

ABOUT YOUR MEDICINE

Pimozide (PIM-oh-zide) is used to treat the symptoms of Gilles de la Tourette's syndrome. It is meant only for patients with severe symptoms who cannot take or have not been helped by other medicine. Pimozide may also be used for other conditions as determined by your doctor.

If any of the information in this leaflet causes you special concern or if you want additional information about your medicine and its use, check with your doctor, nurse, or pharmacist. **Remember, keep this and all other medicines out of the reach of children and never share your medicines with others.**

BEFORE USING THIS MEDICINE

Discuss with your doctor possible side effects of this medicine. Some may be serious and/or permanent. For example, tardive dyskinesia (a movement disorder) may occur and may not go away after you stop using the medicine.

Tell your doctor, nurse, and pharmacist if you . . .
- are allergic to any medicine, either prescription or nonprescription (OTC);
- are pregnant or intend to become pregnant while using this medicine;
- are breast-feeding;
- are taking **any** other prescription or nonprescription (OTC) medicine;
- have **any** other medical problems.

PROPER USE OF THIS MEDICINE

Use pimozide only as directed by your doctor. Do not use more of it, do not use it more often, and do not use it for a longer time than ordered.

If you miss a dose of this medicine, take it as soon as possible. Then take any remaining doses for that day at regularly spaced times. Do not double doses.

PRECAUTIONS WHILE USING THIS MEDICINE

Your doctor should check your progress at regular visits, especially during the first few months of treatment with this medicine.

Do not suddenly stop taking this medicine without first checking with your doctor. Your doctor may want you to reduce the amount gradually.

This medicine will add to the effects of alcohol and other CNS depressants (medicines that slow down the nervous system). **Check with your doctor before taking any such depressants while you are taking this medicine.**

This medicine may cause some people to become drowsy or less alert or to have blurred vision or muscle stiffness, especially as the amount of medicine is increased. Even if you take pimozide at bedtime, you may feel drowsy or less alert on arising. **Make sure you know how you react to this medicine before you drive, use machines, or do other jobs that require you to see clearly, be alert, and have good muscle control.**

Although not a problem for many patients, dizziness, light-headedness, or fainting may occur, especially when you get up from a lying or sitting position. Getting up slowly may help. If the problem continues, check with your doctor.

Before having any kind of surgery or dental or emergency treatment, tell the physician or dentist in charge that you are using this medicine.

Pimozide may cause dryness of the mouth. For temporary relief, use sugarless gum or candy, melt bits of ice in your mouth, or use a saliva substitute. If dry mouth continues for more than 2 weeks, check with your physician or dentist.

POSSIBLE SIDE EFFECTS OF THIS MEDICINE
Side Effects That Should Be Reported To Your Doctor Immediately

Stop taking this medicine and get emergency help immediately if any of the following side effects occur:

Rare—Convulsions (seizures); difficult or fast breathing; fast heartbeat or irregular pulse; fever (high); high or low (irregular) blood pressure; increased sweating; loss of bladder control; muscle stiffness (severe); tiredness or weakness; unusually pale skin

Other Side Effects That Should Be Reported To Your Doctor

More common—Difficulty in speaking or swallowing; loss of balance control; mask-like face; mood or behavior changes; restlessness or need to keep moving; shuffling walk; slowed movements; stiff arms and legs; trembling of fingers and hands

Less common or rare—Inability to move eyes; increased blinking or spasms of eyelids; lip smacking or puckering; muscle spasms, especially of the face, neck, or back; puffing of cheeks; rapid or worm-like movements of tongue; sore throat and fever; uncontrolled chewing or twisting movements of neck, trunk, arms, or legs; unusual bleeding or bruising; unusual facial expressions or body positions; yellow eyes or skin

Side Effects That Usually Do Not Require Medical Attention

These possible side effects may go away during treatment; however, if they continue or are bothersome, check with your doctor, nurse, or pharmacist.

More common—Blurred vision or other vision problems; constipation; dizziness, lightheadedness, or fainting; drowsiness; dry mouth; skin rash, itching, or discoloration; swelling or soreness of breasts; unusual secretion of milk

Other side effects not listed above may also occur in some patients. If you notice any other effects, check with your doctor, nurse, or pharmacist.

After you stop using pimozide, it may still produce some side effects that need attention. During this time, check with your doctor as soon as possible if you notice lip smacking or puckering, puffing of cheeks, rapid or worm-like movements of the tongue, or uncontrolled chewing or arm or leg movements.

POTASSIUM SUPPLEMENTS   Systemic

Including Potassium Acetate; Potassium Bicarbonate; Potassium Bicarbonate and Potassium Chloride; Potassium Bicarbonate and Potassium Citrate; Potassium Chloride; Potassium Chloride, Potassium Bicarbonate, and Potassium Citrate; Potassium Gluconate; Potassium Gluconate and Potassium Chloride; Potassium Gluconate and Potassium Citrate; Potassium Gluconate, Potassium Citrate, and Ammonium Chloride; Trikates.

■For the Pharmacist■

In providing consultation, consider emphasizing the following selected information (» = major clinical significance):

Description of use
> Description should include function in the body; signs of deficiency

Importance of diet
> Food sources may be preferable to supplements for intake of potassium
>
> Supplements may be needed because of inadequate dietary intake or increased requirements
>
> Potassium content of selected foods; recommended intake for potassium
>
> Not exceeding recommended amounts of potassium

Before using this medication
» Conditions affecting use, especially:
> Sensitivity to potassium
>
> Use in the elderly—Risk of developing hyperkalemia due to age-related changes in ability of kidneys to excrete potassium
>
> Other medications, especially beta adrenergic blocking agents, nonsteroidal anti-inflammatory drugs, anticholinergics, potassium-sparing and thiazide diuretics, low-salt milk, other potassium-containing medications, ACE inhibitors, digitalis glycosides, or heparin
>
> Other medical problems, especially delayed gastric emptying, esophageal compression, or intestinal obstruction or stricture, peptic ulcer; heart block; hyperkalemia or conditions predisposing to hyperkalemia for all potassium supplements; metabolic or respiratory acidosis for potassium acetate

Proper use of this medication
> Proper administration technique:
> Necessary dilution of liquid dosage forms
>
> Taking tablets and capsules with adequate liquids
>
> Complete dissolution of effervescent dosage forms prior to taking
>
> Not using tomato juice for dilution if on a sodium-restricted diet
>
> Not crushing or chewing extended-release dosage forms, unless otherwise directed
>
> Sprinkling contents of some extended-release capsules and some tablets over soft food such as applesauce or mixing with fruit juice, if unable to swallow whole, but only when directed to do so
» Taking each dose immediately after a meal or with food
» Compliance with therapy, especially when taking diuretics and digitalis
» Proper dosing

Missed dose: Taking as soon as possible if remembered within 2 hours; going back to regular dosage schedule; not doubling doses
» Proper storage

Precautions while using this medication
Regular visits to physician to check progress of therapy; serum potassium monitoring may be necessary
» Not taking salt substitutes or low-salt milk or food unless approved by physician; importance of carefully reading labels of all low-salt foods to prevent excess intake of potassium
Checking with physician before beginning strenuous physical exercise if out of condition, to prevent possible hyperkalemia
» Checking with physician at once if signs of gastrointestinal bleeding are observed

Side/adverse effects
Expended wax matrix from some potassium chloride extended-release tablets may be seen in stool and be alarming to patient, although not necessarily an indication of improper dissolution of tablet or lack of bioavailability of potassium chloride
Signs of potential side effects, especially hyperkalemia or contact irritation of the alimentary tract

---

▲ For the Patient ▲

912576

ABOUT YOUR MEDICINE

Potassium (poe-TASS-ee-um) is needed to maintain good health. A balanced diet usually supplies all the potassium a person needs. However, potassium supplements may be needed by patients who do not have enough potassium in their regular diet. Potassium supplements are also used in patients who have lost too much potassium because of illness or treatment with certain medicines.

If any of the information in this leaflet causes you special concern or if you want additional information about your medicine and its use, check with your doctor, nurse, or pharmacist. **Remember, keep this and all other medicines out of the reach of children and never share your medicines with others.**

BEFORE USING THIS MEDICINE

If you are taking this medicine without a prescription, carefully read and follow any precautions on the label. You should be especially careful if you . . .
- are allergic to any medicine, either prescription or nonprescription (OTC);
- are pregnant, intend to become pregnant, or are breast-feeding;
- are taking any other prescription or nonprescription (OTC) medicine, especially captopril, cortisone-like medicine, digitalis glycosides (heart medicine), enalapril, heparin, medicine for inflammation or pain, medicine for stomach pain or cramps, other medicine containing potassium, potassium-sparing diuretics

(amiloride, spironolactone, triamterene), or thiazide diuretics;
- have any other medical problems, especially Addison's disease, diarrhea (continuing or severe), heart disease, intestinal blockage, kidney disease, difficulty in urination, or stomach ulcer.

If you have any questions, check with your doctor, nurse, or pharmacist.

PROPER USE OF THIS MEDICINE

Take this medicine only as directed. Do not take more of it, do not take it more often, and do not take it for a longer time than your doctor ordered. **This is especially important if you are also taking diuretics (water pills) and digitalis medicines for your heart.**

Take this medicine immediately after meals or with food to lessen possible stomach upset or laxative action. Follow each dose, whether liquid, tablet, or capsule, with a glass of water.

If you miss a dose of this medicine and remember within 2 hours, take it as soon as possible. However, if you do not remember until later, skip the missed dose and go back to your regular dosing schedule. Do not double doses.

PRECAUTIONS WHILE USING THIS MEDICINE

Your doctor should check your progress at regular visits to make sure the medicine is working properly and that possible side effects are avoided. Laboratory tests may be necessary.

Since salt substitutes, low-sodium foods (especially some breads and canned foods), and low-sodium milk may contain potassium, do not use them unless told to do so by your doctor. It is important to read the labels carefully on all low-sodium food products.

Check with your doctor at once if you notice blackish stools or other signs of stomach or intestinal bleeding. This medicine, especially when taken in tablet form, may cause such a condition to become worse.

POSSIBLE SIDE EFFECTS OF THIS MEDICINE

Side Effects That Should Be Reported To Your Doctor Immediately

Stop taking this medicine and check with your doctor immediately if any of the following side effects occur:

Rare—Confusion; irregular or slow heartbeat; numbness or tingling in hands, feet, or lips; shortness of breath or difficult breathing; unexplained anxiety; unusual tiredness or weakness; weakness or heaviness of legs

Other Side Effects That Should Be Reported To Your Doctor

Rare—Abdominal or stomach pain, cramping, or soreness (continuing); chest or throat pain, especially when swallowing; stools with signs of blood (red or black color)

Side Effects That Usually Do Not Require Medical Attention

These possible side effects may go away during treatment; however, if they continue or are bothersome, check with your doctor, nurse, or pharmacist.

More common—Diarrhea; nausea; stomach pain, discomfort, or gas (mild); vomiting

Other side effects not listed above may also occur in some patients. If you notice any other effects, check with your doctor, nurse, or pharmacist.

PRAZOSIN   Systemic

■ For the Pharmacist ■

In providing consultation, consider emphasizing the following selected information (» = major clinical significance):

Before using this medication
» Conditions affecting use, especially:
  Sensitivity to quinazolines
  Breast-feeding—Distributed into breast milk in small amounts
  Use in the elderly—Increased sensitivity to hypotensive effects and increased risk of prazosin-induced hypothermia
  Other medical problems, especially severe cardiac disease

Proper use of this medication
  Getting into the habit of taking at same times each day to help increase compliance
» Proper dosing
  Missed dose: Taking as soon as possible; not taking if almost time for next dose; not doubling doses
» Proper storage
For use as an antihypertensive
  Possible need for control of weight and diet, especially sodium intake
» Patient may not experience symptoms of hypertension; importance of taking medication even if feeling well
» Does not cure, but helps control hypertension; possible need for lifelong therapy; serious consequences of untreated hypertension
For use in benign prostatic hyperplasia (BPH)
  Relieves symptoms of BPH but does not change the size of the prostate; may not prevent the need for surgery in the future

Precautions while using this medication
  Regular visits to physician to check progress
» Caution if dizziness, lightheadedness, or sudden fainting occurs, especially after initial dose; taking first dose at bedtime
» Caution when getting up suddenly from a lying or sitting position
» Caution in using alcohol, while standing for long periods or exercising, and during hot weather because of enhanced orthostatic hypotensive effects
» Possibility of drowsiness
» Caution when driving or doing anything else requiring alertness because of possible drowsiness, dizziness, or lightheadedness
» Not taking other medications, especially nonprescription sympathomimetics, unless discussed with physician

Side/adverse effects
  Signs of potential side effects, especially dizziness, orthostatic hypotension, edema, palpitations, urinary incontinence, angina, dyspnea, and priapism

▲ For the Patient ▲

912587

ALPHA₁-BLOCKERS (Oral): *Including Doxazosin; Prazosin; Terazosin.*

ABOUT YOUR MEDICINE

Alpha₁-blockers are used to treat high blood pressure (hypertension). Terazosin is also used to treat benign enlargement of the prostate (benign prostatic hyperplasia [BPH]). These medicines may also be used for other conditions as determined by your doctor.

If any of the information in this leaflet causes you special concern or if you want additional information about your medicine and its use, check with your doctor, nurse, or pharmacist. **Remember, keep this and all other medicines out of the reach of children and never share your medicines with others.**

BEFORE USING THIS MEDICINE

Tell your doctor, nurse, and pharmacist if you . . .
- are allergic to any medicine, either prescription or nonprescription (OTC);
- are pregnant or intend to become pregnant while using this medicine;
- are breast-feeding;
- are taking any other prescription or nonprescription (OTC) medicine, especially medicines for appetite control, asthma, colds, cough, hay fever, or sinus;
- have any other medical problems, especially heart disease.

PROPER USE OF THIS MEDICINE

For patients taking this medicine for high blood pressure:
- This medicine will not cure your high blood pressure but it does help control it. You must continue to take it—even if you feel well—if you expect to keep your blood pressure down. **You may have to take high blood pressure medicine for the rest of your life.**

For patients taking terazosin for benign enlargement of the prostate:
- Remember that terazosin will not shrink the size of your prostate, but it does help to relieve the symptoms.
- It may take up to 6 weeks before your symptoms get better.

If you miss a dose of this medicine, take it as soon as possible. However, if it is almost time for your next dose, skip the missed dose and go back to your regular dosing schedule. Do not double doses.

PRECAUTIONS WHILE USING THIS MEDICINE

Dizziness, lightheadedness, or sudden fainting may occur after you take this medicine, especially when you get up from a sitting or lying position. These effects are more likely to occur when you take the first dose of this medicine. Taking the first dose at bedtime may prevent problems. However, **be especially careful if you need to get up during the night.** These effects may also occur with any doses you take after the first dose. Getting up slowly may help lessen this problem. **If you feel dizzy, lie down so that you do not faint.** Then sit for a few minutes before standing to prevent the dizziness from returning.

The dizziness, lightheadedness, or fainting is more likely to occur if you drink alcohol, stand for long periods of time, exercise, or if the weather is hot. **While you are taking this medicine, be careful to limit the amount of alcohol you drink. Also, use extra care during exercise or hot weather or if you must stand for long periods of time.**

This medicine may cause some people to become drowsy or less alert than they are normally. **Make sure you know how you react to this medicine before you drive, use machines, or do other jobs that could be dangerous if you are dizzy, drowsy, or are not alert.** After you have taken several doses of this medicine, these effects should lessen.

POSSIBLE SIDE EFFECTS OF THIS MEDICINE

The following side effects may occur more or less often than listed, depending on which medicine you are taking.

Side Effects That Should Be Reported To Your Doctor

Less common—Dizziness; dizziness or lightheadedness when standing up; fainting (sudden); fast, irregular, or pounding heartbeat; loss of bladder control (prazosin only); shortness of breath; swelling of feet or lower legs

Rare—Chest pain; continuing, painful, inappropriate erection of the penis (prazosin only); shortness of breath (prazosin only)

Side Effects That Usually Do Not Require Medical Attention

These possible side effects may go away during treatment; however, if they continue or are bothersome, check with your doctor, nurse, or pharmacist.

More common—Drowsiness; headache; unusual tiredness or weakness

Less common—Dryness of mouth (prazosin only); nausea; nervousness (doxazosin and prazosin only)

For doxazosin only (in addition to those listed above)— Restlessness; runny nose; unusual irritability

For prazosin only—rare (in addition to those listed above)—Frequent urge to urinate

For terazosin only (in addition to those listed above)— Back or joint pain; blurred vision; stuffy nose

Other side effects not listed above may also occur in some patients. If you notice any other effects, check with your doctor, nurse, or pharmacist.

PRIMIDONE Systemic

■ For the Pharmacist ■

In providing consultation, consider emphasizing the following selected
information (» = major clinical significance):

Before using this medication
» Conditions affecting use, especially:
    Sensitivity to primidone or barbiturates
    Pregnancy—Abnormalities similar to fetal hydantoin syndrome
      may occur; neonatal hemorrhaging may occur at delivery
    Breast-feeding—Distributed into breast milk, causing drowsiness
      in the baby
    Use in children—Paradoxical excitement and restlessness may
      occur
    Use in the elderly—Paradoxical excitement and restlessness may
      occur
    Other medications, especially adrenocorticoids, anticoagulants,
      estrogens, estrogen-containing contraceptives, CNS depres-
      sion–producing medications, other anticonvulsants, or mono-
      amine oxidase inhibitors
    Other medical problems, especially acute intermittent porphyria,
      or respiratory diseases

Proper use of this medication
» Compliance with therapy; taking every day in doses spaced as di-
    rected
» Proper dosing
    Missed dose: Taking as soon as possible, unless within an hour of
      next scheduled dose; not doubling doses
» Proper storage

Precautions while using this medication
    Regular visits to physician to check progress of therapy
    Checking with physician before discontinuing medication; gradual
      dosage reduction may be needed
    Caution if any kind of surgery, dental treatment, or emergency
      treatment is required
» Avoiding use of alcoholic beverages; not taking other CNS depres-
    sants unless prescribed by physician
» Possible drowsiness; caution when driving or doing other things re-
    quiring alertness
» Possible dizziness or lightheadedness; caution when getting up sud-
    denly from a lying or sitting position
    Caution if any laboratory tests required; possible interference with
      results of cyanocobalamin Co 57, metyrapone, or phentolamine
      tests.

Side/adverse effects
    Signs of potential side effects, especially excitement or restlessness,
      allergic reaction, or megaloblastic anemia

▲ For the Patient ▲

914742

ABOUT YOUR MEDICINE

Primidone (PRYE-mih-done) belongs to the group of medicines called anticonvulsants. It is used in the treatment of

epilepsy to manage certain types of seizures. Primidone may be used alone or in combination with other anticonvulsants.

If any of the information in this leaflet causes you special concern or if you want additional information about your medicine and its use, check with your doctor, nurse, or pharmacist. **Remember, keep this and all other medicines out of the reach of children and never share your medicines with others.**

BEFORE USING THIS MEDICINE

Tell your doctor, nurse, and pharmacist if you . . .
- are allergic to any medicine, either prescription or non-prescription (OTC);
- are pregnant or intend to become pregnant while using this medicine;
- are breast-feeding;
- compete in athletics;
- are taking any other prescription or nonprescription (OTC) medicine, especially adrenocorticoids (cortisone-like medicines), anticoagulants (blood thinners), CNS depressants, MAO inhibitors, other seizure medicine, or oral contraceptives (birth control pills) containing estrogen;
- have any other medical problems, especially asthma, emphysema, or chronic lung disease; or history of porphyria.

PROPER USE OF THIS MEDICINE

Take primidone every day in regularly spaced doses as ordered by your doctor. This will provide the proper amount of medicine needed to prevent seizures.

If you miss a dose of this medicine, take it as soon as possible. However, if it is within an hour of your next dose, skip the missed dose and go back to your regular dosing schedule. Do not double doses.

PRECAUTIONS WHILE USING THIS MEDICINE

It is very important that your doctor check your progress at regular visits, especially during the first few months of treatment with primidone. This will allow your doctor to adjust the amount of medicine you are taking to meet your needs.

If you have been taking primidone regularly for several weeks, you should not suddenly stop taking it. Your doctor may want you to reduce gradually the amount you are taking before stopping completely.

Before having any kind of surgery, dental treatment, or emergency treatment, tell the physician or dentist in charge that you are using this medicine.

This medicine will add to the effects of alcohol and other CNS depressants (medicines that slow down the nervous system, possibly causing drowsiness). **Check with your doctor** before taking any such depressants while you are using this medicine.

Primidone may cause some people to become dizzy, light-headed, drowsy, or less alert than they are normally. Even if taken at bedtime, it may cause some people to feel drowsy or less alert on arising. **Make sure you know how you react to this medicine before you drive, use machines, or do other jobs that require you to be alert.**

Oral contraceptives (birth control pills) containing estrogen may not work properly if you take them while you are taking primidone. Unplanned pregnancies may occur. You should use a different or additional means of birth control while you are taking primidone. If you have any questions about this, check with your doctor or pharmacist.

POSSIBLE SIDE EFFECTS OF THIS MEDICINE
Side Effects That Should Be Reported To Your Doctor

> *Less common*—Unusual excitement or restlessness (especially in children and sometimes in the elderly)

> *Rare*—Skin rash or hives; swelling of eyelids; unusual tiredness or weakness; wheezing or tightness in chest

Side Effects That Usually Do Not Require Medical Attention

These possible side effects may go away during treatment; however, if they continue or are bothersome, check with your doctor, nurse, or pharmacist.

> *More common*—Clumsiness or unsteadiness; dizziness; drowsiness

> *Less common*—Decreased sexual ability; headache; loss of appetite; nausea or vomiting

Other side effects not listed above may also occur in some patients. If you notice any other effects, check with your doctor, nurse, or pharmacist.

PROBENECID   Systemic

■ For the Pharmacist ■

In providing consultation, consider emphasizing the following selected information (» = major clinical significance):

Before using this medication
» Conditions affecting use, especially:
    Allergic reaction to probenecid, history of
    Pregnancy—Probenecid crosses the placenta
    Other medications, especially antibiotics, antivirals, indomethacin, ketoprofen, antineoplastic agents, aspirin or other salicylates, including bismuth subsalicylate (when probenecid used as antihyperuricemic or antigout agent), heparin, methotrexate, nitrofurantoin, or zidovudine
    Other medical problems, especially cancer being treated by cytolytic medication or radiation (x-ray) therapy; kidney stones or other kidney problems, especially if caused by uric acid, or history of; renal function impairment; and blood dyscrasias

Proper use of this medication
    Taking with food or an antacid to minimize gastric irritation
    Missed dose: Taking as soon as possible; not taking if almost time for next dose; not doubling doses
» Proper dosing
» Proper storage
For use as antigout agent
    Several months of continuous therapy may be required for maximum effectiveness
» Medication does not relieve acute attacks but rather helps to prevent them; need to continue taking probenecid with medication prescribed for gout attacks
For use as antihyperuricemic (including gout therapy)
    Importance of high fluid intake and compliance with therapy for alkalinization of urine, if prescribed

Precautions while using this medication
    Regular visits to physician to check progress during long-term therapy
    Caution if any laboratory tests required; possible interference with test results
    Diabetics: May cause false results with copper sulfate urine sugar tests, but not with glucose enzymatic urine sugar tests
For use as antihyperuricemic (including gout therapy)
» Aspirin or other salicylates may decrease uricosuric effects of probenecid; checking with physician regarding concurrent use, since effect is dependent on salicylate dose and duration of use
» Possibility that alcohol taken in large amounts may increase blood uric acid concentration and reduce effectiveness of medication

Side/adverse effects
    Signs and symptoms of potential side effects, especially renal calculi, allergic dermatitis, anaphylaxis, anemia, aplastic anemia, hemolytic anemia, fever, hepatic necrosis, leukopenia, nephrotic syndrome, pain in back and/or ribs, renal colic, and urate nephropathy

---

▲ For the Patient ▲

914753

ABOUT YOUR MEDICINE

Probenecid (proe-BEN-e-sid) is used in the treatment of chronic gout or gouty arthritis. It does not cure gout but after you have been taking it for a few months, it will help prevent gout attacks. Probenecid will help prevent gout attacks only as long as you continue to take it. Probenecid is also used to prevent or treat other medical problems that may occur if too much uric acid is present in the body. In addition, probenecid is sometimes used with certain kinds of antibiotics to make them more effective in the treatment of infections.

If any of the information in this leaflet causes you special concern or if you want additional information about your medicine and its use, check with your doctor, nurse, or pharmacist. **Remember, keep this and all other medicines out of the reach of children and never share your medicines with others.**

BEFORE USING THIS MEDICINE

Tell your doctor, nurse, and pharmacist if you . . .
- are allergic to any medicine, either prescription or nonprescription (OTC);
- are pregnant or intend to become pregnant while using this medicine;
- are breast-feeding;
- are taking **any** other prescription or nonprescription (OTC) medicine;
- have any other medical problems, especially blood or kidney disease or kidney stones.

PROPER USE OF THIS MEDICINE

If probenecid upsets your stomach, it may be taken with food. If this does not work, an antacid may be taken. If stomach upset (nausea, vomiting, or loss of appetite) continues, check with your doctor.

For patients taking probenecid for gout:
- After you begin to take probenecid, gout attacks may continue for a while. However, if you take this medicine regularly as directed by your doctor, the attacks will gradually become less frequent and less painful than before.
- This medicine will help prevent gout attacks but it will not relieve an attack that has already started. **Even if you take another medicine for gout attacks, continue to take this medicine also.**

For patients taking probenecid for gout or to help remove uric acid from the body:
- When you first begin taking probenecid, the amount of uric acid in the kidneys is greatly increased. This may

cause kidney stones in some people. To help prevent this, your doctor may want you to drink at least 10 to 12 full glasses (8 ounces each) of fluids each day, or to take another medicine to make your urine less acid. It is important that you follow your doctor's instructions very carefully.

If you are taking probenecid regularly and you miss a dose, take the missed dose as soon as possible. However, if you do not remember until it is almost time for the next dose, skip the missed dose. Do not double doses.

PRECAUTIONS WHILE USING THIS MEDICINE

If you will be taking probenecid for more than a few weeks, your doctor should check your progress at regular visits.

For patients taking probenecid for gout or to remove uric acid from the body:
- Taking aspirin or other salicylates will lessen the effects of probenecid. Also, drinking too much alcohol may increase the amount of uric acid in the blood and lessen the effects of this medicine. Therefore, **do not take aspirin or other salicylates or drink alcoholic beverages while taking this medicine,** unless you have first checked with your doctor.

POSSIBLE SIDE EFFECTS OF THIS MEDICINE
Side Effects That Should Be Reported To Your Doctor

Less common—Bloody urine; lower back pain; painful urination

Rare—Difficulty in breathing; fever; skin rash or itching; sore throat, fever, and chills; sudden decrease in amount of urine; swelling of feet, lower legs, or face; unusual bleeding or bruising; unusual tiredness or weakness; weight gain; yellow eyes or skin

Signs of overdose—Convulsions (seizures); vomiting (severe and continuing)

Side Effects That Usually Do Not Require Medical Attention

These possible side effects may go away during treatment; however, if they continue or are bothersome, check with your doctor, nurse, or pharmacist.

More common—Headache; loss of appetite; nausea or vomiting (mild)

Other side effects not listed above may also occur in some patients. If you notice any other effects, check with your doctor, nurse, or pharmacist.

PROBENECID AND COLCHICINE   Systemic

■ For the Pharmacist ■

In providing consultation, consider emphasizing the following selected information (» = major clinical significance):

Before using this medication
» Conditions affecting use, especially:
   Allergic reaction to probenecid or sensitivity to colchicine, history of
   Pregnancy—Probenecid crosses the placenta; colchicine reported to be teratogenic in humans
   Use in the elderly—Increased susceptibility to cumulative colchicine toxicity
   Other medications, especially antibiotics, antivirals, bone marrow depressants or blood dyscrasia–causing medications, indomethacin, ketoprofen, antineoplastic agents, aspirin or other salicylates, including bismuth subsalicylate, heparin, methotrexate, nitrofurantoin, or zidovudine
   Other medical problems, especially alcohol abuse, severe cardiac or gastrointestinal disorders; cancer being treated by cytolytic medication or radiation (x-ray) therapy; kidney stones or other kidney problems, especially if caused by uric acid, or history of; renal function impairment; hepatic function impairment; stomach ulcer or other stomach problems, and blood dyscrasias

Proper use of this medication
   Taking with food or an antacid to minimize gastric irritation
   Importance of not taking more medication than the amount prescribed
   Several months of continuous therapy may be required for maximum effectiveness
» Medication does not relieve acute attacks of gout but rather helps to prevent them; need to continue taking probenecid and colchicine with medication prescribed for gout attacks
   Importance of high fluid intake and compliance with therapy for alkalinization of urine, if prescribed
» Proper dosing
   Missed dose: Taking as soon as possible; not taking if almost time for next dose; not doubling doses
» Proper storage

Precautions while using this medication
   Regular visits to physician to check progress during therapy
   Caution if any laboratory tests required; possible interference with test results
   Diabetics: May cause false results with copper sulfate urine sugar tests, but not with glucose enzymatic urine sugar tests
» Aspirin or other salicylates may decrease uricosuric effects of probenecid; checking with physician regarding concurrent use, since effect is dependent on salicylate dose and duration of use
» Possibility that alcohol taken in large amounts may increase the risk of colchicine-induced gastrointestinal toxicity; also, may increase uric acid concentrations and thereby reduce effectiveness of medication

» For patients taking high doses (4 tablets a day): Discontinuing at once and notifying physician as soon as possible if symptoms of gastrointestinal toxicity occur

Side/adverse effects

Signs and symptoms of potential side effects, especially renal calculi, allergic dermatitis, anaphylaxis, anemia, aplastic anemia, hemolytic anemia, fever, hepatic necrosis, leukopenia, nephrotic syndrome, pain in back and/or ribs, renal colic, urate nephropathy, colchicine-induced gastrointestinal toxicity, and peripheral neuritis

---

▲ For the Patient ▲

914764

ABOUT YOUR MEDICINE

Probenecid (proe-BEN-e-sid) and **colchicine** (KOL-chi-seen) combination is used to treat gout or gouty arthritis.

This medicine helps to prevent gout attacks. Although colchicine may also be used to relieve an attack of gout, this requires more colchicine than this combination medicine contains. This medicine will help prevent gout attacks only as long as you continue to take it.

If any of the information in this leaflet causes you special concern or if you want additional information about your medicine and its use, check with your doctor, nurse, or pharmacist. **Remember, keep this and all other medicines out of the reach of children and never share your medicines with others.**

BEFORE USING THIS MEDICINE

Tell your doctor, nurse, and pharmacist if you . . .
- are allergic to any medicine, either prescription or nonprescription (OTC);
- are pregnant or intend to become pregnant while using this medicine;
- are breast-feeding;
- are taking **any** other prescription or nonprescription (OTC) medicine;
- have any other medical problems, especially blood disease, heart disease, intestinal disease, kidney disease or stones (or history of), or liver disease.

PROPER USE OF THIS MEDICINE

If this medicine upsets your stomach, it may be taken with food or an antacid. If stomach upset continues, check with your doctor.

Take this medicine only as directed by your doctor. Do not take more of it and do not take it more often than your doctor ordered. The colchicine in this combination medicine may cause serious side effects if too much is taken.

This medicine will help prevent gout attacks, but it will not relieve an attack that has already started. **Even if you take** another medicine for gout attacks, continue to take this medicine also.

When you first begin taking this medicine, the amount of uric acid in the kidneys is greatly increased. This may cause kidney stones or other kidney problems. To help prevent this, your doctor may want you to drink at least 10 to 12 glasses (8 ounces each) of fluids each day, or to take another medicine to make your urine less acid. It is important that you follow your doctor's instructions.

If you miss a dose of this medicine, take it as soon as possible. However, if it is almost time for your next dose, skip the missed dose and go back to your regular dosing schedule. Do not double doses.

PRECAUTIONS WHILE USING THIS MEDICINE

Do not take aspirin or other salicylates or drink alcoholic beverages while you are taking this medicine, unless you have first checked with your doctor.

For patients taking 4 tablets or more of this medicine a day:
• **Stop taking this medicine immediately and check with your doctor as soon as possible if severe diarrhea, nausea or vomiting, or stomach pain occurs while you are taking this medicine.**

POSSIBLE SIDE EFFECTS OF THIS MEDICINE

Side Effects That Should Be Reported To Your Doctor Immediately

*Signs of an allergic reaction—rare—*Fast or irregular breathing; puffiness or swelling of the eyelids or around the eyes; shortness of breath, troubled breathing, tightness in chest, or wheezing; changes in the skin color of the face occurring together with any of the other side effects listed here; skin rash, hives, or itching occurring together with any other of the side effects listed here

Other Side Effects That Should Be Reported To Your Doctor

*Less common—*Lower back pain (severe or sharp); painful urination; skin rash, hives, or itching (without other signs of an allergic reaction)

*Rare—*Black, tarry stools; cloudy urine; cough or hoarseness; numbness, tingling, pain, or weakness in hands or feet; sores, ulcers or white spots on lips or in mouth; sore throat, fever, and chills; swelling of face, fingers, feet, and/or lower legs; swollen and/or painful glands; sudden decrease in amount of urine; unusual bleeding or bruising; unusual tiredness or weakness; weight gain; yellow eyes or skin

Side Effects That Usually Do Not Require Medical Attention

These possible side effects may go away during treatment; however, if they continue or are bothersome, check with your doctor, nurse, or pharmacist.

> *More common*—Diarrhea (mild); headache; loss of appetite; nausea or vomiting (mild); stomach pain

Other side effects not listed above may also occur in some patients. If you notice any other effects, check with your doctor, nurse, or pharmacist.

PROBUCOL   Systemic

■ For the Pharmacist ■

In providing consultation, consider emphasizing the following selected information (» = major clinical significance):

Before using this medication
Diet as preferred therapy; importance of following prescribed diet
» Conditions affecting use, especially:
Sensitivity to probucol
Breast-feeding—Use not recommended because of potentially serious adverse effects on nursing infants
Use in children—Not recommended in children under 2 years of age since cholesterol is required for normal development
Other medical problems, especially primary biliary cirrhosis, and cardiac abnormalities including congestive heart failure and QT interval prolongation

Proper use of this medication
» Importance of not taking more or less medication than the amount prescribed
This medication does not cure the condition but rather helps control it
» Compliance with prescribed diet
Taking with meals, since medication is more effective with food
» Proper dosing
Missed dose: Taking as soon as possible; not taking if almost time for next dose; not doubling doses
» Proper storage

Precautions while using this medication
» Importance of close monitoring by the physician
» Checking with physician before discontinuing medication; blood lipid concentrations may increase significantly

Side/adverse effects
Signs of potential side effects, especially angioneurotic edema, blood dyscrasias, QT interval prolongation, and tachycardia

▲ For the Patient ▲

914775

ABOUT YOUR MEDICINE

Probucol (proe-BYOO-kole) is used to lower levels of cholesterol (a fat-like substance) in the blood. This may help prevent medical problems caused by cholesterol clogging the blood vessels.

If any of the information in this leaflet causes you special concern or if you want additional information about your medicine and its use, check with your doctor, nurse, or pharmacist. **Remember, keep this and all other medicines out of the reach of children and never share your medicines with others.**

BEFORE USING THIS MEDICINE

Importance of diet—Before prescribing medicine for your condition, your doctor will probably try to control your condition by prescribing a personal diet for you. Such a diet may be low in fats, sugars, and/or cholesterol. Many people are able to control their condition by carefully following their doctor's orders for proper diet and exercise. Medicine is prescribed only when additional help is needed and is effective only when a schedule of diet and exercise is properly followed. **Follow carefully the special diet your doctor gave you.**

Also, this medicine is less effective if you are greatly overweight. It may be very important for you to go on a reducing diet. However, check with your doctor before going on any diet.

Tell your doctor, nurse, and pharmacist if you . . .
- are allergic to any medicine, either prescription or non-prescription (OTC);
- are pregnant or intend to become pregnant while using this medicine;
- are breast-feeding;
- are taking any other prescription or nonprescription (OTC) medicine;
- have any other medical problems, especially heart, liver, or gallbladder disease.

PROPER USE OF THIS MEDICINE

Many patients who have high cholesterol levels will not notice any signs of the problem. In fact, many may feel normal. **Take this medicine exactly as directed by your doctor, even though you may feel well.** Try not to miss any doses and do not take more medicine than your doctor ordered.

Remember that this medicine will not cure your condition but it does help control it. Therefore, you must continue to take this medicine as directed if you expect to keep your cholesterol levels down.

This medicine works better when taken with meals.

If you miss a dose of this medicine, take it as soon as possible. However, if it is almost time for your next dose, skip the missed dose and go back to your regular dosing schedule. Do not double doses.

PRECAUTIONS WHILE USING THIS MEDICINE

It is very important that your doctor check your progress at regular visits. This will allow your doctor to see if the medicine is working properly to lower your cholesterol levels and if you should continue to take it.

Do not stop taking this medicine without first checking with your doctor. When you stop taking this medicine, your blood fat levels may increase again. Your doctor may want you to follow a special diet to help prevent this.

POSSIBLE SIDE EFFECTS OF THIS MEDICINE
Side Effects That Should Be Reported To Your Doctor

> *More common*—Dizziness or fainting; fast or irregular heartbeat
>
> *Rare*—Swellings on face, hands, or feet, or in mouth; unusual bleeding or bruising; unusual tiredness or weakness

Side Effects That Usually Do Not Require Medical Attention

These possible side effects may go away during treatment; however, if they continue or are bothersome, check with your doctor, nurse, or pharmacist.

> *More common*—Bloating; diarrhea; nausea and vomiting; stomach pain
>
> *Less common*—Headache; numbness or tingling of fingers, toes, or face

Other side effects not listed above may also occur in some patients. If you notice any other effects, check with your doctor, nurse, or pharmacist.

PROCAINAMIDE   Systemic

▣ For the Pharmacist ▣

In providing consultation, consider emphasizing the following selected information (» = major clinical significance):

Before using this medication
» Conditions affecting use, especially:
    Sensitivity to procaine or other related agents
    Pregnancy—Procainamide crosses the placenta
    Breast-feeding—Procainamide and NAPA are distributed into breast milk
    Use in children—Higher doses may be needed to maintain adequate therapeutic concentrations in some patients
    Use in the elderly—May be more susceptible to hypotension
    Dental—May be more susceptible to microbial infection, delayed healing, and gingival bleeding because of risk of leukopenia and thrombocytopenia; may cause dryness of mouth
    Other medications, especially other antiarrhythmics, antihypertensives, antimyasthenics, neuromuscular blocking agents, and pimozide
    Other medical problems, especially atrioventricular block, torsades de pointes, severe digitalis intoxication, congestive heart failure, renal function impairment, lupus erythematosus, myasthenia gravis, or ventricular tachycardia during an occlusive coronary episode

Proper use of this medication
» Taking exactly as directed even if feeling well
    Taking on empty stomach for faster absorption, or with food or milk to reduce stomach irritation
    Proper administration of extended-release tablets: Swallowing tablets whole, without breaking, crushing, or chewing
» Importance of not missing doses and of taking at evenly spaced intervals
» Proper dosing
    Missed dose: Taking as soon as possible if remembered within 2 hours (4 hours for extended-release tablets); not taking if remembered later; not doubling doses
» Proper storage

Precautions while using this medication
    Regular visits to physician to check progress
» Checking with physician before discontinuing medication; gradual dosage reduction may be necessary to avoid worsening of condition
» Caution if any kind of surgery (including dental surgery) or emergency treatment is required
    Carrying medical identification card or bracelet
» Possibility of dizziness with high dosage, especially in elderly; caution when driving or doing things requiring alertness
    Caution if any laboratory tests required; possible interference with test results

Side/adverse effects
    Signs of potential side effects, especially allergic reaction, SLE-like syndrome, CNS effects, Coombs' positive hemolytic anemia, leukopenia, and thrombocytopenia

Extended-release tablet matrix may be seen in stool and is to be expected

---

▲ For the Patient ▲

913036

ANTIARRHYTHMICS, TYPE I (Oral): *Including Disopyramide; Encainide; Flecainide; Mexiletine; Moricizine; Procainamide; Propafenone; Quinidine; Tocainide.*

ABOUT YOUR MEDICINE

Type I antiarrhythmics are used to correct irregular heartbeats to a normal rhythm and to slow an overactive heart.

There is a chance that these medicines may cause new heart rhythm problems when they are used. Usually this effect is rare and mild. However, some of these medicines are more likely than others to cause this effect. For example, encainide and flecainide have been shown to cause severe problems in some patients, and so they are only used to treat serious heart rhythm problems. Discuss this possible effect with your doctor.

If any of the information in this leaflet causes you special concern or if you want additional information about your medicine and its use, check with your doctor, nurse, or pharmacist. **Remember, keep this and all other medicines out of the reach of children and never share your medicines with others.**

BEFORE USING THIS MEDICINE

Tell your doctor, nurse, and pharmacist if you . . .
- are allergic to any medicine, either prescription or non-prescription (OTC);
- are pregnant or intend to become pregnant while using this medicine;
- are breast-feeding;
- are taking **any** other prescription or nonprescription (OTC) medicine;
- have **any** other medical problems.

PROPER USE OF THIS MEDICINE

Take this medicine exactly as directed by your doctor, even though you may feel well. Do not take more medicine than ordered.

For patients taking the extended-release capsules or tablets:
- Swallow whole without breaking, crushing, or chewing.

It is best to take each dose at evenly spaced times day and night.

For patients taking mexiletine:
- To lessen the possibility of stomach upset, this medicine should be taken with food or immediately after meals or with milk or an antacid.

If you miss a dose of this medicine, take it as soon as possible. However, if you do not remember until it is almost time for the next dose, skip the missed dose and go back to your regular dosing schedule. Do not double doses.

PRECAUTIONS WHILE USING THIS MEDICINE

It is important that your doctor check your progress at regular visits to make sure the medicine is working properly to help your heart.

Do not suddenly stop taking this medicine without first checking with your doctor. Stopping it suddenly may cause a serious change in heart activity.

Dizziness or lightheadedness or blurred vision may occur. **Make sure you know how you react to this medicine before you drive, use machines, or do other jobs that require you to be alert and able to see well.**

For patients taking disopyramide:
- **If signs of hypoglycemia (low blood sugar) such as chills, hunger, nausea, nervousness, or sweating appear, eat or drink a food containing sugar and call your doctor right away.**
- **Use extra care not to become overheated during exercise or hot weather,** since this medicine will often make you sweat less and could possibly result in heatstroke.

POSSIBLE SIDE EFFECTS OF THIS MEDICINE

Side Effects That Should Be Reported To Your Doctor Immediately

> *For quinidine only, especially after the first dose or first few doses*—Breathing difficulty; changes in vision; dizziness, lightheadedness, or fainting; fever; severe headache; ringing in ears; skin rash

Other Side Effects That Should Be Reported To Your Doctor

> *For all antiarrhythmics*—Chest pain; fast or irregular heartbeat; fever or chills; shortness of breath or painful breathing; skin rash or itching; unusual bleeding or bruising

> *For disopyramide (in addition to above)*—Difficult urination; swelling of feet or lower legs

> *For encainide, flecainide, moricizine, and propafenone (in addition to above)*—Swelling of feet or lower legs; trembling or shaking

Side Effects That Usually Do Not Require Medical Attention

These possible side effects may go away during treatment; however, if they continue or are bothersome, check with your doctor, nurse, or pharmacist.

> *For all antiarrhythmics*—Blurred or double vision; dizziness or lightheadedness

For disopyramide (in addition to above)—Dry mouth and
   throat

For flecainide (in addition to above)—Seeing spots

For mexiletine (in addition to above)—Heartburn; nausea and vomiting; nervousness; trembling or shaking
   of hands; unsteadiness or trouble walking

For procainamide (in addition to above)—Diarrhea; loss
   of appetite

For propafenone (in addition to above)—Change in taste

For quinidine (in addition to above)—Bitter taste; diarrhea; flushing of skin with itching; loss of appetite;
   nausea or vomiting; stomach pain or cramps

For tocainide (in addition to above)—Loss of appetite;
   nausea

Other side effects not listed above may also occur in some
patients. If you notice any other effects, check with your
doctor, nurse, or pharmacist.

PROCARBAZINE   Systemic

■ For the Pharmacist ■

In providing consultation, consider emphasizing the following selected information (» = major clinical significance):

Before using this medication
» Conditions affecting use, especially:

   Sensitivity to procarbazine

   Pregnancy—Use not recommended because of mutagenic, teratogenic, and carcinogenic potential; advisability of using contraception; telling physician immediately if pregnancy is suspected

   Breast-feeding—Not recommended because of risk of serious side effects

   Other medications, especially alcohol, local anesthetics, spinal anesthetics, anticholinergics, tricyclic antidepressants, oral antidiabetic agents, antihistamines, other bone marrow depressants, buspirone, caffeine-containing preparations, carbamazepine, other CNS depressants, cocaine, cyclobenzaprine, dextromethorphan, doxapram, fluoxetine, guanadrel, guanethidine, insulin, levodopa, other MAO inhibitors, maprotiline, meperidine and possibly other opioid analgesics, methyldopa, methylphenidate, rauwolfia alkaloids, sympathomimetics, tryptophan, tyramine- or other high pressor amine–containing foods and beverages, or previous cytotoxic drug therapy or radiation therapy

   Other medical problems, especially active alcoholism, bone marrow depression, cardiac arrhythmias, cardiovascular disease or coronary insufficiency, chickenpox, congestive heart failure, severe or frequent headaches, hepatic function impairment, herpes zoster, infection, paranoid schizophrenia or other hyperexcitable personality states, pheochromocytoma, or renal function impairment

Proper use of this medication
» Importance of not taking more or less medication than the amount prescribed

   Caution in taking combination chemotherapy; taking each medication at the right time
» Frequency of nausea and vomiting; importance of continuing medication despite stomach upset

   Checking with physician if vomiting occurs shortly after dose is taken
» Proper dosing

   Missed dose: Taking as soon as remembered if within a few hours; not taking if several hours have passed or if almost time for next dose; not doubling doses
» Proper storage

Precautions while using this medication
» Importance of close monitoring by the physician
» Checking with hospital emergency room or physician if symptoms of hypertensive crisis develop
» Avoiding use of tyramine-containing foods, alcoholic beverages and large quantities of caffeine-containing beverages, over-the-counter cold and cough medicines, and other medication unless prescribed; having list of such for reference

» Obeying rules of caution during 14 days after discontinuing medication

» Caution in taking alcohol or other CNS depressants

» Caution if drowsiness occurs, especially when driving or doing things requiring alertness

» Avoiding immunizations unless approved by physician; other persons in patient's household should avoid immunizations with oral poliovirus vaccine; avoiding other persons who have taken oral poliovirus vaccine or wearing a protective mask that covers nose and mouth

Caution if bone marrow depression occurs:

» Avoiding exposure to persons with bacterial infections, especially during periods of low blood counts; checking with physician immediately if fever or chills, cough or hoarseness, lower back or side pain, or painful or difficult urination occur

» Checking with physician immediately if unusual bleeding or bruising; black, tarry stools; blood in urine or stools; or pinpoint red spots on skin occur

Caution in use of regular toothbrush, dental floss, or toothpick; physician, dentist, or nurse may suggest alternatives; checking with physician before having dental work done

Not touching eyes or inside of nose unless hands washed immediately before

Using caution to avoid accidental cuts with use of sharp objects such as safety razor or fingernail or toenail cutters

Avoiding contact sports or other situations where bruising or injury could occur

Diabetics: Checking urine or blood sugar levels

» Caution if any kind of surgery (including dental surgery) or emergency treatment is required

Carrying medical identification card

Side/adverse effects

May cause adverse effects such as blood problems, loss of hair, hypertensive crisis, and cancer; importance of discussing possible effects with physician

Signs of potential side effects, especially anemia, excessive CNS stimulation, immunosuppression, infection, leukopenia, thrombocytopenia, hemolytic anemia, missing menstrual periods, pneumonitis, gastrointestinal toxicity, hepatotoxicity, peripheral neuropathy, stomatitis, allergic reaction, hypertensive crisis, and orthostatic hypotension

Physician or nurse can help in dealing with side effects

▲ For the Patient ▲

916420

ABOUT YOUR MEDICINE

Procarbazine (pro-KAR-ba-zeen) is an alkylating agent. It is used to treat some kinds of cancer.

If any of the information in this leaflet causes you special concern or if you want additional information about your medicine and its use, check with your doctor, nurse, or pharmacist. **Remember, keep this and all other medicines out of the reach of children and never share your medicines with others.**

BEFORE USING THIS MEDICINE

Discuss with your doctor the possible side effects that may be caused by this medicine. Some of them may be serious and/or long-term.

Tell your doctor, nurse, and pharmacist if you . . .
- are allergic to any medicine, either prescription or non-prescription (OTC);
- are pregnant or intend to have children;
- are breast-feeding;
- are taking **any** other prescription or nonprescription (OTC) medicine;
- have **any** other medical problems;
- have ever been treated with x-rays or cancer medicines.

PROPER USE OF THIS MEDICINE

Use this medicine only as directed. Do not use more or less of it and do not use it more often than ordered.

If you miss a dose of this medicine and you remember within a few hours, take it as soon as you remember. However, if it is almost time for your next dose, skip the missed dose and do not double the next one. Instead, check with your doctor.

PRECAUTIONS WHILE USING THIS MEDICINE

It is very important that your doctor check your progress at regular visits.

When taken with certain foods, drinks, or other medicines, procarbazine can cause very dangerous reactions. **To avoid such reactions:**
- Do not eat foods that have a high tyramine content (most common in foods that are aged to increase their flavor).
- Do not drink alcoholic beverages, or alcohol-free or reduced-alcohol beer or wine.
- Do not eat or drink large amounts of caffeine-containing food or beverages such as chocolate, coffee, tea, or cola.
- Do not take any other medicine unless prescribed by your doctor.

After you stop using this medicine you must continue to obey the above rules of caution for at least 2 weeks.

This medicine may cause some people to become drowsy or less alert than they are normally. **Make sure you know how you react to this medicine before you drive, use machines, or do other jobs that require you to be alert.**

While you are taking procarbazine, and for several weeks after treatment:
- **Do not have any immunizations (vaccinations) without your doctor's approval.**
- If you are going to have surgery or dental or emergency treatment, **tell the physician or dentist in charge that you have been taking this medicine.**

Procarbazine can temporarily lower the number of white
blood cells in your blood, increasing the chance of getting
an infection. It can also lower the number of platelets, which
are necessary for proper blood clotting. If this occurs:
- Avoid people with infections.
- Be careful when using a regular toothbrush, dental floss,
  or toothpick.
- Do not touch your eyes or the inside of your nose unless
  you have just washed your hands and have not touched
  anything else in the meantime.
- Be careful not to cut, bruise, or injure yourself.

POSSIBLE SIDE EFFECTS OF THIS MEDICINE

Side Effects That Should Be Reported To Your Doctor Immediately

Less common—Black, tarry stools; blood in urine or stools;
bloody vomit; cough or hoarseness; fever or chills; lower
back or side pain; painful or difficult urination; pinpoint red spots on skin; unusual bleeding or bruising

Rare—Chest pains; enlarged pupils of eyes; fast or slow
heartbeat; headache (severe or pounding); increased
sensitivity of eyes to light; increased sweating (possibly
with fever or cold, clammy skin); stiff neck

Other Side Effects That Should Be Reported To Your Doctor

More common—Confusion; convulsions; cough; hallucinations; missing periods; shortness of breath; thickening of bronchial secretions; tiredness or weakness
(continuing)

Less common—Diarrhea; sores in mouth and on lips; tingling or numb fingers or toes; unsteadiness; yellow eyes
or skin

Rare—Fainting; skin rash or itching; wheezing

Side Effects That Usually Do Not Require Medical Attention

These possible side effects may go away during treatment;
however, if they continue or are bothersome, check with your
doctor, nurse, or pharmacist.

More common—Drowsiness; joint pain; muscle pain or
twitching; nausea and vomiting; nervousness; nightmares; trouble in sleeping; unusual tiredness or weakness

Other side effects not listed above may also occur in some
patients. If you notice any other effects, check with your
doctor, nurse, or pharmacist.

PROGESTINS   Systemic
Including Hydroxyprogesterone; Medroxyprogesterone;
Megestrol; Norethindrone; Norgestrel; Progesterone.

■ For the Pharmacist ■

In providing consultation, consider emphasizing the following selected
information (》 = major clinical significance):

Before using this medication
》 Conditions affecting use, especially:
  Pregnancy—With the exception of progesterone, use is not rec-
    ommended during pregnancy
  Breast-feeding—Breast-feeding is not recommended during use,
    since progestins are distributed into breast milk in variable
    amounts
  Dental—May predispose patient to bleeding of gingival tissues,
    gingival hyperplasia, gingivitis, or gum inflammation
  Other medications, especially bromocriptine
  Other medical problems, especially some cases of carcinoma of
    the breast or reproductive organs; hepatic disease or dys-
    function; incomplete abortion; suspected pregnancy; abnor-
    mal or undiagnosed vaginal bleeding; or active or history of
    thrombophlebitis, thromboembolic disorders, or cerebral apo-
    plexy

Proper use of this medication
》 Compliance with therapy; taking medication at the same time each
  day, every day of the year if used for contraception
》 Proper dosing
  Missed dose:
    When used other than as contraceptive—Taking missed dose as
      soon as possible; not taking at all if almost time for next dose;
      not doubling doses
    When used as contraceptive—Discontinuing medication when a
      dose is missed and using alternative birth control method
      until menstrual period begins or pregnancy is ruled out
》 Proper storage

Precautions while using this medication
》 Importance of close monitoring by physician
  Checking with physician as soon as possible if menstrual period is
    missed or unusual bleeding occurs, especially if using progestin
    as a contraceptive
》 Stopping medication immediately and checking with physician if
  pregnancy is suspected
  If scheduled for laboratory tests, telling physician if taking proges-
    tins; certain blood tests may be affected by progestins
  Possibility of dental problems, such as tenderness, swelling, or bleed-
    ing of gums; brushing and flossing teeth, massaging gums, and
    having dentist clean teeth regularly; checking with dentist if
    there are questions about care of teeth or gums or if tenderness,
    swelling, or bleeding of gums is noticed
  Keeping an extra 1-month supply available when using as oral con-
    traceptive
  Keeping tablets in original container especially when using as oral
    contraceptive
  Importance of not giving medication to anyone else

Side/adverse effects

Signs of potential side effects, especially changes in vaginal bleeding pattern, blood clots, galactorrhea, hepatitis or gallbladder obstruction, hypersensitivity, mental depression, or neuro-ocular lesions

---

▲ For the Patient ▲

915199

ABOUT YOUR MEDICINE

Progestins (proe-JESS-tins) are produced by the body and are necessary during the childbearing years for the development of the milk-producing glands, and for the proper regulation of the menstrual cycle. They are also prescribed:

- to treat a certain type of disorder of the uterus known as endometriosis.
- to prevent pregnancy, when used in birth-control pills.
- to help treat selected cases of cancer of the breast, kidney, or uterus.
- for testing the body's production of certain hormones.

Progestins may also be used for other conditions as determined by your doctor.

If any of the information in this leaflet causes you special concern or if you want additional information about your medicine and its use, check with your doctor, nurse, or pharmacist. **Remember, keep this and all other medicines out of the reach of children and never share your medicines with others.**

BEFORE USING THIS MEDICINE

Tell your doctor, nurse, and pharmacist if you . . .

- are allergic to any medicine, either prescription or non-prescription (OTC);
- are pregnant or intend to become pregnant while using this medicine;
- are breast-feeding;
- are taking any other prescription or nonprescription (OTC) medicine, especially one that contains bromocriptine;
- have any other medical problems, especially blood clots, stroke, or cancer (or history of); changes in vaginal bleeding; or liver or gallbladder disease.

PROPER USE OF THIS MEDICINE

Most patients should receive with this medicine an information sheet regarding the benefits and risks specific to the product dispensed. **Be sure you have read and understand that information.** This leaflet does not replace that information sheet.

Take this medicine only as directed. Do not take more of it and do not take it for a longer time than ordered. To do so may increase the chance of side effects. When used for birth control, this medicine should be taken every day of the year, with doses taken 24 hours apart.

If you miss a dose of this medicine and you are:
- *not* **taking it for birth control,** take the missed dose as soon as possible. However, if it is almost time for your next dose, skip the missed dose. Do not double doses.

- **taking it for birth control,** the safest thing to do is to stop taking the medicine immediately and use another method of birth control until your period begins or until your doctor determines that you are not pregnant.

PRECAUTIONS WHILE USING THIS MEDICINE

It is very important that your doctor check your progress at regular visits. These visits will usually be every 6 to 12 months, but may be more often.

Check with your doctor right away:
- if vaginal bleeding continues for an unusually long time.
- if your menstrual period has not started within 45 days of your last period.
- **if you suspect that you may have become pregnant. You should stop taking this medicine immediately.**

If you are taking this medicine for birth control:
- **When you begin to use birth control tablets** your body will need time to adjust before pregnancy will be prevented. **Use a second method of birth control for at least the first 3 weeks to ensure full protection.**

POSSIBLE SIDE EFFECTS OF THIS MEDICINE

Side Effects That Should Be Reported To Your Doctor Immediately

Along with their needed effects, **progestins sometimes cause some unwanted effects,** such as blood clots, heart attack and stroke, and problems of the liver and eyes. Although these effects are rare, they can be very serious and may cause death. **Get emergency help immediately** if you have sudden or severe headache, loss of coordination, loss of or change in vision, shortness of breath, or slurred speech; pains in chest, groin, or leg (especially in calf of leg); or weakness, numbness, or pain in arm or leg.

Other Side Effects That Should Be Reported To Your Doctor

More common—Changes in vaginal bleeding

Less common or rare—Bulging eyes; discharge from breasts; double vision; loss of vision (gradual, partial, or complete); mental depression; pains in stomach, side, or abdomen; skin rash or itching; yellow eyes or skin

Side Effects That Usually Do Not Require Medical Attention

These possible side effects may go away during treatment; however, if they continue or are bothersome, check with your doctor, nurse, or pharmacist.

> *More common*—Changes in appetite; changes in weight; swelling of ankles and feet; unusual tiredness or weakness

Other side effects not listed above may also occur in some patients. If you notice any other effects, check with your doctor, nurse, or pharmacist.

PROPAFENONE Systemic

■ For the Pharmacist ■

In providing consultation, consider emphasizing the following selected information (» = major clinical significance):

Before using this medication
» Conditions affecting use, especially:
  Sensitivity to propafenone
  Pregnancy—Reduces fertility in monkeys, dogs, and rabbits; in rats, causes increased maternal and neonatal mortality, decreased maternal and infant weight gain, and reduced neonatal development
  Other medications, especially digoxin or warfarin
  Other medical problems, especially second or third degree atrioventricular (AV) block, right bundle branch block associated with a left hemiblock, cardiogenic shock, congestive heart failure, sick sinus syndrome, or sinus bradycardia

Proper use of this medication
» Compliance with therapy; taking as directed even if feeling well
» Importance of not missing doses and taking at evenly spaced intervals
  Missed dose: Taking as soon as possible if remembered within 4 hours; not taking if remembered later; not doubling doses
» Proper storage

Precautions while using this medication
  Regular visits to physician to check progress
  Carrying medical identification card or bracelet
» Caution if any kind of surgery (including dental surgery) or emergency treatment is required
  Caution when driving or doing things requiring alertness because of possible dizziness

Side/adverse effects
  Signs of potential side effects, especially ventricular tachyarrhythmias, angina, congestive heart failure, agranulocytosis, bradycardia, conduction abnormalities, hypotension, joint pain, and trembling or shaking

▲ For the Patient ▲

913036

ANTIARRHYTHMICS, TYPE I (Oral): *Including Disopyramide; Encainide; Flecainide; Mexiletine; Moricizine; Procainamide; Propafenone; Quinidine; Tocainide.*

ABOUT YOUR MEDICINE

Type I antiarrhythmics are used to correct irregular heartbeats to a normal rhythm and to slow an overactive heart.

There is a chance that these medicines may cause new heart rhythm problems when they are used. Usually this effect is rare and mild. However, some of these medicines are more likely than others to cause this effect. For example, encainide and flecainide have been shown to cause severe problems in some patients, and so they are only used to treat serious heart rhythm problems. Discuss this possible effect with your doctor.

If any of the information in this leaflet causes you special concern or if you want additional information about your medicine and its use, check with your doctor, nurse, or pharmacist. **Remember, keep this and all other medicines out of the reach of children and never share your medicines with others.**

BEFORE USING THIS MEDICINE

Tell your doctor, nurse, and pharmacist if you . . .
- are allergic to any medicine, either prescription or non-prescription (OTC);
- are pregnant or intend to become pregnant while using this medicine;
- are breast-feeding;
- are taking **any** other prescription or nonprescription (OTC) medicine;
- have **any** other medical problems.

PROPER USE OF THIS MEDICINE

Take this medicine exactly as directed by your doctor, even though you may feel well. Do not take more medicine than ordered.

For patients taking the extended-release capsules or tablets:
- Swallow whole without breaking, crushing, or chewing.

It is best to take each dose at evenly spaced times day and night.

For patients taking mexiletine:
- To lessen the possibility of stomach upset, this medicine should be taken with food or immediately after meals or with milk or an antacid.

If you miss a dose of this medicine, take it as soon as possible. However, if you do not remember until it is almost time for the next dose, skip the missed dose and go back to your regular dosing schedule. Do not double doses.

PRECAUTIONS WHILE USING THIS MEDICINE

It is important that your doctor check your progress at regular visits to make sure the medicine is working properly to help your heart.

Do not suddenly stop taking this medicine without first checking with your doctor. Stopping it suddenly may cause a serious change in heart activity.

Dizziness or lightheadedness or blurred vision may occur. **Make sure you know how you react to this medicine before you drive, use machines, or do other jobs that require you to be alert and able to see well.**

For patients taking disopyramide:
- **If signs of hypoglycemia (low blood sugar) such as chills, hunger, nausea, nervousness, or sweating appear, eat or drink a food containing sugar and call your doctor right away.**

- **Use extra care not to become overheated during exercise or hot weather,** since this medicine will often make you sweat less and could possibly result in heatstroke.

POSSIBLE SIDE EFFECTS OF THIS MEDICINE

Side Effects That Should Be Reported To Your Doctor Immediately

For quinidine only, especially after the first dose or first few doses—Breathing difficulty; changes in vision; dizziness, lightheadedness, or fainting; fever; severe headache; ringing in ears; skin rash

Other Side Effects That Should Be Reported To Your Doctor

For all antiarrhythmics—Chest pain; fast or irregular heartbeat; fever or chills; shortness of breath or painful breathing; skin rash or itching; unusual bleeding or bruising

For disopyramide (in addition to above)—Difficult urination; swelling of feet or lower legs

For encainide, flecainide, moricizine, and propafenone (in addition to above)—Swelling of feet or lower legs; trembling or shaking

Side Effects That Usually Do Not Require Medical Attention

These possible side effects may go away during treatment; however, if they continue or are bothersome, check with your doctor, nurse, or pharmacist.

For all antiarrhythmics—Blurred or double vision; dizziness or lightheadedness

For disopyramide (in addition to above)—Dry mouth and throat

For flecainide (in addition to above)—Seeing spots

For mexiletine (in addition to above)—Heartburn; nausea and vomiting; nervousness; trembling or shaking of hands; unsteadiness or trouble walking

For procainamide (in addition to above)—Diarrhea; loss of appetite

For propafenone (in addition to above)—Change in taste

For quinidine (in addition to above)—Bitter taste; diarrhea; flushing of skin with itching; loss of appetite; nausea or vomiting; stomach pain or cramps

For tocainide (in addition to above)—Loss of appetite; nausea

Other side effects not listed above may also occur in some patients. If you notice any other effects, check with your doctor, nurse, or pharmacist.

PYRAZINAMIDE   Systemic

■For the Pharmacist■

In providing consultation, consider emphasizing the following selected
information (» = major clinical significance):

Before using this medication
» Conditions affecting use, especially:
  Hypersensitivity to pyrazinamide, ethionamide, isoniazid, niacin
    (nicotinic acid), or other chemically related medications
  Breast-feeding—Pyrazinamide is distributed into breast milk
  Other medical problems, especially severe hepatic function im-
    pairment

Proper use of this medication
» Compliance with full course of therapy, which may take months
» Proper dosing
  Missed dose: Taking as soon as possible; not taking if almost time
    for next dose; not doubling doses
» Proper storage

Precautions while using this medication
  Regular visits to physician to check progress
  Checking with physician if no improvement within 2 to 3 weeks
» Diabetics: May interfere with urine ketone determinations

Side/adverse effects
  Signs of side effects, especially arthralgia, gouty arthritis, and hep-
    atotoxicity

▲ For the Patient ▲

914833

ABOUT YOUR MEDICINE

Pyrazinamide (peer-a-ZIN-a-mide) belongs to the general
family of medicines called anti-infectives. It is used, along
with other medicines, to help the body overcome tuberculosis
(TB).

**To help clear up your tuberculosis (TB) completely, you must
keep taking this medicine for the full time of treatment, even
if you begin to feel better. This is very important. It is also
important that you do not miss any doses.**

If any of the information in this leaflet causes you special
concern or if you want additional information about your
medicine and its use, check with your doctor, nurse, or pharmacist. **Remember, keep this and all other medicines out of
the reach of children and never share your medicines with
others.**

BEFORE USING THIS MEDICINE

Tell your doctor, nurse, and pharmacist if you . . .
  • are allergic to any medicine, either prescription or non-
    prescription (OTC);

- are pregnant or intend to become pregnant while using this medicine;
- are breast-feeding;
- are taking any other prescription or nonprescription (OTC) medicine;
- have any other medical problems, especially severe liver disease.

PROPER USE OF THIS MEDICINE

To help clear up your tuberculosis (TB) completely, **it is important that you keep taking this medicine for the full time of treatment** even if you begin to feel better after a few weeks. **It is important that you do not miss any doses.**

If you do miss a dose of this medicine, take it as soon as possible. However, if it is almost time for your next dose, skip the missed dose and go back to your regular dosing schedule. Do not double doses.

PRECAUTIONS WHILE USING THIS MEDICINE

It is very important that your doctor check your progress at regular visits.

If your symptoms do not improve within 2 to 3 weeks, or if they become worse, check with your doctor.

Diabetics—This medicine may cause false test results with urine ketone tests. Check with your doctor before changing your diet or the dosage of your diabetes medicine.

This medicine must not be given to other people or used for other infections unless you are otherwise directed by your doctor.

POSSIBLE SIDE EFFECTS OF THIS MEDICINE

Side Effects That Should Be Reported To Your Doctor Immediately

   More common—Pain and swelling of joints, especially big toe, ankle, and knee; tense, hot skin over affected joints

   Rare—Loss of appetite; unusual tiredness or weakness; yellow eyes or skin

Side Effects That Usually Do Not Require Medical Attention

These possible side effects may go away during treatment; however, if they continue or are bothersome, check with your doctor, nurse, or pharmacist.

   Rare—Itching; skin rash

Other side effects not listed above may also occur in some patients. If you notice any other effects, check with your doctor, nurse, or pharmacist.

QUINIDINE   Systemic

■ For the Pharmacist ■

In providing consultation, consider emphasizing the following selected
  information (» = major clinical significance):

Before using this medication
» Conditions affecting use, especially:
      Sensitivity to quinine
      Breast-feeding—Distributed into breast milk
      Use in children—Use of extended-release dosage form not rec-
        ommended
      Dental—May decrease or inhibit salivary flow
      Other medications, especially antiarrhythmics, anticoagulants,
        neuromuscular blocking agents, pimozide, and urinary al-
        kalizers
      Other medical problems, especially complete or incomplete atrio-
        ventricular block, digitalis toxicity, severe intraventricular
        conduction defects, hepatic or renal function impairment,
        myasthenia gravis, or thrombocytopenia

Proper use of this medication
      Taking medication with water at least 1 hour before or 2 hours after
        meals for better absorption; may be taken with food or milk to
        lessen gastrointestinal irritation
      Proper administration of extended-release tablets: Swallowing tablet
        whole; not breaking, crushing, or chewing before swallowing
» Compliance with therapy; taking as directed even if feeling well
» Proper dosing
      Missed dose: Taking as soon as possible if remembered within
        2 hours; if remembered later, not taking at all; not doubling
        doses
» Proper storage

Precautions while using this medication
      Regular visits to physician to check progress
» Checking with physician before discontinuing medication
» Caution if any kind of surgery (including dental surgery) or emer-
        gency treatment is required
      Carrying medical identification card
» Checking with physician if symptoms of quinidine intolerance occur

Side/adverse effects
      Signs of potential side effects, especially allergic reaction, cincho-
        nism, hypotension or extreme CNS effects, anemia, paradoxical
        tachycardia, and thrombocytopenia

▲ For the Patient ▲

913036

ANTIARRHYTHMICS, TYPE I (Oral): *Including
Disopyramide; Encainide; Flecainide; Mexiletine;
Moricizine; Procainamide; Propafenone; Quinidine;
Tocainide.*

ABOUT YOUR MEDICINE

Type I antiarrhythmics are used to correct irregular heart-beats to a normal rhythm and to slow an overactive heart.

There is a chance that these medicines may cause new heart rhythm problems when they are used. Usually this effect is rare and mild. However, some of these medicines are more likely than others to cause this effect. For example, encainide and flecainide have been shown to cause severe problems in some patients, and so they are only used to treat serious heart rhythm problems. Discuss this possible effect with your doctor.

If any of the information in this leaflet causes you special concern or if you want additional information about your medicine and its use, check with your doctor, nurse, or pharmacist. **Remember, keep this and all other medicines out of the reach of children and never share your medicines with others.**

BEFORE USING THIS MEDICINE

Tell your doctor, nurse, and pharmacist if you . . .
- are allergic to any medicine, either prescription or non-prescription (OTC);
- are pregnant or intend to become pregnant while using this medicine;
- are breast-feeding;
- are taking **any** other prescription or nonprescription (OTC) medicine;
- have **any** other medical problems.

PROPER USE OF THIS MEDICINE

Take this medicine exactly as directed by your doctor, even though you may feel well. Do not take more medicine than ordered.

For patients taking the extended-release capsules or tablets:
- Swallow whole without breaking, crushing, or chewing.

It is best to take each dose at evenly spaced times day and night.

For patients taking mexiletine:
- To lessen the possibility of stomach upset, this medicine should be taken with food or immediately after meals or with milk or an antacid.

If you miss a dose of this medicine, take it as soon as possible. However, if you do not remember until it is almost time for the next dose, skip the missed dose and go back to your regular dosing schedule. Do not double doses.

PRECAUTIONS WHILE USING THIS MEDICINE

It is important that your doctor check your progress at regular visits to make sure the medicine is working properly to help your heart.

Do not suddenly stop taking this medicine without first checking with your doctor. Stopping it suddenly may cause a serious change in heart activity.

Dizziness or lightheadedness or blurred vision may occur. **Make sure you know how you react to this medicine before you drive, use machines, or do other jobs that require you to be alert and able to see well.**

For patients taking disopyramide:

- **If signs of hypoglycemia (low blood sugar) such as chills, hunger, nausea, nervousness, or sweating appear, eat or drink a food containing sugar and call your doctor right away.**

- **Use extra care not to become overheated during exercise or hot weather,** since this medicine will often make you sweat less and could possibly result in heatstroke.

POSSIBLE SIDE EFFECTS OF THIS MEDICINE

Side Effects That Should Be Reported To Your Doctor Immediately

For quinidine only, especially after the first dose or first few doses—Breathing difficulty; changes in vision; dizziness, lightheadedness, or fainting; fever; severe headache; ringing in ears; skin rash

Other Side Effects That Should Be Reported To Your Doctor

For all antiarrhythmics—Chest pain; fast or irregular heartbeat; fever or chills; shortness of breath or painful breathing; skin rash or itching; unusual bleeding or bruising

For disopyramide (in addition to above)—Difficult urination; swelling of feet or lower legs

For encainide, flecainide, moricizine, and propafenone (in addition to above)—Swelling of feet or lower legs; trembling or shaking

Side Effects That Usually Do Not Require Medical Attention

These possible side effects may go away during treatment; however, if they continue or are bothersome, check with your doctor, nurse, or pharmacist.

For all antiarrhythmics—Blurred or double vision; dizziness or lightheadedness

For disopyramide (in addition to above)—Dry mouth and throat

For flecainide (in addition to above)—Seeing spots

For mexiletine (in addition to above)—Heartburn; nausea and vomiting; nervousness; trembling or shaking of hands; unsteadiness or trouble walking

For procainamide (in addition to above)—Diarrhea; loss of appetite

For propafenone (in addition to above)—Change in taste

For quinidine (in addition to above)—Bitter taste; diarrhea; flushing of skin with itching; loss of appetite; nausea or vomiting; stomach pain or cramps

For tocainide (in addition to above)—Loss of appetite; nausea

Other side effects not listed above may also occur in some patients. If you notice any other effects, check with your doctor, nurse, or pharmacist.

RAUWOLFIA ALKALOIDS   Systemic

Including Alseroxylon; Deserpidine; Rauwolfia Serpentina; Reserpine.

■For the Pharmacist■

In providing consultation, consider emphasizing the following selected
  information (» = major clinical significance):

Before using this medication
» Conditions affecting use, especially:
    Sensitivity to any of the rauwolfia alkaloids
    Pregnancy—Teratogenic in animals
    Breast-feeding—Distributed into breast milk
    Use in the elderly—May be more sensitive to the CNS depres-
      sant and hypotensive effects
    Dental—May decrease or inhibit salivary flow
    Other medications, especially monoamine oxidase (MAO) in-
      hibitors
    Other medical problems, especially gallstones, peptic ulcer, ul-
      cerative colitis, or mental depression

Proper use of this medication
    Possible need for control of weight and diet, especially sodium intake
» Patient may not experience symptoms of hypertension; importance
    of taking medication even if feeling well
» Does not cure but helps control hypertension; possible need for life-
    long therapy; serious consequences of untreated hypertension
    Getting into the habit of taking at same time each day to help
      increase compliance
    Caution in taking combination therapy; taking each medication at
      the right time
    Taking with meals or milk to reduce gastrointestinal irritation
» Proper dosing
    Missed dose: Not taking missed dose at all and not doubling doses
» Proper storage

Precautions while using this medication
    Regular visits to physician to check progress
» Not taking other medications, especially nonprescription sympatho-
    mimetics, unless discussed with physician
» Caution if any kind of surgery (including dental surgery) or emer-
    gency treatment is required
» Caution if depression or changes in sleep pattern occur
» Caution in taking alcohol or other CNS depressants
» Caution when driving or doing things requiring alertness because of
    possible drowsiness or dizziness
    Possible dryness of mouth; using sugarless candy or gum, ice, or
      saliva substitute for relief; checking with physician or dentist if
      dry mouth continues for more than 2 weeks
    Nasal stuffiness may occur; nasal decongestants or other OTC prep-
      arations containing sympathomimetics should not be used with-
      out first consulting physician or pharmacist

Side/adverse effects
    Dizziness, arrhythmias, bradycardia, black, tarry stools, bloody vomit,
      chest pain, drowsiness or faintness, headache, impotence or de-
      creased sexual interest, lack of energy or weakness, mental
      depression or inability to concentrate, nervousness or anxiety,

vivid dreams or nightmares or early-morning sleeplessness, shortness of breath

---

▲ For the Patient ▲

914866

ABOUT YOUR MEDICINE

Rauwolfia alkaloids are used to treat high blood pressure
(hypertension). They may also be used to treat other conditions as determined by your doctor.

If any of the information in this leaflet causes you special
concern or if you want additional information about your
medicine and its use, check with your doctor, nurse, or pharmacist. **Remember, keep this and all other medicines out of
the reach of children and never share your medicines with
others.**

BEFORE USING THIS MEDICINE

Tell your doctor, nurse, and pharmacist if you . . .
- are allergic to any medicine, either prescription or nonprescription (OTC);
- are pregnant or intend to become pregnant while using
  this medicine;
- are breast-feeding;
- are taking any other prescription or nonprescription
  (OTC) medicine, especially MAO inhibitors;
- have any other medical problems, especially gallstones,
  mental depression (or history of), stomach ulcer, or ulcerative colitis.

PROPER USE OF THIS MEDICINE

Many patients who have high blood pressure will not notice
any signs of the problem. In fact, many may feel normal.
Take your medicine exactly as directed and keep your doctor's appointments even if you feel well.

This medicine will not cure your high blood pressure but it
does help control it. You must continue to take it—even if
you feel well—if you expect to keep your blood pressure
down. **You may have to take high blood pressure medicine
for the rest of your life.**

If this medicine upsets your stomach, it may be taken with
meals or milk. If stomach upset continues or gets worse,
check with your doctor.

If you miss a dose of this medicine, do not take the missed
dose at all and do not double the next one. Instead, go back
to your regular dosing schedule.

PRECAUTIONS WHILE USING THIS MEDICINE

For patients taking this medicine for high blood pressure:
- **Do not take other medicines unless they have been discussed with your doctor.** This especially includes over-
  the-counter (nonprescription) medicines for appetite

control, asthma, colds, cough, hay fever, or sinus problems, since they may tend to increase your blood pressure.

Before having any kind of surgery or dental or emergency treatment, **tell the physician or dentist in charge that you are taking this medicine.**

This medicine may cause mental depression. **Tell your doctor right away:**
- if you or anyone else notices unusual changes in your mood.
- if you start having early-morning sleeplessness or unusually vivid dreams or nightmares.

This medicine will add to the depressant effects of alcohol and other medicines (CNS depressants) that slow down the nervous system. **Check with your doctor before taking any such depressants while taking this medicine.**

This medicine may cause some people to become drowsy or less alert than normal. This is more likely to happen when you begin to take it or when you increase the dose. **Make sure you know how you react before you drive, use machines, or do other jobs that require you to be alert.**

POSSIBLE SIDE EFFECTS OF THIS MEDICINE
Side Effects That Should Be Reported To Your Doctor Immediately

> *Less common*—Drowsiness or faintness; impotence or decreased sexual interest; lack of energy or weakness; mental depression or inability to concentrate; nervousness or anxiety; vivid dreams or nightmares or early-morning sleeplessness

Other Side Effects That Should Be Reported To Your Doctor

> *More common*—Dizziness

> *Less common*—Black tarry stools; bloody vomit; chest pain; headache; irregular or slow heartbeat; shortness of breath; stomach cramps or pain

> *Rare*—Painful or difficult urination; skin rash or itching; stiffness; trembling and shaking of hands and fingers; unusual bleeding or bruising

Side Effects That Usually Do Not Require Medical Attention

These possible side effects may go away during treatment; however, if they continue or are bothersome, check with your doctor, nurse, or pharmacist.

> *More common*—Diarrhea; dry mouth; loss of appetite; nausea and vomiting; stuffy nose

Other side effects not listed above may also occur in some patients. If you notice any other effects, check with your doctor, nurse, or pharmacist.

After you stop using this medicine, it may still produce some side effects that need attention. **Check with your doctor immediately** if you notice drowsiness or faintness; impotence or decreased sexual interest; irregular or slow heartbeat; lack of energy or weakness; mental depression or inability to concentrate; nervousness or anxiety; vivid dreams, nightmares, or early-morning sleeplessness.

RESERPINE, HYDRALAZINE, AND HYDROCHLOROTHIAZIDE   Systemic

■ For the Pharmacist ■

In providing consultation, consider emphasizing the following selected information (» = major clinical significance):

Before using this medication
»   Conditions affecting use, especially:

Sensitivity to any of the rauwolfia alkaloids, hydralazine, thiazide diuretics, other sulfonamide-type medications, bumetanide, furosemide, or carbonic anhydrase inhibitors

Pregnancy—Reserpine teratogenic in animals; hydralazine reported to cause blood problems in infants of mothers who took hydralazine and causes birth defects in animals; hydrochlorothiazide not recommended for routine use and may cause jaundice, thrombocytopenia, hypokalemia in infant

Breast-feeding—Reserpine and hydrochlorothiazide distributed into breast milk; recommended that nursing mothers avoid hydrochlorothiazide during first month of breast-feeding because of reports of suppression of lactation

Use in the elderly—May be more sensitive to the CNS depressant, hypotensive, and electrolyte effects

Dental—May decrease or inhibit salivary flow

Other medications, especially monoamine oxidase (MAO) inhibitors, diazoxide, cholestyramine, colestipol, digitalis glycosides, or lithium

Other medical problems, especially gallstones, peptic ulcer, ulcerative colitis, mental depression, coronary artery disease, rheumatic heart disease, or anuria or severe renal function impairment

Proper use of this medication
Possible need for control of weight and diet, especially sodium intake
»   Patient may not experience symptoms of hypertension; importance of taking medication even if feeling well
»   Does not cure, but helps control hypertension; possible need for lifelong therapy; serious consequences of untreated hypertension
Diuretic effects of medication and timing of doses to minimize inconvenience of diuresis
Getting into habit of taking at same time each day to help increase compliance
Taking with meals or milk to reduce gastrointestinal irritation
»   Proper dosing
Missed dose: Taking as soon as possible; not taking if almost time for next dose; not doubling doses
»   Proper storage

Precautions while using this medication
Regular visits to physician to check progress
»   Not taking other medications, especially nonprescription sympathomimetics, unless discussed with physician
»   Caution if any kind of surgery (including dental surgery) or emergency treatment is required
»   Caution when driving or doing things requiring alertness because of possible headache, drowsiness, or dizziness
Caution if orthostatic hypotension occurs
»   Caution if depression or changes in sleep pattern occur

» Caution in taking alcohol or other central nervous system (CNS)
    depressants
  Possibility of hypokalemia; possible need for additional potassium
    in diet; not changing diet without first checking with physician
  To prevent dehydration, checking with physician if severe nausea,
    vomiting, or diarrhea occurs and continues
  Diabetics: May increase blood sugar levels
  Possible photosensitivity; avoiding unprotected exposure to sun; us-
    ing protective clothing and sun block product; avoiding use of
    sunlamp, tanning bed, or tanning booth
  Nasal stuffiness may occur; nasal decongestants or other OTC prep-
    arations containing sympathomimetics should not be used with-
    out first consulting physician or pharmacist
  Possible dryness of mouth; using sugarless candy or gum, ice, or
    saliva substitute for relief; checking with physician or dentist if
    dry mouth continues for more than 2 weeks

Side/adverse effects
  Signs and symptoms of potential side effects, especially electrolyte
    imbalance, agranulocytosis, allergic reaction, angina pectoris,
    cutaneous vasculitis, lymphadenopathy, peripheral neuritis, SLE-
    like syndrome, cholecystitis, pancreatitis, hepatic function im-
    pairment, hyperuricemia, gout, thrombocytopenia, dizziness, ar-
    rhythmias, bradycardia, black tarry stools, bloody vomit, drows-
    iness or faintness, headache, impotence or decreased sexual
    interest, lack of energy or weakness, mental depression or in-
    ability to concentrate, nervousness or anxiety, vivid dreams or
    nightmares or early-morning sleeplessness, and shortness of breath

---

▲ For the Patient ▲

912612

ABOUT YOUR MEDICINE

Reserpine, hydralazine, and **hydrochlorothiazide** combination is used to treat high blood pressure (hypertension).

If any of the information in this leaflet causes you special
concern or if you want additional information about your
medicine and its use, check with your doctor, nurse, or pharmacist. **Remember, keep this and all other medicines out of
the reach of children and never share your medicines with
others.**

BEFORE USING THIS MEDICINE
Tell your doctor, nurse, and pharmacist if you . . .
  • are allergic to any medicine, either prescription or non-
    prescription (OTC);
  • are pregnant or intend to become pregnant while using
    this medicine;
  • are breast-feeding;
  • are taking any other prescription or nonprescription
    (OTC) medicine, especially cortisone-like medicines;
    digitalis glycosides (heart medicine); lithium; MAO in-
    hibitors; methenamine; or medicines for appetite con-
    trol, asthma, colds, cough, hay fever, or sinus;
  • have any other medical problems, especially colitis, gall-
    stones, heart or blood vessel disease, kidney disease,
    mental depression, or stomach ulcer.

PROPER USE OF THIS MEDICINE

This medicine may cause an unusual feeling of tiredness when you begin taking it. You may also notice an increase in urine or in frequency of urination. To keep this from affecting nighttime sleep:

- if you are to take a single dose a day, take it in the morning after breakfast.
- if you are to take more than one dose, take the last one no later than 6 p.m.

This medicine will not cure your high blood pressure but it does help control it. You must continue to take it—even if you feel well—if you expect to keep your blood pressure down. **You may have to take high blood pressure medicine for the rest of your life.**

If you miss a dose of this medicine, take it as soon as possible. However, if it is almost time for your next dose, skip the missed dose and go back to your regular dosing schedule. Do not double doses.

PRECAUTIONS WHILE USING THIS MEDICINE

This medicine may cause headaches, dizziness, or drowsiness. **Make sure you know how you react to this medicine before you drive or do jobs that require you to be alert.**

This medicine may cause mental depression. **Tell your doctor right away:**

- if you or anyone else notices unusual changes in your moods.
- if you start having early-morning sleeplessness or vivid dreams.

This medicine will add to the effects of alcohol and other CNS depressants (medicines that slow down the nervous system). **Check with your doctor before taking any such depressants while you are taking this medicine.**

POSSIBLE SIDE EFFECTS OF THIS MEDICINE

Side Effects That Should Be Reported To Your Doctor Immediately

More common—General feeling of discomfort or weakness

Less common—Drowsiness or faintness; impotence or decreased sexual interest; inability to concentrate; mental depression; nervousness or anxiety; vivid dreams, nightmares, or early-morning sleeplessness

Other Side Effects That Should Be Reported To Your Doctor

Less common—Black tarry stools; blisters on skin; bloody vomit; chest pain; headache; irregular heartbeat; joint pain; numbness, tingling, pain, or weakness in hands or feet; shortness of breath; skin rash or itching; sore throat and fever; swelling of lymph glands

Rare—Painful or difficult urination; stiffness; stomach pain (severe) with nausea and vomiting; trembling of hands; unusual bleeding or bruising; yellow eyes or skin

Side Effects That Usually Do Not Require Medical Attention

These possible side effects may go away during treatment; however, if they continue or are bothersome, check with your doctor, nurse, or pharmacist.

More common—Diarrhea; dizziness when standing up; loss of appetite; nausea or vomiting; stuffy nose

Other side effects not listed above may also occur in some patients. If you notice any other effects, check with your doctor, nurse, or pharmacist.

After you stop using this medicine, it may still produce some side effects that need attention. **Check with your doctor immediately** if you notice drowsiness or faintness; general feeling of body discomfort or weakness; impotence or decreased sexual interest; irregular heartbeat; mental depression or inability to concentrate; nervousness or anxiety; vivid dreams, nightmares, or sleeplessness.

RIFABUTIN   Systemic

■ For the Pharmacist ■

In providing consultation, consider emphasizing the following selected
information (» = major clinical significance):

Before using this medication
» Conditions affecting use, especially:
    Hypersensitivity to rifabutin or rifampin
    Other medications, especially zidovudine
    Other medical problems, especially active tuberculosis

Proper use of this medication
    Taking on an empty stomach, or with food if gastrointestinal irri-
        tation occurs
» Compliance with full course of therapy, which may take months
» Proper dosing
» Missed dose: Taking as soon as possible; not taking if almost time
        for next dose; not doubling doses
» Proper storage

Precautions while using this medication
» Regular visits to physician to check progress
» Medication causes tears to turn reddish orange to reddish brown
        and may also permanently discolor soft contact lenses; avoiding
        the use of soft contact lenses during treatment

Side/adverse effects
    Signs of potential side effects, especially skin rash, arthralgia, dys-
        geusia, myalgia, neutropenia, pseudojaundice, and uveitis
    Reddish orange to reddish brown discoloration of urine, stools, sa-
        liva, skin, sputum, sweat, and tears may be alarming to patient,
        although medically insignificant

▲ For the Patient ▲

919371

ABOUT YOUR MEDICINE

Rifabutin (rif-a-BUE-tin) is used to help prevent *Mycobacterium avium* complex (MAC) disease from spreading
throughout the body in patients with advanced human immunodeficiency virus (HIV) infection. MAC is an infection
caused by two similar bacteria, *Mycobacterium avium* and
Mycobacterium intracellulare. Mycobacterium avium is
more common in patients with HIV infection. MAC may
also occur in other patients whose immune system is not
working properly. Symptoms of MAC in people with AIDS
(acquired immunodeficiency syndrome) include fever, night
sweats, chills, weight loss, and weakness. Rifabutin will not
work for colds, flu, or other virus infections.

If any of the information in this leaflet causes you special
concern or if you want additional information about your
medicine and its use, check with your doctor, nurse, or pharmacist. **Remember, keep this and all other medicines out of**

the reach of children and never share your medicines with others.

BEFORE USING THIS MEDICINE

Tell your doctor, nurse, and pharmacist if you . . .
- are allergic to any medicine, either prescription or non-prescription (OTC);
- are pregnant or intend to become pregnant while using this medicine;
- are breast-feeding;
- are taking any other prescription or nonprescription (OTC) medicine, especially zidovudine;
- have any other medical problems, especially active tuberculosis.

PROPER USE OF THIS MEDICINE

Rifabutin may be taken on an empty stomach (either 1 hour before or 2 hours after a meal). However, if this medicine upsets your stomach, you may want to take it with food.

For patients unable to swallow capsules:
- Contents of the capsules may be mixed with applesauce. Be sure to eat all the food to get the full dose of medicine.

To help prevent MAC disease, **it is very important that you keep taking this medicine for the full time of treatment.** You may have to take it every day for many months. **It is important that you do not miss any doses.**

If you do miss a dose of this medicine, take it as soon as possible. However, if it is almost time for your next dose, skip the missed dose and go back to your regular dosing schedule. Do not double doses. **If this medicine is taken on an irregular schedule, side effects may occur more often and may be more serious than usual.** If you have any questions about this, check with your doctor or pharmacist.

PRECAUTIONS WHILE USING THIS MEDICINE

It is very important that your doctor check your progress at regular visits.

Rifabutin will cause your urine, stool, saliva, skin, sputum, sweat, and tears to turn reddish orange to reddish brown. This is to be expected while you are taking this medicine. This effect may cause soft contact lenses to become permanently discolored. Standard cleaning solutions may not take out all the discoloration. Therefore, **it is best not to wear soft contact lenses while taking this medicine.** Hard contact lenses are not discolored by rifabutin. If you have any questions about this, check with your doctor.

POSSIBLE SIDE EFFECTS OF THIS MEDICINE

Side Effects That Should Be Reported To Your Doctor Immediately

   More common—Skin rash

Rare—Change in taste; eye pain; fever and sore throat; joint pain; loss of vision; muscle pain; yellow skin

Side Effects That Usually Do Not Require Medical Attention

These possible side effects may go away during treatment; however, if they continue or are bothersome, check with your doctor, nurse, or pharmacist.

More common—Nausea; vomiting

This medicine commonly causes reddish orange to reddish brown discoloration of urine, stools, saliva, skin, sputum, sweat, and tears. This side effect does not usually need medical attention. However, tears that have been discolored by this medicine may permanently discolor contact lenses.

Other side effects not listed above may also occur in some patients. If you notice any other effects, check with your doctor, nurse, or pharmacist.

RIFAMPIN   Systemic

■For the Pharmacist■

In providing consultation, consider emphasizing the following selected information (» = major clinical significance):

Before using this medication
» Conditions affecting use, especially:
  Hypersensitivity to rifampin
  Pregnancy—Rifampin crosses the placenta and has rarely caused post-natal hemorrhages in the mother and infant when administered during the last few weeks of pregnancy
  Breast-feeding—Rifampin is distributed into breast milk
  Dental—Patients who develop blood dyscrasias may be at increased risk of microbial infections, delayed healing, and gingival bleeding
  Other medications, especially azole antifungals, corticosteroids, coumarin- or indandione-derivative anticoagulants, oral antidiabetic agents, chloramphenicol, estrogen-containing oral contraceptives, digitalis glycosides, disopyramide, estramustine, estrogens, hepatotoxic medications, isoniazid, methadone, mexiletine, tocainide, phenytoin, quinidine, aminophylline, oxtriphylline, theophylline, or oral verapamil
  Other medical problems, especially alcoholism, active or in remission, or impairment of hepatic function

Proper use of this medication
  Taking with a full glass (240 mL) of water on an empty stomach, 1 hour before or 2 hours after a meal, or with food if gastrointestinal irritation occurs
  Proper administration technique for patients unable to swallow capsules
» Compliance with full course of therapy, which may take months or years
» Proper dosing
» Missed dose: Taking as soon as possible; not taking if almost time for next dose; not doubling doses; intermittent dosing may result in more frequent and/or severe side effects
» Proper storage

Precautions while using this medication
» Regular visits to physician to check progress
  Checking with physician if no improvement within 2 to 3 weeks
» Using an additional method of contraception if taking estrogen-containing oral contraceptives concurrently
» Avoiding alcoholic beverages concurrently with this medication
» Need to report prodromal signs of hepatotoxicity to physician
» Medication causes urine, feces, saliva, sputum, sweat, and tears to turn reddish orange to reddish brown and may also permanently discolor soft contact lenses; avoiding the wearing of soft contact lenses
  Using caution in use of regular toothbrushes, dental floss, and toothpicks; deferring dental work until blood counts have returned to normal; checking with physician or dentist concerning proper oral hygiene
  Possible interference with laboratory values

Side/adverse effects

Reddish orange to reddish brown discoloration of urine, stools, saliva, sputum, sweat, and tears may be alarming to patient, although medically insignificant; however, tears discolored by rifampin may also discolor soft contact lenses

Signs of potential side effects, especially "flu-like" syndrome, hypersensitivity, blood dyscrasias, hepatitis, hepatitis prodromal symptoms, and interstitial nephritis

---

▲ For the Patient ▲

914888

ABOUT YOUR MEDICINE

Rifampin (rif-AM-pin) is used with one or more other medicines to treat tuberculosis (TB). Rifampin is also taken alone by patients who may carry meningitis bacteria in their nose and throat (without feeling sick) and may spread these bacteria to others. This medicine may also be used for other problems as determined by your doctor. However, rifampin will not work for colds, flu, or other virus infections.

If any of the information in this leaflet causes you special concern or if you want additional information about your medicine and its use, check with your doctor, nurse, or pharmacist. **Remember, keep this and all other medicines out of the reach of children and never share your medicines with others.**

BEFORE USING THIS MEDICINE

Tell your doctor, nurse, and pharmacist if you . . .
- are allergic to any medicine, either prescription or nonprescription (OTC);
- are pregnant or intend to become pregnant while using this medicine;
- are breast-feeding;
- are taking **any** other prescription or nonprescription (OTC) medicine;
- have any other medical problems, especially alcohol abuse (or history of) or liver disease.

PROPER USE OF THIS MEDICINE

Rifampin is best taken with a full glass (8 ounces) of water on an empty stomach (either 1 hour before or 2 hours after a meal). However, if this medicine upsets your stomach, your doctor may want you to take it with food.

To help clear up your tuberculosis (TB) completely, **it is very important that you keep taking this medicine for the full time of treatment.** You may have to take it every day for 1 to 2 years or more. **Do not miss any doses.**

If you do miss a dose of this medicine, take it as soon as possible. However, if it is almost time for your next dose, skip the missed dose and go back to your regular schedule. Do not double doses. **If rifampin is taken on an irregular**

schedule, side effects may occur more often and may be more serious than usual.

PRECAUTIONS WHILE USING THIS MEDICINE

Rifampin will cause the urine, stool, saliva, sputum, sweat, and tears to turn reddish orange to reddish brown. This is to be expected and does not usually need medical attention. This effect may cause soft contact lenses (but not hard contact lenses) to become permanently discolored. **Therefore, it is best not to wear soft contact lenses while taking rifampin.**

Oral contraceptives (birth control pills) containing estrogen may not work properly if you take them while you are taking rifampin. Unplanned pregnancies may occur. Use a different means of birth control while taking rifampin.

If your symptoms do not improve within 2 or 3 weeks, or if they become worse, check with your doctor.

If rifampin causes you to feel very tired or weak or causes a loss of appetite, nausea, or vomiting, stop taking it and check with your doctor immediately.

The regular use of alcohol may keep rifampin from working as well. Also, liver problems may be more likely to occur. Therefore, **you should not drink alcoholic beverages while you are taking this medicine.**

Rifampin can lower the number of white blood cells in your blood temporarily, increasing the chance of getting an infection. It can also lower the number of platelets, which are necessary for proper blood clotting. These problems may result in a greater chance of getting certain infections, slow healing, and bleeding of the gums. Be careful when using a regular toothbrush, dental floss, or a toothpick. Dental work should be delayed until your blood counts have returned to normal. Check with your physician or dentist if you have any questions.

This medicine must not be given to other people or used for other infections unless you are otherwise directed by your doctor.

POSSIBLE SIDE EFFECTS OF THIS MEDICINE
Side Effects That Should Be Reported To Your Doctor Immediately

Less common—Chills; difficult breathing; dizziness; fever; headache; itching; muscle and bone pain; shivering; skin rash and redness

Rare—Bloody or cloudy urine; greatly decreased frequency of urination or amount of urine; loss of appetite; nausea or vomiting; sore throat; unusual bruising or bleeding; unusual tiredness or weakness; yellow eyes or skin

Side Effects That Usually Do Not Require Medical Attention

These possible side effects may go away during treatment; however, if they continue or are bothersome, check with your doctor, nurse, or pharmacist.

More common—Diarrhea; stomach cramps

Other side effects not listed above may also occur in some patients. If you notice any other effects, check with your doctor, nurse, or pharmacist.

RIFAMPIN AND ISONIAZID   Systemic

■For the Pharmacist■

In providing consultation, consider emphasizing the following selected information (» = major clinical significance):

Before using this medication
» Conditions affecting use, especially:
>> Hypersensitivity to rifampin, isoniazid, ethionamide, pyrazinamide, niacin (nicotinic acid), or other chemically related medications
>> Pregnancy—Isoniazid and rifampin cross the placenta. It is recommended that isoniazid and rifampin be used to treat pregnant women with tuberculosis; however, rifampin has rarely caused postnatal hemorrhage in the mother and infant when administered during the last few weeks of pregnancy
>> Breast-feeding—Isoniazid and rifampin are distributed into breast milk
>> Dental—Patients who develop blood dyscrasias may be at increased risk of microbial infections, delayed healing, and gingival bleeding
>> Use in children—Use of the fixed-dose combination is not recommended in pediatric patients
>> Use in the elderly—Patients over the age of 50 have the highest incidence of hepatitis
>> Other medicines, especially daily alcohol use, alfentanil, aminophylline, oral antidiabetic agents, coumarin- or indandione-derivative anticoagulants, carbamazepine, chloramphenicol, corticosteroids, digitalis glycosides, disopyramide, disulfiram, estrogens, estramustine, fluconazole, other hepatotoxic medications, itraconazole, ketoconazole, methadone, mexiletine, oral contraceptives oxtriphylline, phenytoin, quinidine, tocainide, theophylline, or verapamil
>> Other medical problems, especially alcoholism, active or in remission, or hepatic function impairment

Proper use of this medication
>> Taking this medication with food or antacids, but not within 1 hour of aluminum-containing antacids, if gastrointestinal irritation occurs
» Compliance with full course of therapy, which may take months or years
» Taking pyridoxine concurrently to prevent or minimize symptoms of peripheral neuritis
» Proper dosing
» Missed dose: Taking as soon as possible; not taking if almost time for next dose; not doubling doses; intermittent dosing may result in more frequent and/or severe side effects
» Proper storage

Precautions while using this medication
» Regular visits to physician to check progress, as well as ophthalmologic examinations if signs of optic neuritis occur
>> Checking with physician if no improvement within 2 to 3 weeks
» Using an alternate method of contraception if taking estrogen-containing oral contraceptives concurrently
» Avoiding alcoholic beverages concurrently with this medication

Checking with physician if vascular reactions occur following concurrent ingestion of cheese or fish with isoniazid-containing medications
» Medication causes urine, feces, saliva, sputum, sweat, and tears to
turn reddish orange to reddish brown and may also permanently
discolor soft contact lenses; avoiding the wearing of soft contact
lenses
» Need to report to physician promptly prodromal signs of hepatitis
or peripheral neuritis
Using caution in use of regular toothbrushes, dental floss, and toothpicks; deferring dental work until blood counts have returned to
normal; checking with physician or dentist concerning proper
oral hygiene
Possible interference with diagnostic tests

Side/adverse effects
Hepatitis may be more likely to occur in patients over 50 years of
age
Reddish orange to reddish brown discoloration of urine, stools, saliva, sputum, sweat, and tears may be alarming to patient, although medically insignificant; however, tears discolored by rifampin may also discolor soft contact lenses
Signs of potential side effects, especially blood dyscrasias, hepatitis,
hepatitis-prodromal symptoms, hypersensitivity, neurotoxicity,
optic neuritis, peripheral neuritis, "flu-like" syndrome, and interstitial nephritis

---

▲ For the Patient ▲

914899

ABOUT YOUR MEDICINE

Rifampin (rif-AM-pin) and **isoniazid** (eye-soe-NYE-a-zid) is
a combination antibiotic medicine. It is used to treat tuberculosis (TB). It may be taken alone or with one or more
other medicines for TB.

**To help clear up your tuberculosis (TB) completely, you must
keep taking this medicine for the full time of treatment, even
if you begin to feel better. This is very important. It is also
important that you do not miss any doses.**

If any of the information in this leaflet causes you special
concern or if you want additional information about your
medicine and its use, check with your doctor, nurse, or pharmacist. **Remember, keep this and all other medicines out of
the reach of children and never share your medicines with
others.**

BEFORE USING THIS MEDICINE

Tell your doctor, nurse, and pharmacist if you . . .
- are allergic to any medicine, either prescription or nonprescription (OTC);
- are pregnant or intend to become pregnant while using
this medicine;
- are breast-feeding;
- are taking **any** other prescription or nonprescription
(OTC) medicine;

- have any other medical problems, especially alcohol
  abuse (or history of) or liver disease.

PROPER USE OF THIS MEDICINE

If this medicine upsets your stomach, take it with food.
Antacids may also help. However, do not take aluminum-
containing antacids within 1 hour of the time you take rifampin and isoniazid combination.

To help clear up your tuberculosis (TB) completely, **it is
very important that you keep taking this medicine for the full
time of treatment** even if you begin to feel better after a few
weeks.

Your doctor may also want you to take pyridoxine (vitamin
B$_6$) every day to help prevent or lessen some of the side
effects of isoniazid. If it is needed, **it is very important to
take pyridoxine every day along with this medicine. Do not
miss any doses.**

If you miss a dose of either of these medicines, take it as
soon as possible. However, if it is almost time for your next
dose, skip the missed dose and go back to your regular dosing
schedule. Do not double doses. **If rifampin and isoniazid
combination is taken on an irregular schedule, side effects
may occur more often and may be more serious than usual.**

PRECAUTIONS WHILE USING THIS MEDICINE

This medicine will cause the urine, stool, saliva, sputum,
sweat, and tears to turn reddish orange to reddish brown.
This is to be expected and does not usually require medical
attention. This effect may cause soft contact lenses to become permanently discolored. **Therefore, it is best not to
wear soft contact lenses while taking this medicine.** Hard
contact lenses are not discolored by this medicine.

**Oral contraceptives (birth control pills) containing estrogen
may not work properly if you take them while you are taking
rifampin and isoniazid combination. Unplanned pregnancies
may occur. You should use a different means of birth control
while you are taking this medicine.**

If your symptoms do not improve within 2 to 3 weeks, or if
they become worse, check with your doctor.

It is very important that your doctor check your progress at
regular visits. In addition, you should **check with your doctor
immediately if blurred vision or loss of vision, with or without
eye pain, occurs during treatment.**

Liver problems may be more likely to occur if you drink
alcoholic beverages regularly while you are taking this medicine. Also, the regular use of alcohol may keep this medicine
from working properly. Therefore, **you should strictly limit
the amount of alcoholic beverages you drink while you are
taking this medicine.**

This medicine must not be given to other people or used for other infections unless you are otherwise directed by your doctor.

POSSIBLE SIDE EFFECTS OF THIS MEDICINE
Side Effects That Should Be Reported To Your Doctor Immediately

> *More common*—Clumsiness or unsteadiness; dark urine; loss of appetite; nausea or vomiting; numbness, tingling, burning, or pain in hands and feet; unusual tiredness or weakness; yellow eyes or skin

> *Less common*—Chills; difficult breathing; dizziness; fever; headache; itching; muscle and bone pain; shivering; skin rash and redness

> *Rare*—Bloody or cloudy urine; blurred vision or loss of vision, with or without eye pain; convulsions (seizures); depression; greatly decreased frequency of urination or amount of urine; joint pain; mood or mental changes; sore throat; unusual bruising or bleeding

Side Effects That Usually Do Not Require Medical Attention

These possible side effects may go away during treatment; however, if they continue or are bothersome, check with your doctor, nurse, or pharmacist.

> *More common*—Diarrhea; stomach cramps or upset

Dark urine and yellowing of the eyes or skin (signs of liver problems) are more likely to occur in patients over 50 years of age.

Other side effects not listed above may also occur in some patients. If you notice any other effects, check with your doctor, nurse, or pharmacist.

RIMANTADINE   Systemic

■ For the Pharmacist ■

In providing consultation, consider emphasizing the following selected information (») = major clinical significance):

Before using this medication
» Conditions affecting use, especially:
  Hypersensitivity to amantadine or rimantadine
  Pregnancy—High doses were embryotoxic and maternotoxic in rats
  Other medical problems, especially epilepsy or a history of seizures, liver function impairment and renal function impairment

Proper use of this medication
» Receiving a flu shot if recommended by your doctor
» Taking before exposure or as soon as possible after exposure
» Compliance with full course of therapy
» Importance of not missing doses and taking at evenly spaced times
  Proper administration technique for oral liquid
» Proper dosing
  Missed dose: Taking as soon as possible; not taking if almost time for next dose; not doubling doses
» Proper storage

Precautions while using this medication
  Caution if dizziness occurs
  Checking with physician if no improvement within a few days

▲ For the Patient ▲

919429

ABOUT YOUR MEDICINE

Rimantadine (ri-MAN-ta-deen) is an antiviral. It is used to help prevent or treat certain types of influenza (flu) infections (type A). It may be given alone or along with flu shots. Rimantadine will not work for colds, other types of flu, or other virus infections.

If any of the information in this leaflet causes you special concern or if you want additional information about your medicine and its use, check with your doctor, nurse, or pharmacist. **Remember, keep this and all other medicines out of the reach of children and never share your medicines with others.**

BEFORE USING THIS MEDICINE

Tell your doctor, nurse, and pharmacist if you . . .
  • are allergic to any medicine, either prescription or nonprescription (OTC);
  • are pregnant or intend to become pregnant while using this medicine;
  • are breast-feeding;

- are taking any other prescription or nonprescription (OTC) medicine;
- have any other medical problems, especially epilepsy or other seizures (or history of), kidney disease, or liver disease.

PROPER USE OF THIS MEDICINE

Talk to your doctor about **getting a flu shot** if you have not had one yet.

This medicine is **best taken before exposure, or as soon as possible after exposure**, to people who have the flu.

To help keep yourself from getting the flu, **keep taking this medicine for the full time of treatment.**

If you already have the flu, **continue taking this medicine for the full time of treatment even if you begin to feel better after a few days.** This will help to clear up your infection completely. If you stop taking this medicine to soon, your symptoms may return. This medicine should be taken for at least 5 to 7 days.

This medicine works best when there is a constant amount in the blood. **To help keep the amount constant, do not miss any doses. Also, it is best to take the doses at evenly spaced times day and night.**

If you are using the oral liquid form of rimantadine, use a specially marked measuring spoon or other device to measure each dose accurately. The average household teaspoon may not hold the right amount of liquid.

If you do miss a dose of the medicine, take it as soon as possible. This will help to keep a constant amount of medicine in the blood. However, if it is almost time for your next dose, skip the missed dose and go back to your regular dosing schedule. Do not double doses.

PRECAUTIONS WHILE USING THIS MEDICINE

This medicine may cause some people to become dizzy or confused, or to have trouble concentrating. **Make sure you know how you react to this medicine before you drive, use machines, or do other jobs that require you to be alert.** If these reactions are especially bothersome, check with your doctor.

If you symptoms do not improve within a few days, or if they become worse, check with your doctor.

POSSIBLE SIDE EFFECTS OF THIS MEDICINE
Side Effects That Usually Do Not Require Medical Attention

These possible side effects may go away during treatment; however, if they continue or are bothersome, check with your doctor, nurse, or pharmacist.

    Less common—Difficulty in concentrating; dizziness; dryness of mouth; headache; loss of appetite; nausea;

nervousness; stomach pain; trouble in sleeping; unusual tiredness; vomiting

Other side effects not listed above may also occur in some
patients. If you notice any other effects, check with your
doctor, nurse, or pharmacist.

SELEGILINE   Systemic

■ For the Pharmacist ■

In providing consultation, consider emphasizing the following selected
information ($\gg$ = major clinical significance):

Before using this medication
$\gg$ Conditions affecting use, especially:
        Sensitivity to selegiline
        Other medications, especially fluoxetine or meperidine and pos-
          sibly other narcotic (opioid) analgesics
        Other medical problems, especially a history of peptic ulcer dis-
          ease

Proper use of this medication
$\gg$ Importance of not taking more medication than the amount pre-
    scribed; to do so may increase the risk of side effects
    Missed dose: Taking as soon as possible; not taking in the late after-
      noon or evening; not taking if almost time for next dose; not
      doubling doses.
$\gg$ Proper storage

Precautions while using this medication
$\gg$ If taking 20 mg or more of selegiline a day, avoiding tyramine-
    containing foods, alcoholic beverages, and large quantities of
    caffeine-containing beverages, over-the-counter cold and cough
    medicines, and other medications, unless prescribed
$\gg$ Checking with hospital emergency room or physician if symptoms
    of hypertensive crisis develop
$\gg$ Possibility of orthostatic hypotension; caution when getting up sud-
    denly from a lying or sitting position
    Possible dryness of mouth; using sugarless candy or gum, ice, or
    saliva substitute for relief; checking with physician or dentist if
    dryness of mouth continues for more than 2 weeks

Side/adverse effects
    Signs of potential side effects, especially dyskinesias, mood or men-
    tal changes, angina pectoris, arrhythmias, asthma, bradycardia,
    peripheral edema, extrapyramidal effects, hallucinations, severe
    headache, severe hypertension, gastrointestinal bleeding, ortho-
    static hypotension, prostatic hypertrophy, and tardive dyskinesia

▲ For the Patient ▲

917106

ABOUT YOUR MEDICINE

Selegiline (seh-LEDGE-ah-leen) is used in combination with
levodopa or levodopa and carbidopa combination to treat
Parkinson's disease, sometimes called shaking palsy or paralysis agitans.

If any of the information in this leaflet causes you special
concern or if you want additional information about your
medicine and its use, check with your doctor, nurse, or pharmacist. **Remember, keep this and all other medicines out of
the reach of children and never share your medicines with
others.**

BEFORE USING THIS MEDICINE

Discuss with your doctor possible side effects of this medicine. Some may be serious and/or permanent.

Tell your doctor, nurse, and pharmacist if you . . .
- are allergic to any medicine, either prescription or non-prescription (OTC);
- are pregnant or intend to become pregnant while using this medicine;
- are breast-feeding;
- are taking any other prescription or nonprescription (OTC) medicine, especially fluoxetine or meperidine;
- have any other medical problems, especially stomach ulcer (history of).

PROPER USE OF THIS MEDICINE

Take this medicine only as directed. Do not take more of it, do not take it more often, and do not take it for a longer time than your doctor ordered.

If you miss a dose of this medicine, take it as soon as possible. However, if you do not remember the missed dose until late afternoon or evening, skip it and go back to your regular dosing schedule. Do not double doses.

PRECAUTIONS WHILE USING THIS MEDICINE

When selegiline is taken at doses of 10 mg or less per day for the treatment of Parkinson's disease, there are no restrictions on food or beverages you eat or drink.
For patients using higher than usual doses of selegiline:
- **Dangerous reactions, such as sudden high blood pressure, may occur if doses higher than 10 mg per day are taken with certain foods, beverages, or other medicines.** Ask your doctor, nurse, or pharmacist for a list of these foods, drinks, and medicines.

- **Check with your doctor immediately** if you have severe chest pain, headache, nausea, or vomiting; enlarged pupils; fast or slow heartbeat; increased sensitivity of eyes to light; increased sweating (possibly with fever or cold, clammy skin); or stiff or sore neck. These may be signs of unusually high blood pressure.

- Also, for at least 2 weeks after you stop taking this medicine, these foods, beverages, and other medicines may continue to react with selegiline if it was taken in high doses.

Dizziness, lightheadedness, or fainting may occur, especially when you get up from a lying or sitting position. Getting up slowly may help. If the problem continues or gets worse, check with your doctor.

POSSIBLE SIDE EFFECTS OF THIS MEDICINE
Side Effects That Should Be Reported To Your Doctor

More common—Increase in unusual movements of body; mood or mental changes

Less common or rare—Bloody or black, tarry stools; difficulty in speaking; difficult or frequent urination; dizziness or lightheadedness, especially when getting up from a lying or sitting position; hallucinations; irregular heartbeat; lip smacking or puckering, puffing of cheeks, rapid or worm-like movements of tongue, uncontrolled chewing movements, or uncontrolled movements of arms, legs, face, neck, and back; loss of balance control; restlessness or desire to keep moving; severe stomach pain; swelling of feet or lower legs; twisting movements of body; vomiting of blood or material that looks like coffee grounds; wheezing, difficulty in breathing, or tightness in chest

Side Effects That Usually Do Not Require Medical Attention

These possible side effects may go away during treatment; however, if they continue or are bothersome, check with your doctor, nurse, or pharmacist.

More common—Abdominal or stomach pain; dizziness or feeling faint; dry mouth; nausea or vomiting; trouble in sleeping

Other side effects not listed above may also occur in some patients. If you notice any other effects, check with your doctor, nurse, or pharmacist.

SERTRALINE   Systemic

■For the Pharmacist■

In providing consultation, consider emphasizing the following selected
information (» = major clinical significance):

Before using this medication
» Conditions affecting use, especially:
>>> Sensitivity to sertraline
>>> Pregnancy—Animal studies using higher than maximum human
mg/kg doses have shown delayed ossification in fetuses and
decreased pup survival, probably due to *in utero* exposure to
sertraline; clinical significance is unknown
>>> Dental—Decreased salivary flow may contribute to caries, per-
iodontal disease, candidiasis, and discomfort
>>> Other medications, especially digitoxin, warfarin, and MAO in-
hibitors
>>> Other medical problems, especially hepatic or renal dysfunction
or history of drug dependence

Proper use of this medication
» Compliance with therapy; not taking more or less medicine than
prescribed
» Up to 4 weeks or more of therapy may be required before antide-
pressant effects are achieved
» Proper dosing
>> Missed dose: Discussing with doctor what to do about any missed
doses
» Proper storage

Precautions while using this medication
>> Regular visits to physician to check progress of therapy
» Avoiding use of alcoholic beverages; not taking other CNS depressants unless prescribed by physician
» Possible drowsiness, impairment of judgment, thinking, or motor
skills; caution when driving or doing jobs requiring alertness
» Possible dryness of mouth; using sugarless gum or candy, ice, or
saliva substitute for relief; checking with physician or dentist if
dry mouth continues for more than 2 weeks

Side/adverse effects
>> Fever; mania or hypomania; or skin rash, hives, or itching

▲ For the Patient ▲

918936

ABOUT YOUR MEDICINE

Sertraline (SER-tra-leen) is used to treat mental depression.

If any of the information in this leaflet causes you special
concern or if you want additional information about your
medicine and its use, check with your doctor, nurse, or pharmacist. **Remember, keep this and all other medicines out of
the reach of children and never share your medicines with
others.**

BEFORE USING THIS MEDICINE

Tell your doctor, nurse, and pharmacist if you . . .
- are allergic to any medicine, either prescription or non-prescription (OTC);
- are pregnant or intend to become pregnant while using this medicine;
- are breast-feeding;
- are taking any other prescription or nonprescription (OTC) medicine, especially digitoxin, MAO inhibitors, or warfarin;
- have any other medical problems.

PROPER USE OF THIS MEDICINE

Take this medicine only as directed by your doctor, to benefit your condition as much as possible. Do not take more of it, do not take it more often, and do not take it for a longer time than your doctor ordered.

You may have to take sertraline for up to 4 weeks or longer before you begin to feel better. Your doctor should check your progress at regular visits during this time.

Always take this medicine at the same time in relation to meals and snacks. You may take it on a full or empty stomach, but always take it the same way. This is to make sure that your body absorbs the medicine the same way.

Because sertraline is taken by different patients at different times of the day, you and your doctor should discuss what to do about any missed doses.

PRECAUTIONS WHILE USING THIS MEDICINE

It is important that your doctor check your progress at regular visits, to allow for changes in your dose and help reduce any side effects.

This medicine may add to the effects of alcohol and other CNS depressants (medicines that slow down the nervous system). **Check with your doctor before taking any such depressants while you are using this medicine.**

This medicine may cause some people to become drowsy. **Make sure you know how you react to this medicine before you drive, use machines, or do other jobs that require you to be alert.**

This medicine may cause dryness of the mouth. For temporary relief, use sugarless gum or candy, melt bits of ice in your mouth, or use a saliva substitute. However, if your mouth feels dry for more than 2 weeks, check with your physician or dentist. Continuing dryness of the mouth may increase the chance of dental disease, including tooth decay, gum disease, and fungus infections.

POSSIBLE SIDE EFFECTS OF THIS MEDICINE
Side Effects That Should Be Reported To Your Doctor

Less common or rare—Fast talking and excited feelings or actions that are out of control; fever; skin rash, hives, or itching

Side Effects That Usually Do Not Require Medical Attention

These possible side effects may go away during treatment; however, if they continue or are bothersome, check with your doctor, nurse, or pharmacist.

More common—Decreased appetite or weight loss; decreased sexual drive or ability; diarrhea; drowsiness; dryness of mouth; headache; nausea; stomach cramps, gas, or pain; tiredness or weakness; tremor; trouble in sleeping

Other side effects not listed above may also occur in some patients. If you notice any other effects, check with your doctor, nurse, or pharmacist.

SKELETAL MUSCLE
RELAXANTS   Systemic
Including Orphenadrine; Carisoprodol; Chlorphenesin;
Chlorzoxazone; Metaxalone; Methocarbamol.

■For the Pharmacist■

In providing consultation, consider emphasizing the following selected
information (» = major clinical significance):

Before using this medication
» Conditions affecting use, especially:
Sensitivity to—
For all muscle relaxants
The muscle relaxant considered for use, history of
In addition to the above, the following specific information may
apply:
For carisoprodol
Other carbamate derivatives
Breast-feeding—
For carisoprodol only
Excreted in breast milk; may cause sedation and gastroin-
testinal upset in the infant
Other medications, especially—
For all skeletal muscle relaxants
Other CNS depression–producing medications
Other medical problems, especially—
For all skeletal muscle relaxants
Hepatic function impairment or disease or renal function
impairment or disease
In addition to the above, the following specific information may
apply:
For carisoprodol
Acute intermittent porphyria (known or suspected)
For orphenadrine
Conditions that may be adversely affected by anticholi-
nergic activity
For metaxalone
Hemolytic anemia or history of

Proper use of this medication
For all skeletal muscle relaxants
Missed dose: Taking if remembered within an hour or so; not taking
if remembered later; not doubling doses
» Proper storage
In addition to the above, the following specific information may apply:
For chlorzoxazone, metaxalone, and methocarbamol
Tablets may be crushed and mixed with food or liquid for ease of
administration

Precautions while using this medication
For all skeletal muscle relaxants
Regular visits to physician to check progress during prolonged ther-
apy
» Avoiding use of alcohol or other CNS depressants during therapy
unless prescribed or otherwise approved by physician
» Caution if dizziness, drowsiness, or lightheadedness occurs
In addition to the above, the following specific information may apply:

For carisoprodol and methocarbamol
» Caution if blurred vision, other vision problems, or feeling faint occurs
» Caution if clumsiness or unsteadiness occurs
For metaxalone
   Diabetics: May cause false-positive urine sugar tests
For orphenadrine
» Caution if blurred vision, other vision problems, or feeling faint occurs
» Caution if muscle weakness occurs
   Possible dryness of mouth; using sugarless gum or candy, ice, or saliva substitute for relief; checking with dentist if dry mouth continues for more than 2 weeks

Side/adverse effects
   Signs and symptoms of potential side effects, especially:
   For all skeletal muscle relaxants
      Allergic reactions
   In addition to the above, the following specific information may apply:
      For carisoprodol
      Fainting, fast heartbeat, or mental depression
      For chlorphenesin
      Blood dyscrasias
      For chlorzoxazone
      Blood dyscrasias or gastrointestinal bleeding
      May color urine orange or reddish purple
      For metaxalone
      Blood dyscrasias or hepatotoxicity
      For methocarbamol
      Blood dyscrasias
      May color urine black, brown, or green, especially if sample allowed to stand
      With parenteral use only—Convulsions, fainting, or slow heartbeat
      For orphenadrine
      Anticholinergic effects, blood dyscrasias, fainting, fast heartbeat, hallucinations, or pounding heartbeat

---

▲ For the Patient ▲

914582

ORPHENADRINE (Oral)

ABOUT YOUR MEDICINE

Orphenadrine (or-FEN-a-dreen) is a medicine that is used to help relax certain muscles in your body and relieve the pain and discomfort caused by strains, sprains, or other injury to your muscles. One form of orphenadrine is also used to relieve trembling caused by Parkinson's disease. However, this medicine does not take the place of rest, exercise or physical therapy, or other treatment that your doctor may recommend for your medical problem.

If any of the information in this leaflet causes you special concern or if you want additional information about your medicine and its use, check with your doctor, nurse, or pharmacist. **Remember, keep this and all other medicines out of**

the reach of children and never share your medicines with others.

BEFORE USING THIS MEDICINE

Tell your doctor, nurse, and pharmacist if you . . .
- are allergic to any medicine, either prescription or non-prescription (OTC);
- are pregnant or intend to become pregnant while using this medicine;
- are breast-feeding;
- are taking any other prescription or nonprescription (OTC) medicine, especially CNS depressants or narcotics;
- have any other medical problems, especially disease of the digestive tract such as esophagus disease, stomach ulcer, or intestinal blockage; enlarged prostate; glaucoma; myasthenia gravis; or urinary tract blockage.

PROPER USE OF THIS MEDICINE

If you miss a dose of this medicine and remember within an hour or so of the missed dose, take it right away. But if you do not remember until later, skip the missed dose and go back to your regular dosing schedule. Do not double doses.

PRECAUTIONS WHILE USING THIS MEDICINE

If you will be taking orphenadrine for a long period of time (for example, more than a few weeks), your doctor should check your progress at regular visits.

This medicine may add to the effects of alcohol and other CNS depressants (medicines that slow down the nervous system). **Check with your doctor before taking any such depressants while you are using this medicine.**

Orphenadrine may cause some people to have blurred vision or to become drowsy, dizzy, lightheaded, faint, or less alert than they are normally. It may also cause muscle weakness in some people. **Make sure you know how you react to this medicine before you drive, use machines, or do other jobs that require you to be alert.**

Orphenadrine may cause dryness of the mouth. For temporary relief, use sugarless candy or gum, melt bits of ice in your mouth, or use a saliva substitute. However, if dry mouth continues for more than 2 weeks, check with your dentist. Continuing dryness of the mouth may increase the chance of dental disease, including tooth decay, gum disease, and fungal infections.

POSSIBLE SIDE EFFECTS OF THIS MEDICINE
Side Effects That Should Be Reported To Your Doctor

Less common—Fainting; fast or pounding heartbeat

Rare—Hallucinations; skin rash, hives, itching, or redness; unusual tiredness or weakness

*Side Effects That Usually Do Not Require Medical
Attention*

These possible side effects may go away during treatment;
however, if they continue or are bothersome, check with your
doctor, nurse, or pharmacist.

> *More common*—Dry mouth

> *Less common or rare*—Abdominal or stomach cramps or
> pain; blurred or double vision or other vision problems;
> confusion; constipation; difficult urination; dizziness
> or lightheadedness; drowsiness; excitement, irritabil-
> ity, nervousness, or restlessness; headache; muscle
> weakness; nausea or vomiting; trembling

Other side effects not listed above may also occur in some
patients. If you notice any other effects, check with your
doctor, nurse, or pharmacist.

▲ For the Patient ▲

912634

SKELETAL MUSCLE RELAXANTS (Oral): *Including
Carisoprodol; Chlorphenesin; Chlorzoxazone;
Metaxalone; Methocarbamol.*

ABOUT YOUR MEDICINE

Skeletal muscle relaxants are used to relax certain muscles
in your body and relieve the pain and discomfort caused by
strains, sprains, or other injury to your muscles. However,
these medicines do not take the place of rest, exercise or
physical therapy, or other treatment that your doctor may
recommend. Methocarbamol is also used to relieve muscle
problems caused by tetanus.

If any of the information in this leaflet causes you special
concern or if you want additional information about your
medicine and its use, check with your doctor, nurse, or pharmacist. **Remember, keep this and all other medicines out of
the reach of children and never share your medicines with
others.**

BEFORE USING THIS MEDICINE

Tell your doctor, nurse, and pharmacist if you . . .
- are allergic to any medicine, either prescription or nonprescription (OTC);
- are pregnant or intend to become pregnant while using
  this medicine;
- are breast-feeding;
- are taking any other prescription or nonprescription
  (OTC) medicine, especially narcotics or other CNS depressants;
- have any other medical problems, especially kidney disease, liver disease, or porphyria (for carisoprodol only).

PROPER USE OF THIS MEDICINE

Chlorzoxazone, metaxalone, or methocarbamol tablets may be crushed and mixed with a little food or liquid if needed to make the tablets easier to swallow.

If you miss a dose of this medicine and remember within an hour or so of the missed dose, take it right away. However, if you do not remember until later, skip the missed dose and go back to your regular schedule. Do not double doses.

PRECAUTIONS WHILE USING THIS MEDICINE

If you will be taking this medicine for a long time (for example, more than a few weeks), your doctor should check your progress at regular visits.

This medicine will add to the effects of alcohol and other CNS depressants (medicines that slow down the nervous system). **Check with your doctor before taking any such depressants while you are taking this medicine.**

Skeletal muscle relaxants may cause blurred vision, or clumsiness or unsteadiness in some people. They may also cause some people to feel drowsy, dizzy, lightheaded, faint, or less alert than they are normally. **Make sure you know how you react to this medicine before you drive, use machines, or do other jobs that require you to be alert, well-coordinated, and able to see well.**

POSSIBLE SIDE EFFECTS OF THIS MEDICINE
Side Effects That Should Be Reported To Your Doctor

Less common—Fainting; fast heartbeat; fever; hive-like swellings (large) on face, eyelids, mouth, lips, and/or tongue; mental depression; shortness of breath, troubled breathing, tightness in chest, and/or wheezing; skin rash, hives, itching, or redness; stinging or burning of eyes; stuffy nose and red or bloodshot eyes

Rare—Blood in urine; bloody or black tarry stools; cough or hoarseness; fast or irregular breathing; lower back or side pain; muscle cramps or pain (not present before treatment or more painful than before treatment); painful or difficult urination; pinpoint red spots on skin; puffiness or swelling of the eyelids or around the eyes; sores, ulcers, or white spots on lips or in mouth; sore throat and fever with or without chills; swollen and/or painful glands; unusual bleeding or bruising; unusual tiredness or weakness; vomiting of blood or material that looks like coffee grounds; yellow eyes or skin

Side Effects That Usually Do Not Require Medical Attention

These possible side effects may go away during treatment; however, if they continue or are bothersome, check with your doctor, nurse, or pharmacist.

More common—Blurred or double vision or any change
in vision; dizziness or lightheadedness; drowsiness

Chlorzoxazone may cause your urine to turn orange or reddish purple, while methocarbamol may cause it to turn black,
brown, or green. These effects are harmless and will go away
when you stop taking the medicine.

Other side effects not listed above may also occur in some
patients. If you notice any other effects, check with your
doctor, nurse, or pharmacist.

SUCCIMER   Systemic

■ For the Pharmacist ■

In providing consultation, consider emphasizing the following selected information (» = major clinical significance):

Before using this medication
» Conditions affecting use, especially:
    Sensitivity to succimer
    Other medical problems, especially dehydration and renal function impairment

Proper use of this medication
» Removal of child from lead-contaminated environment
    Possible need for hospitalization of child during succimer therapy
    Unpleasant odor of capsules
    Contents of capsule may be sprinkled on food and eaten immediately or given by spoon and followed immediately by a fruit drink
» Proper dosing
    Missed dose: Taking as soon as possible; not taking if almost time for next dose; not doubling doses
» Proper storage

Precautions while using this medication
» Regular visits to physician to check progress of therapy and to prevent adverse effects

Side/adverse effects
    Signs of potential side effects, especially neutropenia

▲ For the Patient ▲

919225

ABOUT YOUR MEDICINE

Succimer (SUX-i-mer) is used to remove excess lead from the body. It is used to treat acute lead poisoning, especially in small children.

If any of the information in this leaflet causes you special concern or if you want additional information about your medicine and its use, check with your doctor, nurse, or pharmacist. **Remember, keep this and all other medicines out of the reach of children and never share your medicines with others.**

BEFORE USING THIS MEDICINE

Tell your doctor, nurse, and pharmacist if you . . .
* are allergic to any medicine, either prescription or nonprescription (OTC);
* are pregnant or intend to become pregnant while using this medicine;
* are breast-feeding;
* are taking any other prescription or nonprescription (OTC) medicine;
* have any other medical problems, especially dehydration or kidney disease.

PROPER USE OF THIS MEDICINE

Children who have too much lead in their bodies should be removed from the lead-containing surroundings (for example, home, school, or other areas where the child has been exposed to lead) until the lead has been removed from the surroundings.

The child may need to be put in the hospital while he or she is receiving succimer. This will allow the doctor to check the child's condition while the lead is being removed from the child's surroundings.

When opening the bottle of succimer, you may notice an unpleasant odor. However, this is a normal odor for these capsules and does not affect the way the medicine works.

If the capsules cannot be swallowed, the contents of the capsule may be sprinkled on food and eaten immediately. The contents may also be given on a spoon and followed by a fruit drink.

If you miss a dose of this medicine, take it as soon as possible. However, if it is almost time for your next dose, skip the missed dose and go back to your regular dosing schedule. Do not double doses.

PRECAUTIONS WHILE USING THIS MEDICINE

It is important that your doctor check your progress at regular visits to make sure that this medicine is working properly and to check for unwanted effects. Certain blood and urine tests must be done regularly to make sure you are taking the correct dose of succimer.

POSSIBLE SIDE EFFECTS OF THIS MEDICINE
Side Effects That Should Be Reported To Your Doctor

   Less common—Fever and chills

Side Effects That Usually Do Not Require Medical Attention

These possible side effects may go away during treatment; however, if they continue or are bothersome, check with your doctor, nurse, or pharmacist.

   More common—Diarrhea; loose stools; loss of appetite; nausea and vomiting; skin rash

Succimer may cause your urine, sweat, and feces to have an unpleasant odor.

Other side effects not listed above may also occur in some patients. If you notice any other effects, check with your doctor, nurse, or pharmacist.

SUCRALFATE   Oral-Local

■For the Pharmacist■

In providing consultation, consider emphasizing the following selected
information (》 = major clinical significance):

Before using this medication
》 Conditions affecting use, especially:
  Sensitivity to sucralfate
  Other medications, especially ciprofloxacin, digoxin, norfloxa-
  cin, ofloxacin, phenytoin, and theophylline

Proper use of this medication
  Taking on empty stomach 1 hour before meals and at bedtime
  Compliance with full course of therapy and keeping appointments
  for check-ups
》 Proper dosing
  Missed dose: Taking as soon as possible; not taking if almost time
  for next dose; not doubling doses
》 Proper storage

Precautions while using this medication
》 Not taking antacids within ½ hour before or after sucralfate

Side/adverse effects
  Signs of potential side effects, especially aluminum toxicity

▲ For the Patient ▲

913150

ABOUT YOUR MEDICINE

Sucralfate (soo-KRAL-fate) is used to treat and prevent duodenal ulcer. It may also be used for other conditions as
determined by your doctor.

Sucralfate contains an aluminum salt.

If any of the information in this leaflet causes you special
concern or if you want additional information about your
medicine and its use, check with your doctor, nurse, or pharmacist. **Remember, keep this and all other medicines out of
the reach of children and never share your medicines with
others.**

BEFORE USING THIS MEDICINE

Tell your doctor, nurse, and pharmacist if you . . .
  • are allergic to any medicine, either prescription or nonprescription (OTC);
  • are pregnant or intend to become pregnant while using
  this medicine;
  • are breast-feeding;
  • are taking any other prescription or nonprescription
  (OTC) medicine, especially ciprofloxacin, norfloxacin,
  or ofloxacin;
  • have any other medical problems.

PROPER USE OF THIS MEDICINE

Sucralfate is best taken with water on an empty stomach 1 hour before meals and at bedtime, unless otherwise directed by your doctor.

Take this medicine for the full time of treatment, even if you begin to feel better. Also, it is important that you keep your doctor's appointments for check-ups so that your doctor will be better able to tell you when to stop taking this medicine.

If you miss a dose of this medicine, take it as soon as possible. However, if it is almost time for your next dose, skip the missed dose and go back to your regular dosing schedule. Do not double doses.

PRECAUTIONS WHILE USING THIS MEDICINE

Antacids may be taken with sucralfate to help relieve any stomach pain, unless your doctor has told you not to use them. **However, antacids should not be taken within 30 minutes before or after sucralfate.** Taking these medicines too close together may keep sucralfate from working properly.

POSSIBLE SIDE EFFECTS OF THIS MEDICINE

Side Effects That Should Be Reported To Your Doctor Immediately

>   *Signs of too much aluminum in the body*—Drowsiness; seizures

Side Effects That Usually Do Not Require Medical Attention

These possible side effects may go away during treatment; however, if they continue or are bothersome, check with your doctor, nurse, or pharmacist.

>   *More common*—Constipation

>   *Less common or rare*—Backache; diarrhea; dizziness or lightheadedness; dryness of mouth; indigestion; nausea; skin rash, hives, or itching; stomach cramps or pain

Other side effects not listed above may also occur in some patients. If you notice any other effects, check with your doctor, nurse, or pharmacist.

SULCONAZOLE Topical

■For the Pharmacist■

In providing consultation, consider emphasizing the following selected information (» = major clinical significance):

Before using this medication
» Conditions affecting use, especially:
  Hypersensitivity to sulconazole or other imidazole derivatives such as miconazole or econazole

Proper use of this medication
  Applying sufficient medication to cover affected and surrounding areas, and rubbing in gently
» Avoiding contact with the eyes
» Not applying occlusive dressing over this medication unless directed to do so by physician
» Using medication for the full time of treatment; fungal infections may require prolonged therapy
» Proper dosing
  Missed dose: Applying as soon as possible; not applying if almost time for the next dose
» Proper storage

Precautions while using this medication
  Checking with physician if no improvement seen within 4 to 6 weeks
  Observing hygienic measures to help cure infection and to help prevent reinfection
  For tinea cruris
    Avoiding underwear that is tight-fitting or made from synthetic materials; wearing loose-fitting cotton underwear instead
  For tinea pedis
    Carefully drying feet, especially between toes, after bathing
    Avoiding socks made from wool or synthetic materials; wearing clean, cotton socks and changing them daily or more often if feet perspire excessively
    Wearing well-ventilated shoes or sandals
  For tinea corporis
    Carefully drying body after bathing
    Avoiding too much heat and humidity if possible
    Wearing well-ventilated, loose-fitting clothing

Side/adverse effects
  Signs of potential side effects, especially hypersensitivity

▲ For the Patient ▲

919407

ABOUT YOUR MEDICINE

Sulconazole (sul-KON-a-zole) is used to treat infections caused by a fungus.

Sulconazole is applied to the skin to treat ringworm of the body (tinea corporis); ringworm of the foot (tinea pedis, athlete's foot); ringworm of the groin (tinea cruris; jock itch); and "sun fungus" (tinea versicolor; pityriasis versicolor). Sulconazole may also be used for other conditions as determined by your doctor.

If any of the information in this leaflet causes you special concern or if you want additional information about your medicine and its use, check with your doctor, nurse, or pharmacist. **Remember, keep this and all other medicines out of the reach of children and never share your medicines with others.**

BEFORE USING THIS MEDICINE

Tell your doctor, nurse, and pharmacist if you . . .
- are allergic to any medicine, either prescription or non-prescription (OTC);
- are pregnant or intend to become pregnant while using this medicine;
- are breast-feeding;
- are taking any other prescription or nonprescription (OTC) medicine;
- have any other medical problems.

PROPER USE OF THIS MEDICINE

Apply enough sulconazole to cover the affected and surrounding skin areas and rub in gently.

Keep this medicine away from the eyes.

When sulconazole is used to treat certain types of fungus infections of the skin, an occlusive dressing (airtight covering, such as kitchen plastic wrap) should *not* be applied over the medicine. To do so may irritate the skin. **Do not apply an airtight covering over this medicine unless you have been directed to do so by your doctor.**

To help clear up your infection completely, **it is very important that you keep using sulconazole for the full time of treatment,** even if your symptoms begin to clear up after a few days. Since fungus infections may be very slow to clear up, you may have to continue using this medicine every day for several weeks or more. If you stop using this medicine too soon, your symptoms may return. **Do not miss any doses.**

If you do miss a dose of this medicine, apply it as soon as possible. However, if it is almost time for your next dose, skip the missed dose and go back to your regular dosing schedule.

PRECAUTIONS WHILE USING THIS MEDICINE

If your skin problem does not improve within 4 to 6 weeks, or if it becomes worse, check with your doctor.

To help clear up your infection completely and to help make sure it does not return, good health habits are also required. The following measures will help reduce chafing and irritation and will keep the area cool and dry:
- For patients who have ringworm of the groin: Wear loose-fitting, cotton underwear.
- For patients who have ringworm of the foot: After bathing, carefully dry the feet, especially between the toes. Wear clean cotton socks and change them daily or more

often if feet sweat freely. It is best to wear sandals or well-ventilated shoes.
- For patients who have ringworm of the body: Carefully dry yourself after bathing. Avoid too much heat and humidity if possible. Wear well-ventilated, loose-fitting clothing.

If you have any questions about this, check with your doctor, nurse, or pharmacist.

POSSIBLE SIDE EFFECTS OF THIS MEDICINE
Side Effects That Should Be Reported To Your Doctor

Less common—Burning or stinging, itching, redness of the skin or other sign of irritation not present before use of this medicine

Other side effects not listed above may also occur in some patients. If you notice any other effects, check with your doctor, nurse, or pharmacist.

SULFAMETHOXAZOLE AND TRIMETHOPRIM   Systemic

■For the Pharmacist■

In providing consultation, consider emphasizing the following selected information (» = major clinical significance):

Before using this medication
» Conditions affecting use, especially:
  Allergy to sulfonamides, furosemide, thiazide diuretics, sulfonylureas, carbonic anhydrase inhibitors, or trimethoprim
  Pregnancy—Sulfamethoxazole and trimethoprim cross the placenta; trimethoprim may interfere with folic acid metabolism
  Breast-feeding—Sulfamethoxazole and trimethoprim are distributed into breast milk; sulfamethoxazole may cause kernicterus in nursing infants; trimethoprim may interfere with folic acid metabolism
  Use in children—Sulfamethoxazole and trimethoprim combination is contraindicated in infants up to 2 months of age for most indications since sulfonamides may cause kernicterus in neonates; the fixed ratio (1:5) combination of sulfamethoxazole and trimethoprim is inappropriate in neonates and older infants because of the altered disposition of sulfamethoxazole and trimethoprim in these patients
  Use in the elderly—Elderly patients may be at increased risk of severe side/adverse effects
  Other medications, especially coumarin- or indandione-derivative anticoagulants, hydantoin anticonvulsants, oral antidiabetic agents, other hemolytics, other hepatotoxic medications, or methotrexate
  Other medical problems, especially blood dyscrasias, G6PD deficiency, hepatic function impairment, megaloblastic anemia due to folic acid deficiency, porphyria, and renal function impairment

Proper use of this medication
» Maintaining adequate fluid intake
  Proper administration technique for oral liquids
» Compliance with full course of therapy
» Importance of not missing doses and taking at evenly spaced times
» Proper dosing
  Missed dose: Taking as soon as possible; not taking if almost time for next dose; not doubling doses
» Proper storage

Precautions while using this medication
» Regular visits to physician to check blood counts
  Checking with physician if no improvement within a few days
  Using caution in use of regular toothbrushes, dental floss, and toothpicks; deferring dental work until blood counts have returned to normal; checking with physician or dentist concerning proper oral hygiene
» Possible skin photosensitivity; avoiding unprotected exposure to sun; using protective clothing; using a sun block product that includes protection against both UVA-caused photosensitivity reactions and UVB-caused sunburn reactions; avoiding use of sunlamp, tanning bed, or tanning booth
» Caution if dizziness occurs

Side/adverse effects

Severe skin problems and blood problems may be more likely to occur in elderly patients who are taking sulfamethoxazole and trimethoprim combination, especially if diuretics are being taken concurrently

Signs of potential side effects, especially blood dyscrasias, crystalluria, goiter, hematuria, hepatitis, hypersensitivity, interstitial nephritis, methemoglobinemia, photosensitivity, Stevens-Johnson syndrome, thyroid function disturbance, toxic epidermal necrolysis, and tubular necrosis

---

▲ For the Patient ▲

918030

ABOUT YOUR MEDICINE

Sulfamethoxazole and **trimethoprim** (sul-fa-meth-OX-a-zole and trye-METH-oh-prim) combination is used to treat infections such as bronchitis, middle ear infection, urinary tract infection, and traveler's diarrhea. It is also used for the prevention and treatment of *Pneumocystis carinii* (noo-moe-siss-tis ka-RIN-ee-eye) pneumonia (PCP). However, it will not work for colds, flu, or other virus infections. Sulfamethoxazole and trimethoprim may also be used for other conditions as determined by your doctor.

If any of the information in this leaflet causes you special concern or if you want additional information about your medicine and its use, check with your doctor, nurse, or pharmacist. **Remember, keep this and all other medicines out of the reach of children and never share your medicines with others.**

BEFORE USING THIS MEDICINE

Tell your doctor, nurse, and pharmacist if you . . .
- are allergic to any medicine, either prescription or nonprescription (OTC);
- are pregnant or intend to become pregnant while using this medicine;
- are breast-feeding;
- are taking **any** other prescription or nonprescription (OTC) medicine;
- have any other medical problems, especially anemia or other blood problems, glucose-6-phosphate dehydrogenase (G6PD) deficiency, kidney disease, liver disease, or porphyria.

PROPER USE OF THIS MEDICINE

Sulfamethoxazole and trimethoprim is best taken with a full glass (8 ounces) of water. Several additional glasses of water should be taken every day, unless otherwise directed by your doctor. Drinking extra water will help to prevent some unwanted effects of sulfamethoxazole and trimethoprim.

To help clear up your infection completely, **keep taking this medicine for the full time of treatment** even if you feel better after a few days; **do not miss any doses.**

If you do miss a dose of this medicine, take it as soon as possible. However, if it is almost time for your next dose, skip the missed dose and go back to your regular dosing schedule. Do not double doses.

PRECAUTIONS WHILE USING THIS MEDICINE

It is very important that your doctor check your progress at regular visits. This medicine may cause blood problems, especially if it is taken for a long time.

If your symptoms do not improve within a few days, or if they become worse, check with your doctor.

Some people who take this medicine may become more sensitive to sunlight than they are normally. **When you begin taking this medicine, avoid too much sun and do not use a sunlamp until you see how you react to the sun,** especially if you tend to burn easily. This sensitivity may last for many months after you stop taking this medicine. **If you have a severe reaction, check with your doctor.**

This medicine may also cause some people to become dizzy. **Make sure you know how you react to this medicine before you drive, use machines, or do other jobs that require you to be alert.** If this reaction is especially bothersome, check with your doctor.

This medicine must not be given to other people or used for other infections unless you are otherwise directed by your doctor.

POSSIBLE SIDE EFFECTS OF THIS MEDICINE
Side Effects That Should Be Reported To Your Doctor Immediately

> *More common*—Itching or skin rash

> *Less common*—Aching of joints and muscles; difficulty in swallowing; pale skin; redness, blistering, peeling, or loosening of skin; sore throat and fever; unusual bleeding or bruising; unusual tiredness or weakness; yellow eyes or skin

> *Rare*—Blood in urine; bluish fingernails, lips, or skin; difficult breathing; greatly increased or decreased frequency of urination or amount of urine; increased thirst; lower back pain; pain or burning while urinating; swelling of front part of neck

Other Side Effects That Should Be Reported To Your Doctor

> *More common*—Increased sensitivity of skin to sunlight

Side Effects That Usually Do Not Require Medical Attention

These possible side effects may go away during treatment; however, if they continue or are bothersome, check with your doctor, nurse, or pharmacist.

More common—Diarrhea; dizziness; headache; loss of
appetite; nausea or vomiting

Other side effects not listed above may also occur in some
patients. If you notice any other effects, check with your
doctor, nurse, or pharmacist.

SULFASALAZINE   Systemic

■ For the Pharmacist ■

In providing consultation, consider emphasizing the following selected information (» = major clinical significance):

Before using this medication
» Conditions affecting use, especially:

Allergies to sulfonamides, salicylates, furosemide, thiazide diuretics, sulfonylureas, carbonic anhydrase inhibitors

Pregnancy—Sulfasalazine and sulfapyridine cross the placenta

Breast-feeding—Sulfasalazine and sulfapyridine are excreted in breast milk

Use in children—Use is contraindicated in infants and children up to 2 years of age since sulfonamides may cause kernicterus

Other medications, especially coumarin- or indandione-derivative anticoagulants, hydantoin anticonvulsants, oral antidiabetic agents, hemolytics, hepatotoxic medications, and methotrexate

Other medical problems, especially blood dyscrasias, G6PD deficiency, hepatic function impairment, porphyria, and renal function impairment

Proper use of this medication
» Not giving to infants up to 2 years of age; sulfasalazine may cause kernicterus

Taking after meals or with food to lessen gastrointestinal irritation
» Maintaining adequate fluid intake

Proper administration technique for enteric-coated tablets
» Compliance with full course of therapy
» Proper dosing

Missed dose: Taking as soon as possible; not taking if almost time for next dose; not doubling doses
» Proper storage

Precautions while using this medication
» Regular visits to physician to check blood counts in patients on long-term therapy

Checking with physician if no improvement within a month or 2

Using caution in use of regular toothbrushes, dental floss, and toothpicks; deferring dental work until blood counts have returned to normal; checking with physician or dentist concerning proper oral hygiene
» Possible photosensitivity reactions
» Caution if dizziness occurs

Possible interference with bentiromide diagnostic test for pancreatic function

Side/adverse effects
Signs of potential side effects, especially blood dyscrasias, headache (continuing), hepatitis, interstitial pneumonitis, hypersensitivity, Lyell's syndrome, photosensitivity, Stevens-Johnson syndrome, and exacerbation of ulcerative colitis

Orange-yellow discoloration of alkaline urine or skin may be alarming to patient although medically insignificant

---

▲ For the Patient ▲

914924

ABOUT YOUR MEDICINE

Sulfasalazine (sul-fa-SAL-a-zeen), a sulfa medicine, is used to prevent and treat inflammatory bowel disease, such as ulcerative colitis. Sulfasalazine is sometimes given with other medicines to treat inflammatory bowel disease. Sulfasalazine may also be used for other conditions as determined by your doctor. However, this medicine will not work for all kinds of infection the way other sulfa medicines do.

If any of the information in this leaflet causes you special concern or if you want additional information about your medicine and its use, check with your doctor, nurse, or pharmacist. **Remember, keep this and all other medicines out of the reach of children and never share your medicines with others.**

BEFORE USING THIS MEDICINE

Tell your doctor, nurse, and pharmacist if you . . .
- are allergic to any medicine, either prescription or nonprescription (OTC);
- are pregnant or intend to become pregnant while using this medicine;
- are breast-feeding;
- are taking **any** other prescription or nonprescription (OTC) medicine;
- have any other medical problems, especially blood problems; glucose-6-phosphate dehydrogenase (G6PD) deficiency; kidney disease; liver disease; or porphyria.

PROPER USE OF THIS MEDICINE

Do not give sulfasalazine to infants up to 2 years of age unless otherwise directed by your doctor. It may cause brain problems.

Sulfasalazine is best taken after meals or with food to lessen stomach upset. If stomach upset continues or is bothersome, check with your doctor.

Each dose of sulfasalazine should also be taken with a full glass (8 ounces) of water. Several additional glasses of water should be taken every day, unless otherwise directed by your doctor. Drinking extra water will help to prevent some unwanted effects (e.g., kidney stones) of the sulfa medicine.

If you are taking the enteric-coated tablet form of this medicine, swallow the tablets whole. Do not break or crush them.

Keep taking this medicine for the full time of treatment even if you begin to feel better after a few days; **do not miss any doses.**

If you do miss a dose of this medicine, take it as soon as possible. However, if it is almost time for your next dose, skip the missed dose and go back to your regular dosing schedule. Do not double doses.

PRECAUTIONS WHILE USING THIS MEDICINE

If your symptoms (including diarrhea) do not improve within a month or 2, or if they become worse, check with your doctor.

It is very important that your doctor check your progress at regular visits. This medicine may cause blood problems, especially if it is taken for a long time. These problems may result in a greater chance of certain infections, slow healing, and bleeding of the gums. Be careful when using regular toothbrushes, dental floss, and toothpicks. Dental work should be delayed until your blood counts have returned to normal. Check with your medical doctor or dentist if you have any questions.

Sulfasalazine may cause your skin to be more sensitive to sunlight than it is normally. Avoid too much sun and do not use a sunlamp until you see how you react. You may still be more sensitive to sunlight or sunlamps for many months after you stop taking this medicine. **If you have a severe reaction, check with your doctor.**

This medicine may also cause some people to become dizzy. **Make sure you know how you react to this medicine before you drive, use machines, or do other jobs that require you to be alert.** If this reaction is especially bothersome, check with your doctor.

POSSIBLE SIDE EFFECTS OF THIS MEDICINE
Side Effects That Should Be Reported To Your Doctor Immediately

More common—Aching of joints and muscles; headache (continuing); itching; skin rash

Less common—Back, leg, or stomach pains; difficulty in swallowing; fever and sore throat; pale skin; redness, blistering, peeling, or loosening of skin; unusual bleeding or bruising; unusual tiredness or weakness; yellow eyes or skin

Rare—Bloody diarrhea, fever, and rash; cough; difficult breathing

Other Side Effects That Should Be Reported To Your Doctor

More common—Increased sensitivity of skin to sunlight

Side Effects That Usually Do Not Require Medical Attention

These possible side effects may go away during treatment; however, if they continue or are bothersome, check with your doctor, nurse, or pharmacist.

More common—Abdominal or stomach pain or upset; diarrhea; dizziness; loss of appetite; nausea or vomiting

In some patients, this medicine may also cause the urine or skin to become orange-yellow. This side effect does not need medical attention.

Other side effects not listed above may also occur in some patients. If you notice any other effects, check with your doctor, nurse, or pharmacist.

SULFINPYRAZONE Systemic

■ For the Pharmacist ■

In providing consultation, consider emphasizing the following selected
information (» = major clinical significance):

Before using this medication
» Conditions affecting use, especially:
    Sensitivity to sulfinpyrazone or NSAIDs, especially aspirin, ox-
        yphenbutazone, or phenylbutazone, history of
    Other medications, especially anticoagulants, rapidly cytolytic
        antineoplastic agents, aspirin or other salicylates, hypopro-
        thrombinemia-inducing cephalosporins, moxalactam, nitro-
        furantoin, platelet aggregation inhibitors, plicamycin, and
        valproic acid
    Other medical problems, especially cancer treated with rapidly
        cytolytic antineoplastic agents or radiation therapy, renal cal-
        culi or history of (especially uric acid calculi), renal function
        impairment, blood dyscrasias, gastrointestinal inflammation
        or ulceration, and active peptic ulcer

Proper use of this medication
» Taking with food or an antacid to minimize gastrointestinal irritation
» Compliance with therapy
    Importance of high fluid intake and compliance with therapy for
        alkalinization of urine, if prescribed, to minimize kidney stone
        formation
» Proper dosing
    Missed dose: Taking as soon as possible; not taking if almost time
        for next dose; not doubling doses
» Proper storage
For use as antigout agent
    Several months of continuous therapy may be required for maximum
        effectiveness
» Medication does not relieve acute gout attacks but rather helps to
    prevent them; need to continue taking sulfinpyrazone with med-
    ication prescribed for gout attacks

Precautions while using this medication
    Regular visits to physician to check progress during therapy
    Caution if any laboratory tests required; possible interference with
        test results
For use as antihyperuricemic (including gout therapy)
» Aspirin or other salicylates may decrease the uricosuric effects of
    sulfinpyrazone; checking with physician regarding concurrent
    use, since effect is dependent on salicylate dose and duration of
    use
» Possibility that alcohol taken in large amounts may increase blood
    uric acid concentration and reduce effectiveness of medication

Side/adverse effects
    Signs and symptoms of potential side effects, especially renal calculi,
        dermatitis, blood dyscrasias, fever, gastrointestinal bleeding, and
        renal failure

▲ For the Patient ▲

914935

ABOUT YOUR MEDICINE

Sulfinpyrazone (sul-fin-PEER-a-zone) is used in the treatment of chronic gout or gouty arthritis, which is caused by too much uric acid in the blood. Sulfinpyrazone does not cure gout, but after you have been taking it for a few months, it may help prevent gout attacks. This medicine will help prevent gout attacks only as long as you continue to take it.

Sulfinpyrazone is sometimes used to prevent or treat other medical problems that may occur if too much uric acid is present in the body. It may also be used for other conditions as determined by your doctor.

If any of the information in this leaflet causes you special concern or if you want additional information about your medicine and its use, check with your doctor, nurse, or pharmacist. **Remember, keep this and all other medicines out of the reach of children and never share your medicines with others.**

BEFORE USING THIS MEDICINE

Tell your doctor, nurse, and pharmacist if you . . .
* are allergic to any medicine, either prescription or non-prescription (OTC);
* are pregnant or intend to become pregnant while using this medicine;
* are breast-feeding;
* are taking **any** other prescription or nonprescription (OTC) medicine;
* have any other medical problems, especially a history of blood disease, kidney stones, or stomach problems; or kidney disease;
* are being treated with x-rays or cancer medicines.

PROPER USE OF THIS MEDICINE

If this medicine upsets your stomach, it may be taken with food. If this does not work, an antacid may be taken. If stomach upset (nausea, vomiting, or stomach pain) continues, check with your doctor.

In order for sulfinpyrazone to help you, it must be taken regularly as ordered by your doctor.

When you first begin taking sulfinpyrazone, the amount of uric acid in the kidneys is greatly increased. This may cause kidney stones. To help prevent this, your doctor may want you to drink at least 10 to 12 glasses (8 ounces each) of fluids each day, or to take another medicine to make your urine less acid. **It is important that you follow your doctor's instructions carefully.**

For patients taking sulfinpyrazone for gout:
- After you begin to take sulfinpyrazone, gout attacks may continue to occur. However, if you take this medicine regularly as directed, the attacks will become less frequent and less painful. After you have been taking sulfinpyrazone for several months, they may stop completely.
- Sulfinpyrazone helps to prevent gout attacks. It will not relieve an attack that has already started. **Even if you take another medicine for gout attacks, continue to take this medicine also.**

If you miss a dose of this medicine, take it as soon as possible. However, if it is almost time for your next dose, skip the missed dose and go back to your regular dosing schedule. Do not double doses.

PRECAUTIONS WHILE USING THIS MEDICINE

Your doctor should check your progress at regular visits in order to make sure that this medicine does not cause unwanted effects.

Taking aspirin or other salicylates may lessen the effects of sulfinpyrazone. This will depend on the dose of aspirin or other salicylate that you take, and how often you take it. Also, drinking too much alcohol may increase the amount of uric acid in the blood and lessen the effects of sulfinpyrazone. Therefore, **do not take aspirin or other salicylates or drink alcoholic beverages while taking this medicine,** unless you have first checked with your doctor.

POSSIBLE SIDE EFFECTS OF THIS MEDICINE

Side Effects That Should Be Reported To Your Doctor Immediately

Rare—Shortness of breath, troubled breathing, tightness in chest, or wheezing; sore throat and fever; sores, ulcers, or white spots on lips or in mouth; swollen or painful glands; unusual bleeding or bruising

Other Side Effects That Should Be Reported To Your Doctor

More common—Lower back or side pain; painful urination (possibly with blood)

Less common—Skin rash

Rare—Bloody or black, tarry stools; fever; increased blood pressure; pinpoint red spots on skin; sudden decrease in amount of urine; swelling of face, fingers, feet, or lower legs; unusual tiredness or weakness; vomiting of blood or material that looks like coffee grounds; weight gain

Side Effects That Usually Do Not Require Medical Attention

These possible side effects may go away during treatment; however, if they continue or are bothersome, check with your doctor, nurse, or pharmacist.

More common—Joint pain, redness, or swelling; nausea or vomiting; stomach pain

Other side effects not listed above may also occur in some patients. If you notice any other effects, check with your doctor, nurse, or pharmacist.

SULFONAMIDES   Systemic

Including Sulfacytine; Sulfadiazine; Sulfamethizole;
Sulfamethoxazole; Sulfisoxazole.

■For the Pharmacist■

In providing consultation, consider emphasizing the following selected
   information (» = major clinical significance):

Before using this medication
» Conditions affecting use, especially:
   Allergy to sulfonamides, furosemide, thiazide diuretics, sulfon-
      ylureas, carbonic anhydrase inhibitors
   Pregnancy—Sulfonamides cross the placenta
   Breast-feeding—Sulfonamides are excreted in breast milk; may
      cause kernicterus in nursing infants
   Use in children—Sulfamethoxazole and sulfisoxazole are con-
      traindicated in infants up to 2 months of age since sulfon-
      amides may cause kernicterus in neonates; sulfacytine is not
      recommended in children up to 14 years of age
   Other medications, especially coumarin- or indandione-deriva-
      tive anticoagulants, hydantoin anticonvulsants, oral antidi-
      abetic agents, other hemolytics, other hepatotoxic medica-
      tions, methenamine, or methotrexate
   Other medical problems, especially blood dyscrasias, G6PD de-
      ficiency, hepatic function impairment, megaloblastic anemia,
      porphyria, and renal function impairment

Proper use of this medication
» Not giving to children under 14 years of age (sulfacytine) or to
      infants under 2 months of age (other sulfonamides)
» Maintaining adequate fluid intake
   Proper administration technique for oral liquids
» Compliance with full course of therapy
» Importance of not missing doses and taking at evenly spaced times
» Proper dosing
   Missed dose: Taking as soon as possible; not taking if almost time
      for next dose; not doubling doses
» Proper storage

Precautions while using this medication
» Regular visits to physician to check blood counts
   Checking with physician if no improvement within a few days
   Using caution in use of regular toothbrushes, dental floss, and tooth-
      picks; deferring dental work until blood counts have returned to
      normal; checking with physician or dentist concerning proper
      oral hygiene
» Possible photosensitivity reactions
» Caution if dizziness occurs

Side/adverse effects
   Severe skin problems and blood problems may be more likely to
      occur in the elderly who are taking sulfamethoxazole and tri-
      methoprim combination, especially if taking diuretics concur-
      rently
   Signs of potential side effects, especially blood dyscrasias, crystal-
      luria, goiter, hematuria, hepatitis, hypersensitivity, interstitial
      nephritis, Lyell's syndrome, photosensitivity, Stevens-Johnson
      syndrome, thyroid function disturbance, and tubular necrosis

▲ For the Patient ▲

912667

ABOUT YOUR MEDICINE

Sulfonamides (sul-FON-a-mides) are used to treat infections. However, they will not work for colds, flu, or other virus infections.

If any of the information in this leaflet causes you special concern or if you want additional information about your medicine and its use, check with your doctor, nurse, or pharmacist. **Remember, keep this and all other medicines out of the reach of children and never share your medicines with others.**

BEFORE USING THIS MEDICINE

Tell your doctor, nurse, and pharmacist if you . . .
- are allergic to any medicine, either prescription or nonprescription (OTC);
- are pregnant or intend to become pregnant while using this medicine;
- are breast-feeding;
- are taking **any** other prescription or nonprescription (OTC) medicine;
- have any other medical problems, especially anemia or other blood problems, glucose-6-phosphate dehydrogenase (G6PD) deficiency, kidney disease, liver disease, or porphyria.

PROPER USE OF THIS MEDICINE

Sulfonamides are best taken with a full glass (8 ounces) of water. Several additional glasses of water should be taken every day, unless otherwise directed by your doctor. Drinking extra water will help to prevent some unwanted effects of sulfonamides.

To help clear up your infection completely, **keep taking this medicine for the full time of treatment** even if you feel better after a few days; **do not miss any doses**.

If you do miss a dose of this medicine, take it as soon as possible. However, if it is almost time for your next dose, skip the missed dose and go back to your regular dosing schedule. Do not double doses.

PRECAUTIONS WHILE USING THIS MEDICINE

It is very important that your doctor check your progress at regular visits. This medicine may cause blood problems, especially if it is taken for a long time.

If your symptoms do not improve within a few days, or if they become worse, check with your doctor.

Some people who take sulfonamides may become more sensitive to sunlight than they are normally. **When you begin taking this medicine, avoid too much sun and do not use a**

sunlamp until you see how you react to the sun, especially if you tend to burn easily. This sensitivity may last for many months after you stop taking this medicine. **If you have a severe reaction, check with your doctor.**

This medicine may also cause some people to become dizzy. **Make sure you know how you react to this medicine before you drive, use machines, or do other jobs that require you to be alert.** If this reaction is especially bothersome, check with your doctor.

This medicine must not be given to other people or used for other infections unless you are otherwise directed by your doctor.

POSSIBLE SIDE EFFECTS OF THIS MEDICINE

Side Effects That Should Be Reported To Your Doctor Immediately

More common—Itching or skin rash

Less common—Aching of joints and muscles; difficulty in swallowing; pale skin; redness, blistering, peeling, or loosening of skin; sore throat and fever; unusual bleeding or bruising; unusual tiredness or weakness; yellow eyes or skin

Rare—Blood in urine; bluish fingernails, lips, or skin; difficult breathing; greatly increased or decreased frequency of urination or amount of urine; increased thirst; lower back pain; pain or burning while urinating; swelling of front part of neck

Other Side Effects That Should Be Reported To Your Doctor

More common—Increased sensitivity of skin to sunlight

Side Effects That Usually Do Not Require Medical Attention

These possible side effects may go away during treatment; however, if they continue or are bothersome, check with your doctor, nurse, or pharmacist.

More common—Diarrhea; dizziness; headache; loss of appetite; nausea or vomiting; tiredness

Other side effects not listed above may also occur in some patients. If you notice any other effects, check with your doctor, nurse, or pharmacist.

SULFONAMIDES AND PHENAZOPYRIDINE Systemic

Including Sulfamethoxazole and Phenazopyridine;
Sulfisoxazole and Phenazopyridine.

■ For the Pharmacist ■

In providing consultation, consider emphasizing the following selected
information (» = major clinical significance):

Before using this medication
» Conditions affecting use, especially:

> Allergies to sulfonamides, furosemide, thiazide diuretics, sul-
> fonylureas, carbonic anhydrase inhibitors, or phenazopyr-
> idine

> Pregnancy—Sulfonamides cross the placenta; use is contrain-
> dicated at term since sulfonamides may cause kernicterus

> Breast-feeding—Sulfonamides are excreted in breast milk; may
> cause kernicterus in the nursing infant

> Use in children—Use is contraindicated in children up to 12
> years of age

> Other medications, especially coumarin- or indandione-deriva-
> tive anticoagulants, hydantoin anticonvulsants, oral antidi-
> abetic agents, hemolytics, hepatotoxic medications, meth-
> enamine, and methotrexate

> Other medical problems, especially blood dyscrasias, G6PD de-
> ficiency, hepatic function impairment, hepatitis, megalo-
> blastic anemia due to folate deficiency, porphyria, and renal
> function impairment

Proper use of this medication
» Maintaining adequate fluid intake; taking with or following meals
   if gastrointestinal irritation occurs
» Compliance with full course of therapy
» Importance of not missing doses and taking at evenly spaced times
» Proper dosing; not giving to infants and children up to 12 years of
   age

> Missed dose: Taking as soon as possible; not taking if almost time
> for next dose; not doubling doses

» Proper storage

Precautions while using this medication

> Checking with physician if no improvement within a few days or if
> symptoms become worse

> Using caution with regular toothbrushes, dental floss, and tooth-
> picks; deferring dental work until blood counts have returned to
> normal; checking with physician or dentist concerning proper
> oral hygiene

» Possible photosensitivity reactions
» Caution if dizziness occurs
» Medication causes urine to turn reddish orange and may stain cloth-
   ing
» Diabetics: May cause false urine sugar and urine ketone test results

Side/adverse effects

> Reddish orange discoloration of urine may be alarming to patient
> although medically insignificant

> Signs of potential side effects, especially blood dyscrasias, crystal-
> luria, goiter, headache, hematuria, hemolytic anemia, hepatitis,

hypersensitivity, interstitial nephritis, Lyell's syndrome, methemoglobinemia, photosensitivity, Stevens-Johnson syndrome, thyroid function disturbance, and tubular necrosis

▲ For the Patient ▲

914968

ABOUT YOUR MEDICINE

Sulfonamide (sul-FON-a-mide) and **phenazopyridine** (fen-az-oh-PEER-i-deen) combinations are used to treat infections of the urinary tract and to help relieve the pain, burning, and irritation of these infections.

If any of the information in this leaflet causes you special concern or if you want additional information about your medicine and its use, check with your doctor, nurse, or pharmacist. **Remember, keep this and all other medicines out of the reach of children and never share your medicines with others.**

BEFORE USING THIS MEDICINE

Tell your doctor, nurse, and pharmacist if you . . .
- are allergic to any medicine, either prescription or nonprescription (OTC);
- are pregnant or intend to become pregnant while using this medicine;
- are breast-feeding;
- are taking **any** other prescription or nonprescription (OTC) medicine;
- have any other medical problems, especially anemia or other blood problems, glucose-6-phosphate dehydrogenase (G6PD) deficiency, hepatitis or other liver disease, kidney disease, or porphyria.

PROPER USE OF THIS MEDICINE

Sulfonamides and phenazopyridine combinations are best taken with a full glass (8 ounces) of water. This medicine may be taken with meals or following meals if it upsets your stomach.

Several additional glasses of water should be taken every day, unless you are otherwise directed by your doctor. Drinking extra water will help to prevent some unwanted effects (e.g., kidney stones) of the sulfonamide.

To help clear up your infection completely, **keep taking this medicine for the full time of treatment** even if you begin to feel better after a few days. If you stop taking this medicine too soon, your symptoms may return.

If you miss a dose of this medicine, take it as soon as possible. This will help to keep a constant amount of medicine in the urine. However, if it is almost time for your next dose, skip the missed dose and go back to your regular dosing schedule. Do not double doses.

PRECAUTIONS WHILE USING THIS MEDICINE

This medicine causes the urine to turn reddish orange. This is to be expected while you are using this medicine and is not harmful. Also, the medicine may stain clothing.

Diabetics—This medicine may cause false test results with some urine sugar tests and urine ketone tests. Check with your doctor before changing your diet or the dosage of your diabetes medicine.

If your symptoms do not improve within a few days, or if they become worse, check with your doctor.

Sulfonamides may cause your skin to be more sensitive to sunlight than it is normally. When you first begin taking this medicine, avoid too much sun and do not use a sunlamp until you see how you react to the sun, especially if you tend to burn easily. You may still be more sensitive to sunlight or sunlamps for many months after stopping this medicine. **If you have a severe reaction, check with your doctor.**

Make sure you know how you react to this medicine before you drive, use machines, or do other jobs that require you to be alert.

This medicine must not be given to other people or used for other infections unless you are otherwise directed by your doctor.

POSSIBLE SIDE EFFECTS OF THIS MEDICINE

Side Effects That Should Be Reported To Your Doctor Immediately

   More common—Itching; skin rash

   Less common—Aching of joints and muscles; blue or blue-purple discoloration of skin; difficulty in swallowing; pale skin; redness, blistering, peeling, or loosening of skin; shortness of breath; sore throat and fever; unusual bleeding or bruising; unusual tiredness or weakness; yellow eyes or skin

   Rare—Blood in urine; greatly increased or decreased frequency of urination; increased thirst; lower back pain; pain or burning while urinating; swelling of front part of neck

Other Side Effects That Should Be Reported To Your Doctor

   More common—Increased sensitivity of skin to sunlight

Side Effects That Usually Do Not Require Medical Attention

These possible side effects may go away during treatment; however, if they continue or are bothersome, check with your doctor, nurse, or pharmacist.

   More common—Diarrhea; dizziness; headache; loss of appetite; nausea or vomiting; tiredness

Other side effects not listed above may also occur in some patients. If you notice any other effects, check with your doctor, nurse, or pharmacist.

SUMATRIPTAN   Systemic

Including Sumatriptan (Injection); Sumatriptan (Oral).

■For the Pharmacist■

In providing consultation, consider emphasizing the following selected information (» = major clinical significance):

Before using this medication
» Conditions affecting use, especially:
   Sensitivity to sumatriptan
   Other medical problems, especially conditions that may be adversely affected by coronary artery constriction, uncontrolled hypertension, tachycardia, and history of cerebrovascular accident

Proper use of this medication
   Administering at first sign of headache (aura or pain)
   Additional benefit may be obtained if the patient lies down in a quiet, dark room after administering medication
» Not using additional doses if a first dose does not provide substantial relief; additional sumatriptan is not likely to be effective in these circumstances; taking alternate medication as previously advised by physician instead
» Taking additional doses, if needed, for return of migraine after initial relief was obtained, provided that prescribed limits (quantity used and frequency of administration) are not exceeded
» Compliance with prophylactic therapy, if prescribed
» Proper administration of
   Tablets—Swallowing whole; not breaking, crushing or chewing before taking
   Injection—
      Reading patient instructions provided with medication
      Proper injection technique
      Discarding used cartridge as directed in patient instructions, using container provided; not discarding autoinjector unit because refill cartridges are available
» Proper dosing
» Proper storage

Precautions while using this medication
   Checking with physician if usual dose fails to relieve 3 consecutive headaches, or if frequency and/or severity of headaches increases
   Avoiding alcohol, which aggravates headache
» Caution if drowsiness or dizziness occurs

Side/adverse effects
   Contacting physician immediately if severe chest pain or signs and symptoms of anaphylactoid reaction occur
   Contacting physician at once if mild pain or tightness in chest or throat occurs and persists for more than 1 hour; even if symptoms are of shorter duration, not using medication again without first consulting physician
   Signs and symptoms of other potential side effects, including dysphagia, palpitation, and skin rash or eruptions

▲ For the Patient ▲

919123

SUMATRIPTAN (Injection)

ABOUT YOUR MEDICINE

Sumatriptan (soo-ma-TRIP-tan) is used to treat severe migraine headaches. It will not relieve any kind of pain other than headaches. However, sumatriptan often relieves other symptoms that occur together with a migraine headache, such as nausea, vomiting, sensitivity to light, and sensitivity to sound.

If any of the information in this leaflet causes you special concern or if you want additional information about your medicine and its use, check with your doctor, nurse, or pharmacist. **Remember, keep this and all other medicines out of the reach of children and never share your medicines with others.**

BEFORE USING THIS MEDICINE

Tell your doctor, nurse, and pharmacist if you . . .
- are allergic to any medicine, either prescription or non-prescription (OTC);
- are pregnant or intend to become pregnant while using this medicine;
- are breast-feeding;
- are taking any other prescription or nonprescription (OTC) medicine;
- have any other medical problems, especially heart or blood vessel disease.

PROPER USE OF THIS MEDICINE

To relieve your migraine as soon as possible, use sumatriptan at the first sign that the headache is coming. If you get warning signals of a coming migraine (an aura), you may use the medicine before the headache pain actually starts. However, even if you do not use sumatriptan until your migraine has been present for several hours, the medicine will still work.

Lying down in a quiet, dark room for a while after you use this medicine may help relieve your migraine.

If you do not feel much better in 1 to 2 hours after an injection of sumatriptan, **do not use any more of this medicine for the same migraine.** A migraine that is not relieved by the first dose of sumatriptan will probably not be relieved by a second dose, either. Ask your doctor ahead of time about other medicine to be used if sumatriptan does not work. However, even if sumatriptan does not relieve one migraine, it may still relieve the next one.

If you feel much better after a dose of sumatriptan, but your headache comes back or gets worse after a while, you may use more sumatriptan. However, **use this medicine only as** directed by your doctor. **Do not use more of it, and do not use it more often than directed.** Using too much sumatriptan may increase the chance of side effects.

Your doctor may direct you to use another medicine to help prevent headaches. **It is important that you follow your doctor's directions, even if your headaches continue to occur.**

This medicine comes with patient directions. **Read them carefully before using the medicine,** and check with your doctor or pharmacist if you have any questions.

Your doctor or nurse will teach you how to inject yourself with the medicine. **Be sure to follow the directions carefully. Check with your doctor or nurse if you have any problems using the medicine.**

Be sure to follow the patient directions about safely discarding the empty cartridge and the needle. Keep the autoinjector unit, because refills are available.

PRECAUTIONS WHILE USING THIS MEDICINE

Check with your doctor if you have used sumatriptan for 3 headaches, and have not had good relief. Also, check with your doctor if your migraine headaches are worse, or if they occur more often, than before you started using sumatriptan.

Drinking alcoholic beverages can cause headaches or make them worse. People who suffer from severe headaches should probably avoid alcoholic beverages, especially during a headache.

Some people feel drowsy or dizzy during or after a migraine, or after using sumatriptan. As long as you are feeling drowsy or dizzy, **do not drive, use machines, or do other jobs that require you to be alert and clearheaded.**

POSSIBLE SIDE EFFECTS OF THIS MEDICINE

Side Effects That Should Be Reported To Your Doctor Immediately

Stop using this medicine and check with your doctor immediately if any of the following side effects occur:

Rare—Chest pain (severe); swelling of eyelids, face, or lips; wheezing

Check with your doctor right away if any of the following side effects continue for more than 1 hour. Even if they go away in less than 1 hour, **check with your doctor before using any more sumatriptan if the following side effects occur:**

Less common—Chest pain (mild); heaviness, tightness, or pressure in chest or neck

Side Effects That Should Be Reported To Your Doctor

Less common—Difficulty in swallowing; pounding heartbeat; skin rash or bumps on skin

Side Effects That Usually Do Not Require Medical Attention

These possible side effects may go away during treatment; however, if they continue or are bothersome, check with your doctor, nurse, or pharmacist.

> *More common*—Burning, pain, or redness at place of injection; discomfort in jaw, mouth, tongue, throat, nose, or sinuses; dizziness; drowsiness; feeling cold, "strange," or weak; feeling of burning, warmth, heat, numbness, tightness, or tingling; flushing; lightheadedness; muscle aches, cramps, or stiffness; nausea or vomiting

Other side effects not listed above may also occur in some patients. If you notice any other effects, check with your doctor, nurse, or pharmacist.

▲ For the Patient ▲

919134

SUMATRIPTAN (Oral)

ABOUT YOUR MEDICINE

Sumatriptan (soo-ma-TRIP-tan) is used to treat severe migraine headaches. It will not relieve any kind of pain other than headaches. However, sumatriptan often relieves other symptoms that occur together with a migraine headache, such as nausea, vomiting, sensitivity to light, and sensitivity to sound.

If any of the information in this leaflet causes you special concern or if you want additional information about your medicine and its use, check with your doctor, nurse, or pharmacist. **Remember, keep this and all other medicines out of the reach of children and never share your medicines with others.**

BEFORE USING THIS MEDICINE

Tell your doctor, nurse, and pharmacist if you . . .
- are allergic to any medicine, either prescription or nonprescription (OTC);
- are pregnant or intend to become pregnant while using this medicine;
- are breast-feeding;
- are taking any other prescription or nonprescription (OTC) medicine;
- have any other medical problems, especially heart or blood vessel disease.

PROPER USE OF THIS MEDICINE

To relieve your migraine as soon as possible, take sumatriptan at the first sign that the headache is coming. If you get warning signals of a coming migraine (an aura), you may take the medicine before the headache pain actually starts. However, even if you do not take sumatriptan until your migraine has been present for several hours, the medicine will still work.

Lying down in a quiet, dark room for a while after you take this medicine may help relieve your migraine.

If you do not feel much better in 2 to 4 hours after a tablet is taken, **do not take any more of this medicine for the same migraine.** A migraine that is not relieved by the first dose of sumatriptan will probably not be relieved by a second dose, either. Ask your doctor ahead of time about other medicine to be taken if sumatriptan does not work. However, even if sumatriptan does not relieve one migraine, it may still relieve the next one.

If you feel much better after a dose of sumatriptan, but your headache comes back or gets worse after a while, you may take more sumatriptan. However, **take this medicine only as directed by your doctor. Do not take more of it, and do not take it more often than directed.** Using too much sumatriptan may increase the chance of side effects.

Your doctor may direct you to take another medicine to help prevent headaches. **It is important that you follow your doctor's directions, even if your headaches continue to occur.**

Sumatriptan tablets are to be swallowed whole. **Do not break, crush, or chew the tablets before swallowing them.**

PRECAUTIONS WHILE USING THIS MEDICINE

Check with your doctor if you have taken sumatriptan for 3 headaches, and have not had good relief. Also, check with your doctor if your migraine headaches are worse, or if they occur more often, than before you started taking sumatriptan.

Drinking alcoholic beverages can cause headaches or make them worse. People who suffer from severe headaches should probably avoid alcoholic beverages, especially during a headache.

Some people feel drowsy or dizzy during or after a migraine, or after taking sumatriptan. As long as you are feeling drowsy or dizzy, **do not drive, use machines, or do other jobs that require you to be alert and clearheaded.**

POSSIBLE SIDE EFFECTS OF THIS MEDICINE
Side Effects That Should Be Reported To Your Doctor Immediately

Stop taking this medicine and check with your doctor immediately if any of the following side effects occur:

Rare—Chest pain (severe); swelling of eyelids, face, or lips; wheezing

Check with your doctor right away if any of the following side effects continue for more than 1 hour. Even if they go away in less than 1 hour, **check with your doctor before using any more sumatriptan if the following side effects occur:**

> *Less common*—Chest pain (mild); heaviness, tightness, or pressure in chest or neck

Side Effects That Should Be Reported To Your Doctor

> *Less common*—Difficulty in swallowing; pounding heartbeat; skin rash or bumps on skin

Side Effects That Usually Do Not Require Medical Attention

These possible side effects may go away during treatment; however, if they continue or are bothersome, check with your doctor, nurse, or pharmacist.

> *More common*—Discomfort in jaw, mouth, tongue, throat, nose, or sinuses; dizziness; drowsiness; feeling cold, "strange," or weak; feeling of burning, warmth, heat, numbness, tightness, or tingling; flushing; lightheadedness; muscle aches, cramps, or stiffness; nausea or vomiting

Other side effects not listed above may also occur in some patients. If you notice any other effects, check with your doctor, nurse, or pharmacist.

TACRINE   Systemic

■ For the Pharmacist ■

In providing consultation, consider emphasizing the following selected information (» = major clinical significance):

Before using this medication
» Conditions affecting use, especially:
Hypersensitivity to tacrine or other acridine derivatives
Other medications, especially cimetidine, neuromuscular blocking agents, NSAIDs, smoking tobacco, and theophylline
Other medical problems, especially asthma, cardiovascular conditions (such as bradycardia, hypotension, or sick sinus syndrome), epilepsy or history of seizures, gastrointestinal or urinary tract obstruction, head injury with loss of consciousness, hepatic function impairment, increased intracranial pressure, intracranial lesions, Parkinson's disease, peptic ulcer, and unstable metabolic disorders

Proper use of this medication
» Not taking more medication than the amount prescribed because of increased risk of adverse effects
Taking tacrine on empty stomach if tolerated
Taking doses at regular intervals for maximum efficacy
» Proper dosing
Missed dose: taking as soon as possible; not taking if within 2 hours of time for next dose; not doubling doses
» Proper storage

Precautions while using this medication
» Importance of complying with monitoring schedule and keeping appointments with physician and/or laboratory
Informing physician when new symptoms arise or when previously noted symptoms increase in severity
Caution if any kind of surgery or emergency treatment is required; informing physician or dentist in charge that tacrine is being taken
Caution if dizziness, clumsiness, or unsteadiness occurs
» Not decreasing dose or discontinuing treatment without consulting physician because of possible decline in cognitive function and behavioral disturbances
» Suspected overdose: Getting emergency help at once

Side/adverse effects
Ataxia; gastrointestinal toxicity, specifically anorexia, diarrhea, nausea, or vomiting; hepatotoxicity; cardiovascular effects, specifically bradycardia, hypertension, hypotension, or palpitation; convulsions; skin rash; syncope; asthma; mood or mental changes, specifically aggression, irritability, or nervousness; parkinsonian extrapyramidal effects; tachycardia; urinary obstruction

▲ For the Patient ▲

919611

ABOUT YOUR MEDICINE

Tacrine (TA-crin) is used to treat the symptoms of mild to moderate Alzheimer's disease. Tacrine will not cure Alzheimer's disease, and it will not stop the disease from getting worse. However, tacrine can improve thinking ability in some patients.

If any of the information in this leaflet causes you special concern or if you want additional information about your medicine and its use, check with your doctor, nurse, or pharmacist. **Remember, keep this and all other medicines out of the reach of children and never share your medicines with others.**

BEFORE USING THIS MEDICINE

Tell your doctor, nurse, and pharmacist if you . . .
- are allergic to any medicine, either prescription or non-prescription (OTC);
- are pregnant or intend to become pregnant while using this medicine;
- are breast-feeding;
- are taking any other prescription or nonprescription (OTC) medicine, especially cimetidine; medicine for pain or inflammation, except narcotics; or theophyllline;
- have **any** other medical problems;
- smoke tobacco.

PROPER USE OF THIS MEDICINE

Take this medicine only as directed by your doctor. Do not take more or less of it, and do not take it more or less often than your doctor ordered. Tacrine seems to work better when it is taken at regularly spaced times, usually four times a day between meals. However, your doctor may want you to take tacrine with food if this medicine upsets your stomach.

PRECAUTIONS WHILE USING THIS MEDICINE

It is important that your doctor check your progress at regular visits. Also, you must have your blood tested regularly to see if this medicine is affecting your liver.

Before having any surgery (including dental surgery) or emergency treatment, tell the medical doctor or dentist in charge that you are taking this medicine.

POSSIBLE SIDE EFFECTS OF THIS MEDICINE

Side Effects That Should Be Reported To Your Doctor

More common—Clumsiness or unsteadiness; diarrhea; loss of appetite; nausea; vomiting

Less common—Fainting; fast or pounding heartbeat; fever; high or low blood pressure; skin rash; slow heartbeat

Rare—Aggression, irritability, or nervousness; change in stool color; convulsions (seizures); cough, tightness in chest, troubled breathing, or wheezing; stiffness of arms or legs, slow movement, or trembling and shaking hands and fingers; trouble in urinating; yellow eyes or skin

Signs of overdose—Convulsions (seizures); greatly increased sweating; greatly increased watering of mouth;

increasing muscle weakness; low blood pressure; nausea (severe); shock (fast weak pulse, irregular breathing, large pupils); slow heartbeat; vomiting (severe)

Side Effects That Usually Do Not Require Medical Attention

These possible side effects may go away during treatment; however, if they continue or are bothersome, check with your doctor, nurse, or pharmacist.

More common—Abdominal or stomach pain or cramping; dizziness; headache; indigestion; muscle aches or pain

Other side effects not listed above may also occur in some patients. If you notice any other effects, check with your doctor, nurse, or pharmacist.

TAMOXIFEN   Systemic

■ For the Pharmacist ■

In providing consultation, consider emphasizing the following selected
information (» = major clinical significance):

Before using this medication
» Conditions affecting use, especially:
    Sensitivity to tamoxifen
    Pregnancy—Use not recommended because of risk of miscar-
    riage, death of the fetus, birth defects, and vaginal bleeding;
    advisability of using nonhormonal contraception during (and
    for about 2 months following) therapy; telling physician im-
    mediately if pregnancy is suspected
    Breast-feeding—Not recommended because of risk of serious
    side effects

Proper use of this medication
» Importance of not taking more or less medication than the amount
    prescribed
    Proper administration of enteric-coated tablets: Swallowing whole
    without crushing or breaking
» Frequency of nausea and vomiting; importance of continuing med-
    ication despite stomach upset
    Checking with physician if vomiting occurs shortly after dose is
    taken
» Proper dosing
    Missed dose: Not taking at all; not doubling doses
» Proper storage

Precautions while using this medication
» Importance of close monitoring by the physician
    For women: May increase fertility; advisability of using nonhor-
    monal contraception during therapy; telling physician immedi-
    ately if pregnancy is suspected
    Not taking an antacid within 1 or 2 hours of taking enteric-coated
    dosage form of tamoxifen

Side/adverse effects
For women: Increased risk of endometrial carcinoma
Signs of potential side effects, especially confusion, hepatotoxicity,
    retinopathy, corneal opacities, pulmonary embolus, thrombosis,
    and weakness or sleepiness
Asymptomatic side effects, including hepatotoxicity and ocular tox-
    icity
Physician or nurse can help in dealing with side effects

▲ For the Patient ▲

916442

ABOUT YOUR MEDICINE

Tamoxifen (ta-MOX-i-fen) is a medicine that blocks the effects of the hormone estrogen in the body. It is used to treat
some cases of breast cancer in females.

If any of the information in this leaflet causes you special
concern or if you want additional information about your

medicine and its use, check with your doctor, nurse, or pharmacist. **Remember, keep this and all other medicines out of the reach of children and never share your medicines with others.**

BEFORE USING THIS MEDICINE

Discuss with your doctor the possible side effects that may be caused by this medicine. Some of them may be serious and/or long-term.

Tell your doctor, nurse, and pharmacist if you . . .
- are allergic to any medicine, either prescription or nonprescription (OTC);
- are pregnant or intend to become pregnant while using this medicine;
- are breast-feeding;
- are taking **any** other prescription or nonprescription (OTC) medicine;
- have any other medical problems.

PROPER USE OF THIS MEDICINE

Use this medicine only as directed by your doctor. Do not use more or less of it, and do not use it more often than your doctor ordered.

Tamoxifen commonly causes nausea and vomiting. However, it is very important that you continue to use the medicine, even if you begin to feel ill. Ask your doctor, nurse, or pharmacist for ways to lessen these effects.

If you vomit shortly after taking a dose of tamoxifen, check with your doctor.

If you miss a dose of this medicine, do not take the missed dose at all and do not double the next one. Instead, go back to your regular dosing schedule and check with your doctor.

PRECAUTIONS WHILE USING THIS MEDICINE

It is very important that your doctor check your progress at regular visits to make sure this medicine is working properly and to check for unwanted effects.

Tamoxifen may make you more fertile. It is best to use some type of birth control while you are taking it. However, do not use oral contraceptives (the "Pill") since they may change the effects of tamoxifen. Tell your doctor right away if you think you have become pregnant while taking this medicine.

POSSIBLE SIDE EFFECTS OF THIS MEDICINE

Tamoxifen has been reported to increase the chance of cancer of the uterus (womb) in some women taking it. Discuss this possible effect with your doctor.

Side Effects That Should Be Reported To Your Doctor

Rare—Blurred vision; confusion; pain or swelling in legs; shortness of breath; vaginal bleeding; weakness or sleepiness; yellow eyes or skin

Side Effects That Usually Do Not Require Medical Attention

These possible side effects may go away during treatment; however, if they continue or are bothersome, check with your doctor, nurse, or pharmacist.

> *More common*—Hot flashes; nausea or vomiting; weight gain
>
> *Less common*—Bone pain; changes in periods; headache; itching in genital area; skin rash or dryness; vaginal discharge

Other side effects not listed above may also occur in some patients. If you notice any other effects, check with your doctor, nurse, or pharmacist.

TERAZOSIN   Systemic

■ For the Pharmacist ■

In providing consultation, consider emphasizing the following selected information (» = major clinical significance):

Before using this medication
» Conditions affecting use, especially:
   Sensitivity to quinazolines
   Use in the elderly—Increased sensitivity to hypotensive effects
   Other medical problems, especially angina, severe cardiac disease, hepatic function impairment, or renal function impairment

Proper use of this medication
   Getting into the habit of taking at same time each day to help increase compliance
» Proper dosing
   Missed dose: Taking as soon as possible the same day; not taking if not remembered until next day; not doubling doses
» Proper storage
For use as an antihypertensive
   Possible need for control of weight and diet, especially sodium intake
» Patient may not experience symptoms of hypertension; importance of taking medication even if feeling well
» Does not cure, but helps control hypertension; possible need for lifelong therapy; serious consequences of untreated hypertension
For use in benign prostatic hyperplasia (BPH)
   Relieves symptoms of BPH but does not change the size of the prostate; may not prevent the need for surgery in the future
   May require 2 to 6 weeks of therapy before patient experiences improvement of symptoms

Precautions while using this medication
   Regular visits to physician to check progress
» Caution if dizziness, lightheadedness, or sudden fainting occurs, especially after initial dose; taking first dose at bedtime
» Caution when getting up suddenly from a lying or sitting position
» Caution in using alcohol, while standing for long periods or exercising, and during hot weather because of enhanced orthostatic hypotensive effects
» Possibility of drowsiness
» Caution when driving or doing anything else requiring alertness because of possible drowsiness, dizziness, or lightheadedness
» Not taking other medication, especially nonprescription sympathomimetics, unless discussed with physician

Side/adverse effects
   Signs of potential side effects, especially angina, dizziness, dyspnea, orthostatic hypotension, palpitations, peripheral edema, and tachycardia

▲ For the Patient ▲

912587

ALPHA₁-BLOCKERS (Oral): *Including Doxazosin; Prazosin; Terazosin.*

ABOUT YOUR MEDICINE

Alpha$_1$-blockers are used to treat high blood pressure (hypertension). Terazosin is also used to treat benign enlargement of the prostate (benign prostatic hyperplasia [BPH]). These medicines may also be used for other conditions as determined by your doctor.

If any of the information in this leaflet causes you special concern or if you want additional information about your medicine and its use, check with your doctor, nurse, or pharmacist. **Remember, keep this and all other medicines out of the reach of children and never share your medicines with others.**

BEFORE USING THIS MEDICINE

Tell your doctor, nurse, and pharmacist if you . . .
- are allergic to any medicine, either prescription or non-prescription (OTC);
- are pregnant or intend to become pregnant while using this medicine;
- are breast-feeding;
- are taking any other prescription or nonprescription (OTC) medicine, especially medicines for appetite control, asthma, colds, cough, hay fever, or sinus;
- have any other medical problems, especially heart disease.

PROPER USE OF THIS MEDICINE

For patients taking this medicine for high blood pressure:
- This medicine will not cure your high blood pressure but it does help control it. You must continue to take it—even if you feel well—if you expect to keep your blood pressure down. **You may have to take high blood pressure medicine for the rest of your life.**

For patients taking terazosin for benign enlargement of the prostate:
- Remember that terazosin will not shrink the size of your prostate, but it does help to relieve the symptoms.
- It may take up to 6 weeks before your symptoms get better.

If you miss a dose of this medicine, take it as soon as possible. However, if it is almost time for your next dose, skip the missed dose and go back to your regular dosing schedule. Do not double doses.

PRECAUTIONS WHILE USING THIS MEDICINE

Dizziness, lightheadedness, or sudden fainting may occur after you take this medicine, especially when you get up from a sitting or lying position. These effects are more likely to occur when you take the first dose of this medicine. Taking the first dose at bedtime may prevent problems. However, **be especially careful if you need to get up during the night.** These effects may also occur with any doses you take after the first dose. Getting up slowly may help lessen this problem. **If you feel dizzy, lie down so that you do not faint.** Then sit for a few minutes before standing to prevent the dizziness from returning.

The dizziness, lightheadedness, or fainting is more likely to occur if you drink alcohol, stand for long periods of time, exercise, or if the weather is hot. **While you are taking this medicine, be careful to limit the amount of alcohol you drink. Also, use extra care during exercise or hot weather or if you must stand for long periods of time.**

This medicine may cause some people to become drowsy or less alert than they are normally. **Make sure you know how you react to this medicine before you drive, use machines, or do other jobs that could be dangerous if you are dizzy, drowsy, or are not alert.** After you have taken several doses of this medicine, these effects should lessen.

POSSIBLE SIDE EFFECTS OF THIS MEDICINE

The following side effects may occur more or less often than listed, depending on which medicine you are taking.

Side Effects That Should Be Reported To Your Doctor

Less common—Dizziness; dizziness or lightheadedness when standing up; fainting (sudden); fast, irregular, or pounding heartbeat; loss of bladder control (prazosin only); shortness of breath; swelling of feet or lower legs

Rare—Chest pain; continuing, painful, inappropriate erection of the penis (prazosin only); shortness of breath (prazosin only)

Side Effects That Usually Do Not Require Medical Attention

These possible side effects may go away during treatment; however, if they continue or are bothersome, check with your doctor, nurse, or pharmacist.

More common—Drowsiness; headache; unusual tiredness or weakness

Less common—Dryness of mouth (prazosin only); nausea; nervousness (doxazosin and prazosin only)

For doxazosin only (in addition to those listed above)—Restlessness; runny nose; unusual irritability

For prazosin only—rare (in addition to those listed above)—Frequent urge to urinate

For terazosin only (in addition to those listed above)—Back or joint pain; blurred vision; stuffy nose

Other side effects not listed above may also occur in some patients. If you notice any other effects, check with your doctor, nurse, or pharmacist.

TERBINAFINE   Topical

■For the Pharmacist■

In providing consultation, consider emphasizing the following selected information (» = major clinical significance):

Before using this medication
» Conditions affecting use, especially:
   Sensitivity to terbinafine

Proper use of this medication
   Applying sufficient medication to cover affected and surrounding areas, and rubbing in gently
» Avoiding contact with the eyes
» Not applying occlusive dressing over this medication unless directed to do so by physician
» Proper dosing
» Compliance with full course of therapy; fungal infections may require prolonged therapy
   Missed dose: Applying as soon as possible; not applying if almost time for next dose
» Proper storage

Precautions while using this medication
   Checking with physician if no improvement within 4 weeks
» Using hygienic measures to help cure infection and prevent reinfection:
   For tinea corporis
      Carefully drying the body after bathing
      Avoiding excess heat and humidity if possible; keeping moisture from accumulating on affected areas of the body
      Wearing well-ventilated, loose-fitting clothing
      Using a bland, absorbent powder once or twice daily; using the powder after the cream has been applied and has disappeared into the skin
   For tinea cruris
      Avoiding underwear that is tight-fitting or made from synthetic materials; wearing loose-fitting cotton underwear instead
      Using a bland, absorbent powder on the skin; using the powder between administration times for terbinafine
   For tinea pedis
      Carefully drying feet, especially between toes, after bathing
      Avoiding socks made from wool or synthetic materials; wearing clean, cotton socks and changing them daily or more often if feet perspire excessively
      Wearing sandals or well-ventilated shoes
      Using a bland, absorbent powder between toes, on feet, and in socks and shoes liberally once or twice daily; using the powder between administration times for terbinafine

Side/adverse effects
   Signs of potential side effects, especially hypersensitivity

---

▲ For the Patient ▲

919247

ABOUT YOUR MEDICINE

Terbinafine is used to treat infections caused by a fungus.

Terbinafine is applied to the skin to treat ringworm of the body (tinea corporis); ringworm of the foot (tinea pedis; athlete's foot); and ringworm of the groin (tinea cruris; jock itch).

If any of the information in this leaflet causes you special concern or if you want additional information about your medicine and its use, check with your doctor, nurse, or pharmacist. **Remember, keep this and all other medicines out of the reach of children and never share your medicines with others.**

BEFORE USING THIS MEDICINE

Tell your doctor, nurse, and pharmacist if you . . .
- are allergic to any medicine, either prescription or non-prescription (OTC);
- are pregnant or intend to become pregnant while using this medicine;
- are breast-feeding;
- are taking any other prescription or nonprescription (OTC) medicine;
- have any other medical problems.

PROPER USE OF THIS MEDICINE

Apply enough terbinafine to cover the affected and surrounding skin areas and rub in gently.

Keep this medicine away from the eyes.

Do not apply an occlusive dressing (airtight covering, such as a tight bandage or plastic kitchen wrap) over this medicine unless you have been directed to do so by your doctor.

To help clear up your infection completely, it is **very important that you keep using terbinafine for the full time of treatment,** even if your symptoms begin to clear up after a few days. Since fungus infections may be very slow to clear up, you may have to continue using this medicine every day for several weeks or more. If you stop using this medicine too soon, your symptoms may return. **Do not miss any doses.**

If you do miss a dose of this medicine, apply it as soon as possible. However, if it is almost time for your next dose, skip the missed dose and go back to your regular dosing schedule.

PRECAUTIONS WHILE USING THIS MEDICINE

If your skin problem does not improve within 4 weeks, or if it becomes worse, check with your doctor.

To help clear up your infection completely and to help make sure it does not return, good health habits are also needed.

The following measures will help reduce chafing and irritation and will also help keep the area cool and dry.

- **For patients using terbinafine for ringworm of the body:** Carefully dry yourself after bathing. Avoid too much heat and humidity if possible. Try to keep moisture from building up on affected areas of the body. Wear well-ventilated, loose-fitting clothing. Use a bland, absorbent powder (for example, talcum powder) once or twice a day. Be sure to use the powder after terbinafine cream has been applied and has disappeared into the skin.

- **For patients using terbinafine for ringworm of the groin:** Wear loose-fitting, cotton underwear. Use a bland, absorbent powder (for example, talcum powder) on the skin. It is best to use the powder between the times you use terbinafine.

- **For patients using terbinafine for ringworm of the foot:** After bathing, carefully dry the feet, especially between the toes. Wear clean, cotton socks and change them daily or more often if the feet sweat a lot. It is best to wear sandals or well-ventilated shoes. Use a bland, absorbent powder or a nonprescription antifungal powder between the toes, on the feet, and in socks and shoes once or twice a day. It is best to use the powder between the times you use terbinafine.

If you have any questions about these measures, check with your doctor, nurse, or pharmacist.

POSSIBLE SIDE EFFECTS OF THIS MEDICINE
Side Effects That Should Be Reported To Your Doctor

Rare—Redness, itching, burning, blistering, swelling, oozing, or other signs of skin irritation not present before use of this medicine

Other side effects not listed above may also occur in some patients. If you notice any other effects, check with your doctor, nurse, or pharmacist.

TETRACYCLINES   Systemic

Including Demeclocycline; Doxycycline; Methacycline; Minocycline; Oxytetracycline; Tetracycline.

■ For the Pharmacist ■

In providing consultation, consider emphasizing the following selected information (» = major clinical significance):

Before using this medication
» Conditions affecting use, especially:
   Sensitivity to tetracyclines
   Pregnancy—Tetracyclines cross the placenta; use is not recommended during the last half of pregnancy since tetracyclines may cause permanent discoloration of teeth, enamel hypoplasia, and inhibition of skeletal growth in the fetus; also, fatty infiltration of the liver may occur in pregnant women, especially with high intravenous doses
   Breast-feeding—Tetracyclines are excreted in breast milk; although tetracyclines may form nonabsorbable complexes with breast-milk calcium, use is not recommended because of the possibility of their causing permanent discoloration of teeth, enamel hypoplasia, inhibition of linear skeletal growth, photosensitivity reactions, and oral and vaginal thrush in infants
   Use in children—In infants and children up to 8 years of age, tetracyclines may cause permanent discoloration of teeth, enamel hypoplasia, and a decrease in linear skeletal growth rate
   Other medications, especially antacids, calcium supplements, cholestyramine, choline and magnesium salicylates, colestipol, estrogen-containing oral contraceptives, iron supplements, magnesium salicylate, or magnesium-containing laxatives
   Other medical problems, especially nephrogenic diabetes insipidus or renal function impairment

Proper use of this medication
» Not giving to children up to 8 years of age
   Taking with at least a full glass of water while in an upright position to avoid esophageal ulceration or to decrease gastrointestinal irritation
» Avoiding concurrent use of milk or other dairy products when taking oral demeclocycline, oxytetracycline, and tetracycline; if gastrointestinal irritation still occurs, these medicines may be taken with food
   Oral doxycycline and minocycline may be taken with food or milk if gastric irritation occurs
» Discarding outdated or decomposed tetracyclines (decomposed products may be toxic)
» Compliance with full course of therapy
» Importance of not missing doses and taking at evenly spaced times
» Proper dosing
   Missed dose: Taking as soon as possible; not taking if almost time for next dose; not doubling doses
» Proper storage

Precautions while using this medication
   Checking with physician if no improvement within a few days (or a few weeks or months for acne patients)

» Avoiding antacids, calcium supplements, choline and magnesium salicylates, iron supplements, magnesium salicylate, magnesium-containing laxatives, sodium bicarbonate within 1 to 3 hours of oral tetracyclines

» Use of an alternate or additional method of contraception if concurrently taking estrogen-containing oral contraceptives
   Caution if surgery with general anesthesia is required

» Possible photosensitivity reactions

» Caution if dizziness, lightheadedness, or unsteadiness occurs

Side/adverse effects

Signs of potential side effects such as discoloration of infant's or children's teeth, nephrogenic diabetes insipidus—with demeclocycline, pigmentation of skin and mucous membranes—with minocycline, benign intracranial hypertension, hepatotoxicity, pancreatitis, and photosensitivity

---

▲ For the Patient ▲

912689

ABOUT YOUR MEDICINE

Tetracyclines (te-tra-SYE-kleens) are used to treat certain infections and also to help control acne. Demeclocycline and doxycycline may also be used for other problems as determined by your doctor. Tetracyclines will not work for colds, flu, or other virus infections.

If any of the information in this leaflet causes you special concern or if you want additional information about your medicine and its use, check with your doctor, nurse, or pharmacist. **Remember, keep this and all other medicines out of the reach of children and never share your medicines with others.**

BEFORE USING THIS MEDICINE

Tell your doctor, nurse, and pharmacist if you . . .
* are allergic to any medicine, either prescription or non-prescription (OTC);
* are pregnant or intend to become pregnant while using this medicine; tetracyclines should not be used during the last half of pregnancy;
* are breast-feeding;
* are taking any other prescription or nonprescription (OTC) medicine, especially antacids, calcium or iron supplements, cholestyramine, colestipol, magnesium-containing laxatives, oral contraceptives (birth control pills) containing estrogen, or other medicines containing calcium, iron, or magnesium;
* have any other medical problems, especially diabetes insipidus (water diabetes—demeclocycline only), or kidney disease.

PROPER USE OF THIS MEDICINE

Tetracyclines should be taken with a full glass (8 ounces) of water to prevent irritation of the esophagus or stomach. In addition, most tetracyclines are best taken on an empty stomach (either 1 hour before or 2 hours after meals). However, if this medicine upsets your stomach, your doctor may want you to take it with food; **but do not take milk or other dairy products within 1 or 2 hours of the time you take tetracyclines** (except doxycycline or minocycline).

Do not give tetracyclines to infants or children under 8 years of age unless directed by your doctor. Tetracyclines may cause permanently discolored teeth and other problems in this age group.

To help clear up your infection completely, **keep taking this medicine for the full time of treatment** even if you begin to feel better; **do not miss any doses.**

If you do miss a dose of this medicine, take it as soon as possible. However, if it is almost time for your next dose, skip the missed dose and go back to your regular dosing schedule. Do not double doses.

PRECAUTIONS WHILE USING THIS MEDICINE

If your symptoms do not improve within a few days (or a few weeks or months for acne patients), or if they become worse, check with your doctor.

Oral contraceptives (birth control pills) containing estrogen may not work properly if you take them while you are taking tetracyclines. Unplanned pregnancies may occur. You should use a different or additional means of birth control while you are taking tetracyclines. If you have any questions about this, check with your doctor or pharmacist.

Tetracyclines may cause your skin to be more sensitive to sunlight than it is normally. When you begin taking this medicine, avoid too much sun and do not use a sunlamp until you see how you react. This sensitivity may last for 2 weeks to several months or more after you stop taking this medicine. **If you have a severe reaction, check with your doctor.**

This medicine must not be given to other people or used for other infections unless you are otherwise directed by your doctor.

POSSIBLE SIDE EFFECTS OF THIS MEDICINE
Side Effects That Should Be Reported To Your Doctor

*For all tetracyclines—More common—*Increased sensitivity of skin to sunlight (rare with minocycline)

*Rare—*Abdominal pain; bulging fontanel (soft spot on head) of infants; discolored teeth (in infants and children); headache; loss of appetite; nausea and vomiting; yellow skin; visual changes

*For demeclocycline (in addition to the above)—*Greatly increased frequency of urination or amount of urine; increased thirst; unusual tiredness or weakness

For minocycline (in addition to the above)—Discoloration of skin and mucous membranes

Side Effects That Usually Do Not Require Medical Attention

These possible side effects may go away during treatment; however, if they continue or are bothersome, check with your doctor, nurse, or pharmacist.

More common—Cramps or burning of the stomach; diarrhea; dizziness, lightheadedness, or unsteadiness (minocycline only); nausea or vomiting

Less common—Itching of the rectal or genital (sex organ) areas; sore mouth or tongue

In some patients tetracyclines may cause the tongue to become darkened or discolored. This will go away when you stop taking this medicine.

Other side effects not listed above may also occur in some patients. If you notice any other effects, check with your doctor, nurse, or pharmacist.

THIOXANTHENES   Systemic
Including Chlorprothixene; Flupenthixol; Thiothixene.

▉For the Pharmacist▉

In providing consultation, consider emphasizing the following selected
information (» = major clinical significance):

Before using this medication
» Conditions affecting use, especially:
   Sensitivity to thioxanthenes or phenothiazines
   Pregnancy—Reports of hyperreflexia in neonates when phar-
      macologically related phenothiazines were used during preg-
      nancy; animal studies have shown an increase in resorption
      rates and decreased fertility with phenothiazines
   Breast-feeding—Pharmacologically related phenothiazines are
      distributed into breast milk causing tardive dyskinesia and
      possible drowsiness in nursing baby
   Use in children—Children are more prone to extrapyramidal
      symptoms
   Use in the elderly—Elderly patients are more likely to develop
      extrapyramidal, anticholinergic, hypotensive, and sedative
      effects; reduced dosage recommended
   Dental—Thioxanthene-induced blood dyscrasias may result in
      infections, delayed healing, and bleeding; dry mouth may
      cause caries and candidiasis; increased motor activity of face,
      head, and neck may interfere with some dental procedures
   Other medications, especially alcohol or other CNS depression–
      producing medications, epinephrine, other extrapyramidal
      reaction–causing medications, levodopa, or quinidine
   Other medical problems, especially blood dyscrasias, bone mar-
      row depression, circulatory collapse, CNS depression, alco-
      holism, cardiovascular disease, hepatic function impairment,
      or Reye's syndrome

Proper use of this medication
   Taking with food or milk to reduce gastrointestinal irritation
» Diluting thiothixene oral solution with recommended beverages prior
      to use
» Compliance with therapy; not taking more medication or more often
      than directed
» May require several weeks of therapy to obtain desired effects
» Proper dosing
   Missed dose: Taking as soon as possible; not taking if within 2 hours
      of next scheduled dose; continuing on regular schedule; not dou-
      bling doses
» Proper storage

Precautions while using this medication
   Regular visits to physician to check progress of therapy
   Checking with physician before discontinuing medication; gradual
      dosage reduction may be needed
» Avoiding use of alcoholic beverages or other CNS depressants dur-
      ing therapy
   Avoiding use of antacids or medicine for diarrhea within 2 hours of
      taking thioxanthenes
» Caution if any kind of surgery, dental treatment, or emergency
      treatment is required

» Possible drowsiness; caution when driving, using machines, or doing other things requiring alertness
» Possible dizziness or lightheadedness; caution when getting up suddenly from a lying or sitting position
» Possible heatstroke: caution during exercise or hot weather, or when taking hot baths
» Possible skin photosensitivity; avoiding unprotected exposure to sun; using protective clothing; using a sun block product that includes protection against both UVA-caused photosensitivity reactions and UVB-caused sunburn reactions; avoiding use of sunlamp, tanning bed, or tanning booth

Possible dryness of mouth; using sugarless gum or candy, ice, or saliva substitute for relief; checking with physician or dentist if dry mouth continues for more than 2 weeks
» Avoiding spilling liquid medication on skin or clothing; may cause contact dermatitis

Observing precautions for long-acting parenteral form for up to 3 weeks

Side/adverse effects
» Stopping medication and notifying physician immediately if symptoms of neuroleptic malignant syndrome (NMS) appear
» Notifying physician as soon as possible if early signs of tardive dyskinesia appear

Possibility of withdrawal symptoms

Signs of potential side effects, especially akathisia, dystonias, parkinsonian effects, tardive dyskinesia or dystonia, allergic reactions, anticholinergic effects, deposition of opaque substances in lens and cornea or retinopathy, hypotension, skin discoloration, blood dyscrasias, heat stroke, obstructive jaundice, and NMS

▲ For the Patient ▲

915042

ABOUT YOUR MEDICINE

Thioxanthenes (thye-oh-ZAN-theens) are used in the treatment of nervous, mental, and emotional conditions.

If any of the information in this leaflet causes you special concern or if you want additional information about your medicine and its use, check with your doctor, nurse, or pharmacist. **Remember, keep this and all other medicines out of the reach of children and never share your medicines with others.**

BEFORE USING THIS MEDICINE

Discuss with your doctor possible side effects of this medicine. Some may be serious and/or permanent. For example, tardive dyskinesia (a movement disorder) may occur and may not go away after you stop using the medicine.

Tell your doctor, nurse, and pharmacist if you . . .
• are allergic to any medicine, either prescription or non-prescription (OTC);
• are pregnant or intend to become pregnant while using this medicine;
• are breast-feeding;

- are taking **any** other prescription or nonprescription (OTC) medicine;
- have **any** other medical problems.

PROPER USE OF THIS MEDICINE

This medicine may be taken with food or a full glass (8 ounces) of water or milk to reduce stomach irritation.

Do not take more of this medicine or take it more often than ordered.

Sometimes this medicine must be taken for several weeks before its full effect is reached.

If you miss a dose of this medicine, take it as soon as possible. However, if it is almost time for your next dose, skip the missed dose. Do not double doses.

PRECAUTIONS WHILE USING THIS MEDICINE

This medicine will add to the effects of alcohol and other CNS depressants (medicines that slow down the nervous system). **Check with your doctor before taking any such depressants while you are using this medicine.**

This medicine may cause some people to become drowsy or less alert than they are normally. Even if taken at bedtime, you may feel drowsy or less alert on arising. **Make sure you know how you react to this medicine before you drive, use machines, or do other jobs that require you to be alert.**

Dizziness, lightheadedness, or fainting may occur while taking this medicine, especially when you get up. Getting up slowly may help.

This medicine will often make you sweat less, allowing your body temperature to increase. **Use extra care not to become overheated during exercise, hot baths or saunas, or hot weather while you are taking this medicine. Overheating may make you feel dizzy or faint and can result in heatstroke.**

Some people who take this medicine may become more sensitive to sunlight than they are normally. **When you first begin taking this medicine, avoid too much sun and do not use a sunlamp until you see how you react to the sun,** especially if you tend to burn easily. **If you have a severe reaction, check with your doctor.**

POSSIBLE SIDE EFFECTS OF THIS MEDICINE

Side Effects That Should Be Reported To Your Doctor Immediately

Stop taking this medicine and get emergency help immediately if you notice:

Rare—Convulsions (seizures); difficulty in breathing; fast heartbeat; high fever; high or low (irregular) blood pressure; increased sweating; loss of bladder control; muscle stiffness (severe); unusual tiredness; unusually pale skin

Other Side Effects That Should Be Reported To Your Doctor

> *More common*—Difficulty in talking or swallowing; inability to move eyes; lip smacking or puckering; loss of balance control; mask-like face; muscle spasms, especially of neck and back; puffing of cheeks; rapid or worm-like movements of tongue; restlessness or need to keep moving (severe); shuffling walk; stiffness of arms and legs; trembling and shaking of hands; unusual twisting movements of body; uncontrolled chewing movements; uncontrolled movements of the arms and legs
>
> *Less common*—Blurred vision or other eye problems; difficult urination; fainting; skin discoloration; skin rash
>
> *Rare*—Hot, dry skin or lack of sweating; increased blinking or spasms of eyelid; muscle weakness; sore throat and fever; unusual bleeding or bruising; unusual facial expressions or body positions; yellow eyes or skin

Side Effects That Usually Do Not Require Medical Attention

These possible side effects may go away during treatment; however, if they continue or are bothersome, check with your doctor, nurse, or pharmacist.

> *More common*—Constipation; decreased sweating; dizziness, lightheadedness, or fainting; drowsiness (mild); dry mouth; increased appetite and weight; increased sensitivity of skin to sunlight; nasal congestion

Some side effects may occur after you have stopped taking this medicine. Check with your doctor as soon as possible if you notice dizziness, nausea and vomiting, stomach pain, trembling of fingers and hands, or uncontrolled continuing movements of mouth, tongue, or jaw.

Other side effects not listed above may also occur in some patients. If you notice any other effects, check with your doctor, nurse, or pharmacist.

THYROID HORMONES   Systemic

Including Levothyroxine; Liothyronine; Liotrix; Thyroglobulin; Thyroid.

■ For the Pharmacist ■

In providing consultation, consider emphasizing the following selected information (» = major clinical significance):

Before using this medication
» Conditions affecting use, especially:
   Allergy to thyroid hormones
   Pregnancy—Crosses the placenta to a limited extent; regular monitoring is necessary as maternal dose may change during pregnancy
   Breast-feeding—Small amounts are distributed into breast milk
   Use in the elderly—Sensitivity to thyroid effects is greater in the elderly than in younger age groups and dose adjustment is necessary
   Other medications, especially coumarin- or indandione-derivative anticoagulants, cholestyramine, colestipol, sympathomimetics
   Other medical problems, especially adrenocorticol insufficiency, cardiovascular disease, history of hyperthyroidism, pituitary insufficiency, thyroid sensitivity with long-standing hypothyroidism or myxedema, or thyrotoxicosis

Proper use of this medication
» Importance of not taking more or less medication than the amount prescribed; taking medication at the same time every day for consistent effect
» Possible need for lifelong therapy; checking with physician before discontinuing medication
» Proper dosing
   Missed dose: Taking as soon as possible; not taking if almost time for next dose and not doubling doses; notifying physician if two or more doses in a row are missed
» Proper storage

Precautions while using this medication
» Importance of close monitoring by the physician
   Caution with angina or coronary artery disease; heavy exercise or exertion may precipitate angina
» Caution if any kind of surgery (including dental surgery) or emergency treatment is required
   Avoiding other medications unless prescribed by physician because of possible interference with effects of thyroid hormone

Side/adverse effects
   Signs of potential side effects, especially allergic reaction and pseudotumor cerebri

▲ For the Patient ▲

912703

ABOUT YOUR MEDICINE

Thyroid medicines belong to the general group of medicines called hormones. They are used when the thyroid gland does

not produce enough hormone. They are also used to help
decrease the size of enlarged thyroid glands (known as goiter)
and to treat thyroid cancer.

If any of the information in this leaflet causes you special
concern or if you want additional information about your
medicine and its use, check with your doctor, nurse, or pharmacist. **Remember, keep this and all other medicines out of
the reach of children and never share your medicines with
others.**

BEFORE USING THIS MEDICINE

Tell your doctor, nurse, and pharmacist if you . . .
* are allergic to any medicine, either prescription or nonprescription (OTC);
* are pregnant or intend to become pregnant while using
  this medicine;
* are breast-feeding;
* are taking any other prescription or nonprescription
  (OTC) medicine, especially anticoagulants (blood thinners); cholestyramine; colestipol; or medicines for appetite control, asthma, colds, cough, hay fever, or sinus;
* have any other medical problems, especially hardening
  of the arteries, heart disease, high blood pressure, history of overactive thyroid, underactive adrenal gland,
  or underactive pituitary gland.

PROPER USE OF THIS MEDICINE

Use this medicine only as directed by your doctor. Do not
use more or less of it, and do not use it more often than your
doctor ordered. Your doctor has prescribed the exact amount
your body needs. If you take different amounts, you may
experience symptoms of an overactive or underactive thyroid. Take this medicine at the same time each day to make
sure it always has the same effect.

Do not change brands of thyroid medicine without first
checking with your doctor.

If your condition is due to a lack of thyroid hormone, you
may have to take this medicine for the rest of your life. It
is very important that you **do not stop taking this medicine
without first checking with your doctor.**

If you miss a dose of this medicine, take it as soon as possible.
However, if it is almost time for your next dose, skip the
missed dose and go back to your regular dosing schedule.
Do not double doses. If you miss 2 or more doses in a row
or if you have any questions about this, check with your
doctor.

PRECAUTIONS WHILE USING THIS MEDICINE

This medicine may take a few days or weeks to have a
noticeable effect on your condition. Until it begins to work,
you may experience no change in your symptoms. Check
with your doctor if the symptoms of clumsiness, coldness,

constipation, dry puffy skin, listlessness, muscle aches, sleepiness, tiredness, unusual weight gain, or weakness continue.

If you have a certain type of heart disease, this medicine may cause chest pain or shortness of breath when you exert yourself. Do not overdo exercise or physical work. If you have any questions about this, check with your doctor.

Before having any kind of surgery or dental or emergency treatment, **tell the physician or dentist in charge that you are taking this medicine.**

POSSIBLE SIDE EFFECTS OF THIS MEDICINE
Side Effects That Should Be Reported To Your Doctor

Rare—Headache (severe) in children; hives; skin rash

Signs of overdose—Chest pain; rapid or irregular heartbeat; shortness of breath

Signs that your dosage may need adjusting—Changes in appetite; changes in menstrual periods; diarrhea; fever; hand tremors; headache; irritability; leg cramps; nervousness; sensitivity to heat; trouble in sleeping; sweating; vomiting; weight loss

Other side effects not listed above may also occur in some patients. If you notice any other effects, check with your doctor, nurse, or pharmacist.

■For the Pharmacist■

In providing consultation, consider emphasizing the following selected information (》 = major clinical significance):

Before using this medication
》 Conditions affecting use, especially:
  Sensitivity to ticlopidine
  Dental—Risk of increased blood loss during dental procedures
  Surgical—Risk of increased blood loss during surgical procedures
  Other medications, especially aspirin or anticoagulants
  Other medical problems, especially bleeding (active), medical problems in which there is a significant risk of bleeding, and hematopoietic disorders

Proper use of this medication
  Taking medication with food to increase absorption and to reduce the risk of gastrointestinal irritation
  Compliance with prescribed treatment regimen
  Proper dosing
  Missed dose: Taking as soon as possible; not taking if almost time for next dose; not doubling doses
》 Proper storage

Precautions while using this medication
》 Importance of regular blood tests to detect potential adverse effects during the first 3 months of treatment
》 Need to inform all health care providers of use of medication; medication should be discontinued 10 to 14 days prior to elective procedures with a risk of bleeding
》 Because of risk of bleeding, obtaining physician's opinion before participating in activities with substantial risk of injury and contacting physician immediately if injury occurs
》 Notifying physician immediately if signs and symptoms of bleeding, infection, or thrombocytopenia occur
  Possibility that risk of bleeding may continue for 1 to 2 weeks after treatment is discontinued

Side/adverse effects
  Consulting physician immediately if any signs and symptoms of bleeding, agranulocytosis, or thrombocytopenia occur
  Signs and symptoms of other potential adverse effects, especially hepatitis or cholestatic jaundice; skin rash, hives, or itching; or ringing or buzzing in the ears

▲ For the Patient ▲

918390

ABOUT YOUR MEDICINE

Ticlopidine (tye-KLOE-pi-deen) is used to lower the chance of having a stroke. It is given to people who have already had a stroke and to people with certain medical problems that may lead to a stroke. Because ticlopidine can cause serious side effects, especially during the first three months of treatment, it is used mostly for people who cannot take aspirin to prevent strokes.

If any of the information in this leaflet causes you special concern or if you want additional information about your medicine and its use, check with your doctor, nurse, or pharmacist. **Remember, keep this and all other medicines out of the reach of children and never share your medicines with others.**

BEFORE USING THIS MEDICINE

Tell your doctor, nurse, and pharmacist if you . . .
- are allergic to any medicine, either prescription or non-prescription (OTC);
- are pregnant or intend to become pregnant while using this medicine;
- are breast-feeding;
- are taking any other prescription or nonprescription (OTC) medicine, especially anticoagulants (blood thinners), aspirin, or heparin;
- have any other medical problems, especially blood clotting problems, such as hemophilia; blood disease; kidney disease (severe); or stomach ulcers.

PROPER USE OF THIS MEDICINE

Ticlopidine should be taken with food. This helps more of the medicine to be absorbed into the body. It may also lessen the chance of stomach upset.

Take this medicine only as directed. It will not work properly if you take less of it than directed. Taking more than directed may increase the chance of bleeding or other serious side effects without increasing the helpful effects.

If you miss a dose of this medicine, take it as soon as possible. However, if it is almost time for your next dose, skip the missed dose and go back to your regular dosing schedule. Do not double doses.

PRECAUTIONS WHILE USING THIS MEDICINE

It is very important that blood tests be done every 2 weeks for at least the first 3 months of treatment. The tests are needed to find out whether certain side effects are occurring. Finding these side effects early helps to prevent them from becoming serious. Your doctor will arrange for the blood tests to be done. **Be sure that you do not miss any of these tests.**

Tell all medical doctors, dentists, nurses, and pharmacists you go to that you are taking this medicine. Ticlopidine may increase the risk of serious bleeding during an operation or some kinds of dental work. Therefore, treatment may have to be stopped about 10 days to 2 weeks ahead of time.

Ticlopidine may cause serious bleeding, especially after an injury. Sometimes, bleeding inside the body can occur without your knowing about it. Ask your doctor whether there are certain activities you should avoid while taking this medicine, and **check with your doctor immediately if you are injured while being treated with ticlopidine.**

Check with your doctor immediately if you notice bleeding or bruising, especially bleeding that is hard to stop; any sign of infection, such as fever, chills, or sore throat; or sores, ulcers, or white spots in the mouth.

After you stop taking ticlopidine, the chance of bleeding may continue for 1 or 2 weeks. During this time, continue to follow the same precautions that you followed while you were taking the medicine.

POSSIBLE SIDE EFFECTS OF THIS MEDICINE
Side Effects That Should Be Reported To Your Doctor Immediately

> *Less common or rare*—Abdominal or stomach pain (severe) or swelling; back pain; blood in eyes; blood in urine; bloody or black, tarry stools; bruising or purple areas on skin; coughing up blood; decreased alertness; dizziness; fever, chills, or sore throat; headache (severe); joint pain or swelling; nosebleeds; paralysis or problems with coordination; pinpoint red spots on skin; sores, ulcers, or white spots in mouth; stammering or other difficulty in speaking; unusually heavy bleeding or oozing from cuts or wounds; unusually heavy or unexpected menstrual bleeding; vomiting of blood or material that looks like coffee grounds

Other Side Effects That Should Be Reported To Your Doctor

> *More common*—Skin rash

> *Less common or rare*—Hives or itching of skin; ringing or buzzing in ears; yellow eyes or skin

Side Effects That Usually Do Not Require Medical Attention

These possible side effects may go away during treatment; however, if they continue or are bothersome, check with your doctor, nurse, or pharmacist.

> *More common*—Abdominal or stomach pain (mild); bloating or gas; diarrhea; nausea

Other side effects not listed above may also occur in some patients. If you notice any other effects, check with your doctor, nurse, or pharmacist.

TOBRAMYCIN   Ophthalmic

■ For the Pharmacist ■

In providing consultation, consider emphasizing the following selected
information (» = major clinical significance):

Before using this medication
» Conditions affecting use, especially:
Sensitivity to tobramycin or other aminoglycosides

Proper use of this medication
Proper administration technique for ophthalmic solution and oint-
ment
» Compliance with full course of therapy
» Proper dosing
Missed dose: Applying as soon as possible; not applying if almost
time for next dose
» Proper storage

Precautions while using this medication
Checking with physician if no improvement within a few days

Side/adverse effects
Ophthalmic ointments may cause blurred vision for a few minutes
after application
Signs of potential side effects, especially hypersensitivity

▲ For the Patient ▲

917208

ABOUT YOUR MEDICINE

Ophthalmic tobramycin (toe-bra-MYE-sin) is used in the eye
to treat bacterial infections of the eye.

Ophthalmic tobramycin may be used alone or with other
medicines for eye infections. Either the drops or ointment
form of this medicine may be used alone during the day. In
addition, both forms may be used together, with the drops
being used during the day and the ointment at night.

If any of the information in this leaflet causes you special
concern or if you want additional information about your
medicine and its use, check with your doctor, nurse, or pharmacist. **Remember, keep this and all other medicines out of
the reach of children and never share your medicines with
others.**

BEFORE USING THIS MEDICINE

Tell your doctor, nurse, and pharmacist if you . . .
  • are allergic to any medicine, either prescription or non-
    prescription (OTC);
  • are pregnant or intend to become pregnant while using
    this medicine;
  • are breast-feeding;
  • are taking any other prescription or nonprescription
    (OTC) medicine;

- have any other medical problems.

PROPER USE OF THIS MEDICINE

For patients using tobramycin ophthalmic solution (eye drops):

- The bottle is only partially full to provide proper drop control.

- To use:
    —First, wash your hands. Tilt the head back and, pressing your finger gently on the skin just beneath the lower eyelid, pull the lower eyelid away from the eye to make a space. Drop the medicine into this space. Let go of the eyelid and gently close the eyes. Do not blink. Keep the eyes closed for 1 or 2 minutes to allow the medicine to come into contact with the infection.
    —If you think you did not get the drop of medicine into your eye properly, use another drop.
    —To keep the medicine as germ-free as possible, do not touch the applicator tip to any surface (including the eye). Also, keep the container tightly closed.

- If your doctor ordered two different ophthalmic solutions to be used together, wait at least 5 minutes between the times you apply the medicines. This will help to keep the second medicine from "washing out" the first one.

For patients using tobramycin ophthalmic ointment (eye ointment):

- To use:
    —First, wash your hands. Tilt the head back and, pressing your finger gently on the skin just beneath the lower eyelid, pull the lower eyelid away from the eye to make a space. Squeeze a thin strip of ointment into this space. A 1.25-cm (approximately 1/2-inch) strip of ointment is usually enough, unless you have been told by your doctor to use a different amount. Let go of the eyelid and gently close the eyes. Keep the eyes closed for 1 or 2 minutes to allow the medicine to come into contact with the infection.
    —To keep the medicine as germ-free as possible, do not touch the applicator tip to any surface (including the eye). After using tobramycin eye ointment, wipe the tip of the ointment tube with a clean tissue and keep the tube tightly closed.

To help clear up your eye infection completely, **keep using tobramycin for the full time of treatment,** even if your symptoms have disappeared. **Do not miss any doses.**

If you do miss a dose of this medicine, use it as soon as possible. However, if it is almost time for your next dose,

skip the missed dose and go back to your regular dosing
schedule.

PRECAUTIONS WHILE USING THIS MEDICINE

If your eye infection does not improve within a few days, or
if it becomes worse, check with your doctor.

**This medicine must not be given to other people or used for
other infections** unless you are otherwise directed by your
doctor.

POSSIBLE SIDE EFFECTS OF THIS MEDICINE

*Side Effects That Should Be Reported To Your Doctor
Immediately*

> *Less common*—Itching, redness, swelling, or other sign
> of eye or eyelid irritation not present before use of this
> medicine

> *Signs of overdose*—Increased watering of the eyes; itch-
> ing, redness, or swelling of the eyes or eyelids

Eye ointments usually cause your vision to blur for a few
minutes after application.

Other side effects not listed above may also occur in some
patients. If you notice any other effects, check with your
doctor, nurse, or pharmacist.

TOCAINIDE   Systemic

■ For the Pharmacist ■

In providing consultation, consider emphasizing the following selected
information (» = major clinical significance):

Before using this medication
» Conditions affecting use, especially:
   Sensitivity to tocainide or amide-type anesthetics
   Pregnancy—Increased possibility of death in animal fetuses
   Use in elderly—Elderly may be more prone to dizziness and
       hypotension
   Other medical problems, especially second or third degree atrio-
       ventricular (AV) block

Proper use of this medication
» Compliance with therapy; taking as directed even if feeling well
   May be taken with food or milk to reduce stomach upset
» Importance of not missing doses and taking at evenly spaced inter-
   vals
» Proper dosing
   Missed dose: Taking as soon as possible if remembered within
       4 hours; not taking if remembered later; not doubling doses
» Proper storage

Precautions while using this medication
   Regular visits to physician to check progress
   Carrying medical identification card or bracelet
» Caution when driving or doing things requiring alertness because of
   possible dizziness
» Caution if any kind of surgery (including dental surgery) or emer-
   gency treatment is required

Side/adverse effects
   Signs of potential side effects, especially trembling or shaking, leu-
       kopenia or agranulocytosis, thrombocytopenia, pulmonary prob-
       lems, severe skin reactions, and ventricular arrhythmias

▲ For the Patient ▲

913036

ANTIARRHYTHMICS, TYPE I (Oral): *Including
Disopyramide; Encainide; Flecainide; Mexiletine;
Moricizine; Procainamide; Propafenone; Quinidine;
Tocainide.*

ABOUT YOUR MEDICINE

Type I antiarrhythmics are used to correct irregular heartbeats to a normal rhythm and to slow an overactive heart.

There is a chance that these medicines may cause new heart
rhythm problems when they are used. Usually this effect is
rare and mild. However, some of these medicines are more
likely than others to cause this effect. For example, encainide
and flecainide have been shown to cause severe problems in
some patients, and so they are only used to treat serious

heart rhythm problems. Discuss this possible effect with your doctor.

If any of the information in this leaflet causes you special concern or if you want additional information about your medicine and its use, check with your doctor, nurse, or pharmacist. **Remember, keep this and all other medicines out of the reach of children and never share your medicines with others.**

BEFORE USING THIS MEDICINE

Tell your doctor, nurse, and pharmacist if you . . .
- are allergic to any medicine, either prescription or nonprescription (OTC);
- are pregnant or intend to become pregnant while using this medicine;
- are breast-feeding;
- are taking **any** other prescription or nonprescription (OTC) medicine;
- have **any** other medical problems.

PROPER USE OF THIS MEDICINE

Take this medicine exactly as directed by your doctor, even though you may feel well. Do not take more medicine than ordered.

For patients taking the extended-release capsules or tablets:
- Swallow whole without breaking, crushing, or chewing.

It is best to take each dose at evenly spaced times day and night.

For patients taking mexiletine:
- To lessen the possibility of stomach upset, this medicine should be taken with food or immediately after meals or with milk or an antacid.

If you miss a dose of this medicine, take it as soon as possible. However, if you do not remember until it is almost time for the next dose, skip the missed dose and go back to your regular dosing schedule. Do not double doses.

PRECAUTIONS WHILE USING THIS MEDICINE

It is important that your doctor check your progress at regular visits to make sure the medicine is working properly to help your heart.

Do not suddenly stop taking this medicine without first checking with your doctor. Stopping it suddenly may cause a serious change in heart activity.

Dizziness or lightheadedness or blurred vision may occur. **Make sure you know how you react to this medicine before you drive, use machines, or do other jobs that require you to be alert and able to see well.**

For patients taking disopyramide:
- **If signs of hypoglycemia (low blood sugar) such as chills, hunger, nausea, nervousness, or sweating appear, eat or**

drink a food containing sugar and call your doctor right
away.

- **Use extra care not to become overheated during exercise
or hot weather,** since this medicine will often make you
sweat less and could possibly result in heatstroke.

POSSIBLE SIDE EFFECTS OF THIS MEDICINE
*Side Effects That Should Be Reported To Your Doctor
Immediately*

    *For quinidine only, especially after the first dose or first
few doses*—Breathing difficulty; changes in vision;
dizziness, lightheadedness, or fainting; fever; severe
headache; ringing in ears; skin rash

*Other Side Effects That Should Be Reported To Your
Doctor*

    For all antiarrhythmics—Chest pain; fast or irregular
heartbeat; fever or chills; shortness of breath or painful
breathing; skin rash or itching; unusual bleeding or
bruising

    For disopyramide (in addition to above)—Difficult uri-
nation; swelling of feet or lower legs

    *For encainide, flecainide, moricizine, and propafenone
(in addition to above)*—Swelling of feet or lower legs;
trembling or shaking

*Side Effects That Usually Do Not Require Medical
Attention*

These possible side effects may go away during treatment;
however, if they continue or are bothersome, check with your
doctor, nurse, or pharmacist.

    For all antiarrhythmics—Blurred or double vision; diz-
ziness or lightheadedness

    For disopyramide (in addition to above)—Dry mouth and
throat

    For flecainide (in addition to above)—Seeing spots

    For mexiletine (in addition to above)—Heartburn; nau-
sea and vomiting; nervousness; trembling or shaking
of hands; unsteadiness or trouble walking

    For procainamide (in addition to above)—Diarrhea; loss
of appetite

    For propafenone (in addition to above)—Change in taste

    For quinidine (in addition to above)—Bitter taste; diar-
rhea; flushing of skin with itching; loss of appetite;
nausea or vomiting; stomach pain or cramps

    For tocainide (in addition to above)—Loss of appetite;
nausea

Other side effects not listed above may also occur in some
patients. If you notice any other effects, check with your
doctor, nurse, or pharmacist.

TRAZODONE   Systemic

■For the Pharmacist■

In providing consultation, consider emphasizing the following selected information (» = major clinical significance):

Before using this medication
» Conditions affecting use, especially:
> Sensitivity to trazodone
> Pregnancy—Animal studies have shown congenital anomalies and increased fetal resorptions with large doses
> Breast-feeding—Excreted in breast milk
> Use in the elderly—Elderly are more prone to develop sedative and hypotensive effects
> Dental—Dry mouth may result in caries, periodontal disease, oral candidiasis, and discomfort
> Other medications, especially alcohol or other CNS depression–producing medications, or antihypertensives
> Other medical problems, especially myocardial infarction, arrhythmias or other cardiac disease, hepatic function impairment, or renal function impairment

Proper use of this medication
> Taking with or soon after a meal or light snack to minimize stomach upset and dizziness or lightheadedness
» Compliance with therapy
» May require up to 4 weeks to produce significant therapeutic results, although 75% of responding patients benefit within 2 weeks
» Proper dosing
> Missed dose: Taking as soon as possible; not taking if within 4 hours of next scheduled dose; not doubling doses
» Proper storage

Precautions while using this medication
> Regular visits to physician to check progress during therapy
» Checking with physician before discontinuing medication; gradual dosage reduction may be needed
» Caution if any kind of surgery, dental treatment, or emergency treatment is required
» Avoiding use of alcohol or other CNS depressants during therapy
» Possible drowsiness; caution when driving or doing other things requiring alertness
» Possible dizziness; caution when getting up suddenly from a lying or sitting position
> Possible dryness of mouth; using sugarless gum or candy, ice, or saliva substitute for relief; checking with physician or dentist if dry mouth continues for more than 2 weeks

Side/adverse effects
> Sedative and hypotensive side effects more likely to occur in the elderly
> Priapism may occur; discontinuing medication and checking with physician immediately
> Signs of potential side effects, especially CNS effects, fast or slow heartbeat, hypotension, priapism, unusual excitement, or allergic reaction

▲ For the Patient ▲

915053

ABOUT YOUR MEDICINE

Trazodone (TRAZ-oh-done) belongs to the group of medicines known as antidepressants or "mood elevators." It is used to relieve mental depression and depression that sometimes occurs with anxiety.

If any of the information in this leaflet causes you special concern or if you want additional information about your medicine and its use, check with your doctor, nurse, or pharmacist. **Remember, keep this and all other medicines out of the reach of children and never share your medicines with others.**

BEFORE USING THIS MEDICINE

Tell your doctor, nurse, and pharmacist if you . . .
- are allergic to any medicine, either prescription or non-prescription (OTC);
- are pregnant or intend to become pregnant while using this medicine;
- are breast-feeding;
- are taking any other prescription or nonprescription (OTC) medicine, especially CNS depressants or anti-hypertensives (medicine for high blood pressure);
- have any other medical problems, especially heart, kidney, or liver disease.

PROPER USE OF THIS MEDICINE

Take trazodone only as directed by your doctor.

To lessen stomach upset and to reduce dizziness and light-headedness, take this medicine with or shortly after a meal or light snack, even for a daily bedtime dose, unless your doctor has told you to take it on an empty stomach.

Sometimes trazodone must be taken for up to 4 weeks before you begin to feel better, although most people notice improvement within 2 weeks.

If you miss a dose of this medicine, take it as soon as possible. However, if it is within 4 hours of your next dose, skip the missed dose and go back to your regular dosing schedule. Do not double doses.

PRECAUTIONS WHILE USING THIS MEDICINE

It is very important that your doctor check your progress at regular visits. This will allow your doctor to check the medicine's effects and to change the dose if needed.

Do not stop taking this medicine without first checking with your doctor. Your doctor may want you to reduce gradually the amount you are using before stopping completely, to prevent a possible return of your medical problem.

Before having any kind of surgery, dental treatment, or emergency treatment, tell the physician or dentist in charge that you are using this medicine.

Trazodone will add to the effects of alcohol and other CNS depressants (medicines that slow down the nervous system). **Check with your doctor before taking any such depressants while using this medicine.**

Trazodone may cause some people to become drowsy or less alert than they are normally. **Make sure you know how you react to this medicine before you drive, use machines, or do other jobs that require you to be alert.**

Dizziness, lightheadedness, or fainting may occur, especially when you get up from a lying or sitting position. Getting up slowly may help. If this problem continues or gets worse, check with your doctor.

Trazodone may cause dryness of the mouth. For temporary relief, use sugarless gum or candy, melt bits of ice in your mouth, or use a saliva substitute. However, if your mouth continues to feel dry for more than 2 weeks, check with your physician or dentist. Continuing dryness of the mouth may increase the chance of dental disease, including tooth decay, gum disease, and fungal infections.

POSSIBLE SIDE EFFECTS OF THIS MEDICINE

Side Effects That Should Be Reported To Your Doctor Immediately

Stop taking this medicine and check with your doctor immediately if the following side effect occurs:

   Rare—Painful, inappropriate erection of the penis (continuing)

Other Side Effects That Should Be Reported To Your Doctor

   Less common—Confusion; muscle tremors

   Rare—Fainting; fast or slow heartbeat; skin rash; unusual excitement

Side Effects That Usually Do Not Require Medical Attention

These possible side effects may go away during treatment; however, if they continue or are bothersome, check with your doctor, nurse, or pharmacist.

   More common—Dizziness or lightheadedness; drowsiness; dryness of mouth (usually mild); headache; nausea and vomiting; unpleasant taste

Other side effects not listed above may also occur in some patients. If you notice any other effects, check with your doctor, nurse, or pharmacist.

TRETINOIN   Topical

■ For the Pharmacist ■

In providing consultation, consider emphasizing the following selected information (» = major clinical significance):

Before using this medication
» Conditions affecting use, especially:
> Sensitivity to etretinate, isotretinoin, tretinoin, or vitamin A derivatives
> Pregnancy—Topical tretinoin has been shown to cause delayed ossification in a number of bones in some animal fetuses
> Other medical problems, especially eczema and sunburn

Proper use of this medication
» Importance of not using more medication than the amount prescribed
» Not applying medication to windburned or sunburned skin or on open wounds
» Avoiding contact with the eyes, mouth, and nose
> Proper administration technique:
> Reading patient directions carefully before use
> Before applying—Washing with mild or nonallergic soap and warm water; gently patting dry; waiting 20 to 30 minutes for complete drying of skin
> *For cream or gel dosage form*
> Applying enough to cover affected areas and rubbing in gently
> *For solution dosage form*
> Using fingertips, gauze pad, or cotton swab and applying enough to cover affected areas
> Not oversaturating gauze pad or cotton swab to prevent medication from running into areas not intended for treatment
» Proper dosing
> Missed dose: Applying next dose at regularly scheduled time; not doubling doses
» Proper storage

Precautions while using this medication
> Possibility that acne may appear to worsen during the first 2 or 3 weeks of therapy; not stopping medication unless irritation or other symptoms become severe
> Avoiding too frequent washing of face; washing with mild bland soap 2 or 3 times a day is usually sufficient
» Avoiding simultaneous use with other topical acne preparations or preparations containing peeling agents, alcohol-containing preparations, abrasive soaps or cleansers, cosmetics or soaps with drying effect, medicated cosmetics, or other topical skin medication, unless prescribed by physician
> Cosmetics (nonmedicated) may be used, but skin must be washed thoroughly before applying medication
» Avoiding or minimizing exposure of treated areas to sunlight or a sunlamp to lessen the possibility of sunburn
> Using sunscreen preparations or wearing protective clothing over treated areas if excessive sunlight exposure cannot be avoided
» Possibility of increased sensitivity to wind or cold temperatures

Side/adverse effects

The side/adverse effects of tretinoin are reversible upon discontinuation of therapy; however, hyperpigmentation or hypopigmentation may persist for months

Signs of potential side effects, especially blistering, crusting, severe burning or redness, or swelling of skin or darkening or lightening of the treated skin

---

▲ For the Patient ▲

915064

ABOUT YOUR MEDICINE

Tretinoin (TRET-i-noyn) is used to treat certain types of acne. It may also be used to treat other skin diseases as determined by your doctor. Although tretinoin is being used to treat skin that has been damaged by long-time exposure to sunlight, there is not enough information to show that this treatment is safe and effective.

If any of the information in this leaflet causes you special concern or if you want additional information about your medicine and its use, check with your doctor, nurse, or pharmacist. **Remember, keep this and all other medicines out of the reach of children and never share your medicines with others.**

BEFORE USING THIS MEDICINE

Tell your doctor, nurse, and pharmacist if you . . .
- are allergic to any medicine, either prescription or non-prescription (OTC);
- are pregnant or intend to become pregnant while using this medicine;
- are breast-feeding;
- are taking any other prescription or nonprescription (OTC) medicine;
- have any other medical problems, especially eczema or sunburn.

PROPER USE OF THIS MEDICINE

It is very important that you use this medicine only as directed. Do not use more of it, do not use it more often, and do not use it for a longer time than your doctor ordered. To do so may cause irritation of the skin.

Do not apply this medicine to windburned or sunburned skin or on open wounds.

Do not use this medicine in or around the eyes or mouth, or inside the nose. Spread the medicine away from these areas when applying.

Before applying tretinoin, wash the skin with a mild or non-allergic type of soap and warm water, then gently pat dry. Wait 20 to 30 minutes before applying this medicine to make sure the skin is completely dry.

To use the cream or gel form of this medicine:
- Apply enough medicine to cover the affected areas, and rub in gently.

To use the solution form of this medicine:
- Using your fingertips, a gauze pad, or a cotton swab, apply enough tretinoin solution to cover the affected areas.

If you miss a dose of this medicine, skip the missed dose and go back to your regular dosing schedule. Do not double doses.

PRECAUTIONS WHILE USING THIS MEDICINE

During the first 2 or 3 weeks you are using tretinoin, your acne may seem to get worse before it gets better. However, you should not stop using tretinoin unless irritation or other symptoms become severe.

You should avoid washing your face too often. Washing it with a mild bland soap 2 or 3 times a day should be enough, unless you are otherwise directed by your doctor.

When using tretinoin, do not use abrasive soaps or cleansers; alcohol-containing preparations; any other topical acne preparation or preparation containing a peeling agent (for example, benzoyl peroxide, resorcinol, salicylic acid, or sulfur); cosmetics or soaps that dry the skin; medicated cosmetics; or other topical medicine for the skin on the same affected area as this medicine, unless otherwise directed. To do so may cause severe irritation of the skin.

You may use cosmetics (nonmedicated) while being treated with tretinoin, unless otherwise directed by your doctor. However, the areas to be treated must be washed thoroughly before the medicine is applied.

During treatment with this medicine, **avoid exposing the treated areas to too much sunlight or overuse of a sunlamp,** since the skin may be more prone to sunburn. If exposure to too much sunlight cannot be avoided while you are using this medicine, use sunscreen preparations or wear protective clothing over the treated areas.

Some people who use this medicine may become more sensitive to wind and cold temperatures than they are normally. **When you first begin using this medicine, use protection against wind or cold until you see how you react.** If you notice severe skin irritation, check with your doctor.

POSSIBLE SIDE EFFECTS OF THIS MEDICINE
Side Effects That Should Be Reported To Your Doctor

Blistering, crusting, severe burning or redness, or swelling of skin; darkening or lightening of the treated skin

Side Effects That Usually Do Not Require Medical Attention

These possible side effects may go away during treatment; however, if they continue or are bothersome, check with your doctor, nurse, or pharmacist.

> Feeling of warmth on skin; peeling of skin (may occur after a few days); stinging (mild) or redness of skin

The side effects of tretinoin will go away after you stop using the medicine. However, the side effect of darkening or lightening of the skin may take several months before it goes away.

Other side effects not listed above may also occur in some patients. If you notice any other effects, check with your doctor, nurse, or pharmacist.

TRIMETHOBENZAMIDE   Systemic

■ For the Pharmacist ■

In providing consultation, consider emphasizing the following selected information (» = major clinical significance):

Before using this medication
» Conditions affecting use, especially:
> Sensitivity to trimethobenzamide or to benzocaine (for suppository form)
> Pregnancy—Animal studies have shown increased fetal resorptions and stillbirths
> Use in children—Trimethobenzamide is not recommended for treatment of uncomplicated vomiting, due to the possible contribution of centrally acting antiemetics to the development of Reye's syndrome
> Other medications, especially CNS depressants
> Other medical problems, especially dehydration, electrolyte imbalance, encephalitis, high fever, or gastroenteritis

Proper use of this medication
> Not giving to children unless prescribed; giving medication only as directed
> Taking medication only as directed
> Proper administration of this medication (for suppository dosage form only)
» Proper dosing
> Missed dose: Taking as soon as possible; not taking if almost time for next dose; not doubling doses
» Proper storage

Precautions while using this medication
» Avoiding use of alcohol or other CNS depressants
» Possible dizziness, lightheadedness, or drowsiness; caution when driving or doing anything else requiring alertness
> May mask ototoxic effects of large doses of salicylates

Side/adverse effects
> Signs of potential side effects, especially allergic reactions, blood dyscrasias, convulsions, hepatic function impairment, mental depression, opisthotonus, Parkinson-like syndrome, and Reye's syndrome

▲ For the Patient ▲

915097

ABOUT YOUR MEDICINE

Trimethobenzamide (trye-meth-oh-BEN-za-mide) is used to treat nausea and vomiting.

If any of the information in this leaflet causes you special concern or if you want additional information about your medicine and its use, check with your doctor, nurse, or pharmacist. **Remember, keep this and all other medicines out of the reach of children and never share your medicines with others.**

BEFORE USING THIS MEDICINE
Tell your doctor, nurse, and pharmacist if you . . .
- are allergic to any medicine, either prescription or non-prescription (OTC);
- are pregnant or intend to become pregnant while using this medicine;
- are breast-feeding;
- are taking any other prescription or nonprescription (OTC) medicine, especially CNS depressants or tricyclic antidepressants;
- have any other medical problems.

PROPER USE OF THIS MEDICINE
Do not use this medicine to treat nausea and vomiting in children unless otherwise directed by your doctor. If you are giving this medicine to a child, be especially careful not to give more than is prescribed since side effects may be more serious in children.

Trimethobenzamide is used only to relieve or prevent nausea and vomiting. Use it only as directed. Do not use more of it and do not use it more often than your doctor ordered. To do so may increase the chance of side effects.

If you must use this medicine regularly and you miss a dose, use it as soon as possible. However, if it is almost time for your next dose, skip the missed dose and go back to your regular dosing schedule. Do not double doses.

PRECAUTIONS WHILE USING THIS MEDICINE
Trimethobenzamide will add to the effects of alcohol and other CNS depressants (medicines that slow down the nervous system). **Check with your doctor before taking any such depressants while you are using this medicine.**

This medicine may cause some people to become dizzy, light-headed, drowsy, or less alert than they are normally. **Make sure you know how you react to this medicine before you drive, use machines, or do other jobs that require you to be alert.**

When using trimethobenzamide on a regular basis, make sure your doctor knows if you are taking large amounts of aspirin or other salicylates at the same time (as for arthritis or rheumatism). Effects of too much aspirin, such as ringing in the ears, may be covered up by this medicine.

POSSIBLE SIDE EFFECTS OF THIS MEDICINE
Side Effects That Should Be Reported To Your Doctor

> *Rare*—Back pain; convulsions (seizures); mental depression; shakiness or tremors; skin rash; sore throat and fever; unusual tiredness; vomiting (severe or continuing); yellow eyes or skin

Side Effects That Usually Do Not Require Medical Attention

These possible side effects may go away during treatment; however, if they continue or are bothersome, check with your doctor, nurse, or pharmacist.

   More common—Drowsiness

   Less common—Blurred vision; diarrhea; dizziness; headache; muscle cramps

Other side effects not listed above may also occur in some patients. If you notice any other effects, check with your doctor, nurse, or pharmacist.

TRIMETREXATE   Systemic

■ For the Pharmacist ■

In providing consultation, consider emphasizing the following selected information (» = major clinical significance):

Before using this medication
» Conditions affecting use, especially:
Hypersensitivity to trimetrexate or leucovorin
Pregnancy—Trimetrexate is not recommended, because of potential teratogenic and fetotoxic effects; using contraception during trimetrexate treatment; telling physician immediately if pregnancy is suspected
Breast-feeding—Not recommended, because trimetrexate may cause serious side effects in nursing infants
Other medications, especially other bone marrow depressants, or hepatic enzyme inhibitors
Other medical problems, especially bone marrow depression

Proper use of this medication
» For oral leucovorin
» Importance of taking leucovorin concurrently with trimetrexate, and for 3 days following the end of trimetrexate therapy
» Importance of not missing oral leucovorin doses and taking at evenly spaced times
Missed dose: Taking oral leucovorin as soon as possible; not taking if almost time for next dose; not doubling doses
» Proper storage
» Compliance with full course of therapy
» Proper dosing

Precautions while using this medication
Checking with physician if no improvement
» Importance of close monitoring by physician
Caution if bone marrow depression occurs:
» Avoiding exposure to persons with bacterial infections, especially during periods of low blood counts; checking with physician immediately if fever or chills, cough or hoarseness, lower back or side pain, or painful or difficult urination occurs
» Checking with physician immediately if unusual bleeding or bruising; black, tarry stools; blood in urine or stools; or pinpoint red spots on skin occur
Caution in use of regular toothbrush, dental floss, or toothpick; physician, dentist, or nurse may suggest alternatives; checking with physician before having dental work done
Using caution to avoid accidental cuts with use of sharp objects such as safety razor or fingernail or toenail cutters

Side/adverse effects
Signs of potential side effects, especially neutropenia, thrombocytopenia, anemia, fever, mouth sores or ulcers, and skin rash and itching

---

▲ For the Patient ▲

919713

ABOUT YOUR MEDICINE

Trimetrexate (trye-me-TREX-ate) is used together with leucovorin (loo-koe-VOR-in) to treat *Pneumocystis carinii* (noomoe-SISS-tis ka-RIN-ee-eye) pneumonia (PCP), a very serious kind of pneumonia. This kind of pneumonia occurs in patients whose immune systems are not working normally, such as cancer patients, transplant patients, and patients with acquired immune deficiency syndrome (AIDS).

Trimetrexate may cause some serious side effects. To prevent these effects, **you must taken another medicine, leucovorin, together with trimetrexate,** and for three days after you stop taking trimetrexate.

If any of the information in this leaflet causes you special concern or if you want additional information about your medicine and its use, check with your doctor, nurse, or pharmacist. **Remember, keep this and all other medicines out of the reach of children and never share your medicines with others.**

BEFORE USING THIS MEDICINE

Discuss with your doctor the possible side effects that may be caused by this medicine. Some of them may be serious and/or long-term.

Tell your doctor, nurse, and pharmacist if you . . .
- are allergic to any medicine, either prescription or non-prescription (OTC);
- are pregnant or intend to become pregnant while using this medicine;
- are breast-feeding;
- are taking **any** other prescription or nonprescription (OTC) medicine;
- have any other medical problems, especially anemia, low platelet count, or low white blood cell count.

PROPER USE OF THIS MEDICINE

Some medicines given by injection may sometimes be given at home to patients who do not need to be in the hospital for the full time of treatment. If you are using this medicine at home, **make sure you clearly understand and carefully follow your doctor's instructions.**

Put used syringes and needles in a covered container that the needles cannot punch through, then throw the container away. Otherwise, throw away used syringes as directed by your doctor, nurse, or pharmacist.

When you take leucovorin:
- **Leucovorin must be taken with trimetrexate** to help prevent serious unwanted effects. Leucovorin should be

taken during trimetrexate treatment and for 3 days after trimetrexate is stopped.

- **Take oral leucovorin exactly as directed by your doctor.** Do not take more of it, do not take it more often, and do not take it for a longer time than your doctor ordered. Also, do not stop taking leucovorin without checking with your doctor first.
- Oral leucovorin works best when there is a constant amount in the blood. **To help keep the amount constant, do not miss any doses.** If you need help in planning the best times to take your medicine, check with your doctor, nurse, or pharmacist.

If you do miss a dose of leucovorin, use it as soon as possible. This will help to keep a constant amount in the blood. However, if it is almost time for your next dose, skip the missed dose and go back to your regular dosing schedule. Do not double doses.

PRECAUTIONS WHILE USING THIS MEDICINE

If your symptoms do not improve within a few days, or if they become worse, check with your doctor.

It is important that your doctor check your progress at regular visits to make sure that this medicine is working and to check for unwanted effects.

Trimetrexate can temporarily lower the number of white blood cells in your blood, increasing the chance of getting an infection. It can also lower the number of platelets, which are necessary for proper blood clotting. If this occurs:

- Avoid people with infections.
- Be careful when using a regular toothbrush, dental floss, or toothpick.
- Do not touch your eyes or the inside of your nose unless you have just washed your hands and have not touched anything else in the meantime.
- Be careful not to cut, bruise, or injure yourself.

POSSIBLE SIDE EFFECTS OF THIS MEDICINE

Side Effects That Should Be Reported To Your Doctor Immediately

> *More common*—Fever and sore throat
>
> *Less common*—Unusual bleeding or bruising
>
> *Rare*—Fever; mouth sores or ulcers; skin rash and itching; unusual tiredness or weakness

Side Effects That Usually Do Not Require Medical Attention

These possible side effects may go away during treatment; however, if they continue or are bothersome, check with your doctor, nurse, or pharmacist.

> *Less common*—Confusion; nausea and vomiting; stomach pain

Other side effects not listed above may also occur in some patients. If you notice any other effects, check with your doctor, nurse, or pharmacist.

VALPROIC ACID   Systemic
Including Divalproex; Valproic Acid.

■For the Pharmacist■

In providing consultation, consider emphasizing the following selected
information (» = major clinical significance):

Before using this medication
» Conditions affecting use, especially:
> Sensitivity to valproic acid or divalproex
> Fertility—Fertility studies in animals given large doses have shown
> reduced spermatogenesis and testicular atrophy
> Pregnancy—Pregnancy studies in animals have shown skeletal
> abnormalities involving ribs and vertebrae in offspring of
> mothers given large doses; in humans, crosses placenta in
> first trimester and may cause neural tube defects in fetus
> Breast-feeding—Excreted in breast milk
> Use in children—Children are at an increased risk of serious
> hepatotoxicity
> Use in the elderly—Elderly patients tend to have higher serum
> concentrations of free valproic acid; lower daily dosages rec-
> ommended
> Dental—Prolonged bleeding time and/or hemorrhaging; leuko-
> penia and thrombocytopenia may result in increased inci-
> dence of microbial infection, delayed healing, and gingival
> bleeding
> Other medications, especially alcohol or other CNS depression–
> producing medications, heparin or thrombolytic agents, bar-
> biturates, primidone, carbamazepine, other hepatotoxic med-
> ications, mefloquine, phenytoin, or other platelet aggregation
> inhibitors
> Other medical problems, especially significant hepatic disease
> or hepatic function impairment

Proper use of this medication
> Proper administration:
>> *For valproic acid capsules*
>>> Swallowing capsules whole with water only; not breaking,
>>> chewing, or crushing
>> *For divalproex sodium delayed-release capsules*
>>> Swallowing capsules whole, or sprinkling the contents on a
>>> small amount of cool, soft food (such as applesauce or
>>> pudding) and swallowing, not chewing, immediately after
>>> preparation
>> *For divalproex sodium delayed-release tablets*
>>> Swallowing tablets whole; not breaking, chewing, or crushing
>> *For valproic acid syrup*
>>> Mixing with any liquid or adding to a small amount of food
>>> to enhance palatability
> Taking with food if necessary to reduce gastrointestinal side effects
» Compliance with therapy; taking exactly as directed by physician
» Proper dosing
> Missed dose: If dosing schedule is—
>> One dose a day: Taking as soon as possible; not taking if not
>> remembered until next day; not doubling doses
>> Two or more doses a day: Taking if remembered within 6 hours;
>> taking remaining doses for that day at equally spaced inter-
>> vals; not doubling doses

» Proper storage

Precautions while using this medication
» Regular visits to physician to check progress of therapy
» Checking with physician before discontinuing medication; gradual
    dosage reduction may be necessary
» Possible prolonged bleeding or hemorrhage: caution if any kind of
    surgery, dental treatment, or emergency treatment is required
» Avoiding use of alcoholic beverages or other CNS depressants dur-
    ing therapy
    Diabetic patients: When testing for urine ketones, possible false-
    positive test results
    Caution if any laboratory tests required; possible interference with
    results of metyrapone or thyroid function tests
    Possible need for carrying medical identification card or bracelet
» Possible drowsiness; caution when driving or doing other things re-
    quiring alertness

Side/adverse effects
    Signs of potential side effects, especially behavioral, mood, or mental
    changes; hepatotoxicity; hyperammonemia; ophthalmological ef-
    fects; pancreatitis; platelet aggregation inhibition; or thrombo-
    cytopenia

▲ For the Patient ▲

913160

ABOUT YOUR MEDICINE

Valproic (val-PROE-ik) **acid** and **divalproex** (dye-VAL-pro-
ex) belong to the group of medicines called anticonvulsants.
They are used alone or with other medicines to control certain seizures in the treatment of epilepsy. These medicines
may also be used for other conditions as determined by your
doctor.

If any of the information in this leaflet causes you special
concern or if you want additional information about your
medicine and its use, check with your doctor, nurse, or pharmacist. **Remember, keep this and all other medicines out of
the reach of children and never share your medicines with
others.**

BEFORE USING THIS MEDICINE

Tell your doctor, nurse, and pharmacist if you . . .
  • are allergic to any medicine, either prescription or non-
    prescription (OTC);
  • are pregnant or intend to become pregnant while using
    this medicine, since valproic acid may cause birth de-
    fects;
  • are breast-feeding;
  • are taking **any** other prescription or nonprescription
    (OTC) medicine;
  • have any other medical problems, especially liver dis-
    ease.

PROPER USE OF THIS MEDICINE

For patients taking the capsule form of valproic acid:
- Swallow the capsule whole without chewing or breaking, to prevent irritation of the mouth and throat.

For patients taking the delayed-release form of divalproex:
- Swallow the capsule or tablet whole, or sprinkle the contents of the capsule on a small amount of soft food such as applesauce or pudding and swallow without chewing.

For patients taking the tablet form of this medicine:
- Swallow the tablet whole without chewing, breaking, or crushing. This is to prevent damaging the special coating that helps lessen irritation of the stomach.

For patients taking the syrup form of this medicine:
- The syrup may be mixed with liquid or food for a better taste.

This medicine may be taken with meals or snacks to reduce stomach upset.

This medicine must be taken exactly as directed by your doctor in order to prevent seizures and reduce the possibility of side effects.

If you miss a dose of this medicine and you are to take it:
- Once a day—Take the missed dose as soon as possible. However, if you do not remember until the next day, skip the missed dose and go back to your regular dosing schedule. Do not double doses.
- Two or more times a day—If you remember within 6 hours of the missed dose, take it right away. Then take the rest of the doses for that day at equally spaced time periods. Do not double doses.

PRECAUTIONS WHILE USING THIS MEDICINE

Your doctor should check your progress at regular visits, especially for the first few months you take this medicine. This is necessary to allow dose adjustments and to reduce any unwanted effects.

Do not stop taking this medicine without first checking with your doctor. Your doctor may want you to gradually reduce the amount you are taking before stopping completely. Stopping the medicine suddenly may result in seizures.

Before having any kind of surgery or dental or emergency treatment, tell the physician or dentist in charge that you are taking this medicine.

This medicine will add to the effects of alcohol and other CNS depressants (medicines that slow down the nervous system). **Check with your doctor before taking any such depressants while you are using this medicine.**

This medicine may cause some people to become drowsy or less alert than they are normally. **Make sure you know how** you react to this medicine before you drive, use machines, or do other jobs that require you to be alert.

POSSIBLE SIDE EFFECTS OF THIS MEDICINE
Side Effects That Should Be Reported To Your Doctor

   Less common—Abdominal or stomach cramps (severe); behavioral, mood, or mental changes; continuous, uncontrolled back-and-forth and/or rolling eye movements; double vision; increase in seizures; loss of appetite; nausea or vomiting (continuing); spots before eyes; swelling of face; tiredness and weakness; unusual bleeding or bruising; yellow eyes or skin

Side Effects That Usually Do Not Require Medical Attention

These possible side effects may go away during treatment; however, if they continue or are bothersome, check with your doctor, nurse, or pharmacist.

   More common—Abdominal or stomach cramps (mild); change in menstrual periods; diarrhea; hair loss; indigestion; nausea and vomiting; trembling of hands and arms; unusual weight loss or gain

Other side effects not listed above may also occur in some patients. If you notice any other effects, check with your doctor, nurse, or pharmacist.

VASCULAR HEADACHE SUPPRESSANTS, ERGOT DERIVATIVE–CONTAINING Systemic

Including Dihydroergotamine; Ergotamine; Ergotamine, Belladonna Alkaloids, and Phenobarbital; Ergotamine and Caffeine; Ergotamine, Caffeine, and Belladonna Alkaloids; Ergotamine, Caffeine, Belladonna Alkaloids and Pentobarbital; Ergotamine, Caffeine, and Cyclizine; Ergotamine, Caffeine, and Dimenhydrinate; Ergotamine, Caffeine, and Diphenhydramine.

■For the Pharmacist■

In providing consultation, consider emphasizing the following selected information (» = major clinical significance):

Before using this medication

» Conditions affecting use, especially:

Sensitivity to any ingredient in the product considered for use

Pregnancy—Use is not recommended because ergot derivatives have oxytocic activity, which may lead to miscarriage, and vasoconstrictive activity, which may result in fetotoxicity

Breast-feeding—Ergot alkaloids are distributed into breast milk and may cause adverse effects in the infant; ergot alkaloids and medications having anticholinergic activity (belladonna alkaloids, cyclizine, dimenhydrinate, diphenhydramine) may also inhibit lactation; caffeine and pentobarbital are also distributed into breast milk and may cause CNS stimulation or CNS depression, respectively

Use in children—Pediatrics-specific problems have not been reported in children 6 years of age or older, but dihydroergotamine and ergotamine are recommended only for patients unresponsive to less toxic medications; young children, especially those with spastic paralysis or brain damage, may be especially susceptible to the effects of belladonna alkaloids; also, risk of paradoxical hyperexcitability in children receiving cyclizine, dimenhydrinate, diphenhydramine, or pentobarbital

Use in the elderly—Increased risk of hypothermia and other adverse effects associated with ergot derivative–induced peripheral and coronary vasoconstriction; increased susceptibility to effects of medications with anticholinergic activity and to barbiturates

Other medications, especially other vasoconstrictors (including other ergot alkaloids and vasoconstrictors present in local anesthetic solutions)

Other medical problems, especially angina pectoris or other coronary artery disease, hepatic function impairment, hypertension, severe infection, peripheral vascular disease, pruritus, renal function impairment, and recent or contemplated angioplasty or vascular surgery (for dihydroergotamine and ergotamine); anxiety disorders (e.g., agoraphobia, panic attacks), severe cardiac disease, insomnia, or peptic ulcer (for caffeine-containing formulations)

Proper use of this medication

» Importance of not using more medication than the amount prescribed; risk of habituation with too frequent use and of peripheral vasoconstriction or other signs and symptoms of ergotism
   with acute or chronic overdosage

» Taking at first sign of headache (prodromal stage, for migraine with
   aura)

» Lying down in a quiet, dark room after taking initial dose

» Compliance with prophylactic therapy, if prescribed

   Proper administration techniques for—
   Dihydroergotamine injection
   Ergotamine inhalation: Reading patient directions; shaking con-
      tainer after removing cap; exhaling, placing mouthpiece in
      mouth aimed at back of throat, simultaneously inhaling and
      pressing vial down into the adapter; holding breath as long
      as possible after inhaling medication
   Ergotamine sublingual tablets: Allowing to dissolve under tongue;
      not chewing or swallowing whole; not eating, drinking, or
      smoking while tablet is dissolving
   Ergotamine-containing rectal suppositories
   If dividing suppository dosage form: Dividing lengthwise into pieces
      of equal size; easier to accomplish if suppositories have been
      refrigerated

» Proper dosing

» Proper storage

Precautions while using this medication

» Checking with physician if usual dose fails to relieve headaches, or
   if frequency and/or severity of headaches increases; possibility
   that tolerance to or dependence on the medication has developed,
   leading to withdrawal (rebound) or chronic headaches

   Avoiding alcohol, which aggravates headache

   Avoiding smoking because nicotine constricts blood vessels

   Avoiding exposure to excessive cold, which may intensify peripheral
      vasoconstriction

   Notifying physician if infection develops; severe infection may cause
      increased sensitivity to medication

   For ergotamine inhalation—Possible hoarseness or throat irritation,
      which may be prevented by gargling and rinsing mouth after
      use; checking with physician if continuing or bothersome

   Possible interferences with laboratory tests; not taking caffeine for
      12 hours prior to dipyridamole-assisted myocardial perfusion
      study, belladonna alkaloids for 24 hours prior to gastric acid
      secretion test, and cyclizine, dimenhydrinate, or diphenhydra-
      mine for 72 hours prior to skin tests using allergen extracts

» *For formulations containing cyclizine, dimenhydrinate, diphenhydramine, or pentobarbital*

   Caution when driving or doing jobs requiring alertness because of
      possible dizziness, lightheadedness, or drowsiness, especially if
      taking other CNS depressants concurrently

   *For formulations containing belladonna alkaloids, cyclizine, di-
   menhydrinate, or diphenhydramine*

   Possible dryness of mouth, nose, and throat; using sugarless candy
      or gum, ice, or saliva substitute for relief

Side/adverse effects

   Signs and symptoms of potential side effects, especially edema, fast
      or slow heartbeat, cerebral or peripheral ischemia, gangrene, and
      coronary or ocular vasospasm

▲ For the Patient ▲

913070

ERGOT MEDICINES (Oral): *Including Ergotamine;
Ergotamine, Belladonna Alkaloids, and Phenobarbital;
Ergotamine and Caffeine; Ergotamine, Caffeine,
Belladonna Alkaloids, and Pentobarbital.*

ABOUT YOUR MEDICINE
Ergot medicines are used to treat migraine headaches and
some kinds of throbbing headaches. They are not used to
prevent headaches but are used to relieve a headache once
it has started. Some of these medicines may also be used
for other conditions as determined by your doctor.

If any of the information in this leaflet causes you special
concern or if you want additional information about your
medicine and its use, check with your doctor, nurse, or pharmacist. **Remember, keep this and all other medicines out of
the reach of children and never share your medicines with
others.**

BEFORE USING THIS MEDICINE
Tell your doctor, nurse, and pharmacist if you . . .
- are allergic to any medicine, either prescription or nonprescription (OTC);
- are pregnant or intend to become pregnant while using
  this medicine;
- are breast-feeding;
- are taking **any** other prescription or nonprescription
  (OTC) medicine;
- have **any** other medical problems;
- use cocaine;
- regularly drink large amounts of caffeine-containing
  beverages such as coffee, tea, soft drinks, or cocoa.

PROPER USE OF THIS MEDICINE
Take this medicine only as directed by your doctor. If the
amount you are to take does not relieve your headache, do
not take more than your doctor ordered. Instead, check with
your doctor. Taking too much of this medicine or taking it
too often may cause serious effects such as nausea and vomiting; cold, painful hands or feet; or even gangrene, especially
in elderly patients.

This medicine works best if you:
- **Take it at the first sign of headache or migraine attack.**
- **Lie down in a quiet, dark room for at least 2 hours after
  taking it.**

PRECAUTIONS WHILE USING THIS MEDICINE
Since drinking alcoholic beverages may make headaches
worse, it is best to avoid use of alcohol while you are suffering
from them.

Since smoking may increase some of the harmful effects of this medicine, it is best to avoid smoking while you are using it.

If you have a serious infection or illness of any kind, check with your doctor before taking this medicine, since you may be more sensitive to its effects.

This medicine may make you more sensitive to cold temperatures, especially if you have blood circulation problems. Dress warmly during cold weather and be careful during prolonged exposure to cold, such as in winter sports. This is especially important for elderly people.

Belladonna alkaloids (may be contained in this medicine) also may cause your eyes to become more sensitive to light than they are normally. Wearing sunglasses may help lessen the discomfort from bright light.

The caffeine in this combination medicine may interfere with the results of a test that uses dipyridamole (e.g., Persantine) to help find out how well your blood is flowing through certain blood vessels. You should not have any caffeine for at least 4 hours before the test.

POSSIBLE SIDE EFFECTS OF THIS MEDICINE
Side Effects That Should Be Reported To Your Doctor Immediately

> Changes in vision; confusion; convulsions (seizures); fever; mental depression; muscle twitching; numbness and tingling of fingers, toes, or face; red or violet blisters on skin of hands or feet; ringing or other sounds in ears; seeing flashes of "zig-zag" lights; shortness of breath; stomach pain or bloating; tiredness or weakness; slurred speech; unusually fast, irregular, or slow heartbeat

Other Side Effects That Should Be Reported To Your Doctor

> *More common*—Headaches, more often and/or more severe than before; swelling of feet and lower legs

> *Less common or rare*—Anxiety; chest pain; eye pain; hives or itching of skin; pain in arms, legs, or lower back; pale or cold hands or feet; sore throat and fever; unusual bleeding or bruising; yellow eyes or skin

Side Effects That Usually Do Not Require Medical Attention

These possible side effects may go away during treatment; however, if they continue or are bothersome, check with your doctor, nurse, or pharmacist.

> *More common*—Decreased sweating; diarrhea; dizziness; dryness of mouth, nose, throat, or skin; nausea or vomiting

Other side effects not listed above may also occur in some patients. If you notice any other effects, check with your doctor, nurse, or pharmacist.

After you stop using this medicine, your body may need time to adjust. The length of time this takes depends on the amount of medicine you were using and how long you used it. During this time check with your doctor if your headaches begin again or worsen.

ZIDOVUDINE   Systemic

■ For the Pharmacist ■

In providing consultation, consider emphasizing the following selected information (» = major clinical significance):

Before using this medication
» Conditions affecting use, especially:
Hypersensitivity to zidovudine
Pregnancy—Zidovudine crosses the placenta and reaches concentrations in the fetus similar to those observed in adults; zidovudine has been shown to decrease perinatal transmission of HIV
Breast-feeding—It is not known whether zidovudine is distributed into breast milk; however, breast-feeding is not recommended in HIV-infected mothers where safe infant formula is available and affordable
Dental—The bone marrow–depressant effects of zidovudine may result in an increased incidence of certain microbial infections and delayed healing
Other medications, especially other bone marrow depressants, clarithromycin, ganciclovir, or probenecid
Other medical problems, especially bone marrow depression or hepatic function impairment

Proper use of this medication
Supplying patient information about zidovudine
» Importance of not taking more medication than prescribed; importance of not discontinuing medication without checking with physician
» Compliance with full course of therapy
» Importance of not missing doses and taking at evenly spaced times
» Proper dosing
Missed dose: Taking as soon as possible; not taking if almost time for next dose; not doubling doses
» Proper storage

Precautions while using this medication
» Regular visits to physician for blood tests
» Importance of not taking other medications concurrently without checking with physician
Using caution in use of regular toothbrushes, dental floss, and toothpicks; checking with physician or dentist concerning proper oral hygiene
» Avoiding sexual intercourse or using a condom to help prevent transmission of the AIDS virus to others; not sharing needles with anyone

Side/adverse effects
Signs of potential side effects, especially anemia, leukopenia or neutropenia, changes in platelet count, hepatotoxicity, myopathy, and neurotoxicity

---

▲ For the Patient ▲

915508

ABOUT YOUR MEDICINE

Zidovudine (zye-DOE-vue-deen), also called AZT, is used to treat patients who are infected with the human immuno-deficiency virus (HIV). HIV is the virus that causes acquired immune deficiency syndrome (AIDS). HIV attacks the immune system. This medicine appears to slow down the destruction of the immune system caused by HIV. This may help slow down the progress of HIV disease and the serious infections that occur with AIDS. However, zidovudine will not cure or prevent HIV infection, and it will not keep you from spreading the virus to other people. Patients who are taking this medicine may continue to have the problems usually related to AIDS or HIV disease.

If any of the information in this leaflet causes you special concern or if you want additional information about your medicine and its use, check with your doctor, nurse, or pharmacist. **Remember, keep this and all other medicines out of the reach of children and never share your medicines with others.**

BEFORE USING THIS MEDICINE

Discuss with your doctor the possible side effects that may be caused by this medicine. Some of them may be serious.

Tell your doctor, nurse, and pharmacist if you . . .
- are allergic to any medicine, either prescription or non-prescription (OTC);
- are pregnant or intend to become pregnant while using this medicine;
- are breast-feeding;
- are taking **any** other prescription or nonprescription (OTC) medicine;
- have any other medical problems, especially anemia or liver disease;
- have ever been treated with x-rays or cancer medicines.

PROPER USE OF THIS MEDICINE

Take this medicine exactly as directed by your doctor. Do not take more of it, do not take it more often, and do not take it for a longer time than your doctor ordered. Also, do not stop taking this medicine without checking with your doctor first.

Keep taking zidovudine for the full time of treatment, even if you begin to feel better.

This medicine works best when there is a constant amount in the blood. **To help keep the right amount of medicine in your blood, do not miss any doses.** If you need help in planning the best times to take your medicine, check with your doctor, nurse, or pharmacist.

If you do miss a dose of this medicine, take it as soon as possible. However, if it is almost time for your next dose, skip the missed dose and go back to your regular dosing schedule. Do not double doses.

PRECAUTIONS WHILE USING THIS MEDICINE

It is very important that your doctor check your progress at regular visits. This medicine may cause blood problems.

Do not take any other medicines unless you check with your doctor first. Taking other medicines together with zidovudine can increase the chance of side effects from zidovudine.

HIV is spread to other people through infected body fluids such as blood, vaginal fluid, or semen. **If you are infected with HIV, it is best not to have sex** or do anything which involves an exchange of body fluids with other people.

If you do have sex, always wear (or have your partner wear) a condom ("rubber"). Only use condoms made of latex, and **use them every time you have vaginal, anal, or oral sex.** Using a spermicide (such as nonoxynol-9) may also help keep you from spreading HIV, as long as the spermicide does not irritate the vagina, rectum, or mouth. Do not use oil-based jelly, cold cream, baby oil, or shortening as a lubricant— these products can cause the condom (rubber) to break. Lubricants without oil, such as *K-Y Jelly*, are recommended. **If you inject drugs,** get help to stop. **Do not share needles with anyone.** If you have any questions about this, check with your doctor, nurse, or pharmacist.

POSSIBLE SIDE EFFECTS OF THIS MEDICINE

Side Effects That Should Be Reported To Your Doctor Immediately

   More common—Fever, chills, or sore throat; pale skin; unusual tiredness or weakness

The above side effects may also occur up to weeks or months after you stop taking this medicine.

   Rare—Abdominal discomfort; confusion; convulsions (seizures); general feeling of discomfort; loss of appetite; mood or mental changes; muscle tenderness or weakness; nausea

Side Effects That Usually Do Not Require Medical Attention

These possible side effects may go away during treatment; however, if they continue or are bothersome, check with your doctor, nurse, or pharmacist.

   More common—Headache (severe); muscle soreness; nausea; trouble in sleeping

Other side effects not listed above may also occur in some patients. If you notice any other effects, check with your doctor, nurse, or pharmacist.

ZOLPIDEM Systemic

■ For the Pharmacist ■

In providing consultation, consider emphasizing the following selected information (» = major clinical significance):

Before using this medication
» Conditions affecting use, especially:
    Sensitivity to zolpidem
    Breast-feeding—Small amounts of zolpidem are distributed into breast milk; effect on infant is not known
    Use in the elderly—Elderly patients are usually more sensitive to CNS effects of zolpidem
    Other medications, especially other CNS depression–producing medications
    Other medical problems, especially acute alcohol intoxication or sleep apnea

Proper use of this medication
» Not taking more medication than the amount prescribed, because of habit-forming potential
» Not increasing dose if medication becomes less effective over time; checking with physician
    Being prepared to go to sleep immediately after taking medicine
» Proper dosing
    Missed dose—Skipping missed dose; not doubling doses
» Proper storage

Precautions while using this medication
» Avoiding use of alcohol or other CNS depressants during therapy
» Caution if clumsiness or unsteadiness, drowsiness, dizziness, or visual disturbances occur, especially in the elderly
    Checking with physician before discontinuing medication after more than 1 to 2 weeks use; gradual dosage reduction may be necessary to avoid withdrawal symptoms

Side/adverse effects
    Signs of potential side effects, especially ataxia, confusion, mental depression, allergic reaction or rash, anaphylaxis, falling, hypotension, or paradoxical reactions

▲ For the Patient ▲

919393

ABOUT YOUR MEDICINE

Zolpidem (ZOL-pi-dem) is used to treat insomnia (trouble in sleeping). In most cases, sleep medicine should be used only for short periods of time, such as 1 or 2 days, and generally for no longer than 1 or 2 weeks.

If any of the information in this leaflet causes you special concern or if you want additional information about your medicine and its use, check with your doctor, nurse, or pharmacist. **Remember, keep this and all other medicines out of the reach of children and never share your medicines with others.**

BEFORE USING THIS MEDICINE

Discuss with your doctor the possible side effects that may be caused by this medicine. For example, amnesia (memory loss) may occur for several hours after you take a dose of this medicine.

Tell your doctor, nurse, and pharmacist if you . . .
- are allergic to any medicine, either prescription or non-prescription (OTC);
- are pregnant or intend to become pregnant while using this medicine;
- are breast-feeding;
- are taking **any** other prescription or nonprescription (OTC) medicine;
- have any other medical problems, especially sleep apnea.

PROPER USE OF THIS MEDICINE

Take this medicine only as directed by your doctor. If too much is taken, it may become habit-forming (causing mental or physical dependence).

Take zolpidem just before going to bed, when you are ready to go to sleep. This medicine works very quickly to put you to sleep.

Do not take this medicine when your schedule does not permit you to get a full night's sleep (7 to 8 hours). If you must wake up before this, you may continue to feel drowsy and may have memory problems, because the effects of the medicine have not had time to wear off.

PRECAUTIONS WHILE USING THIS MEDICINE

This medicine will add to the effects of alcohol and other CNS depressants (medicines that cause drowsiness). **Check with your doctor before taking any such depressants while you are taking this medicine.**

This medicine may cause some people, especially older persons, to become drowsy, dizzy, lightheaded, clumsy or unsteady, or less alert than they are normally. Even though zolpidem is taken at bedtime, it may cause some people to feel drowsy or less alert on arising. Also, this medicine may cause double vision or other vision problems. **Make sure you know how you react to zolpidem before you drive, use machines, or do anything else that could be dangerous if you are dizzy, or are not alert or able to see well.**

If you have any unusual or strange thoughts or behavior while you are taking zolpidem, be sure to discuss it with your doctor. Some changes that have occurred in people while taking this medicine are like those seen in people who drink alcohol and then act in a manner that is not normal. Other changes may be more unusual and extreme, such as confusion, hallucinations, and unusual excitement, nervousness, or irritability.

If you will be taking zolpidem for a long time, do not stop taking it without first checking with your doctor.

After taking zolpidem for insomnia, you may have difficulty sleeping (rebound insomnia) for the first few nights after you stop taking it.

If you think you or someone else may have taken an overdose of this medicine, get emergency help at once. Taking an overdose of zolpidem or taking alcohol or other CNS depressants with zolpidem may lead to breathing problems and unconsciousness. Some signs of an overdose are severe drowsiness, severe nausea or vomiting, staggering, and troubled breathing.

POSSIBLE SIDE EFFECTS OF THIS MEDICINE
Side Effects That Should Be Reported To Your Doctor

Less common—Clumsiness or unsteadiness; confusion (more common in older adults); mental depression

Rare—Dizziness, lightheadedness, or fainting; falling (more common in older adults); fast heartbeat; hallucinations; skin rash; swelling of face; trouble in sleeping; unusual excitement, nervousness, or irritability; wheezing or difficult breathing

Side Effects That Usually Do Not Require Medical Attention

These possible side effects may go away during treatment; however, if they continue or are bothersome, check with your doctor, nurse, or pharmacist.

Less common—Abdominal or stomach pain; daytime drowsiness; diarrhea; double vision or other vision problems; drugged feeling; dryness of mouth; general feeling of discomfort or illness; headache; memory problems; nausea; nightmares or unusual dreams; vomiting

Other side effects not listed above may also occur in some patients. If you notice any other effects, check with your doctor, nurse, or pharmacist.

After you stop using this medicine, your body may need time to adjust. During this time check with your doctor if you notice any unusual effects.

848

Index

A selected number of brand names *(italicized)* have been
included. The inclusion of a brand name does not mean the
publishers have any particular knowledge that the brand
listed has properties different from other brands of the same
drug, nor should it be interpreted as an endorsement by the
publishers. Similarly, the fact that a particular brand has
not been included does not indicate that the product has
been judged to be unsatisfactory or unacceptable.

A

Abitrate—Clofibrate (Systemic), 221
Accupril—Quinapril—*See* Angiotensin-converting Enzyme (ACE) Inhibitors (Systemic), 31
Accutane—Isotretinoin (Systemic), 465
Acebutolol—*See* Beta-adrenergic Blocking Agents (Systemic), 125
ACE Inhibitors—*See* Angiotensin-converting Enzyme (ACE) Inhibitors (Systemic), 31
ACE Inhibitors and Hydrochlorothiazide—*See* Angiotensin-converting Enzyme (ACE) Inhibitors and Hydrochlorothiazide (Systemic), 35
Acetaco—Acetaminophen and Codeine—*See* Opioid (Narcotic) Analgesics and Acetaminophen (Systemic), 626
Aceta with Codeine—Acetaminophen and Codeine—*See* Opioid (Narcotic) Analgesics and Acetaminophen (Systemic), 626
Acetaminophen and Codeine—*See* Opioid (Narcotic) Analgesics and Acetaminophen (Systemic), 626
Acetaminophen, Codeine, and Caffeine—*See* Opioid (Narcotic) Analgesics and Acetaminophen (Systemic), 626
Acetohexamide—*See* Antidiabetic Agents, Oral (Systemic), 63
Acetophenazine—*See* Phenothiazines (Systemic), 661
Achromycin—Tetracycline—*See* Tetracyclines (Systemic), 799
Achromycin V—Tetracycline—*See* Tetracyclines (Systemic), 799
Aciclovir—*See* Acyclovir (Systemic), 1; Acyclovir (Topical), 4
Aclophen—Chlorpheniramine, Phenylephrine, and Acetaminophen—*See* Antihistamines, Decongestants, and Analgesics (Systemic), 89

Acrivastine—*See* Antihistamines (Systemic), 81
Acrivastine and Pseudoephedrine—*See* Antihistamines and Decongestants (Systemic), 85
Actagen—Triprolidine and Pseudoephedrine—*See* Antihistamines and Decongestants (Systemic), 85
Actagen-C Cough—Triprolidine, Pseudoephedrine, and Codeine—*See* Cough/Cold Combinations (Systemic), 258
ACTH—Corticotropin—*See* Corticosteroids/Corticotropin—Glucocorticoid Effects (Systemic), 253
Acthar—Corticotropin—*See* Corticosteroids/Corticotropin—Glucocorticoid Effects (Systemic), 253
Actifed—Triprolidine and Pseudoephedrine—*See* Antihistamines and Decongestants (Systemic), 85
Actifed with Codeine Cough—Triprolidine, Pseudoephedrine, and Codeine—*See* Cough/Cold Combinations (Systemic), 258
Actifed Head Cold and Allergy Medicine—Triprolidine and Pseudoephedrine—*See* Antihistamines and Decongestants (Systemic), 85
Actifed Plus—Triprolidine, Pseudoephedrine, and Acetaminophen—*See* Antihistamines, Decongestants, and Analgesics (Systemic), 89
Actifed Plus Caplets—Triprolidine, Pseudoephedrine, and Acetaminophen—*See* Antihistamines, Decongestants, and Analgesics (Systemic), 89
Actifed Sinus Nighttime Caplets—Diphenhydramine, Pseudoephedrine, and Acetaminophen—*See* Antihistamines, Decongestants, and Analgesics (Systemic), 89
Acutrim 16 Hour—Phenylpropanolamine (Systemic), 666
Acutrim Late Day—Phenylpropanolamine (Systemic), 666

Cortifoam—Hydrocortisone—*See* Corticosteroids/Corticotropin—Glucocorticoid Effects (Systemic), 253

Cortisol—Hydrocortisone—*See* Corticosteroids/Corticotropin—Glucocorticoid Effects (Systemic), 253

Cortisone—*See* Corticosteroids/Corticotropin—Glucocorticoid Effects (Systemic), 253

Cortone Acetate—Cortisone—*See* Corticosteroids/Corticotropin—Glucocorticoid Effects (Systemic), 253

Cortrophin-Zinc—Corticotropin—*See* Corticosteroids/Corticotropin—Glucocorticoid Effects (Systemic), 253

Corzide—Nadolol and Bendroflumethiazide—*See* Beta-adrenergic Blocking Agents and Thiazide Diuretics (Systemic), 130

Cotanal-65—Propoxyphene and Aspirin—*See* Opioid (Narcotic) Analgesics and Aspirin (Systemic), 630

Cotranzine—Prochlorperazine—*See* Phenothiazines (Systemic), 661

Co-triamterzide—Triamterene and Hydrochlorothiazide—*See* Diuretics, Potassium-sparing, and Hydrochlorothiazide (Systemic), 333

Cotrim—Sulfamethoxazole and Trimethoprim (Systemic), 762

Cotrim DS—Sulfamethoxazole and Trimethoprim (Systemic), 762

Cotrimoxazole—*See* Sulfamethoxazole and Trimethoprim (Systemic), 762

Co-Tuss V—Hydrocodone and Guaifenesin—*See* Cough/Cold Combinations (Systemic), 258

Cotylbutazone—Phenylbutazone—*See* Nonsteroidal Anti-inflammatory Drugs (Systemic), 606

CoTylenol Cold Medication—Chlorpheniramine, Pseudoephedrine, Dextromethorphan, and Acetaminophen—*See* Cough/Cold Combinations (Systemic), 258

Cough/Cold Combinations (Systemic), 258

Coumadin—Warfarin—*See* Anticoagulants (Systemic), 39

Covangesic—Chlorpheniramine, Pyrilamine, Phenylephrine, Phenylpropanolamine, and Acetaminophen—*See* Antihistamines, Decongestants, and Analgesics (Systemic), 89

Cramp End—Ibuprofen—*See* Nonsteroidal Anti-inflammatory Drugs (Systemic), 606

Cromoglicic acid—*See* Cromolyn (Nasal), 267

Cromoglycic acid—*See* Cromolyn (Nasal), 267

Cromolyn (Inhalation-Local), 264

Cromolyn (Nasal), 267

Crysticillin 300 AS—Penicillin G—*See* Penicillins (Systemic), 649

Crystodigin—Digitoxin—*See* Digitalis Glycosides (Systemic), 308

C-Tussin Expectorant—Pseudoephedrine, Codeine, and Guaifenesin—*See* Cough/Cold Combinations (Systemic), 258

Cuprimine—Penicillamine (Systemic), 646

Curretab—Medroxyprogesterone—*See* Progestins (Systemic), 707

Cyclizine (Systemic), 270

Cyclobenzaprine (Systemic), 273

Cyclophosphamide (Systemic), 276

Cycloserine (Systemic), 280

Cyclosporin A—*See* Cyclosporine (Systemic), 283

Cyclosporine (Systemic), 283

Cyclothiazide—*See* Diuretics, Thiazide (Systemic), 337

Cycoflex—Cyclobenzaprine (Systemic), 273

Cycrin—Medroxyprogesterone—*See* Progestins (Systemic), 707

Cylert—Pemoline (Systemic), 643

Cylert Chewable—Pemoline (Systemic), 643

Cyproheptadine—*See* Antihistamines (Systemic), 81

Cytomel—Liothyronine—*See* Thyroid Hormones (Systemic), 807

Cytotec—Misoprostol (Systemic), 567

Cytoxan—Cyclophosphamide (Systemic), 276

D

D.A. Chewable—Chlorpheniramine, Phenylephrine, and Methscopolamine—*See* Antihistamines, Decongestants, and Anticholinergics (Systemic), 93

Dalalone—Dexamethasone—*See* Corticosteroids/Corticotropin—Glucocorticoid Effects (Systemic), 253

Dalalone D.P.—Dexamethasone—*See* Corticosteroids/Corticotropin—Glucocorticoid Effects (Systemic), 253

Dalalone L.A.—Dexamethasone—*See* Corticosteroids/Corticotropin—Glucocorticoid Effects (Systemic), 253

Dallergy—Chlorpheniramine, Phenylephrine, and Methscopolamine—*See* Antihistamines, Decongestants, and Anticholinergics (Systemic), 93

Hydromine Pediatric—Phenylpropanolamine and Hydrocodone—*See* Cough/Cold Combinations (Systemic), 258

Hydromorphone—*See* Opioid (Narcotic) Analgesics (Systemic), 622

Hydromorphone and Guaifenesin—*See* Cough/Cold Combinations (Systemic), 258

Hydromox—Quinethazone—*See* Diuretics, Thiazide (Systemic), 337

Hydropane—Hydrocodone and Homatropine—*See* Cough/Cold Combinations (Systemic), 258

Hydrophen—Phenylpropanolamine and Hydrocodone—*See* Cough/Cold Combinations (Systemic), 258

Hydroxacen—Hydroxyzine—*See* Antihistamines (Systemic), 81

Hydroxyprogesterone—*See* Progestins (Systemic), 707

Hydroxyzine—*See* Antihistamines (Systemic), 81

Hy/Gestrone—Hydroxyprogesterone—*See* Progestins (Systemic), 707

Hygroton—Chlorthalidone—*See* Diuretics, Thiazide (Systemic), 337

Hylorel—Guanadrel (Systemic), 424

Hylutin—Hydroxyprogesterone—*See* Progestins (Systemic), 707

HY-PHEN—Hydrocodone and Acetaminophen—*See* Opioid (Narcotic) Analgesics and Acetaminophen (Systemic), 626

Hyrexin-50—Diphenhydramine—*See* Antihistamines (Systemic), 81

Hytinic—Iron-Polysaccharide—*See* Iron Supplements (Systemic), 457

Hytrin—Terazosin (Systemic), 793

Hyzine-50—Hydroxyzine—*See* Antihistamines (Systemic), 81

I

Ibifon 600 Caplets—Ibuprofen—*See* Nonsteroidal Anti-inflammatory Drugs (Systemic), 606

Ibren—Ibuprofen—*See* Nonsteroidal Anti-inflammatory Drugs (Systemic), 606

Ibu—Ibuprofen—*See* Nonsteroidal Anti-inflammatory Drugs (Systemic), 606

Ibu-4—Ibuprofen—*See* Nonsteroidal Anti-inflammatory Drugs (Systemic), 606

Ibu-6—Ibuprofen—*See* Nonsteroidal Anti-inflammatory Drugs (Systemic), 606

Ibu-8—Ibuprofen—*See* Nonsteroidal Anti-inflammatory Drugs (Systemic), 606

Ibu 200—Ibuprofen—*See* Nonsteroidal Anti-inflammatory Drugs (Systemic), 606

Ibuprin—Ibuprofen—*See* Nonsteroidal Anti-inflammatory Drugs (Systemic), 606

Ibuprofen—*See* Anti-inflammatory Analgesics, Nonsteroidal (Systemic), 606

Ibuprohm—Ibuprofen—*See* Nonsteroidal Anti-inflammatory Drugs (Systemic), 606

Ibuprohm Caplets—Ibuprofen—*See* Nonsteroidal Anti-inflammatory Drugs (Systemic), 606

Ibu-Tab—Ibuprofen—*See* Nonsteroidal Anti-inflammatory Drugs (Systemic), 606

Ilosone—Erythromycin Estolate—*See* Erythromycins (Systemic), 358

Ilotycin—Erythromycin Base—*See* Erythromycins (Systemic), 358; Erythromycin Gluceptate—*See* Erythromycins (Systemic), 358

IMDUR—Isosorbide Mononitrate—*See* Nitrates (Systemic), 595

Imipramine—*See* Antidepressants, Tricyclic (Systemic), 58

Imitrex—Sumatriptan (Systemic), 781

Imodium—Loperamide (Oral-Local), 487

Imodium A-D—Loperamide (Oral-Local), 487

Imodium A-D Caplets—Loperamide (Oral-Local), 487

Improved Sino-Tuss—Chlorpheniramine, Phenylephrine, Dextromethorphan, Acetaminophen, and Salicylamide—*See* Cough/Cold Combinations (Systemic), 258

Indapamide (Systemic), 442

Inderal—Propranolol—*See* Beta-adrenergic Blocking Agents (Systemic), 125

Inderal LA—Propranolol—*See* Beta-adrenergic Blocking Agents (Systemic), 125

Inderide—Propranolol and Hydrochlorothiazide—*See* Beta-adrenergic Blocking Agents and Thiazide Diuretics (Systemic), 130

Inderide LA—Propranolol and Hydrochlorothiazide—*See* Beta-adrenergic Blocking Agents and Thiazide Diuretics (Systemic), 130

Indocin—Indomethacin—*See* Nonsteroidal Anti-inflammatory Drugs (Systemic), 606

Indocin SR—Indomethacin—*See* Nonsteroidal Anti-inflammatory Drugs (Systemic), 606

N

O

About USP and USP DI®

About USP—The information in this volume is prepared by the United States Pharmacopeial Convention, Inc. (USP), the organization that sets the official standards of strength, quality, purity, packaging, and labeling for medical products used in the United States.

USP is an independent, not-for-profit corporation composed of delegates from the accredited colleges of medicine and pharmacy in the U.S.; state medical and pharmaceutical associations; many national associations concerned with medicines; and various departments of the federal government. In addition, four members of the Convention specifically represent the public. USP was established in 1820, and is the only national body that represents the professions of both pharmacy and medicine.

About USP DI®—The USP DI database provides clinically relevant information for the health care professional and corresponding information in lay language for the consumer. First made available in 1980, the database is continuously reviewed and revised and is accessible by either print or electronic means. The information is developed by the consensus of the USP Committee of Revision and its Advisory Panels.

USP DI Volume I, Drug Information for the Health Care Professional contains drug use information for the pharmacist, physician, dentist, nurse, or other health care provider. *USP DI Volume II, Advice for the Patient* is the lay language counterpart to Volume I and is intended for use in patient education programs. *Volume III, Approved Drug Products and Legal Requirements* reproduces FDA's "Orange Book" of therapeutic equivalence information, as well as selected federal and state requirements that affect the prescribing and dispensing of prescription drugs and controlled substances.

The information included in *USP DI Volume II, Advice for the Patient* serves as the basis for many different consumer/patient education initiatives. For example, USP DI® Patient Education Leaflets® (reproduced in this book) are abstracted from Volume II monographs.

For further information about USP or *USP DI®* or to comment on the information published in this book and how it might better meet your information needs, please contact:

USP Drug Information Division
12601 Twinbrook Parkway
Rockville, Maryland 20852

Telephone: (301) 816-8351
Telefax: (301) 816-8374.

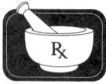

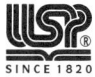

Leaflet Title - $2.35 ea.   # Pads

Cough/Cold Combinations (Oral)**
- 915315 Full Leaflet Text
- 985310 Easy-to-Read

Cyclobenzaprine (Oral)*
- 913648 Full Leaflet Text
- 983643 Easy-to-Read

Digitalis Medicines (Oral)*
- 912248 Full Leaflet Text
- 982243 Easy-to-Read

Diphenoxylate and Atropine (Oral)**
- 912259 Full Leaflet Text
- 982254 Easy-to-Read

Ergot Medicines (Oral)**
- 913070 Full Leaflet Text
- 983075 Easy-to-Read

Erythromycins (Oral)*
- 912827 Full Leaflet Text
- 982822 Easy-to-Read

Estrogens (Oral)*
- 915188 Full Leaflet Text
- 985183 Easy-to-Read

Fluoroquinolones (Oral)*
- 916136 Full Leaflet Text
- 986131 Easy-to-Read

Fluoxetine (Oral)*
- 916147 Full Leaflet Text
- 986142 Easy-to-Read

Gemfibrozil (Oral)*
- 913954 Full Leaflet Text
- 983950 Easy-to-Read

Haloperidol (Oral)*
- 912317 Full Leaflet Text
- 982312 Easy-to-Read

H$_2$-blockers (Oral)*
- 913091 Full Leaflet Text
- 983097 Easy-to-Read

Hydantoin Anticonvulsants (Oral)**
- 912328 Full Leaflet Text
- 982323 Easy-to-Read

Hydralazine (Oral)**
- 912339 Full Leaflet Text
- 982334 Easy-to-Read

Insulin (Injection)**
- 912361 Full Leaflet Text
- 982367 Easy-to-Read

Iron Supplements (Oral)*
- 912372 Full Leaflet Text
- 982378 Easy-to-Read

Levodopa/Carbidopa with Levodopa (Oral)**
- 912383 Full Leaflet Text
- 982389 Easy-to-Read

Lithium (Oral)**
- 913105 Full Leaflet Text
- 983100 Easy-to-Read

Loop Diuretics (Oral)*
- 912850 Full Leaflet Text
- 982855 Easy-to-Read

Lovastatin/Pravastatin/Simvastatin (Oral)*
- 915687 Full Leaflet Text
- 985682 Easy-to-Read

MAO Inhibitor Antidepressants (Oral)**
- 913116 Full Leaflet Text
- 983111 Easy-to-Read

Meclizine/Buclizine/Cyclizine (Oral)**
- 912394 Full Leaflet Text
- 982390 Easy-to-Read

Methyldopa (Oral)**
- 912408 Full Leaflet Text
- 982403 Easy-to-Read

Methylphenidate (Oral)*
- 913127 Full Leaflet Text
- 983122 Easy-to-Read

Metoclopramide (Oral)**
- 914378 Full Leaflet Text
- 984373 Easy-to-Read

Metronidazole (Oral)**
- 912420 Full Leaflet Text
- 982425 Easy-to-Read

Misoprostol (Oral)**
- 916657 Full Leaflet Text
- 986652 Easy-to-Read

Narcotic Analgesics (Oral)*
- 912441 Full Leaflet Text
- 982447 Easy-to-Read

Narcotic Analgesics and Acetaminophen (Oral)*
- 912452 Full Leaflet Text
- 982458 Easy-to-Read

Narcotic Analgesics and Aspirin (Oral)*
- 912463 Full Leaflet Text
- 982469 Easy-to-Read

Nicotine (Transdermal)**
- 918368 Full Leaflet Text
- 988363 Easy-to-Read

*InstaPak I   **InstaPak II

Leaflet Title - $2.35 ea.   # Pads

Nitrates (Oral)*
- 912485 Full Leaflet Text
- 982480 Easy-to-Read

Nitrates (Sublingual)*
- 912860 Full Leaflet Text
- 982866 Easy-to-Read

Nitrofurantoin (Oral)*
- 912496 Full Leaflet Text
- 982491 Easy-to-Read

Nitroglycerin (Topical)**
- 913138 Full Leaflet Text
- 983133 Easy-to-Read

Penicillins (Oral)*
- 912510 Full Leaflet Text
- 982516 Easy-to-Read

Perphenazine and Amitriptyline (Oral)**
- 912521 Full Leaflet Text
- 982527 Easy-to-Read

Phenazopyridine (Oral)**
- 912532 Full Leaflet Text
- 982538 Easy-to-Read

Phenothiazines (Oral)*
- 912554 Full Leaflet Text
- 982550 Easy-to-Read

Platelet Aggregation Inhibitors (Oral)**
- 919167 Full Leaflet Text
- 989162 Easy-to-Read

Potassium-sparing Diuretics (Oral)*
- 912871 Full Leaflet Text
- 982877 Easy-to-Read

Potassium-sparing Diuretics and Hydrochlorothiazide (Oral)*
- 913149 Full Leaflet Text
- 983144 Easy-to-Read

Potassium Supplements (Oral)*
- 912576 Full Leaflet Text
- 982571 Easy-to-Read

Salicylates (Oral)**
- 912623 Full Leaflet Text
- 982629 Easy-to-Read

Sertraline (Oral)**
- 918936 Full Leaflet Text
- 988931 Easy-to-Read

Skeletal Muscle Relaxants (Oral)*
- 912634 Full Leaflet Text
- 982630 Easy-to-Read

Sucralfate (Oral)**
- 913150 Full Leaflet Text
- 983155 Easy-to-Read

Sulfamethoxazole and Trimethoprim (Oral)*
- 918030 Full Leaflet Text
- 988035 Easy-to-Read

Sulfonamides (Oral)*
- 912667 Full Leaflet Text
- 982662 Easy-to-Read

Tetracyclines (Oral)*
- 912689 Full Leaflet Text
- 982684 Easy-to-Read

Thiazide Diuretics (Oral)*
- 912690 Full Leaflet Text
- 982695 Easy-to-Read

Thyroid Hormones (Oral)*
- 912703 Full Leaflet Text
- 982709 Easy-to-Read

Trazodone (Oral)**
- 915053 Full Leaflet Text
- 985059 Easy-to-Read

Tricyclic Antidepressants (Oral)*
- 912736 Full Leaflet Text
- 982731 Easy-to-Read

Valproic Acid (Oral)**
- 913160 Full Leaflet Text
- 983166 Easy-to-Read

Xanthine Bronchodilators (Oral)*
- 912882 Full Leaflet Text
- 982888 Easy-to-Read

Minimum order: 15 pads Subtotal	$
Quantity Discount 5% off orders of at least 200 pads	$
Subtotal	$
Sales tax Maryland residents add 5% sales tax	$
Shipping and handling $.10/pad $4.40/InstaPak $8.80/Complete InstaPak Sets	$
Total	$

Prices subject to change.

Please turn the page
for ordering information
on APhA books.